ERGONOMICS for REHABILITATION PROFESSIONALS

Edited by
SHRAWAN KUMAR

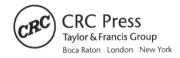

CRC Press
Taylor & Francis Group
Boca Raton London New York

CRC Press is an imprint of the
Taylor & Francis Group, an **informa** business

CRC Press
Taylor & Francis Group
6000 Broken Sound Parkway NW, Suite 300
Boca Raton, FL 33487-2742

First issued in paperback 2017

ISBN 13: 978-1-138-11324-4 (pbk)
ISBN 13: 978-0-8493-8146-1 (hbk)

Library of Congress Cataloging-in-Publication Data

Ergonomics for rehabilitation professionals / Shrawan Kumar.
    p. cm.
Includes bibliographical references and index.
ISBN 978-0-8493-8146-1 (alk. paper)
    1. Medical rehabilitation. 2. Human engineering. I. Kumar, Shrawan. II. Title.

RM930.E74 2009
617'.03--dc22

                                         2008043677

Visit the Taylor & Francis Web site at
http://www.taylorandfrancis.com

and the CRC Press Web site at
http://www.crcpress.com

This book is dedicated to my wife Rita, son Rajesh,
daughter Sheela, and daughter-in-law Zoe.

Contents

SECTION A   *General Concepts*

SECTION B   *Disorders and Disabilities*

SECTION C   Musculoskeletal Disorders

SECTION D   Ergonomics of Selected Interventions

Preface

Ergonomics for Rehabilitation Professionals is an attempt to integrate ergonomics in rehabilitation paradigms toward societal gains. It has been argued before that ergonomics and rehabilitation are complementary disciplines (Kumar 1989, 1992). Despite their apparent distinctly different appearances their constituent components are the same and they deal with the same issues, albeit at different ends of the spectrum. One of the manifested goals of rehabilitation is prevention of the affliction the clinician treats. The latter brings the efforts of rehabilitation beyond the patient group and into the normal population. However, leaving aside severe disability, the definition of disability has blurred significantly. According to the American Disability Act (1990) disability is defined as health condition(s) that significantly impair a major life activity. Interpreting this definition of disability, Fulbright and Jaworski (1990) stated that 20% of the U.S. population has some form of disability.

Aging is a major contributor to disability. Demographic shifts around the world indicate a trend of rapid growth in the senior population. One of the inevitable consequences of the aging process is a progressive decline in functional capacity in most bodily functions, which may vary in rate for different people based on many factors. Some argue that a full tilt progression of technology has shifted the job demands from physical to cognitive and skill realms possibly undermining overall health, and hence promoting impairment and disability. Others counter this with an argument of their own, that technology tends to compensate for functional impairment and disability enabling people to get out of the "disability" umbrella. Regardless of the validity of either argument, the fact remains that functional subnormality, with reference to the standards set some years ago, is on the rise. Regardless of the genesis of functional subnormality of the general population and the disabilities of patient groups, ergonomics can make significant contributions to both the prevention of afflictions and their treatment. It has been argued elsewhere (Kumar 1997) that the ergonomic approach significantly enhances both the accuracy and effectiveness of the rehabilitation regimes in some of the established methodologies and treatment methods. Clearly, as has been stated before (Kumar 1997), both disciplines (ergonomics and rehabilitation) are broad in their scope and have a vast body of knowledge. In this modest effort, I have tried to choose topics that, by example, will serve to blend the two disciplines topic by topic, albeit with differential emphasis. It has been the goal of this volume to reveal the commensalism of the two disciplines for mutual enhancement and not to force one on the other.

In the general section (Section A), to exemplify the philosophical perspective of the book, Kumar presents the conceptual basis of rehabilitation ergonomics. In this chapter, he traces the origin of both fields; explores their philosophy and goals; their parallelism, divergence, and complementarity; the role of ergonomics in rehabilitation; and also defines rehabilitation ergonomics. All human physical activities require motion of the human body involving muscle activities and joint loads. Mechanical activities can be achieved by expenditure of physiological energies. However, the mechanical components and their configuration determine not only the mechanical efficiency but also the physiological efficiency. In Chapter 2, Lin has initially provided the scientific basis of physiological cost consideration and subsequently described the impact of pathologies like orthopedic, neurological, and cardiorespiratory disorders, assistive devices, wheelchair propulsion, aging, and obesity on energy consumption. This interesting chapter has a good citation of relevant literature. In Chapter 3, Moseley and Jones tackle the all-important topic of pain. They provide a broad overview of the field with their perspective of its biology, assessment, and management. The authors have provided a significant list of references, which will help the reader to find more information. In the last chapter (Chapter 4) of the general section, Liu and Lederer have dealt with aging. As aging impacts performance, the role of ergonomics becomes more central. They initially describe the age-related physical, sensory, and cognitive changes and design changes necessary to address these problems. The authors advocate universal design, which will be good for everyone including older adults. They provide a few examples to indicate the manner in which these concepts can be integrated for a practical solution.

The second section, Section B, deals with disorders, disabilities, ways to deal with them, and ergonomic measures to prevent some and reduce others as the case may be. One of the primary needs of every organism in the animal kingdom is that of motion. Given the upright bipedalism of *Homo sapiens*, the kinematics, kinetics, and efficiency of ambulation with any pathology or disorder become a significant challenge to the individual, and their analysis (and understanding) poses additional difficulty. In Chapter 5, Striker describes normal gait and those associated with pathologies. In all these conditions, he considers loading, progression, and stability. However, when one is unable to ambulate on his/her own legs, wheelchair ambulation becomes inevitable. This changes the premise of ambulation profoundly. The biomechanics of the phenomenon becomes totally different as the ambulation is powered by either upper extremities or by a motor. By virtue of incorporation of a device to enable ambulation, ergonomic implications are relevant for both the device and the occupant. In Chapter 6, van der Woude et al. deal with these issues. In manually propelled wheelchairs, there is a transfer from leg to arm work for ambulation. This leads to a host of issues unique to this situation. One aspect deals with the discomfort, overuse, and ultimately injury, while the other deals with the efficiency of the design. The authors of this chapter have discussed vehicle mechanics, human movement system, and the wheelchair interface. One of the consequences of being wheelchair bound is that one is sitting for a much longer period resulting in problems of pressure sores and ulcers. In Chapter 7, Solis and Mushahwar deal with the serious side effect of prolonged seating. The authors give an overview of the etiology of pressure ulcers, their classification, treatment, method of detection, and prevention. They also describe appropriate support surfaces and devices that can dynamically distribute load over seating surfaces. Such approaches have a role in the reduction of pressure localization, which in turn is a causative factor in ulcer formation. In Chapter 8, Haennel and Tomczak describe common cardiac disorder problems and disabilities. The authors look into the problems associated with both myocardial infarction and coronary artery bypass graft surgery.

They examine the typical progression of the patient from an acute event through rehabilitation and various factors that play a critical role in determining the success of the strategy employed in return to work.

Chapters 9 through 12 deal with musculoskeletal disorders. In Chapter 9, Freivalds describes musculoskeletal disorders of the upper extremities and ergonomic interventions for them. He describes the etiology of the common musculoskeletal disorders including tendon, muscle, nerve, vessels, bursa, bone, and cartilage. Subsequently, the author goes on to describe both static and dynamic upper extremity models. Finally, the chapter turns its attention to the intervention strategies of hand tools. Jones and Kumar in Chapter 10 present an entirely original contribution where they examine the methodologies of ergonomic risk assessment for primarily upper extremity disorders. One of the primary difficulties in ergonomic methodologies is that authors of various techniques rely on partial or qualitative validation of their methods. When a person in the field is faced with different methodologies, it becomes a daunting task to determine which to pick. By using clear and objective definitions, the authors have compared five commonly used and cited risk assessment methodologies and demonstrated that each one of them is deficient in predicting risk and injury. They acknowledge that a direct comparison of these methodologies is not possible. This opens up the field for rigorous and objective studies for developing and validating techniques that could be reliably used. In Chapter 11, Maitland considers factors related to musculoskeletal disorders of the neck and shoulders with possible ergonomic interventions. The author concludes that the causative mechanisms for these disorders and effective interventions for these are not yet conclusive. In the last chapter of this section (Chapter 12), van Dieën and van der Beek describe work-related low back pain, focusing on biomechanical factors and primary prevention. It is evident that the subject of low back pain is both vast and complex. The authors describe low back pain and the risk factors associated with it. Finally, they elaborate on a few ergonomic interventions.

The fourth section, Section D, is entirely devoted to selected ergonomic interventions that rehabilitation professionals can use. In Chapter 13, Feney and Harman take a clinical approach to intervention and rehabilitation. The authors provide a critical analysis of therapeutic exercise for subacute low back pain and carpal tunnel syndrome. The authors argue that therapeutic exercise is the foundation for a successful rehabilitation of musculoskeletal dysfunction. However, unfortunately, therapeutic exercise has not been effective on these afflictions. The authors discuss the reasons for this lack of success and suggest approaches to remedy this. Chapter 14 deals with the effective utilization of assistive devices in the workplace. In this chapter, de Jonge has identified the role that assistive devices play in workplace accommodation and has highlighted the value of using a consumer-centered process when selecting and using the technology. Such a selection must also be followed with training where appropriate. Chapter 15 by Bloswick and Howard describes some of the current innovations in assistive technology. Chapter 16 on enabling design by Anderberg et al. discusses universal design at length that will allow an efficient design for all, regardless of their age and disabilities. In Chapter 17 on functional capacity evaluation, Davidson discusses the intricacies of the approach and the challenges faced by rehabilitation professionals. She points out the shortcomings of this approach especially with respect to reliability and validity. However, imperfect as it may be, this tool is in wide use among professionals. Also, it is absolutely essential to determine deficits before they can be compensated. Chapter 18 by Wiker deals with the latter topic. Wiker delves into the concepts, strategies, and techniques of reasonable accommodation to render an individual functional and integrated in the society, who without such accommodation will not be a functional and integrated citizen.

Hopefully, the selection of topics from two vast and seemingly diverse disciplines will initiate the knowledge of some ideas and concepts not only to bridge the gap between the two disciplines but also to spur some activities in the direction that will benefit individual citizens as well as the society at large. This is a lofty dream, but even some activity in this direction will justify the goal of this book.

Shrawan Kumar

REFERENCES

Kumar, S. 1989. Rehabilitation and ergonomics: Complimentary disciplines, *Canadian Journal of Rehabilitation*, 3, 99–111.

Kumar, S. 1992. Rehabilitation: An ergonomic dimension, *International Journal of Industrial Ergonomics*, 9 (2), 97–108.

Kumar, S. 1997. *Perspectives in Rehabilitation Ergonomics*, Taylor & Francis, London.

Editor

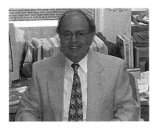

Shrawan Kumar, PhD, DSc, FRS(C), has been a professor of osteopathic manipulative medicine and director of research at the Physical Medicine Institute at the Health Science Center of the University of North Texas at Fort Worth, Texas since September 2007. Prior to taking this position, Dr. Kumar was a professor of physical therapy in the Faculty of Rehabilitation Medicine, and in the Division of Neuroscience, Faculty of Medicine at the University of Alberta, Canada. He joined the Faculty of Rehabilitation Medicine in 1977 and became an associate professor in 1979 and professor in 1982. Dr. Kumar obtained his BSc (zoology, botany, and chemistry) and MSc (zoology) from the University of Allahabad, India, and his PhD (human biology) from the University of Surrey, United Kingdom. He did his postdoctoral work in engineering at Trinity College, Dublin, and worked as a research associate in the Department of Physical Medicine and Rehabilitation at the University of Toronto. In 1994, Dr. Kumar was awarded a peer-reviewed DSc by the University of Surrey in recognition of his lifetime work. He was invited as a visiting professor for the year 1983–1984 at the Center of Ergonomics, Department of Industrial Engineering at the University of Michigan. He was a McCalla Professor during 1984–1985.

Dr. Kumar is an honorary fellow of the Association of Canadian Ergonomists (formerly known as the Human Factors Association of Canada), a fellow of the Human Factors and Ergonomics Society of the United States, and the Ergonomics Society of the United Kingdom. Dr. Kumar was awarded the Sir Frederic Bartlett Medal for excellence in ergonomics research by the Ergonomics Society of the United Kingdom in 1997. The University of Alberta awarded Dr. Kumar one of the seven Killam Annual Professorships for the year 1997–1998 for his distinguished research. The Human Factors and Ergonomics Society of the United States also bestowed its top honor of "Distinguished International Colleague" on Dr. Kumar in 1997. Dr. Kumar was appointed honorary professor of health sciences at the University of Queensland, Brisbane, Australia in 1998. In 2000, he was awarded the Jack Kraft Innovator Award by the Human Factors and Ergonomics Society, United States and the Ergonomics Development Award by the International Ergonomics Association for conceptualizing and developing the subdiscipline of rehabilitation ergonomics. In 2002, he received the highest professional honor from the International Ergonomics Association by being named one of the few IEA fellows. The Ergonomics Society of the United Kingdom invited him to deliver the Society Lecture in 2003. The Royal Society of Canada elected him a fellow in 2004. The 92nd Annual Indian Science Congress invited him to deliver the Professor S. C. Mahalanobish Memorial Oration Lecture in January 2005, which he was unfortunately unable to attend. He has been an invited keynote or plenary speaker at more than 40 national and international conferences in the Americas, Europe, Asia, Africa, and Australia.

Dr. Kumar has published over 450 scientific peer-reviewed publications and studies in the area of musculoskeletal injury causation and prevention with special emphasis on low back pain. He has edited or authored 13 books or monographs. He currently holds grants from the Natural Sciences and Engineering Research Council (NSERC). His work has also been supported by Medical Research Council (MRC), Workers Compensation Board (WCB), and National Research Council (NRC). He has supervised the work of 13 MSc students, 7 PhD students, and 6 postdoctoral students. He was an editor of the *International Journal of Industrial Ergonomics* until 2003, assistant editor of *Transactions of Rehabilitation Engineering*, consulting editor of *Ergonomics* until 2006, and continues to be an associate editor of *Spine* and of *The Spine Journal*. He serves on the editorial boards of six more international journals, and serves as a reviewer of several other international peer-reviewed journals. He also acts as a grant reviewer for NSERC, the Canadian Institute of Health Research (CIHR), Alberta Heritage Foundation for Medical Research (AHFMR), Alberta Occupational Health and Safety, and British Columbia Research in addition to the British Wellcome Foundation and American National Institute of Health (NIH) and National Science Foundation (NSF).

Dr. Shrawan Kumar has organized and chaired regional, national, and international conferences. He has served as the chair of the graduate program in physical therapy from 1979 to 1987; director of research, 1985–1990; chair of the Doctoral Program Development Committee, Faculty of Rehabilitation Medicine; and several other committees. He has served on chair's and dean's selection committees, and as a member of the University of Alberta Planning and Priority Committee and Academic Development Committee as well as chair of the Code of Ethics subcommittee of the International Ergonomics Association.

Contributors

Peter Anderberg
Certec, Department of Design
  Sciences
Lund University
Lund, Sweden

Donald S. Bloswick
Department of Mechanical
  Engineering
University of Utah
Salt Lake City, Utah

and

Department of Family and
  Preventive Medicine
Rocky Mountain Center for
  Occupational and
  Environmental Health
University of Utah
Salt Lake City, Utah

Megan Davidson
School of Physiotherapy
La Trobe University
Melbourne, Victoria, Australia

Sonja de Groot
Rehabilitation Centre
Duyvensz-Nagel Research
  Laboratory
Amsterdam, the Netherlands

and

Center for Human Movement
  Sciences
University Medical Center
  Groningen
University of Groningen
Groningen, the Netherlands

Desleigh de Jonge
School of Health and Rehabilitation
  Sciences
The University of Queensland
St Lucia, Brisbane, Australia

Anne Fenety
School of Physiotherapy
Dalhousie University
Halifax, Nova Scotia, Canada

Andris Freivalds
The Harold and Inge Marcus
  Department of Industrial and
  Manufacturing Engineering
Pennsylvania State University
University Park, Pennsylvania

Libby Gibson
School of Health and Rehabilitation
  Sciences
The University of Queensland
St Lucia, Brisbane, Australia

R. G. Haennel
Department of Physical Therapy
University of Alberta
Edmonton, Alberta, Canada

Katherine Harman
School of Physiotherapy
Dalhousie University
Halifax, Nova Scotia, Canada

Bryan Howard
Department of Mechanical Engineering
University of Utah
Salt Lake City, Utah

Thomas W. J. Janssen
Institute for Fundamental & Clinical
  Human Movement Sciences
Vrije Universiteit
Amsterdam, the Netherlands

and

Rehabilitation Centre
Duyvensz-Nagel Research
  Laboratory
Amsterdam, the Netherlands

Lester Jones
School of Physiotherapy
La Trobe University
Melbourne, Australia

Troy Jones
Department of Physical Therapy
University of Alberta
Edmonton, Alberta, Canada

Bodil Jönsson
Certec, Department of Design
  Sciences
Lund University
Lund, Sweden

Shrawan Kumar
Physical Medicine Institute
Health Science Center
University of North Texas
Fort Worth, Texas

Robert Lederer
Department of Art & Design
University of Alberta
Edmonton, Alberta, Canada

Suh-Jen Lin
School of Physical Therapy
Texas Woman's University
Dallas, Texas

Lili Liu
Department of Occupational
  Therapy
University of Alberta
Edmonton, Alberta, Canada

Murray E. Maitland
Department of Rehabilitation
  Medicine
Division of Physical Therapy
University of Washington
Seattle, Washington

G. Lorimer Moseley
Department of Physiology
  Anatomy & Genetics
University of Oxford
Oxford, United Kingdom

and

Prince of Wales Medical
  Research Institute
Sydney, Australia

Vivian K. Mushahwar
Department of Cell Biology and
  Centre for Neuroscience
University of Alberta
Edmonton, Alberta, Canada

Elin Olander
Industrial Design, Department
  of Design Sciences
Lund University
Lund, Sweden

Leandro R. Solis
Rehabilitation Sciences
University of Alberta
Edmonton, Alberta, Canada

Lena Sperling
Industrial Design, Department
  of Design Sciences
Lund University
Lund, Sweden

Siobhan Strike
Centre for Scientific and Cultural
  Research in Sport
School of Human and
  Life Sciences
Roehampton University
London, United Kingdom

C. R. Tomczak
Department of Physical Therapy
University of Alberta
Edmonton, Alberta, Canada

Allard J. van der Beek
Department of Public and
  Occupational Health
VU University Medical Centre
Amsterdam, the Netherlands

and

Body@Work, Research Centre
  Physical Activity, Work and Health
Amsterdam, the Netherlands

Lucas H. V. van der Woude
Center for Human Movement
  Sciences
University Medical Center
  Groningen
University of Groningen
Groningen, the Netherlands

Jaap H. van Dieën
Research Institute MOVE
Amsterdam, the Netherlands

and

Body@Work, Research Centre
  Physical Activity, Work and Health
Amsterdam, the Netherlands

Stefan van Drongelen
Swiss Paraplegic Research
Nottwil, Switzerland

Dirkjan H. E. J. Veeger
Institute for Fundamental & Clinical
  Human Movement Sciences
Vrije Universiteit
Amsterdam, the Netherlands

and

Man Machine Systems
Technical University Delft
Delft, the Netherlands

Steven F. Wiker
Ergonomics Laboratory
Industrial and Management
  Systems Engineering
  Department
West Virginia University
Morgantown, West Virginia

Section A

General Concepts

1 Rehabilitation Ergonomics: Conceptual Basis

Shrawan Kumar

CONTENTS

1.1 INTRODUCTION

Rehabilitation ergonomics is a young discipline. First proposed in 1979 informally in the literature, rehabilitation ergonomics needs to grow significantly. While the principles of rehabilitation ergonomics may remain stable, undergoing little change, its practice may vary significantly over time. The factor that will be largely responsible for this variation is technology and its evolution. Rehabilitation will continue to concern itself with the restoration of form and function of the human as close to normal as possible. This will be partly achieved by treatment and partly by assistance to the patient. Though the delivery of the treatment may also be modifiable for optimization through ergonomic intervention, it is the external assistance to patients to regain their function that will have the maximal potential of being benefited by incorporation of ergonomics. We have reached a state of development in the fields of rehabilitation and technology that the latter can have a profound effect on the former. However, marriage between these two concepts is not very old. This chapter deals entirely with the theoretical and conceptual aspects of rehabilitation ergonomics, which have been proposed in several publications by Kumar (1989, 1992, 1995) and Davies and Kumar (1996).

1.2 ORIGIN OF REHABILITATION AND ERGONOMICS

A common origin of all human endeavors can be assigned to the rational mind. In a historical sense, however, the same period of human history and the same events therein are known to have shaped and accelerated the development of rehabilitation and ergonomics. A separate but brief consideration follows.

1.2.1 REHABILITATION

The discrete origin of rehabilitation can be traced back to the use of electricity as a medical cure for physical paralysis and mental disease by a German physician, Charles Kratzenstein, in 1744. In the United States, Benjamin Franklin in 1753 stated that electricity produced some uplifting of the spirits. Subsequently, toward the end of the nineteenth century, medical electricity became popular among regular physicians. Its biggest support came from enthusiastic obstetricians and gynecologists (Gritzer and Arluke, 1985). Despite such developments, rehabilitation had not evolved as a prevalent practice. In fact, before World War I, disability was not considered a medical or social problem in America (Gritzer and Arluke, 1985). Such a situation was due to the combination of a lack of demand for expensive medical care and the lack of financial ability of the disabled to pay for lengthy service. However, just before World War I, the issue of permanent disability caused by industrial accidents was getting some attention. Several states in the United States passed workmen's compensation laws, providing medical services and financial aid for the disabled (Mock, 1917). With the outbreak of World War I, the number of the permanently disabled grew rapidly. By May 1919, approximately 123,000 disabled soldiers returned to the United States. Heavy casualties in Europe had forced those European nations to develop medical and rehabilitation services. Therefore, because of the necessity, the profession of rehabilitation emerged and gained support. During those early years, rehabilitation was primarily staffed by orthopedic surgeons and nurses. However, the orthopedic surgeons trained and employed physiotherapy aides to help them deliver the physical part of the treatment. These physiotherapy aides evolved since then, initially into four-year professionally trained physical therapists, and subsequently into postgraduates, with the development of a masters level course for entry professionals. Though occupational therapy has its roots outside World War I, it was the latter which brought it into the rehabilitation fold. The war time territorial struggle over vocational rehabilitation resulted in occupational therapists proclaiming that "vocational training or education per se is not a form of occupational therapy, but when given to reestablish function, to give a more normal view of life, it may well be classed as a form of occupational therapy" (AOTA, 1918). Finally, the specialty of speech therapy, though created as a separate occupation in the 1920s, joined rehabilitation after World War II. The interrelationship between speech therapy and rehabilitation is not as strong as that between physical and occupational therapy.

1.2.2 ERGONOMICS

Human ergonomic instinct can be logically associated with the human endeavors of making simple tools and shelter. The improvements to these endeavors, occurring in discrete steps of technological advancements, were incorporated in subsequent products. No deliberate attention was paid to ergonomics. Subsequently, however, it was necessitated by the Industrial Revolution and accelerated by the two world wars.

According to Christensen (1976), the growth of ergonomics took place in three phases: (a) the age of machines, (b) the power of revolution, and (c) machines for minds. In the first phase, advances in the textile industry and the application of steam power are worth noting. However, a pointed interest in the relationship between humans and their working environment became unmistakably clear during World War I. The productivity of ammunition factories became critical to the war effort. The production pressure and schedule in Great Britain resulted in health problems of workers and necessitated the formation of a health committee in 1915, which was renamed the Industrial Health Research Board in 1929. However, it was not recognized until World War II that some of the newly developed military equipment could not be operated safely or effectively. This started a conscious effort to design tools and tasks for people rather than the other way around. Under such an urgency, diverse research activity was undertaken with one goal in mind—to achieve military superiority. Thus the wars provided impetus to originate, pressure to evolve, and purpose to focus. Such a scenario set the stage for the birth of the science of "ergonomics." In fact, the ongoing activity of professionals involved in this field and their desire to continue to collaborate resulted in formal adoption of the term "ergonomics" in 1950 (Edholm and Murrell, 1973). This term was proposed by Professor Murrell in 1949; Seminara (1979) did, however, point out that the term ergonomics was not new. In fact, it was first used in 1857 by Jastrzebowski, a Polish professor.

1.3 PHILOSOPHY OF REHABILITATION AND ERGONOMICS

The philosophy of any discipline is its guiding force. Initial tentative positions are the subject of considerable discussion, exchange of ideas, and rationalization. Emergence of consensus is an evolutionary landmark and a sign of maturity of the discipline. From such a position, identifiable specific goals ensue. Finally, a circumscribing and delineating definition is formulated to encompass the philosophy and the goals.

1.3.1 REHABILITATION

Rehabilitation is concerned with restoration of functions: physical and psychosocial. This involves the enhancement and optimization of impaired residual human facilities. Where normalcy cannot be restored or recovery has not reached a functional level, a technological intervention, such as augmentative devices, is in order to bring the environment to the patient. Philosophically one may argue that most people are disabled to some extent on a continuum scale of superable to functionless in one or more of the multitude of functions they perform (Figure 1.1). The evidence of such a disability can also be provided in various assistive devices the able-bodied humans use in the multitude of functions they perform in their everyday lives. Nevertheless, the complement of faculties with which most people are born is considered to be the reference point. A decrement from this natural endowment, congenital or caused by disease or accident, is considered functional impairment and this needs rehabilitation. A physical impairment may lead to psychological maladjustment and social problems. Therefore, rehabilitation is concerned with complete reintegration of the disabled individual in the mainstream of the society.

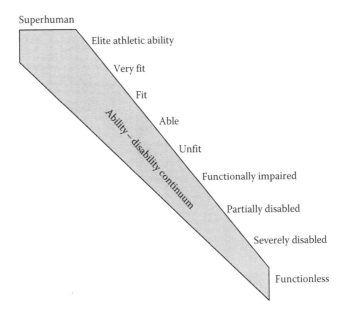

FIGURE 1.1 Scale of functioning.

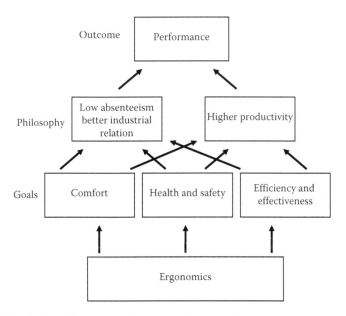

FIGURE 1.2 Goals, philosophy, and outcome of ergonomics.

1.3.2 ERGONOMICS

Philosophically, ergonomics has dual focus—(a) the worker and (b) the work, with the former taking precedence over the latter. Within the discipline, it is recognized that the worker is the performer and is responsible for productivity. A healthy, comfortable, well-adjusted worker with high morale will be optimally productive. In addition, when the job is fitted to the worker, production will be optimized. These two aspects contribute to better industrial relations and productivity. Thus, the complementary nature of the focus of ergonomics on the worker and the work enhance their mutual effectiveness (Figure 1.2).

1.4 GOALS OF REHABILITATION AND ERGONOMICS

1.4.1 REHABILITATION

The most important goal of rehabilitation is the remediation of disability and dysfunction. Motivated by the welfare of the patient, the rehabilitation discipline strives to provide relief and/or liberation from psychophysical limitations. The fulfillment of this goal, though of central relevance to the fields of rehabilitation, can be better accomplished if its necessity could be avoided. Thus, preservation of health becomes an important aspect of rehabilitation. Such goals are realized through education and exercise.

Despite the best efforts of health preservation, diseases do set in (such as arthritis, stroke, nerve entrapment, low back pain, etc.) and accidents do occur. Under these circumstances, it is the role of rehabilitation to arrest dysfunction and prevent deformity first. This is supplemented with functional restoration. The aim is to reach as close to the normal level of function as possible. The emphasis on normal functioning necessitates a clear and good grasp of "normalcy" in qualitative as well as quantitative terms. A quantitative measurement of functional impairment becomes essential for treatment goal setting and regimen selection. At times, due to the nature of the condition or the general health status of the patient, full recovery may be impossible. At such times, preparation of the patient to adapt to the disability and be functional is attempted. This adaptation may mean learning new skills, for example using a different body member to perform the same function. When such endeavors do not lead to independent living and deficiencies remain, augmentative devices are used to compensate for the residual deficits. Such individuals are also given an altered perspective to accept the disability they suffer from. Information on the social support agencies and groups is also provided to fall back upon, if needed.

1.4.2 ERGONOMICS

Ergonomics has three goals: comfort, well-being, and efficiency and effectiveness. Enhancement of comfort or reduction of discomfort reduces the tedium of the job, contributing to higher productivity and worker morale. Ensuring the well-being of workers through hazard elimination from the workplace promotes health on a long-term basis. This optimizes productivity, enhances worker morale, and reduces labor turnover. The latter is of strategic significance in economic terms to the industry and good for the morale and loyalty of the worker. Another benefit arising from this is better industrial relations. Lastly, the increase in efficiency and effectiveness of the industrial operations on the shop floor has economic benefit for all. This goal is achieved by job design, work space layout, and appropriate training.

1.5   DEFINITION OF REHABILITATION AND ERGONOMICS

1.5.1   REHABILITATION

Rehabilitation is a discipline of recent origin. Moreover, it is still evolving. Initially, the discipline primarily consisted of physiatrists and their assistants. Subsequently, physical therapists, occupational therapists, prosthetists, social workers, and rehabilitation engineers joined the field. All of these developments have taken place sequentially in the space of the last 60 years. Perhaps it is due to this constantly changing and expanding scope of the discipline that its position is not entrenched in a formal definition. Furthermore, each class of professional, out of necessity, has a different perspective of the discipline. Such is the case due to difference in training, priority, approach, and course of action. This, therefore, causes different professionals to view the discipline from the perspective of their subspecialty. It may also be for this reason that a clear and concise definition of the discipline has not emerged. A definition, nevertheless, is essential. It was this consideration with which a definition was proposed by Kumar (1989) as stated below:

> Rehabilitation is a science of systematic multi-dimensional study of disorders human neuro-psycho-social and/or musculoskeletal function(s) and its (their) remediation by physico-chemical and/or psycho-social means.

1.5.2 ERGONOMICS

A situation parallel to rehabilitation is evident in ergonomics. Ergonomics, however, is not as well established as rehabilitation among educational and service institutions. Having emerged in the same time period and due to the same evolutionary pressures, rehabilitation and ergonomics have significant commonality. However, they are generally viewed differently. The latter situation is suggested due to the difference in the immediate beneficiary of the knowledge and technology (disabled person versus suboptimal environment or machine). The consequence of good or bad ergonomics will ultimately affect everybody. However, the impression of remoteness created by this difference in the center of activity does not arouse the same passion in argument or similar sympathy in the listener. Though it is possible and likely that bad ergonomics may have resulted in the necessity to rehabilitate many war veterans, this is not generally seen as a direct cause and effect relationship. It is also possible that in spite of good ergonomics in extremely risky and highly demanding situations like war, the outcome in some cases may still have been similar. The need to harness all human faculties, sensory, motor, and psychological, at a heightened level and sustain them for optimum function could not fall within the expertise of any given existing discipline. Different demands on the military personnel on the two sides of the Atlantic during the wars spearheaded the development of this field along two different directions. In Europe, physical and physiological aspects were addressed largely, whereas in the United States, the cognitive factors were considered of supreme significance in their war efforts. As a result, there is a continuing debate as to whether the field is "ergonomics" or "human factors." Some of the professional societies have adapted both terms in their name (Human Factors and Ergonomics Society, USA). However, though not universally agreed, a more generic and universal term, "ergonomics" was coined and defined by Murrell (1949) as follows:

> Ergonomics (Greek), ergon – work; nomos – natural laws "ergonomics is the study of natural laws governing work."

The merit of this definition is that it encompasses all physical, physiological, and cognitive factors without giving superiority to any aspect. It is accepted that this field of study addresses the issues at the human–machine interface.

1.6 PARALLELISM BETWEEN REHABILITATION AND ERGONOMICS

The foregoing review of the origin, philosophies, and goals of the two disciplines indicate significant commonality between these two sciences. The central goal for both is to enable, enhance, and optimize human function. The context and the clientele may, however, be different.

Rehabilitation is concerned with disability prevention, restoration of function, and deficit compensation among patients who have lost some of their faculties. Ergonomics, on the other hand, is driving to increase efficiency and effectiveness by tapping the maximum possible from the existent resources of a normal person. The adaptation and adjustments are made in environment or human–machine interface to optimize the human capability. The central goal for both of them, nonetheless, is to enhance and optimize human function in different regions of the ability scale. Due to the scale difference, the populations for whom these are geared are different,

TABLE 1.1
Goals of Ergonomics and Rehabilitation Compared

Ergonomics	Rehabilitation
Ensure comfort	Health promotion
Achieve well-being	Eliminate pain and suffering
Ensure continued health	Maintenance of ability
Ensure worker safety	Dysfunction prevention
Achieve effectiveness	Restoration of function—treatment Adaptation to environment—exercise
Enhance efficiency	Development of skill—training
	Deficit compensation by augmentative devices
Promote high morale by industrial relations	Social adjustments with counseling and social resources

therefore, creating an impression of exaggerated divergence. The relationship between the goals of these two disciplines is summarized in Table 1.1. It is evident that these two disciplines have shared goals. Rehabilitation generally seems to be content with functional independence, the activities of daily living being the most significant yardstick. For ergonomics, though, industrial production and accident prevention are important measures.

As both, ergonomics and rehabilitation are goal-oriented disciplines, their approach remains open and flexible to ensure the success of the final objective. Both have drawn their relevant concepts from the same established basic and applied sciences and integrated them in an appropriate manner to achieve their desired goals. Therefore, both these sciences are inherently multidisciplinary. Each one has generous contribution from physical sciences, life sciences, behavioral sciences, anthropometry, biomechanics, and kinesiology.

Thus, identical goals, their reliance on the same constituent disciplines, and working toward enhancing and optimizing human function ties these two disciplines very closely.

Various ergonomic concepts and practices interweave through the rehabilitation fabric without a deliberate effort to incorporate these from a different science. A more structured integrated approach will enhance the effectiveness of rehabilitation, it may also be stated here that in many cases a lack of application or regard for ergonomics may precipitate injury and necessitate rehabilitation. The relationship between these is so intimate that one can state:

Rehabilitation is ergonomics for the disabled.

1.7 DIVERGENCE BETWEEN REHABILITATION AND ERGONOMICS

The differences between these two sciences, in addition to the context and clientele, lie in the specific body of knowledge, which may be described and differentiated as clinical and nonclinical. In addition, the major difference lies in the fact that the practitioners and researchers in ergonomics work toward adjusting and optimizing factors external to workers to enhance comfort, well-being, effectiveness, and efficiency. The rehabilitation practitioners and researchers on the other hand work mainly toward enhancing the factors internal to workers for restoration of functions. However, effort is also made to compensate for residual dysfunction by external, augmentative devices. Such activities are mostly undertaken by, among others, rehabilitation or clinical engineers.

1.8 COMPLEMENTARY ROLES OF REHABILITATION

1.8.1 IDENTIFICATION: MAGNITUDE OF THE PROBLEM

An unknown etiology and/or the preventative procedures for many diseases such as arthritis and stroke, do not allow meaningful control over their occurrence. However, a real control on the occurrence of many accidents may be within our grasp. Some accidents occur off-the-job in unstructured activities. These may be difficult to curb. However, a large number of accidents and injuries are occupational in origin. As these accidents occur during structured tasks in a known work environment, it is possible to identify the hazards. A redesign of the task and/or environment may eliminate the hazard and reduce the chances of injury. Though such figures for all of Canada are not available, many other countries do keep statistics. In 1977, there were 2.2 million disabling injuries in the United States resulting in 80,000 permanent impairments (NSC, 1978). Belknap (1985) reported statistics of such injuries in the United States, which have increased by 10% in 1978 over 1945 figures (Table 1.2). A comparative magnitude of these problems in selected countries is presented and extrapolated from the ILO (Geneva) figures (Table 1.3). The magnitude

---

TABLE 1.2
Work-Related Disabling Injuries in the United States

Year	Disabling Injuries On-the-Job
1945	2,000,000
1955	1,950,000
1960	1,950,000
1965	2,100,000
1970	2,200,000
1975	2,200,000
1976	2,200,000
1977	2,300,000
1978	2,200,000
Change (%) from 1945 to 1978	10%

Source: Belknap, R.G., in *Encyclopedia of Occupational Health and Safety*, 3rd edn., International Labour Office, Geneva, 1985.

TABLE 1.3

Number of On-the-Job Disabling Injuries in Selected Countries

Countries	1982	1983
Argentina	61,436	70,586
Egypt	62,312	62,933
France	950,520	N/A
Hong Kong	70,879	70,895
India	322,473	287,776
Switzerland	114,551	114,665
The United Kingdom	396,000	N/A
The United States	2,182,400	2,182,700

Source: After Year Book of Labour Statistics, 1984.

TABLE 1.4

Number of On-the-Job Accidents and Permanent Disabilities in Alberta

Years	Number of Total Injuries (A)	Number of Permanent Disabilities (B)	B as % of A	Musculoskeletal Injuries (C)	C as % of A
1983	57,246	2,165	3.78	N/A	N/A
1984	55,732	2,513	4.50	48,849	87.65
1985	62,626	2,172	3.46	55,155	88.07
1986	58,903	2,547	4.32	52,075	88.40
1987	58,637	2,456	4.18	52,059	88.78

N/A, not available.

Compiled from Alberta WCB annual reports.

of such problems has stayed at a sustained 3.5%–4.5% level in Alberta (Table 1.4). The evidence of the magnitude of the problem in the sector where considerable control can be exercised is evident from these figures. Ensuring workers' comfort and well-being are committed goals of ergonomics. One of the important goals of rehabilitation is health preservation, and disability and dysfunction prevention. Therefore, the role of ergonomics is complementary to the goal of rehabilitation. Mital and Karwowski (1988) emphasize the critical role of thorough application of ergonomics on the job for the success of disability prevention program.

1.8.2 REASON FOR CONSIDERING CHANGE

The usual first response of most employers to a disabling injury of an employee is to invoke long-term disability leave policies. Most employee programs provide for such protection. Such an action adds to the disabled pool. It was estimated that 30% of the entire American population had a disability in the late 1970s (Grall, 1979). Two out of three adults with disability did not work (Memmot, 1987). Such a large percentage falling out of the workforce is a serious loss to the national economy. Not only do these people cease to produce, lose self-worth and self-esteem, but also have to be supported by the public purse. It, therefore, makes strong economic and social sense to try and reintegrate these people into the normal workforce.

In the United States, the landmark legislation passed in 1973 tended to reduce the impact of this problem. This legislation, known as Title V, guarantees the rights of disabled Americans. Section 503 of this Act mandates that all federal contractors and subcontractors, holding $2500 annually in contracts with the government, are required to take affirmative action, steps to recruit, hire, and promote qualified handicapped employees. It also clearly states that federal contractors must make reasonable accommodations to the physical and mental limitations of an applicant for employment. In 1974, the U.S. Congress passed the Vietnam Era Veterans Readjustment Assistance Act. Section 402 of that law states that federal contractors receiving more than $10,000 annually from the government must develop affirmative action programs to recruit, hire, and promote qualified handicapped veterans and Vietnam-era veterans. This section also requires affirmative action and reasonable accommodation.

1.8.3 BENEFITS OF INTEGRATING PEOPLE WITH DISABILITY IN THE WORKFORCE: PROOF AND POTENTIAL

A shrinking labor pool, legal requirements, and the high cost of worker compensation and disability payments make a compelling argument with strong economic sense to maximize human resources. In the United States, in 1984, 25,000 placements of developmentally disabled were made in competitive employment and 50,000 were placed in 1985. This program was guided away from dependency toward goals of productivity, self-sufficiency, and integration into community life. It was estimated that 87,000 handicapped workers will earn about $400 million in gross annual taxable wages (Human Development News, 1987). There is little doubt about the cost-effectiveness of such programs. In an evaluation survey of JAN (1987) with a response rate of 28%, 90% of employers believed that they had benefited from employing handicapped. Of these, 14% thought that their benefit was not economic. Sixty-four percent estimated their benefit to be between $1,000 and $10,000; another 22% estimated their benefit to range between $15,000 and $30,000.

1.8.4 ERGONOMICS COMPLEMENTING REHABILITATION

Looking at the prevalent practice of rehabilitation, it is clearly discernible that rehabilitation had largely been based on physiological and biochemical criteria. It also took into account the functional criteria of activities of daily living, generally in a qualitative manner. The range of motion (ROM) before, during, and after rehabilitation remains one consistent quantitative measure, which was used frequently for the functional assessment. If, however, the primary goal of rehabilitation is functional restoration following injury or disease, a further adaptation of strategy is essential. First, a clear establishment of multifaceted quantitative norms of various human activities is an essential starting point. Many human studies dwell on unidimensional performance of elite athletes. However, the norm of the average population is considered more appropriate for rehabilitation. This starting point will allow both, a quantitative evaluation of the functional impairment and a goal for rehabilitation regimes to work toward. Such a course of action will also allow quantitative evaluation of effectiveness of various unvalidated rehabilitation procedures. The nature and extent of functional deficit and recovery will have to be determined in as many dimensions as possible, which affect the function. Also, a position is advocated here that rehabilitation is not complete until the patient has returned to productive employment, or retrained to enter an alternate profession suitable to his/her capabilities. This will certainly introduce an element of thorough job demands analysis and job modification. For optimization of the productivity, all ergonomic principles will have to be effectively employed. Only such a broadening of the scope of rehabilitation will result in holistic rehabilitation (Figure 1.3).

A disability may be defined as a perturbation, which adversely affects function. An individual with disability who performs multitude of activities may have decrement in one or more variables. In order to continue to perform normally, an individual will have to have normal kinematics, kinetics, ROM, strength, endurance, perception, motor coordination, mobility, no pain, and normal psyche to enumerate more important factors. Decrement in one may significantly affect the performance

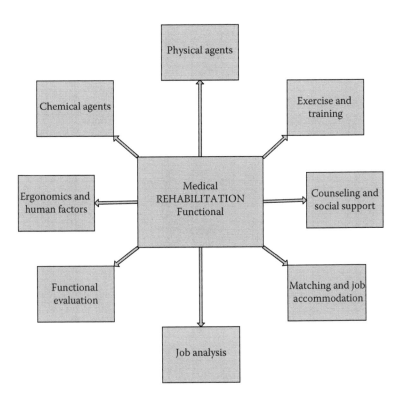

FIGURE 1.3 Holistic model of rehabilitation.

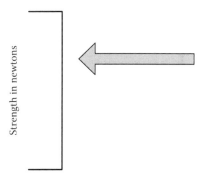

FIGURE 1.4   Functional strength measure.

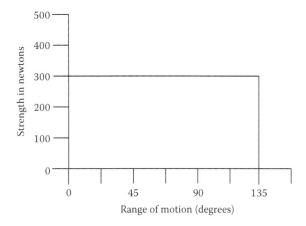

FIGURE 1.5   Performance criteria of strength and motion.

score in others. Therefore, the activities of daily living as well as vocational tasks have to be rated for multidimensional parameters, including all variables that are employed. If in a given activity only the strength of a body member is needed, it can be measured and recorded (Figure 1.4). If strength is required to be exerted through a ROM, both criteria need to be tested (Figure 1.5). For the activity in question, if a certain speed is necessary, it will also have to be assessed (Figure 1.6). The boundary of this graph will represent the functional capacity of the worker for this given task based on the tests conducted. However, these are not the only variables that affect human performance. The combination of strength, ROM, and speed characterize some of the physical demands of activity performed once. The frequency of operation and the duration of work shift will be essential to be considered for vocational rehabilitation. The muscle tone will determine the endurance, and cardiopulmonary fitness will determine the aerobic capacity. The dexterity and precision of the operation are other physical variables, which will need to be accounted for. It is obvious, therefore, that even in physical domain, the task requirements become multidimensional (Figure 1.7).

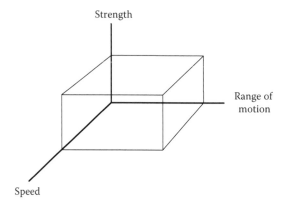

FIGURE 1.6   The boundary of physical functional capability.

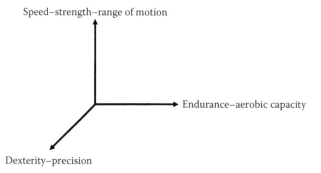

FIGURE 1.7   Profile of physical requirements for a task.

Similar multidimensional requirements in social as well as psychological domains are essential ingredients of work-worthiness of every individual undergoing rehabilitation (Figures 1.8 and 1.9). In the final assessment the patient will have to be tested on all these aspects (Figure 1.10). The decision to return to a given work will have to depend on the demands of the tasks. By overlapping the requirements of the task on the pool of resources that an individual has, one could clearly see the suitability of the patient to the task (Figure 1.11). In this hypothetical case, a high demand on endurance and aerobic capacity is made. It clearly violates the guideline of not exceeding one-third of the aerobic capacity (NIOSH, 1981). As such, while the individual is capable of handling every other aspect, he will not be able to endure the demand of physiological cost. Furthermore, an excessive demand on muscle endurance will prevent the individual from being able to carry on for a significant length of time. A variable by variable quantitative assessment and a separate comparison with design criteria of each variable should be the standard procedure for placement. Clearly, when the task becomes more demanding and requires many more attributes from the patient, the complexity of the situation will increase. It will need a more

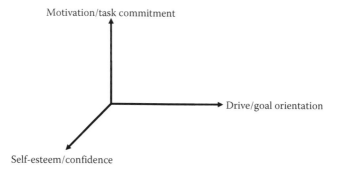

FIGURE 1.8   Profile of social requirements of tasks.

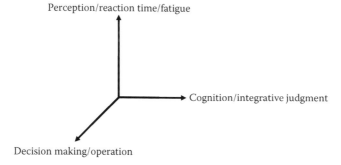

FIGURE 1.9   Profile of psychological requirements for a task.

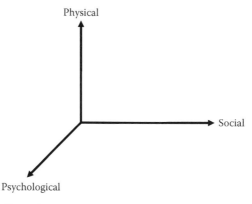

FIGURE 1.10   The dimensions of work-worthiness.

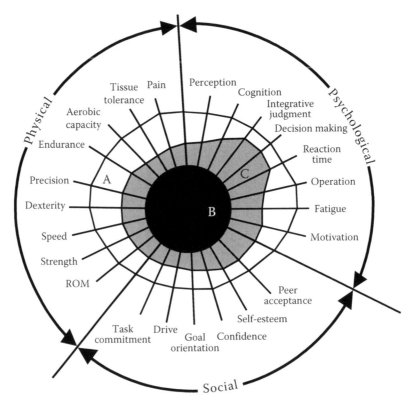

FIGURE 1.11 A hypothetical case showing comparison of job requirements and job capabilities.

sophisticated evaluation and management system. Different variables may have to be assigned separate weights in order to arrive at a realistic and meaningful solution. Such an assessment of a disabled person will allow a comparison with the norms to determine the extent of the deficit. This information will also allow one to plan the strategy of rehabilitation effort and subsequent steps of integration.

1.9 DISABILITY CONTEXT

The description and understanding of the term and concept of disability is somewhat obscured by nonstandardized usage. Conceptually, disability is a reduced functional status resulting from an impairment, giving rise to a handicap. These terms according to the International Classification of Impairments, Disabilities, and Handicaps (ICIDH) proposed by the WHO (1990) are as follows:

- *Impairment*: "Any loss or abnormality of psychological and anatomical structure or function." Therefore, impairments are disturbances at the level of the organ, which include damage or loss in part or whole of a body part or member, as well as derangement or loss of mental function.

- *Disability*: "A restriction or lack of ability (resulting from impairment) to perform an activity in the manner or within the range considered normal for a human being." Therefore, a disability is a functional limitation or activity restriction, probably caused by an impairment.
- *Handicap*: "A disadvantage for a given individual, resulting from an impairment or disability that limits or prevents the fulfilment of a role that is normal (depending on age, sex and social and cultural factors) for that individual." Thus, the term handicap describes the situation of nonfulfillment of social and economic roles of disabled people, which, depending on circumstances, environment, and culture, would be normal for others to do.

From the functional point of view then, Kumar (1989) argued that most people are disabled to some extent in one or more of the multitude of functions the individual performs. The reference is taken from, in such determinations, the normative data, which are obtained from a large group of normal people. The scale of functioning is presented in Figure 1.1. Strictly speaking then, all functions which one is capable of, must fall within this range. However, for any given individual, the extent of a disability and handicap may be dependent on the hierarchy and frequency of use of the given function.

1.10   MEDICAL AND HEALTH MODEL

The inevitability of impairment, ensuing disability, and handicap assured by statistical law of averages has become a fact of life of our socioeconomic structure. The World Health Organization in its World Program of Action has identified three goals to cope with the problem. First is the primary prevention. It is to be accomplished by measures aimed at preventing the onset of mental, physical, and sensory impairments. If impairment has occurred, then negative physical, psychological, and social consequences can be minimized or eliminated. The second goal is rehabilitation. A goal-oriented and time-limited process aimed at enabling the impaired, also strives to reduce and eliminate pain and suffering. The third and final goal is equalization of opportunities; cultural and social life, including sports and recreational facilities, are made accessible to all. Thus, the coping medical and health model has the tripartite goals of prevention, rehabilitation, and equalization (Figure 1.12).

1.11   ERGONOMIC DIMENSION

The dual complimentary emphases of ergonomics are placed on the worker and the work. Work is not just important but, in this context, is the ultimate objective. The "end" of work is achieved through the "means" of the worker. Therefore, the worker by the logic of hierarchy, technical, and social considerations becomes the most important component and strategic focal point for technological considerations. A comfortable, healthy, and well-adjusted worker is more likely to be a motivated worker with high morale. Such a combination of factors is generally known to translate into high productivity and better industrial relations. Thus, the complementarity of the dual focus has a tendency to establish and optimize the gain of a

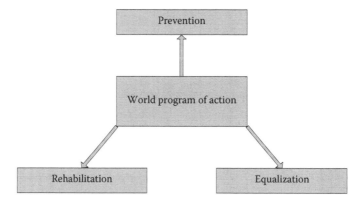

FIGURE 1.12   World program of action.

self-amplifying loop. Under unfavorable circumstances, the converse is also likely to happen (Figure 1.13).

Thus, the tripartite goals of ergonomics are not only mutually complimentary in influencing the outcome measure significantly, but are also parallel to and compatible with the tripartite goals of the coping medical and health model. The complementarity between the prevention of impairment and the comfort of worker, rehabilitation of disability, health and safety, equalization of opportunity, and efficiency and effectiveness are obvious. Ensuring comfort and well-being of the workers through hazard identification and their elimination from the workplace will accomplish the public health goal of prevention of impairment, thereby eliminating the need for rehabilitation. Such a step is likely to optimize productivity, enhance worker morale, and reduce labor turnover. These are strategically significant in economic terms for

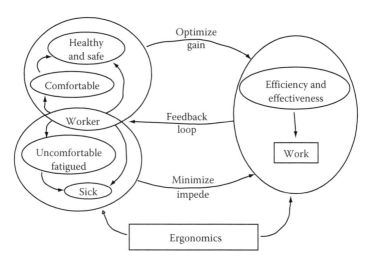

FIGURE 1.13   Interdependence of dual focus of ergonomics.

industry and good for the morale and loyalty of workers. From these emerge better and stable industrial relations. In order to achieve this, the task at hand is ergonomically fitted to the worker. Given the worker characteristic, normal or impaired, the process of fitting the job through adjustment or modification to maximize worker capability is ergonomics, parallel to the process of disability rehabilitation of the medical and health model. The ergonomic principle of enhancing efficiency and effectiveness is complimentary to the equalization of opportunity, which seeks to enhance environmental accessibility to disabled people through reduction in demand.

Ergonomics, however, is not only complimentary to the medical and health model but can also be an effective tool in the realization of its goals. Impairment prevention can be achieved to a large extent through hazard elimination. The process of rehabilitation can be significantly enhanced by incorporation of ergonomics in treatment and management strategies. The role of ergonomics lies not only in provision of normative standards but also in the development of testing and evaluation techniques. The latter provides quantitative measures of success. Furthermore, ergonomics can offer meaningful enhancements of treatment regimes. In the final stage of management with equalization of opportunity, the role of ergonomics is prevalent, pervasive, and extensive. In fact, the equalization of opportunities can be delivered only through the medium of ergonomics. The role of ergonomics integrated in the medical and health model is represented in Figures 1.14 and 1.15.

1.12 APPLICATION OF ERGONOMICS IN REHABILITATION

Rehabilitation of workers to gainful employment is one of the primary goals of Workers' Compensation Boards in the United States. The fulfillment of such a goal is dependent upon the degree of incorporation of principles described above. With these considerations, it is strongly suggested that all Workers' Compensation Boards must have a Work Evaluation Department. The purpose of the Work Evaluation Department should be able to assess a client's capacity to return to employment.

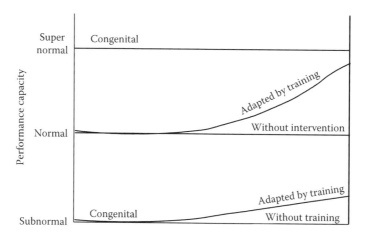

FIGURE 1.14 Congenital and adapted performance endowment.

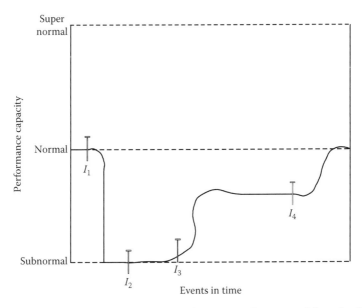

FIGURE 1.15   Generic outcome of normal performance endowment subjected to interventions of impairment, rehabilitation.

The work evaluator must evaluate clients from a multifaceted perspective as it relates to the employment and develops a quantitative inventory of their capabilities. The work evaluator must endeavor to maximize function following impairment to facilitate successful return to work through job analysis and job accommodation where needed, education in optimized work procedures, as well as provision of appropriate assistive devices. The work evaluator should work in cooperation with rehabilitation engineer and vocational counselor to facilitate transition from the rehabilitation phase to gainful employment. In order to achieve this, the following service functions may be essential.

1.12.1   FUNCTIONAL EVALUATION

An assessment to determine a person's physical work capacity, perceptual and cognitive abilities, and work behaviors should be conducted. Within the physical domain, functional activities, for example, sitting, standing, walking, climbing, jumping, running, balancing, kneeling, crouching, crawling, squatting, lifting, carrying, pushing, pulling, reaching, handling, strength, endurance, speed, aerobic capacity, dexterity, and precision, should be given special attention. On the psychological front, the perceptual and cognitive abilities should be tested through tasks of feeling, seeing, hearing, memory, concentration, judgment, decision making, learning ability, and others. The social aspects profile should be rated on motivation, perseverance, adaptability, reliability, goal orientation, self-esteem, confidence, punctuality, appearance, organization, attitude to peers, attitude to supervision, judgment, and others.

1.12.2 JOB-RELATED EVALUATION

An assessment of a person's ability to work in a specific job must be determined on the basis of the criteria stated in previous categories, at least after simulating specific job components. An effort must be made by the work evaluator to make the assessments on the job site during the performance of the tasks in a real work environment.

1.12.2.1 Job Demands Analysis

A systematic study of the physical demands of the job and work site must be performed. Included in this analysis should be work postures, tool use, material handling, environmental factors, and work pacing. This information must then be compared to work methods or work site modifications.

1.12.2.2 Job Accommodation

Based on the previously conducted job analysis, job/job site modification may be implemented, if necessary, to enhance a worker's ability to function. The modifications made should be individual specific to ensure an optimum "worker–work" fit. Such a modification may be augmented by necessary education of the employee and the employer in the ergonomic and related issues of the given case.

1.12.3 OPERATIONAL BLUEPRINT

With the increasing size of the special population, which needs services spanning the traditional territories of rehabilitation and ergonomics, and the intrinsic commonality with overlap between these disciplines, it is a matter of some urgency to develop a plan to operationalize the integrated execution to meet the social needs. In any such activity, multiple levels of effort will be necessary. In order to adequately cover most circumstances, functional divisions are necessary. Some considerations will be more appropriate for people, others for processes, and still others for products. A brief discussion ensues in that order.

1.12.3.1 People-Related

In the functional domain, a clear establishment of multifaceted quantitative norms of various human activities is an essential starting point. A direct transfer of information generated in numerous studies, which dwell on unidimensional performance in athletic activities, is not relevant. First, these levels of activities cannot be sustained on a long-term basis due to their intensity. Second, their influence on other variables, which may also be required in operation (to a varying degree), will not be known. Furthermore, these studies use people who excel in these activities incorporating an elite bias. It is therefore essential to have multidimensional functional evaluation norms of normal and average people of both sexes and different age groups. Such an endeavor will allow us to determine the gender and age factors of ready adjustment in a given population. Such an extensive database, though tedious to develop, will serve as a three-dimensional framework to base functional assessment to determine the nature and extent of functional deficiencies and impairments. One such database has been developed and reported by Kumar (1991). This will also provide a goal for treatment planning and a continuous comparison to determine any progress or remaining deficiency, as the case may be. Thus, the nature and extent of functional impairment and subsequent recovery when determined multidimensionally (in all relevant criteria) will assist holistic rehabilitation (Kumar, 1989). Commonly, patients are released soon after partial rehabilitation (barely functional for activities of daily living) and are not followed to their workplaces. Not only philosophically, but also pragmatically, it is emphasized that rehabilitation is incomplete unless the patient is reintegrated in the work force with or without adjustment and/or augmentation. The independence of a patient is not limited to physical partial functions, but includes economic independence and social adjustment. A disregard for such a holistic rehabilitation may incur significant cost to the society, lost productivity to the economy, and adverse social and psychological impact on the patient. Only a concurrent broadening of scope of ergonomics and rehabilitation and their overlapping application can result in holistic rehabilitation (Figure 1.16).

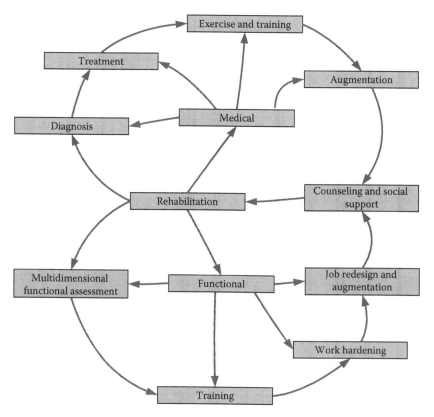

FIGURE 1.16   Component interaction in holistic rehabilitation.

1.12.3.1.1 Physical Work-Worthiness

An impairment is a perturbation, which adversely affects function. An individual with an impairment, during the course of daily living and work, will perform a multitude of activities involving numerous physical traits. Due to interdependence of physical traits and the dependence of more than one trait on one physical or physiological parameter, the functional aberration is likely to be variable in multiple dimensions. In order to maintain normal performance, one will have to have normal ROM, strength, endurance, kinematics, kinetics, perception, and motor coordination. A physical injury causing pain may affect more than one variable in varying amounts, resulting in an entirely different picture compared to preinjury state. Therefore, physical work-worthiness must be rated multidimensionally incorporating all relevant variables. The traditional medical model of rehabilitation generally based the rehabilitation decisions heavily on ROM. Such a practice would be considered sound if the ROM was the sole variable required to be functional. No useful and productive work can be done by just moving body parts. Generally, force application is also essential. Thus, testing of motion for the available range may be the first necessary step (Figures 1.17 and 1.18). Having determined the required motion for a given task, it will be essential to determine the maximum strength required to carry out the task in question. Due to the concurrent requirement of ROM and strength, the job requirement can be presented as in Figure 1.19. Productive work environment

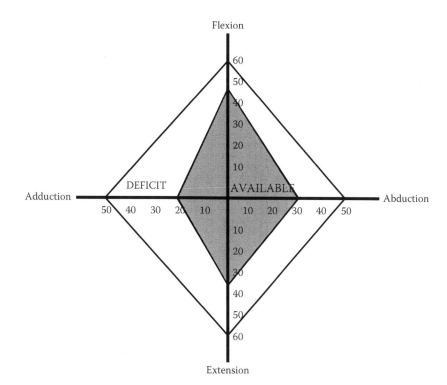

FIGURE 1.17 A quantitative pictorial depiction.

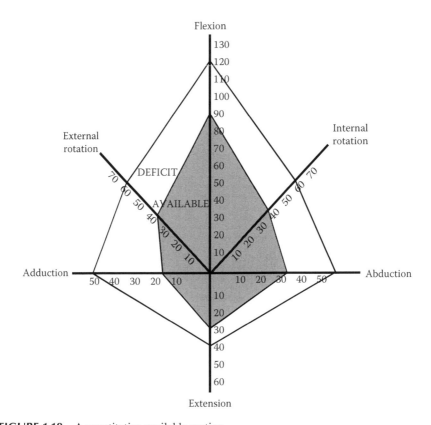

FIGURE 1.18 A quantitative available motion.

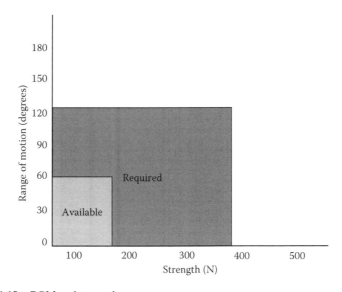

FIGURE 1.19 ROM and strength.

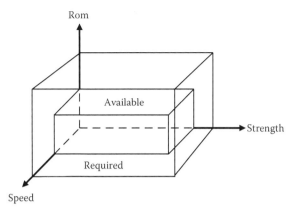

FIGURE 1.20   Physical traits required.

has a constant demand of pacing and/or output. Therefore, the speed of activity with required strength within the established ROM also becomes an essential criterion. Simultaneous consideration of all three factors can provide a complete picture of job requirements (Figure 1.20). An overlap of the patient capability on the job requirement profile will be essential for a quantitative functional assessment and determination of deficiencies. The difference between the boundary lines of job requirement and availability in the patient will be a quantitative measure of deficiency due to impairment for one task cycle. Other physical and physiological variables such as endurance, cardiopulmonary fitness, aerobic capacity, dexterity, precision, tissue tolerance characteristics, and status of pain will all determine full physical workworthiness. All these physical traits will be demanded for work-worthiness due to the repetitive nature of productive industrial work (Figure 1.21). An interaction between the production quota and reasonable human performance capability will determine the frequency of operation and the shift duration.

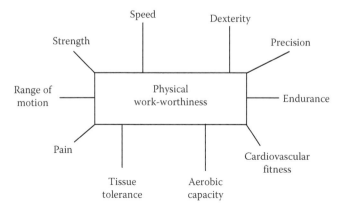

FIGURE 1.21   Major physical traits.

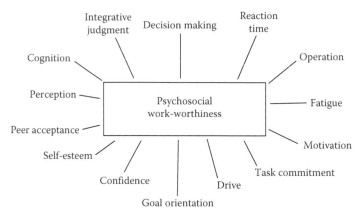

FIGURE 1.22 Major psychosocial traits.

1.12.3.1.2 *Psychosocial Work-Worthiness*

A similar multidimensional requirement in psychosocial domain is essential for optimal functioning of the worker (Figure 1.22). For final assessment, the patient will
have to be quantitatively tested on all affected relevant variables. The decision of
further treatment, training, or returning to work will significantly depend on the job
demand. It will be only through, preferably, a quantitative overlap of the patient's
physical and psychosocial capability over the job requirement that an ergonomically
trained rehabilitation professional will be able to determine the shortfall and select a
strategy to manage (Figure 1.23). This imaginary task requires a great deal of speed,
precision, dexterity, perception, cognition, and fast reaction time. On these criteria,
the hypothetical patient has deficiencies and is, at the time of assessment, unsuitable
to be sent back to this job. A similar deficiency and hence incompatibility could be
found in the physical domain. Under these two sets of conditions, different decisions
will be made for divergent rehabilitation strategies. Furthermore, a comparison of
patients with normative data on all these scales will help determine quantitative
functional impairment or disability, as the case may be.

1.12.3.2 Process-Related

Subsequent to the rehabilitation effort, many patients are left with residual functional impairment, which may inhibit their being gainfully employed. In Canada,
almost one-half (45.6%) of all disabled people required assistance in performing
heavy household chores, while nearly one quarter required assistance to perform
daily housework (22.4%) or to shop (23.2%) (Statistics Canada, 1990). In many cases,
disability impact is compounded due to many people having more than one disability. Statistics Canada (1990) reported that though mobility and agility are the most
common disabilities at 64.4% and 55% respectively, hearing, mental, and visual
disabilities ranked at 30.8%, 27.3%, and 16% in that order. It is also reported that only
40.3% of all disabled persons of working age were gainfully employed in Canada in
contrast to 66.6% of the general population (Statistics Canada, 1990).

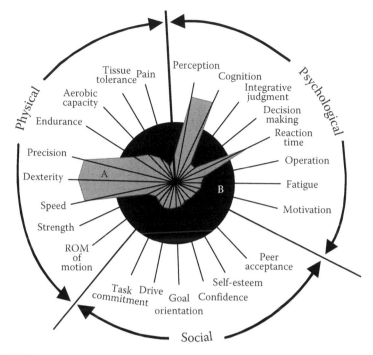

FIGURE 1.23 A conceptual model.

To enable people with disabilities, the first and foremost attention has to be given to job redesign in light of the quantitative functional assessment, as detailed before. To a disabled worker, the components of the job demand falling beyond the person's capability have to be modified to bring the job within the worker's capability. Such job accommodation most frequently may involve modification of hardware as well as the processes. For now, until the categories of generic disabilities along with magnitude of gradations are established, these may have to be dealt with on a case by case basis. In some cases, a job redesign may not be sufficient to enable a disabled worker, for which an assistive or augmentative device may be required. Such a strategy may also be found effective among cases with minor disability, where assistive devices may circumvent a need for hardware modification. Such a strategy of flexible matching with varying extent of job modification and assistive devices will not only give the disabled person a sense of self-worth, but also increase the gross national product.

Assistive devices may range from a simple cane to sophisticated robots. Disabled people require personal attention and care. These individuals rely on family members, friends, or attendants for their daily needs and mobility. The largest cost for these people is not medical care but maintenance, attendant care, nursing home, and home care expenses on top of loss of productivity due to inability to work. Assistive devices offer disabled people a chance to decrease these costs and function more effectively in the society by performing the processes, which they otherwise could not. It is revealing to note that in 1980 in the United States, over 3000 times as much money was spent on people and equipment to care for the disabled than was spent on development of technology that would allow the disabled to care for themselves—$220 billion versus $66 million (McNeal, 1982). LeBlanc and Leifer (1982) also reported that the money spent on the technology of assistive devices was economically beneficial to the society. They stated that every dollar spent on assistive device technology returned $11 in benefit to the society.

Gilbert et al. (1987) reported development of a robot mannequin with 38 degrees of freedom in movement to test the effectiveness of protective clothing in hazardous environment. This mannequin equipped with skin sensors had the ability to replicate ancillary biological systems including sampling of chemical reagents, which would be of immense value to a disabled worker with loss of tactile sense. NASA (1989) reported development of a device, which may improve the vision of people with visual disability of low vision, which cannot be corrected medically, surgically, or with eye glasses. Such a restoration of visual function will allow execution of normal productive life. Tuchi et al. (1985) reported development of a robotic aid for the blind. This robot is designed to replicate the functions of a guide dog. It can be programmed with appropriate landmark information of an area and it has the capability to guide the owner to a desired destination. Such examples clearly indicate that identification and quantification of a needed process or component of a task may allow development and fabrication of an augmentative device, which may enable an otherwise disabled worker. It will, therefore, be of value to analyze many of the tasks in question ergonomically and develop an inventory of generic processes, which may help many disabled individuals.

Since the functional restoration is the final outcome of rehabilitation, the effectiveness and efficiency of the process is the ergonomic concern. In ergonomic terms, the process of rehabilitation involves two interfaces: (1) the interface between the therapist and the patient, which will have a bearing on the effectiveness of treatment and (2) the interface between the patient and the environment surrounding the patient. Both these interfaces will interact in determining the final outcome of the functional normalcy of the patient (Figure 1.24).

1.12.3.2.1 Therapist–Patient Interface

Intense therapist–patient interaction occurs at two levels: (a) psychological and (b) physical. The knowledge, biases, and expectations of therapists may have a significant impact on the final functional outcome of the patient's rehabilitation. These may shape the patient's expectation, motivation, and compliance. To ascertain if such biases do exist among therapists, Simmonds and Kumar (1996) tested a sample of 69 physical therapists. Each therapist viewed three videotaped assessments of patients with low back pain that differed in severity. A brief history of patients containing their Workers Compensation was provided with the videotape to each participating therapist. Another group of therapists was not provided any information on the patient. These therapists were required to make prognoses based on the physical assessment on the videotapes. Although the therapists made similar physical assessments, their prognosis of the patients was significantly different ($p < 0.5$) across the information group. The workers compensation status was deemed to have a negative effect on the outcome in patients even with mild low back pain. On the other hand, the nonworkers compensation status was considered positive by

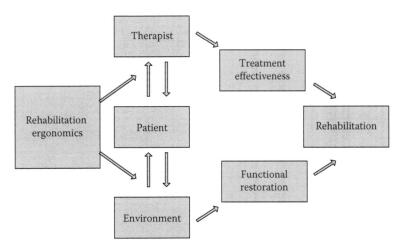

FIGURE 1.24 A theoretical model of rehabilitation ergonomics.

therapists in prognosis of recovery. Thus, such knowledge biased the opinions and expectations of the therapists. Basmajian (1975), Peat (1981), and Harkappa et al. (1991) have all reported that the psychosocial factors may have significant impact on the treatment outcome. Therefore, a preventative ergonomic intervention in the psychological domain at the therapist–patient interface may have a significant impact on the outcome.

At the physical level, more than the validity of the technique, the efficiency and the accuracy of treatment is of paramount importance for an effective treatment. The point will be illustrated by two examples. First, physical medicine and physical therapy are delivered through physical medium; therefore, an accurate location of a physical landmark is essential. These are invariably determined by the technique of palpation before delivering the treatment. An identification of landmark through palpation has been considered accurate and objective (Grieve, 1981; Lee, 1989). This prevalent belief has generally gone unchallenged despite the lack of objective evidence. To test this assumption, Burton et al. (1990) tested reliability of repeated identification of palpable landmarks. He used invisible marking pen and measured the distance between consecutive marks for spinal levels S_2, L_4, and T_{12}. Though the distances between the consecutive marks varied, they remained within 5 mm for S_2 and L_4, and 10 mm for T_{12} landmarks within raters. Between raters, however, for T_{12} this distance was 35 mm. Thus, within rater, these palpation results were considered repeatable and reliable for bony landmarks "easy-to-palpate from surface." In a study, Simmonds and Kumar (1993) investigated the reliability of palpability of (a) the anterior border of lateral collateral ligament at the level of knee joint, (b) the spinous process of L_4, (c) the posterior superior iliac spine, and (d) the transverse process of L_4. Experienced therapists were asked to mark each structure with an invisible ink and repeat the process after lapse of time. While the palpation of L_4 was done accurately, all others were inaccurate. The level of inaccuracy increased with the depth of the tissue ($p < 0.02$). It is conceivable that a poor reliability of many clinical tests may be due to the errors associated with palpation.

Thus standardization of this procedure to enhance accuracy at this interface is of vital importance for an optimal outcome.

The next stage of effective treatment will depend on the delivery of an appropriate dose of a valid treatment. One of the common treatment modalities for the low back pain is spinal mobilization. Four grades of mobilization and their needs have been advocated in the literature (McKenzie, 1987). Therapists commonly administer spinal mobilization subjectively assessing the grade of the treatment they administer. The accuracy of such an assessment needs to be established. Therefore in a study, Simmonds et al. (1995) quantified the forces exerted on and the displacements produced of the vertebral body during mobilization on a spinal model. Kumar (1995) designed and fabricated a therapeutic spinal model (U.S. patent number: 5,441,413). On this model, 10 experienced therapists performed four grades of mobilizations at three different levels of joint stiffness—low, medium, and high stiffness. The mean peak force values recorded were lowest in the least stiff condition across all grades of mobilization (57.6–120 N). For medium and high stiffness, the exerted force values were similar, ranging between 82 and 178 N for medium stiffness and 81–162 N for the high stiffness. Similarly, the peak displacement for each grade of mobilization for low, medium, and high levels of stiffness ranged between 2.2 and 3.4 mm, 1.8 and 2.0 mm, and 1.9 and 2.2 mm respectively. The results showed that there was a significant difference in force exerted due to the stiffness of the spine as well as the grade of mobilization ($p < 0.01$). However, there was a large range of intertherapist variability. The force exerted by different therapists varied between 7 and 380 times, whereas the displacements produced varied between 12 and 112 times. The value of any treatment depends on delivery of a valid treatment in a consistently standardized manner. The degree of variability encountered among seasoned therapists may be a reason for concern. Therefore, it is essential to standardize the treatment. The latter will be achievable through ergonomics. Enhancing this consistency will optimize the outcome of rehabilitation.

1.12.3.2.2   Patient–Environment Interface

There is considerable value in an objective and holistic assessment of patient's performance and a profile of the tasks to be performed. Such matching for determination of deficits as advocated by Kumar (1992) will be essential to focus the rehabilitation attempts for optimizing the rehabilitation outcome.

1.12.3.2.3   Means

The means of successful implementation of the objectives of rehabilitation ergonomics lie in development of methodology, databases, their interpretation and integration. The methodology may be adapted for the purpose from the existing tools and methods. Using these, relevant databases need to be created to develop norms or ranges of samples of interests. These databases then need to be integrated for appropriate use, in this case, design or modification.

With aging, trauma, or disease, there may be decrement in one or more functions of the body. Most functions require motion, force application, and velocity of execution. If one considers these functions in an occupational context, endurance and repetition become important. Therefore, it is essential to determine the job profile in terms of motion, force, velocity, and repetition. For this information to be helpful and relevant, the data must be collected in the occupational milieu and simultaneously. Therefore, the force exerting capacity through the ROM and sustainable velocity and repetition will be essential. Thus, such multidimensional data must be collected in physical, psychological, and social domains (Kumar, 1992). The decision regarding a course of action (treatment, training, return to work, etc.) will depend on the job demand. A quantitative overlap of the patient's physical and psychosocial capability over the job requirement (Figure 1.23) will allow an ergonomically trained rehabilitation professional to determine the deficiencies and select a strategy to manage the case. This hypothetical task requires a great deal of speed, precision, dexterity, perception, cognition, and fast reaction time. On these criteria in this hypothetical example, the identified deficiencies prohibit to return the worker to work. For this job, the patient needs further rehabilitation. However, there may be another job, which this patient may be able to do. Thus, depending on the severity of deficiencies, the patients may be placed either on an alternate job, returned to rehabilitation, or sent for work hardening. Thus, in order to employ rehabilitation ergonomics, one may have to consider a variety of steps and strategies as presented by Kumar (1992) (Figures 1.21 and 1.22).

Although the components of the rehabilitation ergonomics are multiple, they either impact on the "therapist–patient" interface or the "patient–environment" interface. It will be only through a thoughtful and careful application and execution that we may be able to more or less overcome the barriers to a significant segment of our population, and make a positive contribution to the national as well as world economy. Therefore, the following model represents the theoretical framework of rehabilitation ergonomics (Figure 1.3).

1.12.3.3 Product-Related

One of the important tenets of development of any product and its sustained success would be the ability of the market place to be able to support it. A continued state subsidy for such items spells their ultimate demise due to non-affordability rather than lack of usefulness. At first sight, the above statement may appear uncompassionate, contrary to the motive of furtherance of this argument in the first place. If the initial design criteria take this fact into account, the products may last much longer in the market and benefit the disabled population. In exploring such a market, the socioeconomic statistics about disabled people is very pertinent. Statistics Canada (1990) states that only 40% of all disabled people are employed in Canada. While up to 50% of disabled men are gainfully employed, only 30% of women with disability have employment. The Secretary of State stated that over 57% of all persons with disability have an annual income less than $10,000. Grall (1979) reported that in the United States, the chronically disabled were likely to have only one-half of the income of nonhandicapped and were twice as likely not to have health insurance. Disabled people were at least three times more likely to be unemployed. Furthermore, up to 30% of the American population was disabled. This clearly indicates that there are a large number of people needing special products with little money available. Any product developed for this market, therefore, has to be low cost for affordability reason.

Despite the inherent difficulties with the market, there are many groups of people associated with the disabled who will be secondary beneficiaries of such availability and prove to be vocal and powerful advocates. These people will include physiatrists, orthopedists, neurologists, cardiologists, ophthalmologists, and ENT specialists among medical professionals. Almost the entire allied health professionals including nurses, therapists, and rehabilitation engineers will also constitute a strong supporting group. Lastly, the family and friends of disabled people will also be indirect beneficiaries of such products in a big way. Of course, the manufacturers and suppliers will also have a vested interest in success of such an endeavor. Since such developments are likely to touch lives of so many, their consideration in depth is a technical as well as moral responsibility of ergonomists.

In a Health and Activity Limitation survey, the Alberta Bureau of Statistics (1989) and Statistics Canada (1990) have divided the disability types into a total of seven categories: mobility, agility, seeing, hearing, speaking, other, and nature not specified. The first two constituted the bulk of disabilities for Alberta (Table 1.5). The United Nations (1990), in its international survey of disability, identified five broad issues: (a) presence of impairment, (b) presence of disabilities, (c) causes of impairment, (d) social, economic, and environment characteristics, and (e) distribution and use of services and support. For the current discussion, presence of impairments and disabilities are most relevant and are presented in Tables 1.6 and 1.7. A concurrence in classification, description, and definition of impairment and disability between different countries still appears to be a fair distance away. A lack of commonality in classification and description of impairment and disability may be a formidable impediment in universalization of solutions. It may, therefore, be the necessary first step to develop a functional categorization regardless of cause and nature of impairment. The discipline of ergonomics is equipped to commence

TABLE 1.5
Nature and Severity of Disability by Age Group in Alberta

Disability	15–64 Years	65 Years and Older
Nature		
Total	155,725	73,160
Mobility	92,250	56,495
Agility	80,980	49,775
Seeing	18,185	15,560
Hearing	36,655	30,210
Speaking	9,905	3,835
Other	37,575	17,665
Unspecified	15,490	2,145
Severity		
Mild	82,220	26,170
Moderate	52,365	27,085
Severe	21,140	19,910

TABLE 1.6
United Nation's Classification of Impairments

Category	Type	Description
Physical (sensory)	Aural	Auditory sensitivity
	Language	Language functions and speech
	Ocular	Visual acuity
	Visceral	Internal organs and impairments of other special functions, e.g., sexual, mastication, and swallowing
Physical (other)	Skeletal	Head and trunk region, mechanical and motor impairments of limbs and deficiencies of limbs
	Disfiguring	Disfigurement of head and trunk, regions of limbs
Intellectual and psychological	Intellectual and psychological	Intelligence, memory, thinking consciousness, wakefulness, perception and attention, emotive and volitional functions, and behavior patterns
Generalized sensory and others		

TABLE 1.7
United Nations (1990) Classification of Disabilities

Category	Type	Description
Physical (functioning)	Locomotor	Ambulation and confining disabilities
	Communication	Speaking, listening
	Personal Care	Personal hygiene, dressing, feeding, and excretion
	Body disposition	Domestic disabilities, e.g., preparing and serving food and care of dependents, disabilities of body movement, e.g., fingering, gripping, and holding
	Dexterity	Skill in body movements, including manipulative skills and ability to regulate control mechanisms
Social functioning	Behavior	Awareness and disabilities in reactions
	Situational	Dependence and endurance and environmental disabilities relating to tolerance of environmental factor
Other		Disabilities of particular skills and other activity restrictions

the development of a generic functional classification applicable across conditions, which results in similar functional deficiencies. These criteria can then be incorporated in design and development of products for use by disabled consumers. Existing products considered suitable for use by disabled consumers can be tested against the criteria thus generated. Therefore, the scope of ergonomics can readily expand to include rehabilitation, which in fact is a legitimate but relatively unexplored dimension. Thus, rehabilitation ergonomics may be considered to consist of components as shown in Figures 1.21 and 1.22. An extensive need for a category of product universally needed by disabled people is appropriate clothing. Some creativity and innovation in this area can go a long way to make life so much easier for all concerned. An efficient functioning of disabled population is not only a moral nicety, but an economic necessity in newly emerging reality of life.

1.12.3.3.1   A Case Study of Ergonomic Product Design

Rheumatoid arthritis (RA) is a chronic progressive disease that affects men, women, and children of all ages. Even with excellent attention to medicine and rehabilitation, the disease can be disabling to various degrees. A random survey of 15,268 people found an overall prevalence of RA to be 2.7% , with a maximum prevalence of 5.5% among older females and a minimum prevalence of 0.4% among younger males (Issacson et al., 1987). During periods of disease exacerbation, damage can be done to the periarticular soft tissues. Damage to these structures leads to joint deformities. It is therefore important that the joints and their surrounding soft tissues be protected from stress and inherent weakness. Muscle strength and joint ROM must be maintained, however.

MacBain et al. (1981) suggested that, among other things, the following principles are particularly important in the management of rheumatoid hands. First, discretion must be used in exercise and it must be modified appropriately. Second, strong finger flexion should be avoided if there is active synovitis or if laxity is present. A finger load may be magnified from 2.8 to 4.3 times in the effector flexor tendon (Ohtsuki, 1981). Therefore, if violated, movement may aggravate both tenosynovitis and synovitis. Such forces may cause tendons to gradually stretch with repetitive activity (Goldstein, 1981), further increasing the laxity. An exertion of contractile force would also significantly increase the intra-articular pressure of the inflamed joints stretching the joint capsules (Kumar et al., 1976). Such activities may, therefore, increase deformity and dysfunction. Therefore, an assistive device can be used to decrease the amount of stress on the soft and inflamed tissues.

A repetitive task such as wringing or squeezing water out of dishcloths or washcloths is a task that places deforming forces on the rheumatoid hand (strong finger flexion and ulnar deviation of the MCP joints of one hand and radial deviation of the other (Tichauer, 1978), and should be avoided if joint laxity or active synovitis is present. Using an assistive device to avoid the deforming forces and to place the stress on larger muscles and joints would decrease the stress on smaller, less stable joints and protect them.

Older women are the primary target of RA. More often, they are found to be homemakers and do the wringing or squeezing task many times daily. People with RA have decreased grip strength compared to normal individuals, and have inflammation and instability, so this task encourages deformities to occur. It is

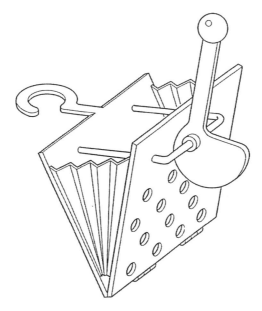

FIGURE 1.25   Domestic dish cloth squeezing device.

likely that an assistive device specifically designed to perform the task of removing water from cloths would be beneficial. The purpose of this study was to determine if there was a need for an aid to assist in the removal of water from cloths, and if so, to develop such an aid.

1.12.3.3.2   The Device

Hard plastic was used for the device. Two $10 \times 15\,cm$ rectangles were cut and joined together on one of the short ends by copper rivets, forming a wedge-shaped receptacle. The angled rectangle was riddled with holes to allow the water to escape. The straight rectangle had a plastic hook riveted to it at a right angle. This hook allowed the device to hand on the spray nozzle on a kitchen sink. A 10 cm long mechanical lever at the end of a 5 cm diameter cam was attached to the front of the device by steel rods. By applying the palm of the hand to the superior aspect of the lever and pulling down, water was squeezed from a cloth placed in the receptacle. The depth of the device (Figure 1.25) that could sit in the sink was 10 cm. The full depth including the hook was 18 cm. A ball of 7.5 cm diameter was attached to the end of the handle to prevent stress concentration at the point of contact with hand.

REFERENCES

Alberta Bureau of Statistics, 1989. Health and Activity Limitation Survey (Adults in Households). Package of Special Tabulations. Edmonton.

American Occupational Therapy Association, 1918. Proceedings of the Second Annual Meeting (cited by Gritzer and Arluke, 1985).

Armstrong, R.D. et al. 1987. Finger flexion function in rheumatoid arthritis: The reliability of eight simple tests. *Br J Rheumatol*, 26, 118–122.

Basmajian, J.V. 1975. Research or retrench. The rehabilitation professions challenged. *Phys Ther*, 55(6), 607–610.

Beals, C.A. et al. 1985. Measurement of exercise tolerance in patients with rheumatoid arthritis and osteoarthritis. *J Rheumatol*, 12, 458–461.

Belknap, R.G. 1985. Accidents off-the-job. *Encyclopedia of Occupational Health and Safety*, 3rd edn. Geneva: International Labour Office.

Burton, K., Edwards, V.A., and Sykes, D.A. 1990. "Invisible" skin marking for testing palpatory reliability. *J Manual Med*, 5, 27–29.

Christensen, J.M. 1976. Ergonomics: Where have we been and where are we going? *Proceedings of the 6th Congress of the International Ergonomics Association*, July 11–16, Santa Monica, CA.

Davies, D. and Kumar, S. 1996. A domestic assistive device for rheumatoid hands. *J Occup Rehabil*, 6, 135–143.

Edholm, O.G. and Murrell, K.H.F. 1973. The Ergonomics Research Society. A history 1949–1970. *Ergonomics*, 1(1), 6–39.

Fernando, M.U. and Robertson, J.C. 1982. Grip "strength" in the healthy. *Rheumatol Rehab*, 21, 179–181.

Gilbert, R.W. et al. 1987. Design of a distributed control system for a robotic mannequin. *International Topical Meeting of Remote Systems and Robotics in Hostile Environments*, March 29, Pasco, Washington.

Goldstein, S. 1981. Biomechanical aspects of cumulative trauma to tendons and tendon sheaths. Unpublished PhD thesis, University of Michigan, Ann Arbor, MI.

Grall, T.B. 1979. A feasibility study of product testing and reporting for handicapped consumers. Consumers Union of United States, Inc. Mount Vernon, NY 10550.

Grieve, G.P. 1981. *Common Vertebral Joint Problems*. Edinburgh, Scotland: Churchill Livingstone.

Gritzer, G. and Arluke, A. 1985. *The Making of Rehabilitation: A Political Economy of Medical Specialization. 1890–1980*. Berkeley, CA: University of California Press.

Harkappa, K. et al. 1991. Health locus of control beliefs and psychological distress as predictors for treatment outcome in low back pain patients: Results of a three-month follow-up of a controlled intervention study. *Pain*, 46, 35–41.

Human Development News. *Special Edition*. 1987, Office of Human Development Services. US Department of Health and Human Services, Washington, DC, 20201.

International Labour Office 1978. *Basic Principles of Vocational Rehabilitation of the Disabled*, 2nd edn. Geneva: International Labour Office.

Issacson, J., Allander, E., and Brostrom, L.A. 1987. A seventeen-year follow-up of a population survey of rheumatoid arthritis. *Scand J Rheum*, 16, 145–152.

JAN 1987. Evaluation Survey. Executive Summary.

Kumar, S. 1989. Rehabilitation and ergonomics: Complimentary disciplines. *Can J Rehabil*, 3, 99–111.

Kumar, S. 1991. A Research Report on Functional Evaluation of Human Back. University of Alberta Press, Edmonton.

Kumar, S. 1992. Rehabilitation: An ergonomic dimension. *Int J Ind Ergon*, 9, 97–108.

Kumar, S. 1995. Therapeutic spinal mobilizer. U.S. Patent.

Kumar, S. et al. 1976. The significance of intra-articular pressure on rehabilitation of rheumatoid joints. *IEEE/EMB 8th Annu Conf Proc.*, pp. 1793–1796.

LeBlanc, M. and Leifer, L. 1982. Environmental control and robotic manipulation aids. Institute of Electrical and Electronics Engineers. *Eng Med Biol*, 15–16.

Lee, D. 1989. *The Pelvic Girdle*. Edinburgh, Scotland: Churchill Livingstone, pp. 15–91.

MacBain, K.P., Galbraith, M., and Brady, F. 1981. Non-operative hand management of adult-onset rheumatoid arthritis. *Arthritis Soc*, Toronto, Canada.

McKenzie, R.A. 1987. Mechanical diagnosis and therapy of low back pain toward a better understanding. In L.T. Towery and J.R. Taylor, eds., *Physical Therapy of Low Back*. New York: Churchill Livingstone, pp. 157–173.

McNeal, D.R. 1982. Applying technology to help the disabled. Institute of Electrical and Electronics Engineers. *Eng Med Biol*, 15–16.

Memmot, M. 1987. More firms adapt to disabilities. *USA Today*, June 9, 1987.

Mital, A. and Karwowski, W. 1988 Rehabilitation: An urgent need? In A. Mital and W. Karwowski, eds., *Ergonomics in Rehabilitation*. London: Taylor & Francis, pp. 1–9.

Mock, H. 1917. Industrial medicine and surgery: The neo specialty. *J Am Med Assoc*, 68, 1.

Murrell, K.H.F. 1949. Cited in Edholm, O.G. and Murrell, K.H.F. (1973). The Ergonomics Research Society. A history 1949–1970. *Ergonomics*, 1, 6–39.

National Aviation and Space Agency, 1989. Space Age vision aids. National Aeronautic and Space Administration Technical Briefs, September.

NIOSH 1981. Work Practices Guide for Manual Lifting. U.S. Department of Health and Human Services, Washington, DC.

National Safety Council 1978. *Accidents Facts*. Chicago, IL: National Safety Council.

Ohtsuki, T. 1981. Inhibition of individual fingers curing grip strength exertion. *Ergonomics* 24, 21–36.

Peat, M. 1981. Physiotherapy: Art or science? *Physiother Canada*, 33(3), 170–176.

Seminara, J.L. 1979. A survey of ergonomics in Poland. *Ergonomics*, 22, 479–505.

Simmonds, M. and Kumar, S. 1993. Location of body structure by palpation: Reliability study. *Int J Ind Ergonom*, 11, 145–151.

Simmonds, M. and Kumar, S. 1996. Does knowledge of a patient's workers compensation status influence clinical judgements? *J Occup Rehabil*, 6(2), 93–107.

Simmonds, M., Kumar, S., and Lechelt, E. 1995. Use of a spinal model to quantify the forces and motion that occur during therapists' tests of spinal motion. *Phys Ther*, 75(3), 212–222.

Statistics Canada 1990. *The Health and Activity Limitation Survey*. Highlights: Disabled Persons in Canada. Catalogue number, 82-602. Ottawa.

Tichauer, E. 1978. *The Biomechanical Basis of Ergonomics*. New York: John Wiley & Sons, pp. 67–69.

Tuchi, S. et al. 1985. Electrocutaneous communication in a guide dog robot (MELDOG). *IEEE Trans Biomed Eng*, 32, 461–469.

United Nations, 1990. Disability Statistics Compendium. Department of International Economic and Social Affairs Statistical Office, New York, Series Y, No. 4.

World Health Organization, 1990. *International Classification of Impairments, Disabilities and Handicaps*. Geneva: WHO.

Workers' Compensation Board (Alberta) 1983. Annual Report.

Workers' Compensation Board (Alberta) 1984. Annual Report.

Workers' Compensation Board (Alberta) 1985. Annual Report.

Workers' Compensation Board (Alberta) 1986. Annual Report.

Workers' Compensation Board (Alberta) 1987. Annual Report.

2 Energy Cost Considerations in Common Disabilities: Scientific Basis and Clinical Perspectives

Suh-Jen Lin

CONTENTS

Independent activities of daily living and walking are important basic functions that most people value in life. Walking is one of the five major activities–walking, breathing, hearing, seeing, and speaking. If any of these functions is severely impaired, the person is considered on disabilities in federal legislation. According to the Americans with Disabilities Act of 1990, significant impairment in at least one of the five major life activities would constitute a disability.

Appropriate energy supply is one of the prerequisites for a person to walk efficiently and independently. Maximum energy efficiency is especially a fundamental phenomenon for all movements and functions. Each daily activity requires a certain amount of energy supply, which comes from the combustion of foods, predominantly carbohydrates and fat, in the body. With appropriate amounts of oxygen delivery through adequate cardiac output, gas exchange in the lung and the working muscles, food combustion produces the amount of energy-carrier molecules, adenosine triphosphates (ATP), required for muscular work. Therefore, any functional activity requires a delicate coordination among cardiorespiratory function, neuromuscular control, and muscular activity. People with disabilities often experience high metabolic demand of physical activities compared to their healthy peers, due to impairments in the cardiorespiratory system, neural control, or musculoskeletal performance. Before a discussion on the energy expenditure in patients with disabilities, some basic terminology in exercise physiology will be reviewed.

2.1 DEFINITIONS OF ENERGY EXPENDITURE AND RELATED TERMS

Total daily energy expenditure comprises three components: resting metabolic rate (RMR), thermic effect of feeding, and thermic effect of physical activity. Within the total daily energy expenditure, thermic effect of feeding accounts for about 10%, thermic effect of physical activity accounts for about 15%–30%, and RMR accounts for about 60%–75%.[1] RMR represents the total metabolism of a body functioning at rest, which is highly related to the fat-free mass in a healthy person, and low RMR is associated with a high risk of weight gain. The thermic effect of physical activity refers to the energy expenditure of all types of physical activities including household, industrial, and recreational activities, and the energy expenditure required for most physical activities in healthy people have been published in a compendium.[2]

Energy is commonly expressed in kilocalories (kcal). However, it is difficult to be directly measured for human activities. Instead, oxygen consumption measured at rest or during activity is used to indicate energy expenditure. Depending on the proportion of foods (carbohydrate, fat, and protein) combusted, the energy equivalent per mole of mixed food combusted approximates 4.82 kcal/L of oxygen consumed.[1] A rounded value of 5 kcal energy output per liter of oxygen consumption consumed is commonly used for estimating the body's energy expenditure under steady-state conditions.[1] The rate of oxygen consumption, or energy expenditure, is usually normalized by the body weight to allow for comparisons across subjects, and is expressed as the amount of oxygen consumed per kilogram of body weight per minute of time (mL/kg/min).

The oxygen consumption is more commonly expressed as a bigger unit, MET, to facilitate communication. The unit MET is defined as multiples of the RMR. One MET is equivalent to 3.5 mL O_2 consumption per unit of body mass per minute (i.e., 3.5 mL/kg/min). Most physical activities use MET to illustrate the energy requirements.

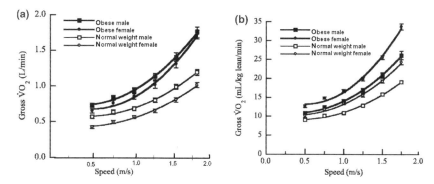

FIGURE 2.1 Illustration of the relationship between gross oxygen consumption and speed. (Modified from Browning, R.C., et al., *J. Appl. Physiol.*, 100, 390, 2006.)

For example, according to the Compendium of Physical Activities, walking at 3 mph (80 m/min) requires 3.3 MET of energy and walking at 2.5 mph (66.67 m/min) requires approximately 3 MET.[2]

Walking is a daily physical activity for everyone. There is a linear relationship between walking speeds (3.0–5.0 km/h, i.e., 1.9–3.1 mph) and oxygen consumption.[1] At higher speeds, the walking economy decreases, so there is a higher proportional increase in oxygen consumption at higher speeds.[1] More accurately, the relationship between oxygen consumption and walking speed is curvilinear across most populations[3] (Figure 2.1). Several quadratic equations were derived to estimate energy expenditure from walking speeds:[4–9]

$VO_2 = 0.00110 \ (speed)^2 + 5.9$ (Ralston),[4]

$VO_2 = 0.336 \ (speed)^2 + 6.15$ (Corcoran and Brengelmann)[8] (*Note*: The oxygen consumption is in the unit of mL/kg/min and speed is in m/min),

$VO_2 = 3.31 \ (\pm 0.58) \ (speed)^2 + 8.51 \ (\pm 0.93)$ (*Note*: speed is in m/s) (Malatesta et al.).[9]

Whereas the relationship between energy expenditure and running speed is linear, several linear equations were reported for running speeds[6] (Table 2.1).

Heart rate is a measure of cardiac workload, and there is a positive linear relationship between heart rate and the oxygen consumption over a wide range of aerobic exercise intensity.[1] Heart rate is commonly used to estimate oxygen consumption clinically, since direct laboratory measurement of oxygen consumption is sophisticated and expensive. Using exercise heart rate to estimate oxygen consumption is reasonably accurate. However, there are other factors affecting heart rate responses, such as the circadian rhythm, environmental temperature, emotions, previous food intake, body position, muscle groups exercised, and whether the exercise is static or dynamic.[1] Heart rate response is commonly expressed as the percentage of age-predicted maximal heart rate to indicate the relative exercise intensity, and used to compare exercise intensity between subjects. The exercise intensity of a person's comfortable walking velocity in general approximates as 50% age-predicted maximal heart rate.[10] Individuals can sustain prolonged physical activity if they are

TABLE 2.1

Predicted Equations for Oxygen Consumption for Walking and Running in Adolescents

	VO$_2$ (mL/kg/min)	
R	0.95	
SEE	3.07	
	mph	**m/min**
Variable		
Constant	2.112	2.1124
Speed	5.856	0.2184
Speed × mode[a]	−4.833	−0.1802
Speed^2 × mode[a]	1.002	0.0014

Source: Modified from Walker, J.L., et al., *Med. Sci. Sports Exerc.*, 31, 311, 1999.

Note: The model includes speed and mode as variables. The coefficients for each variable in the models are listed vertically under either unit of measurement for speed (mph or m/min).

[a] Mode: walk = 1, run = 0.

functioning at an exercise intensity less than 50% of their maximum aerobic capacity.[1] Prolonged period of walking at an exercise intensity greater than 85% of age-predicted maximal hart rate is intolerable for most individuals.[11]

Gait efficiency, or locomotion efficiency, is defined as the energy expenditure per meter of distance traveled (mL/kg/m), which is calculated by dividing the rate of oxygen consumption (mL/kg/min) by the corresponding speed (m/min). A lower computed numerical value of gait efficiency indicates better efficiency, i.e., for the same amount of work, the lower the energy expenditure per unit of work, the higher the efficiency. The human body system, similar to any other mechanical systems, aims to achieve the most economic function as much as possible. The relationship between gait efficiency and walking speeds has been shown to be parabolic (or U-shaped), with the optimal gait efficiency (the minimum value of gait efficiency) occurring around the medium walking speeds, at about 4–5 km/h (1.12–1.38 m/s, or 2.5–3.13 mph).[3,12–15] Figure 2.2 illustrates the relationship between gait efficiency and walking speed. This U-shaped relationship might be a fundamental principle of locomotion. Walking at higher or lower speeds will result in poorer gait efficiency (economy), i.e., increased numerical value of gait efficiency.

Another term, energy expenditure index (EEI) or physiological cost index (PCI), is also commonly used in the literature to indicate efficiency. It is determined by the ratio of net ambulatory heart rate change to the walking speed ((HR_{amb} − HR_{rest})/ speed, with the speed in the unit of m/min). In children and adolescents, the best EEI also corresponds to the comfortable speed of walking.[16] As discussed above, many other factors (such as the circadian rhythm) also affect the heart rate, so the

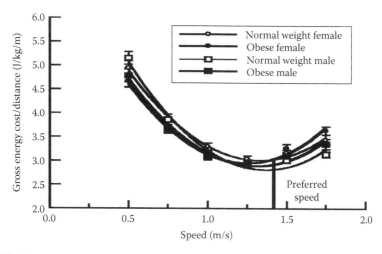

FIGURE 2.2 Illustration of the preferred speed corresponding to the speed with the least energy expenditure per distance of walking. (Modified from Browning, R.C., et al., *J. Appl. Physiol.*, 100, 390, 2006.)

physiologic cost index sometimes may not be as responsive or representative as the gait efficiency.

The self-selected walking velocity (SSWV) is defined as an individual's natural, comfortable walking speed or preferred walking speed. As shown in Table 2.2, the reported SSWV ranges from 74 to 83 m/min,[4,5,8,17–19] which is close to the functional velocity required to cross a traffic intersection from curb to curb (79 m/min), and

TABLE 2.2

Energy Expenditure and Gait Efficiency at Comfortable Walking Speed in Normal Subjects

References	Subjects (Age)	Speed (m/min)	Oxygen Consumption (mL/kg/min)	Gait Efficiency[a] (mL/kg/m)
Waters et al.[21,23–25]	Children (6–12)	70	15.3	0.22
	Teens (13–19)	73	12.9	0.18
	Adults (20–59)	80	12.1	0.15
	Seniors (60–80)	74	12.0	0.16
Fisher and Gullickson;[17]	Adults	74	11.6[b]	0.156
Ralston;[4] Corcoran and		83	12.6[b]	0.152
Brengelmann;[8] Waters		82	12.6[b]	0.154
et al.;[18] Bobbert[5]		81	12.6[b]	0.176
Ulkar et al.[19]	Adults	99.79 ± 10.13	11.71 ± 1.9	0.12 ± 0.02

[a] Gait efficiency is defined as the ratio of oxygen consumption (mL/kg/min) to speed (m/min).

[b] Based on the conversion factor of 5 kcal = 1 L O_2 consumed.

relates to a community ambulation velocity (78 m/min).[15] Several factors affect a person's SSWV, such as maximal aerobic capacity, gender, and age. A person with a higher maximal aerobic capacity was shown to have a higher SSWV.[20] Men have a faster comfortable walking speed than women,[3,15] whereas children and adolescents have lower comfortable walking speeds due to their smaller statues and lower exercise capacities.[21] The SSWV is also found to correspond to the speed with the best gait efficiency, i.e., the lowest energy expenditure per distance of walking.[3,17,22]

Human walking has been modeled as a force-driven harmonic oscillator, which requires a periodic forcing function to maintain its oscillation amplitude in the presence of gravitational, damping, and stiffness forces.[26] When the frequency of the driving force of a harmonic oscillator is equal to the natural frequency of the oscillator (i.e., the leg), resonance occurs and the force required to maintain the same oscillation amplitude is minimized. The stride frequency at the SSWV was found to be predictable by the natural frequency of the pendulum model based on the information of leg mass, center of mass, and moment of inertia of the leg in normal subjects.[26,27] When bilaterally adding mass to the ankles, stride time of walking increased, corresponding to a decreased predicted resonant frequency of the pendulum model.[26] When the stride length was held constant, subjects responded to speed changes by changing their cadences; the energy expenditure did not change much until their cadence exceeded the preferred cadence.[27] Therefore, a change in SSWV away from its normal value would make the system less energy-efficient.

Mechanical efficiency is defined as the ratio of power output relative to its total energy input.[1] The actual work output is expressed as a force acting through a vertical displacement, which is easy to determine during cycle ergometry, stair climbing, or bench stepping. Horizontal walking does not involve vertical displacement and hence does not accomplish any mechanical work. However, muscular movement accomplishes internal work and energy is expended to sustain the muscular contraction. The mechanical efficiency could be reported as the "gross" or "net" mechanical efficiency. The "gross" mechanical efficiency refers to the ratio of mechanical work accomplished to the total energy expenditure, including the resting energy cost as well as any muscular work. For the "net" mechanical efficiency, the resting oxygen consumption is subtracted. The efficiency of human locomotion is low, with the gross mechanical efficiency being about 20%–30% for able-bodied children and adults in walking, running, and cycling.[1] The remainder of the energy input is used to overcome the resistance and friction of movement, or is lost as heat.

Many factors affect the mechanical efficiency of exercise, such as the rate of work (power), speed of movement,[28,29] muscle fiber type,[30] muscle flexibility,[31] age, gender, fitness level, skill level, and disease processes. At a low to moderate rate of work, a pedaling rate of 40–60 rpm was reported to be most energy-efficient for arm or cycle ergometer exercises.[28,29] The comfortable walking velocity for an adult is around 1.33 m/s, which corresponds to the speed with the best gait efficiency.[12,14] Cyclists with greater economy of cycling often have a higher proportion of type I, slow-twitched muscle fibers.[30] Patients with various kinds of chronic diseases or disabilities often have reduced mechanical efficiency.

Maximal physical work capacity, or physical capacity, is defined as the maximal amount of work a person could perform. The criterion measure of a person's physical capacity is the maximal oxygen uptake ($VO_{2\,max}$). It is commonly measured through a graded exercise test protocol (treadmill, cycle ergometer, arm ergometer, or step) by the indirect calorimetry method with a sophisticated stationary metabolic cart or a telemetry metabolic system.[1,32] A healthy person's maximal physical capacity is related to age, gender, and training status. With aging, there is approximately a 1% reduction in $VO_{2\,max}$ per year between 25 and 75 years.[33] In general, for an individual to carry out a full-time job, the physical demand for that job should not exceed 40% of their maximal physical capacity.[34]

Many factors affect the energy expenditure of physical activities in healthy people. Intrinsic factors affecting energy consumption, defined as factors that come from the body itself, include the following: gender, age,[9,13,23] body composition,[3] fitness level (trained versus sedentary),[13] muscle fiber type (oxidative versus glycolytic metabolism), degree of muscle atrophy, muscle strength, range of motion, and hemoglobin content (anemia, polycythemia).[1] With aging, there is a decline in the economy of walking.[8,13,35] Males have a better fitness level than females due to a greater proportion of lean body mass and hemoglobin content,[1] yet both genders are shown to have similar economy of walking.[35] Adolescents have a relative high energy expenditure of walking and a low gait efficiency when compared to adults.[6] Obese people were shown to have a similar gait efficiency as people with normal weight.[3]

Extrinsic factors affecting energy consumption of activities, defined as factors coming from the environment or devices, include the following: mode of exercise (treadmill versus over ground walking),[36,37] speed and grade of treadmill,[5,8,24] floor surface, footwear, the amount and the location of loading,[38] type of device used (e.g., crutch, cane, and walker), patterns of gait (swing through, reciprocal), orthotic use, weight-bearing status, posture, and wheelchair use. Walking on treadmill allows for convenient measurement of physiologic parameters, has a low intercycle variability of gait, and is commonly used for multiple-speed gait studies. Energy expenditure during treadmill walking was shown to underestimate the energy expenditure of floor walking,[36,37] but studies on the difference of energy consumption between floor walking and treadmill walking have been equivocal.[7,36,39,40]

Walking movements are robust against changing loads based on a computer simulation study.[41] Based on the magnitude and the location of the added mass, the movement of the system will convert to a new steady state as described by a limit cycle, which is structurally stable against changes in inertial conditions within a certain range. Specifically, the upper limits of the mass affixed to the parts of the body are 5, 15, 5, 1, and 0.5 kg of the HAT (head, arms, and trunk), pelvis, thigh, shank, and foot, respectively. This might also explain the negligible effects on energy expenditure in some studies when large loads were applied to the center of gravity of the body,[42] or when a small weight was applied to the ankles.[43] This is in contrast to reports that showed a significant effect of a large load on the energy expenditure of walking when placed on distal foot segments.[38,44]

2.2 ENERGY EXPENDITURE IN PEOPLE WITH ORTHOPEDIC DISORDERS

In the literature, many studies have reported the energy expenditure in people with orthopedic disorders, such as amputation, arthrodesis, knee immobilization, knee flexion contracture, and total joint replacement such as total hip replacement.

2.2.1 AMPUTATION

Major lower extremity amputation often is associated with significant mortality and morbidity rate, especially for vascular amputation.[45] Prosthesis fitting and ambulation mark an important milestone for an amputee. With advances in prosthesis design and technology, problems of increased energy expenditure of walking and a slow comfortable walking speed associated with prosthesis have greatly improved.[17,18,25,46–51]

Factors affecting the increased metabolic demand of walking in amputees could again be either intrinsic or extrinsic. The intrinsic factors are related to the level of amputation,[18] length of the residual limb,[52] cause of amputation, gait asymmetry, muscle atrophy in the amputated limb, and physical fitness of the amputee.[53] The extrinsic factors are related to devices of walking, type of prosthesis foot,[54,55] weight of prosthesis,[56] prosthesis components,[57,58] and crutches versus prosthesis use. From a biomechanical perspective, the increased metabolic cost of gait was shown to be related to the increased mechanical work, the disturbance of the sinusoidal changes of the center of body mass and the efficiency of the pendulum-like mechanism.[59]

In general, lower limb amputees who have a higher level of limb amputation will have a higher energy expenditure of walking. The order of energy expenditure for different levels of amputation is generally as follows: transfemoral (above knee) amputation > transtibial (below knee) amputation > Syme (ankle) amputation.[18,60] However, a longitudinal case study showed that the energy expenditure of walking for an amputee using a below-knee prosthesis was not worse than that with a Syme prosthesis, because a dynamic response foot of a below-knee prosthesis enhanced the energy restore at the ankle.[61]

With well-fit prosthesis, muscle strengthening, and gait retraining, a skilled prosthesis user can save the energy of walking much more than walking with crutches,[18,62] but walking with a prosthesis may not provide a better functional outcome if the expense of energy is too high. For example, the use of crutches was shown to provide a faster walking speed and a less amount of energy expenditure in vascular unilateral transfemoral patients.[18] Wheeling was shown to be more practical, having a faster speed of transportation and a lower amount of energy expenditure than walking with a prosthesis or crutches for a bilateral transfemoral amputee.[63]

At the same level of lower limb amputation, traumatic amputees generally have a better economy of gait and require less energy expenditure of walking than that of vascular amputees. This is because the traumatic amputees are generally younger, have a higher fitness level, and fewer cardiovascular comorbidities.[64–66] The success rate for prosthesis fitting and rehabilitation in general is better in traumatic amputees than in vascular amputees.

In recent years, there has been much research on the optimal inertial properties of prosthesis that would improve energy efficiency and gait symmetry. Effects of heavyweight prosthesis on the energy expenditure of walking and gait largely depend on the inertial properties of the prosthesis leg and the type of amputation.[56,67–70] Small amounts of added prosthetic mass[67] or even matching up to the intact limb mass, without shifting the center of mass of the leg, did not increase energy expenditure of walking in below-knee amputees.[56] However, distal loading to the prosthesis,[71] or matching the prosthesis' moment of inertia to the intact leg, had detrimental effects on gait parameters and the energy expenditure.[68] Furthermore, amputees were shown to adopt similar kinematic patterns and adjust joint torques in response to the small prosthetic mass perturbations.[69] Currently, lightweight prosthesis is no longer the trend of prosthesis manufacturing for traumatic amputees. Some advanced suspension systems, such as the suction type of suspension and the suspension sleeve, are designed in a way to tightly hold the heavy prosthesis to the stump or residual limb. It is likely that the optimal inertial properties of a prosthesis leg for amputees could be found in the near future. However, people with vascular amputation often have other comorbidities and poor physical capacity, so they probably could not take advantage of heavy prosthesis without the increased burden of energy expenditure.

Many studies in the literature have documented the effects of prosthesis foot type on the energy expenditure and the biomechanics of gait.[54,55,64,65,72–75] It has been shown that different types of dynamic response foot design incorporated flexibility and force-producing capability in the foot or shank of the prosthesis, which leads to reduced energy expenditure and improved gait efficiency when compared to traditional solid ankle cushion heel (SACH) foot. The dynamic response foot is especially beneficial during faster walking speeds or running.[55] However, it appears that no specific type of dynamic response foot is superior, and this awaits further research.

Walking has been modeled as an inverted pendulum, i.e., energy is exchanged between kinetic energy and gravitational potential energy from one stride to the next stride.[76] However, the human pendulum is not an ideal frictionless pendulum system, so the maximum exchange is only about 65%.[77] For amputee gait, the energy exchange is generally not as good as that of normal subjects. With rehabilitation, amputees showed a better energy exchange, a higher SSWV, and a better gait efficiency.[59] This is similar to the observation that women of East Africa are able to carry heavy head-supported weight, because they have an improved energy transfer from step to step through many years of practice.[78] By adding prosthetic mass in transfemoral amputees, they were also shown to have a better energy exchange between steps (effectively conserving the mechanical work), no increase in metabolic cost of walking, and a faster comfortable walking speed.[79] Table 2.3 shows the energy expenditure and gait efficiency at comfortable speed in amputees.

2.2.2 Joint Immobilization

Immobilization of different lower limb joints was shown to result in increased energy expenditure, reduced walking speed, and reduced economy of walking due to the altered biomechanics of lower limb segments.[17] Among the different joints, ankle immobilization has the least effect on energy expenditure (about a 6% increase), when compared to knee or hip immobilization. The effect of knee immobilization on energy expenditure depends on the knee angle, with a knee angle of 165°, resulting in the lowest (10%) increase in energy expenditure, and a knee angle of 180°, resulting in a 13% increase in energy expenditure.[17]

TABLE 2.3
Energy Expenditure and Gait Efficiency at Comfortable
Speed in Amputees

References	Subjects	Speed (m/min)	Oxygen Consumption (mL/kg/min)	Gait Efficiency (Net O_2 Cost) (mL/kg/m)
Waters et al.[18]	*Prosthesis use*			
	Vascular amputees			
	Above knee	36 ± 15	12.6 ± 2.9	0.35 ± 0.06
	Below knee	45 ± 9	11.7 ± 1.6	0.26 ± 0.05
	Syme	54 ± 10	11.5 ± 1.5	0.21 ± 0.06
	Traumatic amputees			
	Above knee	52 ± 14	12.9 ± 3.4	0.25 ± 0.05
	Below knee	71 ± 10	15.5 ± 2.9	0.20 ± 0.05
	Crutches use			
	Vascular amputees			
	Above knee	48 ± 11	15.0 ± 2.9	
	Below knee	39 ± 13	14.6 ± 1.5	
	Syme	39 ± 14	12.8 ± 4.3	
	Traumatic amputees			
	Above knee	65 ± 16	15.9 ± 5.4	
	Below knee	71 ± 10	22.4 ± 4.3	
Pagliarulo et al.[47]	Traumatic below knee	71	15.5	
Gailey et al.[67]	Traumatic below knee	76	12.8	
	Normal subjects	76	11.2	
Lin-Chan et al.[61]	Traumatic below knee (single case)	79–80	—	—
Hsu et al.[54]	Traumatic below knee	71	—	—

2.3   ENERGY EXPENDITURE IN PEOPLE WITH NEUROLOGICAL DISORDERS

People with neurological impairments often have a slower comfortable walking speed and a higher energy cost of walking when compared to their healthy peers. Both primary and secondary factors affect their functional abilities. The primary factors refer to the impairments resulting from the disorders, such as the severity of muscle paralysis, muscle weakness, spasticity, cocontraction, level of injury, deficit of coordination, and limited range of motion.[80,81] The secondary factors, such as weight gain, contractures, deconditioning,[82–85] fatigue, and breathlessness, further impact the metabolic demand of mobility.[86]

Many studies in the literature have documented the energy expenditure of walking and physical activities in patients with neurological disorders, such as stroke, postpoliomyelitis, spinal cord injury, multiple sclerosis (MS), cerebral palsy (CP), and low lumbar myelomeningocele (a developmental defect of the vertebral column causing hernial protrusion of the spinal cord, meninges, and spinal fluid). Due to advances in functional electrical stimulation and orthosis technology, there have been many more studies on functional ambulation and aerobic endurance in patients with spinal cord injury than there were 30 years ago.

2.3.1 STROKE PATIENTS

Each year, approximately 700,000 people in the United States suffer a stroke, and almost one-third of these strokes are recurrent.[87] Stroke patients often have cardiovascular comorbidities (e.g., hypertension, arteriosclerosis, congestive heart failure, obesity, diabetes, and coronary artery disease) and are usually physically inactive. Reduced exercise capacity and increased metabolic demand with physical activity in them are commonly reported in the literature.[8,81,83,88,89] The increased metabolic demand of physical activity was shown to be related to neuromuscular impairments, musculoskeletal changes, increased mechanical work of muscles, and reduced fitness level.[81]

To accommodate the increased metabolic demand of walking, stroke patients often adopt a slower comfortable walking speed in order to keep their gait efficiency similar to that of healthy subjects.[81,90] The peak exercise capacity for acute stroke patients was found to be about 50%–60% of age- and gender-matched normative values of sedentary individuals, and was highly related to the premorbid physical activity level and the stage of functional recovery.[83,91] The physical capacity in moderate traumatic brain injury patients was also reduced due to neuromuscular sequela.[82]

In addition to therapeutic exercise, use of an ankle–foot orthosis is common in stroke patients, and favorable reduction in the metabolic demand of walking and gait improvement has been reported.[92,93] Gait training with weight-supported treadmill in stroke patients has gained much attention in recent years, and shown positive effects in reducing the metabolic demand of walking and improving SSWV.[94–96] Treadmill aerobic training at slow speed[97] or task-oriented exercise[98] in chronic stoke patients also showed reduced metabolic demand at submaximal workload and improved walking speed and endurance. Physical activity and exercise recommendations for stroke patients were published in 2004 with major goals to increase their aerobic capacity and sensorimotor function, and reduce stroke risks.[99] Table 2.4 shows the energy expenditure at comfortable walking speed and at peak exercise intensity in stroke patients.

2.3.2 SPINAL INJURY PATIENTS

The American Spinal Cord Injury Association (ASIA) established a standard scoring system, Lower Extremity Muscle Score (LEMS), to classify motor paralysis in patients with spinal injury. Higher LEMS scores would indicate better motor abilities of legs.[100–102] International standards for the neurological and functional classifications of spinal injury also coincide with the ASIA standards.[103]

Depending on the level of spinal injury, the need for compensatory upper extremity use with crutches for stabilizing the trunk and swinging both legs would post

TABLE 2.4

Energy Expenditure and Gait Efficiency at Comfortable Walking Speed in Stroke Patients

References	Device	Speed (m/min)	Oxygen Consumption (mL/kg/min)	Gait Efficiency (mL/kg/m)
Cunha-Filho et al.[80]	A mixed group ($n = 20$)	40.2	10.18	0.253
Franceschini et al.[92]	With AFO[a]	21.39 ± 7.30	9.42 ± 1.62	0.49 ± 0.20
	Without AFO	15.47 ± 6.95	9.87 ± 1.92	0.76 ± 0.41
Danielsson and Sunnerhagen[93]	With AFO	20.40 ± 3.60	8.60 ± 0.40	0.51 ± 0.06
	Without AFO	16.20 ± 1.80	8.80 ± 0.50	0.58 ± 0.07

[a] AFO, ankle–foot orthosis.

higher energy demand and lower energy efficiency in spinal injury patients during walking and the negotiation of architectural barriers.[101,104–106] Spinal injury patients who have more preservation in motor abilities of the legs will have a higher level of functional ambulation ability and a lower energy requirement than patients who have a higher degree of leg paralysis. It has been shown that there is a positive linear relationship between LEMS and walking velocity (Figure 2.3), i.e., the higher the motor abilities, the faster the walking velocity. In addition, there also exists a negative linear relationship between LEMS and the energy expenditure of walking[107] (Figure 2.4), i.e., a higher motor score indicates lower energy expenditure of walking.

Heart rate is a good indicator of exercise intensity for spinal injury patients who use functional electrical neuromuscular stimulation.[108] This facilitates the monitoring of exercise intensity during ambulation without having to conduct the cumbersome measurement of oxygen consumption. Blunted heart rate response and

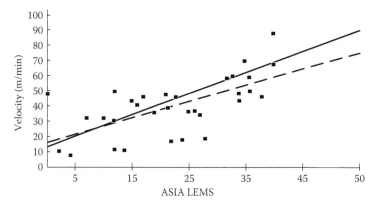

FIGURE 2.3 The relationship between the ASIA LEMS and gait velocity, which is defined by the equation, Velocity = 17.2 + LEMS (solid line). (From Waters, R.L., et al., *Arch. Phys. Med. Rehabil.*, 75, 756, 1994. With permission.)

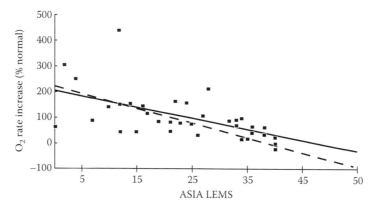

FIGURE 2.4   The relationship between the ASIA LEMS and O_2 rate increase is defined by the equation, O_2 rate increase = $207 - 4.4 \times$ LEMS (solid line). (From Waters, R.L., et al., *Arch. Phys. Med. Rehabil.*, 75, 756, 1994. With permission.)

a slower oxygen uptake were seen in functional electrical stimulation of leg muscles in spinal injury patients, which was thought to be related to the physical deconditioning or reduced leg muscle mass in paraplegic patients.[109] Spinal injury patients with a complete injury under T6 (sixth thoracic vertebra) or an incomplete injury above T6 are commonly prescribed orthotics or walking aids to be trained to walk. With the option to use a walker or crutches, the use of crutches has shown a better gait efficiency and a lower energy expenditure than the use of a walker in incomplete spinal injury patients.[19] For patients with a higher thoracic level of injury, however, the high energy demand of walking often forces them to give up walking with devices after being discharged home, which further compromises their osteoporosis and limb contracture.

Newer orthotic devices in combination with functional neuromuscular stimulation have resulted in much improvement in the ambulation abilities of spinal injury patients. A weight-bearing control orthosis,[110] a reciprocal gait orthosis,[111] and an electrical stimulation combined with orthosis use[112–114] were shown to reduce the energy expenditure of walking, and improve the gait efficiency and the hemodynamic responses for thoracic level paraplegia patients. In addition, the type of orthosis and gait pattern also affect the energy expenditure of walking in spinal injury patients. Table 2.5 shows the energy expenditure and gait efficiency at the comfortable walking speed in spinal injury patients with different types of assistive devices and gait. Walking with swing through gait usually has a higher speed of walking than walking with reciprocal gait, and results in a better gait efficiency in children with lower lumbar myelomeningocele.[115] Besides gait training, pool exercise therapy has also led to improvements in gait characteristics and a reduction in the metabolic demand in patients with spastic paralysis, such as patients with stroke, MS, or spinal cord injury.[116]

The RMR in chronic spinal injury patients was found to be 14%–27% lower than that of able-bodied controls, which was thought to be related to the reduced fat-free mass and altered sympathetic nervous system activity in such patients.[104] Due to the

TABLE 2.5

Energy Expenditure and Gait Efficiency at Comfortable Walking Speed in Spinal Injury Patients

References	Subjects/Devices	Speed (m/min)	Oxygen Consumption (mL/kg/min)	Gait Efficiency (mL/kg/m)
Williams et al.[117]	Myelodysplasia			
	No orthosis (sacral)	48	13.0	0.28
	0 KAFO[a] (lumbar)	38	16.6	0.49
	1 KAFO (lumbar)	29	17.5	0.77
	2 KAFO (thoracic)	19	18.1	1.35
Waters et al.[118]	Spinal cord injury (SCI) ($n = 36$)			
	0 KAFO	48.1	15.1	0.37
	1 KAFO	37.1	14.7	0.46
	2 KAFO	18.9	14.9	1.15
	None	66.5	14.2	0.22
	Cane/crutch	47.9	14.2	0.29
	Crutches	37.8	15.7	0.56
	Walker	11.8	12.7	1.20
Waters et al.[107]	Spinal cord injury ($n = 36$)			
	LEMS[b] ≥ 30	57.5 ± 12.3	14.6 ± 3.0	0.26 ± 0.07
	LEMS 21–29	31.4 ± 11.4	13.2 ± 1.6	0.51 ± 0.25
	LEMS ≤ 20	30.5 ± 15.6	15.2 ± 3.4	0.76 ± 0.61
Moore et al.[115]	Low lumbar myelomeningocele			
	Swing through gait	53.95	17.19	0.342
	Reciprocal gait	40.49	16.81	0.492
	Control group	63.97	10.98	0.171
Cunha-Filho et al.[80]	Cervical and thoracic level SCI ($n = 10$)			
	Devices mixed group	33	13.28	0.40
Ulkar et al.[19]	Incomplete SCI ($n = 9$)			
	Repeated measure			
	Walker	13.84 ± 6.64	13.14 ± 2.49	1.20 ± 0.67
	Lofstrand crutches	28.02 ± 20.97	12.71 ± 2.37	0.84 ± 0.66

TABLE 2.5 (continued)
Energy Expenditure and Gait Efficiency at Comfortable Walking
Speed in Spinal Injury Patients

References	Subjects/Devices	Speed (m/min)	Oxygen Consumption (mL/kg/min)	Gait Efficiency (mL/kg/m)
Kawashima et al.[110]	T_8–T_{12} injury ($n = 4$)			
	Weight-bearing control orthosis	16–22	14.21–18.04	0.82–0.89
Kawashima et al.[101]	T_5–T_{12}	19.88	18.16	0.9965

ª KAFO, knee-ankle-foot-orthosis.
ᵇ LEMS, Lower Extremity Muscle Score from the ASIA.[100]

limited mobility function and the high energy demand of mobility, patients with spinal injury were observed to have reduced physical capacity.[119] Combining a reduced RMR and a reduced physical activity level, spinal injury patients are at a great risk of gaining weight after the period of rehabilitation. This raises an urgent need for promoting physical activities in spinal injury patients, which is also an important issue for all patients with physical disabilities.

2.3.3 CEREBRAL PALSY (CP)

CP is a nonprogressive brain disorder occurring during, before, or soon after birth, and it results in developmental delay and multiple impairments in mentality, vision, hearing, speech, muscle coordination, muscle tone, balance, movements, and physical capacity. The incidence is about 2–2.5 in 1000 live births.[120] The impaired musculoskeletal development in later years also contributes to the disabilities in CP children.

Similar to people with other disabilities, individuals with CP have increased energy expenditure for a given submaximal workload,[121,122] reduced maximal oxygen uptake,[123] decreased gait efficiency, decreased mechanical efficiency,[122] and decreased comfortable walking speed when compared to healthy children and adults.[124–128] Possible causes for the increased energy demand of walking include the following: spasticity, cocontraction,[129] atypical patterns of movements, deficit in motor control, joint contracture, quadriceps muscle weakness, fatiguability, and inefficient energy transfer between body segments. Muscle pathological changes in CP children include decreased blood flow, decreased sarcomeres with hypoextensibility, atrophy of type II fibers, hypertrophy of type I fibers, and increased fat and connective tissue, hence it was suggested that the metabolic inefficiency and fatigue in CP children might be due to local muscle-related factors rather than cardiopulmonary impairments.[130] However, the exact causal relationship between specific impairments and the increased energy expenditure still awaits further multidisciplinary studies.

According to the Gross Motor Function Classification System (GMFCS), a five-level functional grading system, children with CP aged between 1 and 12 years could be classified into five functional classes: I, II, III, IV, and V.[131,132] The severity of the motor function impairment was found to be highly related to the increased energy expenditure and decreased gait efficiency of walking.[121] Therefore, interventions that improve motor function, such as the use of orthosis, assistive devices, muscle strengthening, and gait training, can also improve gait efficiency and reduce the energy expenditure of walking.

Four potential criteria for self-optimization of the preferred walking pattern in healthy children and children with hemiplegic CP have been identified: (1) minimization of physiological cost, (2) maximization of mechanical energy conservation, (3) minimization of gait asymmetry, and (4) minimization of the variability of interlimb and intralimb coordination.[133] These criteria provide a clear direction of comprehensive clinical approaches for children with CP, such as the use of shoe lift for correction of leg discrepancy, muscle strengthening to improve muscle atrophy, stretching, medications, and orthosis to improve ankle spasticity,[134] and motor control and motor learning to improve gait coordination and stability.[135] Each of the above approaches addresses a specific aspect of the optimization criteria, and together they improve the body system in CP children to accomplish gait optimization. Besides, it was identified that the stride frequency of the preferred walking velocity could be predicted by the natural frequency of the force-driven harmonic oscillator, when muscle mass, leg length discrepancy, and increased muscle stiffness of CP children were taken into consideration.[133] It is likely that the natural frequency of the leg might provide a target for gait training to tune the CP children to their energy-efficient gait pattern.

Walking with flexed knee is commonly observed in CP children due to equines deformity and/or knee spasticity and contracture. In normal children, it was found that walking with a brace with progressively increasing knee angle increased the energy expenditure of walking and slowed the walking speed.[136] Specifically, when the knee flexion angle exceeded $15°$, significant increase in energy expenditure was observed due to increased quadriceps, tibiofemoral, and patellofemoral forces.[137,138] Table 2.6 shows the energy expenditure of flexed knee gait.

The physical capacity of individuals with CP is generally lower than that of age-matched able-bodies.[123,127,139–141] Measurement of peak oxygen uptake with a cycle ergometer exercise test in CP children poses challenges to researchers due to spasticity at the ankle and the knee, preventing smooth pedaling. Treadmill testing is

TABLE 2.6
Energy Expenditure of Flexed Knee Gait

Degrees	Velocity (m/min)	O₂ Rate (mL/kg/min)	Gait Efficiency (mL/kg/m)
0	80	11.8	0.16
15	77	12.8	0.17
30	75	14.3	0.19
45	67	14.5	0.22

Source: Modified from Waters, R.L. and Mulroy, S., *Gait Posture*, 9, 207, 1999.

TABLE 2.7

Submaximal Oxygen Consumption (VO_2) Values in Three Treadmill Exercise Studies of Children with Cerebral Palsy (CP) and Able-Bodied Children

References	Treadmill Speed (m/min)	Children with CP		Able-Bodied Children	
		VO_2 (mL/kg/min)	% $VO_2{}_{max}$[a]	VO_2 (mL/kg/min)	% $VO_2{}_{max}$
Unnithan et al.[128]	50.0	16.6 ± 5.90	53.2 ± 26.0	10.2 ± 0.84	22.5 ± 4.93
Rose et al.[140]	51.0	18.00 ± 5.00	—	10.00 ± 0.50	—
Rose et al.[143]	21.5	14.25 ± 3.67	—	8.63 ± 1.27	—
	37.6	19.08 ± 7.20	—	10.55 ± 1.24	—

Source: Modified from Unnithan, V.B., et al., *Sports Med.*, 26, 239, 1998.

[a] $VO_2{}_{max}$ = maximal VO_2 value.

also limited due to balance problems and movement incoordination in CP children. The physiologic cost index provides an alternative as a clinically useful measure of energy demand in disabled children. The within-day and between-day variability of oxygen consumption measurement were reported to be around 8.6% and 13%, respectively, and the variability of the physiologic cost index were even much higher in CP children.[142] Therefore, it was suggested that a longer acclimation to treadmill walking was necessary in children with severe motor function involvement in order to reduce the measurement variability of energy consumption or physiologic cost index. Table 2.7 shows the oxygen consumption in CP children compared with able-bodied children.

Some factors related to the low exercise capacity in CP children have been identified. Spasticity, muscle pathology, musculoskeletal limitations, and a less mobile lifestyle could all contribute to the low physical capacity in children with CP. With increased aerobic activities and exercises in their physical education classes, children with CP were shown improved motor coordination and reduced energy expenditure at submaximal exercise.[144]

2.3.4 Multiple Sclerosis (MS)

MS is a demyelinating disease of the central nervous system, and the motor system is often affected. MS commonly causes general fatigue and dyspnea with physical activity. The neurological impairments in MS patients often lead to a sedentary lifestyle, which then leads to reduced cardiovascular fitness, disuse muscle atrophy, and weakness.[85] This disease is also characterized by periods of exacerbation and remission. During the remission, MS patients are able to walk at slow speeds, but the metabolic demand of walking is high. The increased metabolic demand of walking was found to be related to muscle spasticity,[145] respiratory muscle weakness,[146,147] and reduced quality of life.[147]

2.3.5   Parkinson's Disease and Postpoliomyelitis

The resting energy expenditure in patients with Parkinson's disease was shown increased, and it was thought to relate to a disturbance in the neuroendocrine balance.[148] The increase in resting energy expenditure could cause weight loss in these patients.

Patients with postpoliomyelitis were shown to have a reduced comfortable walking speed, an increased energy expenditure at a given walking speed, and a reduced gait efficiency when compared to their healthy counterparts.[149,150] There is a strong negative relationship between lower extremity muscle strength and the energy expenditure of walking, i.e., the weaker the lower extremity muscle strength, the higher the energy expenditure of walking.

2.4   ENERGY EXPENDITURE IN PEOPLE WITH CARDIORESPIRATORY DISABILITIES

Increased oxygen consumption at rest or during household activities and decreased SSWV have been well reported in patients with chronic obstructive pulmonary disease (COPD),[151] cystic fibrosis,[152] pacemaker,[153] peripheral arterial disease,[154] and coronary artery disease.[155] The possible mechanisms for the increased metabolic demand with physical activity include the following factors: declining pulmonary mechanics, malnutrition, chronic inflammation of the respiratory system, cellular defects, higher energy cost of breathing, impaired cardiac contractility, and decreased physical capacity.[156]

Some energy conservation techniques for pulmonary patients can be applied in activities of daily living, such as not putting things on high shelves or low shelves, sitting in a chair for brushing teeth and washing face, and avoiding bending forward for lifting objects. These conservation techniques have shown to reduce energy consumption.[157] Breathing exercises, such as diaphragmatic breathing, pursed-lip breathing, or a combination of the two exercises showed a reduction in oxygen consumption in COPD patients.[158] The benefits of cardiac rehabilitation have been well documented for improving peak exercise capacity, reducing cardiac risk factors, and improving the quality of life in cardiac patients.[32]

In order to recommend the appropriate physical activities for patients with disabilities, there have been many recent studies on the energy expenditure of physical activities in patients with chronic diseases or disabilities. For example, patients with coronary artery disease or pacemaker were shown to have increased metabolic demand for most household activities.[153] It was suggested that for cardiac patients with a maximal aerobic capacity equal to or greater than 5 METs, they could safely handle ordinary household activities (2–4 METs) because those activities are at about 60% of their peak VO_2, i.e., considered as a moderate exercise intensity.[155] Table 2.8 shows the oxygen consumption and SSWV in some cardiac and pulmonary patients. Table 2.9 shows the measured energy expenditure in some activities of daily living in cardiac patients.

TABLE 2.8

Oxygen Consumption and Self-Selected Walking Velocity in Selected Pulmonary and Cardiac Patients

References	Subjects	Oxygen Consumption (mL/kg/min)	SSWV (m/min)
Menard-Rothe et al.[151]	End-stage emphysema	—	
	Male		44.5 ± 15.0
	Female		39.6 ± 12.3
Marconi et al.[154]	Peripheral artery disease	11.8 ± 2.3	53.33
	Normal subjects	8.4 ± 0.6	53.33

TABLE 2.9

Measured Energy Expenditure in Some Activities of Daily Living in Cardiac Patients

Task	Measured METs ± SD	Compendium[2] (METs)
Vacuuming	3.3 ± 0.7	2.5
Bed linens	3.0 ± 0.6	2.5
Groceries	3.1 ± 0.5	2.5
Laundry	2.5 ± 0.4	2.0
Treadmill (2.6 mph)	3.4 ± 0.3	3.0 (2.5 mph)

Source: Adapted from Skemp, K.M., et al., *Clin. Exerc. Physiol.*, 3, 213, 2001.

2.5 OTHER CONSIDERATIONS

2.5.1 ASSISTIVE DEVICES

It is well known that the use of assistive devices, such as cane or walker, slows the walking velocity and increases the energy demand of walking.[159,160] The energy expenditure for walking with different assistive devices, from the highest to the lowest, has been reported in the following order: walker > crutches > cane or crutch > no device.[161,162] People who require a walker for walking usually have a higher degree of impairment, which might explain the higher energy requirements in their walking compared to those who walk with other devices, or without a device. Walking with a rolling walker was found to require lower energy expenditure than walking with a pickup walker.[163] Among different weight-bearing status and assistive devices, walking with alternating bilateral partial weight bearing, or unilateral partial weight bearing required 33% more energy than normal walking, and walking with nonweight-bearing status required 78% more energy than normal walking.[164]

2.5.2 Wheelchair Propulsion

People with disabilities often use wheelchair for daily mobility, longer distance of transportation, or sports activities. Manual wheelchair propulsion requires good muscle strength of the upper extremity, trunk control, and physical capacity. The metabolic demand for driving a wheelchair is similar to doing an arm crank exercise, but with a lower mechanical efficiency.[165] Exercises with the upper extremity require a higher energy demand than leg exercises at any given submaximal workload, due to the smaller muscle mass, a larger recruitment of type II muscle fibers, a smaller capillary bed, and a higher vascular resistance of the upper extremity.[166] Other factors such as floor surface,[167] propelling speed,[168] and wheelchair design[169] also greatly influence the energy demand of wheelchair propulsion for people with disabilities. Table 2.10 shows the energy expenditure of manual wheelchair propulsion.

2.5.3 Aging with a Disability

With aging, many body systems and functions deteriorate, such as easily fatigable muscles, reduced cardiac output, reduced ventilatory capacity, reduced muscle mass, reduced flexibility, decreased bone mineral density, reduced balance ability, and reduced maximal aerobic power.[170] Problems in energy expenditure and efficiency[171]

TABLE 2.10
Energy Expenditure of Manual Wheelchair Propulsion

References	Subjects/Conditions	Oxygen Consumption (mL/kg/min)	Speed (m/min)
Wolfe et al.[167]	*Concrete*		
	Normal	11.8 ± 2.6	56.6
	Deconditioned	13.0 ± 2.2	53.3
	Paraplegic: Hard tires	15.7 ± 5.3	82.7
	Paraplegic: Pneumatic tires	15.7 ± 3.8	79.8
	Carpet		
	Normal subjects	12.5 ± 2.9	43.3
	Deconditioned	14.0 ± 1.7	37.5
	Paraplegic: Hard tires	16.9 ± 5.0	65.3
	Paraplegic: Pneumatic tires	17.1 ± 4.4	63.6
Mukherjee et al.[168]	Slow speed	9.52 ± 1.14	24.6
	Freely chosen speed	14.02 ± 2.94	56.8
	Fast speed	16.36 ± 3.54	72.3
Mukherjee and Samanta[169]	Arm-crank propelled wheelchair		
	One arm	10.30 ± 1.14	122.8
	Two arms	9.94 ± 0.95	132.5

would only get worse with aging for people with physical disabilities, but there are not many data available in the literature.

Normal aging without any chronic disease is characterized by reduced daily energy expenditure, so elderly people have a higher risk of developing obesity. This is also common in elderly persons with disabilities. Health promotion and wellness programs are needed for this population, with additional factors taken into consideration and with suitable modifications, such as their medical conditions, overload stress on small muscles of the upper extremity, adaptation of equipment to fit the specific types of disability, accessibility of the training facility, and temperature regulation.[170]

On the other hand, some elderly have a few chronic diseases that are associated with an increased resting energy expenditure, such as diabetes, congestive heart failure, Parkinson's disease, Alzheimer's disease, and COPD.[172,173] Poor nutritional intake plus increased resting energy expenditure with chronic diseases were thought to be the possible causes of unexplained weight loss in the elderly.[172,173] Therefore, special attention also has to be paid to specific exercise conditioning and proper nutritional supplement for the elderly with chronic diseases.

2.5.4 Physical Disability and Obesity

In recent years, health care for people with disabilities has been increasingly focused on the prevention of secondary complications arising from the disabilities. The secondary conditions refer to those preventable medical, emotional, or social problems resulting directly or indirectly from the disability, such as obesity, muscle atrophy, pneumonia, urinary tract infection, depression, fatigue, pressure sore, and joint pain.[174] Obesity is not an acute condition, but it has many ramifications.

Physical inactivity often results from the functional limitations of the disability, a feeling of depression, and fatigue, leading to an unhealthy lifestyle and adverse behaviors.[174] Either due to primary deficits or disuse, muscle atrophy leads to a decreased fat-free mass and results in a reduction of the resting energy expenditure. Combining the two factors together, reduced energy expenditure in physical activity and reduced resting energy expenditure lead to reduced total energy expenditure in people with disabilities. Therefore, people with disabilities have a higher tendency to reach a positive energy balance state.

The development of obesity seems to be a vicious cycle for people with disabilities. Obesity compounds the problems of high energy demand of physical activities in people with disabilities, which reduces the likelihood of participation in social activities and exercise, and reduces their ability to care for themselves. Secondary complications such as hypertension, type II diabetes, and coronary disease develop as obesity continues. It can further lead to many health complications, increasing the health care cost for people with disabilities and the health care burden on society.

One of the federal health focus areas of "Healthy People 2010" encourages people to engage regular moderate-intensity exercise in order to curb the health complications arising from the epidemic of obesity and physical inactivity. Promoting physical activity, aerobic exercise, and muscle strengthening in people with disabilities have become even more important than the health promotion for people without disabilities. Improved ergonomic design of exercise equipments to fit people with disabilities would greatly facilitate their participation in leisure physical activities. Improved physical fitness in people with disabilities will then be possibly achieved, and prevention of secondary complications will also be accomplished.

2.6 CONCLUSION

Due to severe impairments in specific body systems, people with disabilities require more energy for most physical activities, such as walking, activities of daily living, leisure activities, and sports activities. Therefore, they tend to walk slower and are less energy-efficient. Rehabilitation with therapeutic exercises, the use of assistive devices and orthosis, modifications of work and home environment, and prosthesis training could all improve the neuromuscular control, movement coordination, muscle performance, and cardiorespiratory functions of their body systems. The overall goal of training is to improve their body systems to become more energy efficient for physical activities. In addition to the treatment of primary impairments, future directions of rehabilitation for people with disabilities should involve health promotion and wellness programs, in order to prevent secondary complications and to improve their health.

ACKNOWLEDGMENTS

I would like to thank Elaine Cox, our librarian, for her help in the literature search, and my husband, Dr. Roger W. Chan, for his thorough review and editorial comments on the manuscript.

REFERENCES

1. McArdle, W., Katch, F., and Katch, V., *Exercise Physiology*, 6th edn., Lippincott Williams & Wilkins, Philadelphia, PA, 2007, Chapters 8 and 9.
2. Ainworth, B. E., et al., Compendium of physical activities: An update of activity codes and MET intensities, *Med Sci Sports Exerc*, 32(9), S498, 2000.
3. Browing, R. C., et al., Effects of obesity and sex on the energetic cost and preferred speed of walking, *J Appl Physiol*, 100, 390, 2006.
4. Ralston, H., Energy–speed relation and optimal speed during level walking, *Int Z Angew Physiol*, 17S, 277, 1958.
5. Bobbert, A., Energy expenditure in level and grade walking, *J Appl Physiol*, 15, 1015, 1960.
6. Walker, J., et al., The energy cost of horizontal walking and running in adolescents, *Med Sci Sports Exerc*, 31(2), 311, 1999.
7. Hall, C., et al., Energy expenditure of walking and running: Comparison with prediction equations, *Med Sci Sports Exerc*, 36(12), 2128, 2004.
8. Corcoran, P. and Brengelmann, G., Oxygen uptake in normal and handicapped subjects, in relation to speed of walking beside velocity-controlled cart, *Arch Phys Med Rehabil*, 51, 78, 1970.
9. Malatesta, D., et al., Energy cost of walking and gait instability in healthy 65- and 80-yr-olds, *J Appl Physiol*, 95, 2248, 2003.
10. Nielsen, D., Comparison of energy cost and gait efficiency during ambulation in below-knee amputees using different prosthetic feet—A preliminary report, *J Prothet Orthot*, 1(1), 24, 1988.

11. Nielsen, D., et al., Energy cost, exercise intensity, and gait efficiency of standard versus rocker-bottom axillary crutch walking, *Phys Ther*, 70, 487, 1990.
12. Inman, V., Ralston, H., and Todd, F., *Human Walking*, Williams & Wilkins, Baltimore, MD, 1981, p. 62.
13. Martin, P., Rothstein, D., and Larish, D., Effects of age and physical activity status on the speed-aerobic demand relationship of walking, *J Appl Physiol*, 73(1), 200, 1992.
14. Zarrugh, M., Todd, F., and Ralston, H., Optimization of energy expenditure during level walking, *Eur J Appl Physiol Occup Physiol*, 33, 293, 1974.
15. Finley, F. and Cody, K., Locomotive characteristics of urban pedestrians, *Arch Phys Med Rehabil*, 51, 423, 1970.
16. Rose, J., et al., The energy expenditure index: A method to quantitate and compare walking energy expenditure for children and adolescents, *J Ped Orthop*, 11(5), 571, 1991.
17. Fisher, S. V. and Gullickson, G., Energy cost of ambulation in health and disability: A literature review, *Arch Phys Med Rehabil*, 59(3), 124, 1978.
18. Waters, R., et al., Energy cost of walking of amputees: The influence of level of amputation, *J Bone Joint Surg Am*, 58A, 42, 1976.
19. Ulkar, B., et al., Energy expenditure of the paraplegic gait: Comparison between different walking aids and normal subjects, *Int J Rehabil Res*, 26, 213, 2003.
20. Cunningham, D., et al., Determinants of self-selected walking pace across ages 19 to 66, *J Geront*, 37, 560, 1982.
21. Waters, R., et al., Energy cost of walking in normal children and teenagers, *Dev Med Child Neurol*, 25, 184, 1983.
22. Jaegers, S., et al., The relationship between comfortable and most metabolically efficient walking speed in persons with unilateral above-knee amputation, *Arch Phys Med Rehabil*, 74, 521, 1993.
23. Waters, R., et al., Comparative cost of walking in young and old adults, *J Orthop Res*, 1(1), 73, 1983.
24. Waters, R., et al., Energy-speed relationship of walking: Standard tables, *J Orthop Res*, 6(2), 215, 1988.
25. Waters, R. and Mulroy, S., The energy expenditure of normal and pathologic gait, *Gait Posture*, 9, 207, 1999.
26. Holt, K., Hamill, J., and Andres, R., The force-driven harmonic oscillator as a model for human locomotion, *Hum Mov Sci*, 9, 55, 1990.
27. Holt, K., Hamill, J., and Andres, R., Predicting the minimal energy costs of human walking, *Med Sci Sports Exerc*, 23, 491, 1991.
28. Ferguson, R. A., et al., Muscle oxygen uptake and energy turnover during dynamic exercise at different contraction frequencies in humans, *J Physiol*, 536, 261, 2001.
29. Powers, S. K., Beadle, R. E., and Mangum, M., Exercise efficiency during arm ergometry: Effects of speed and work rate, *J Appl Physiol*, 56, 495, 1984.
30. Coyle, E., et al., Cycling efficiency is related to the percentage of type I muscle fibers, *Med Sci Sports Exerc*, 24, 782, 1992.
31. Gleim, G., Stachenfeld, N., and Nicholas, J., The influence of flexibility on the economy of walking and jogging, *J Orthop Res*, 8, 814, 1990.
32. American College of Sports Medicine, *ACSM's Guidelines for Exercise Testing and Prescription*, 7th edn., Lippincott Williams & Wilkins, Philadelphia, PA, 2005.
33. Jackson, A., et al., Changes in aerobic power of women, ages 20-64 yr, *Med Sci Sports Exerc*, 28, 844, 1996.
34. Åstrand, P. -O., et al., *Textbook of Work Physiology: Physiological Bases of Exercise*, 4th edn., Human Kinetics, Champaign, IL, 2003, p. 649.
35. Davies, M. and Dalsky, G., Economy of mobility in older adults, *J Orthop Sports Phys Ther*, 26(2), 69, 1997.
36. Pearce, M. E., et al., Energy cost of treadmill and floor walking at self-selected paces, *Eur J Appl Physiol Occup Physiol*, 52, 115, 1983.

37. Bassett, D. J., et al., Aerobic requirements of overground versus treadmill running, *Med Sci Sports Exerc*, 17, 477, 1985.
38. Royer, T. and Martin, P. E., Manipulation of leg mass and moment of inertia: Effects on energy cost of walking, *Med Sci Sports Exerc*, 37(4), 649, 2005.
39. Ralston, H., Comparison of energy expenditure during treadmill walking and floor walking, *J Appl Physiol*, 15, 1156, 1960.
40. Murray, M., et al., Treadmill vs. floor walking: Kinematics, electromyogram, and heart rate, *J Appl Physiol*, 59(1), 87, 1985.
41. Taga, G., A model of the neuro-musculo-skeletal system for human locomotion, *Biol Cybern*, 73, 113, 1995.
42. Saibene, F., The mechanism for minimizing energy expenditure in human locomotion, *Eur J Clin Nutr*, 44(Suppl), 65, 1990.
43. Skinner, H. and Barrack, R., Ankle weighting effect on gait in able-bodied adults, *Arch Phys Med Rehabil*, 71, 112, 1990.
44. Ralston, H. and Lukin, L., Energy level of human body segments during level walking, *Ergonomics*, 12(1), 39, 1969.
45. Aulivola, B., et al., Major lower extremity amputation, *Arch Surg*, 139, 395, 2004.
46. Molen, N., Energy/speed relation of below-knee amputees walking on motor-driven treadmill, *Int Z Angew Physiol*, 31, 173, 1973.
47. Pagliarulo, M., Waters, R., and Hislop, H., Energy cost of walking of below knee amputees having no vascular disease, *Phys Ther*, 59, 538, 1979.
48. James, U., Oxygen uptake and heart rate during prosthetic walking in healthy male unilateral above-knee amputees, *Scan J Rehabil Med*, 5, 71, 1973.
49. Gailey, R., et al., Energy expenditure of trans-tibial amputees during ambulation at self-selected pace, *Prosth Orthot Int*, 18, 84, 1994.
50. Huang, C., et al., Amputation: Energy cost of ambulation, *Arch Phys Med Rehabil*, 60, 18, 1979.
51. Aulivola, B., et al., Major lower extremity amputation: Outcome of a modern series, *Arch Surg*, 139, 395, 2004.
52. Gonzalez, E., Corcoran, P., and Reyes, R., Energy expenditure in below-knee amputees: Correlation with stump length, *Arch Phys Med Rehabil*, 55, 111, 1974.
53. Velzen, J. V., et al., Physical capacity and walking ability after lower limb amputation: A systemic review, *Clin Rehabil*, 20, 999, 2006.
54. Hsu, M., et al., The effects of prosthetic foot design on physiologic measurements, self-selected walking velocity, and physical activity in people with transtibial amputation, *Arch Phys Med Rehabil*, 87(1), 123, 2006.
55. Hsu, M., et al., Physiological measurements of walking and running in people with transtibial amputations with 3 different prostheses, *J Orthop Sports Phys Ther*, 29(9), 526, 1999.
56. Lin-Chan, S., et al., The effect of added prosthetic mass on physiologic responses and stride frequency during multiple speeds of walking in persons with transtibial amputation, *Arch Phys Med Rehabil*, 84(12), 1865, 2003.
57. Buckley, J., Spence, W., and Solomonidis, S., Energy cost of walking: Comparison of 'intelligent prosthesis' with conventional mechanism, *Arch Phys Med Rehabil*, 78, 330, 1997.
58. Gailey, R., et al., The CAT-CAM socket and quadrilateral socket: A comparison of energy cost during ambulation, *Prosth Orthot Int*, 17, 95, 1993.
59. Detrembleur, C., et al., Relationship between energy cost, gait speed, vertical displacement of center of body mass and efficiency of pendulum-like mechanism in unilateral amputee gait, *Gait Posture*, 21(4), 333, 2005.
60. Pinzur, M., et al., Energy demands for walking in dysvascular amputees as related to the level of amputation, *Orthopaedics*, 15, 1033, 1992.
61. Lin-Chan, S., et al., Physiological responses to multiple speed treadmill walking for syme versus transtibial amputation: A case study, *Disabil Rehabil*, 25(23), 1333, 2003.

62. Ganguli, S. and Bose, K., Biomechanical approach to the functional assessment of the use of crutches for ambulation, *Ergonomics*, 17(3), 365, 1974.
63. Wu, Y. -J., et al., Energy expenditure of wheeling and walking during prosthetic rehabilitation in a woman with bilateral transfemoral amputations, *Arch Phys Med Rehabil*, 82(2), 265, 2001.
64. Torburn, L., et al., Energy expenditure during ambulation in dysvascular and traumatic below-knee amputees: A comparison of five prosthetic feet, *J Rehabil Res Dev*, 32(2), 111, 1995.
65. Huang, G., Chou, Y., and Su, F., Gait analysis and energy consumption of below-knee amputees wearing three different prosthetic feet, *Gait Posture*, 12(2), 162, 2000.
66. Bussmann, J., Grootscholten, E., and Stam, H., Daily physical activity and heart rate response in people with a unilateral transtibial amputation for vascular disease, *Arch Phys Med Rehabil*, 85, 240, 2004.
67. Gailey, R., et al., The effects of prosthesis mass on metabolic cost of ambulation in non-vascular trans-tibial amputees, *Prosth Orthot Int*, 21, 9, 1997.
68. Mattes, S., Martin, P., and Royer, T., Walking symmetry and energy cost in persons with unilateral transtibial amputations: Matching prosthetic and intact limb inertial properties, *Arch Phys Med Rehabil*, 81(5), 561, 2000.
69. Selles, R. W., et al., Adaptations to mass perturbations in transtibial amputees: Kinetic or kinematic invariance? *Arch Phys Med Rehabil*, 85(12), 2046, 2004.
70. Selles, R., et al., Effects of prosthetic mass and mass distribution on kinematics and energetics of prosthetic gait: A systematic review, *Arch Phys Med Rehabil*, 80(12), 1593, 1999.
71. Lehmann, J., et al., Mass and mass distribution of below-knee prosthesis: Effect on gait efficacy and self-selected walking speed, *Arch Phys Med Rehabil*, 79, 162, 1998.
72. Torburn, L., et al., Below knee amputee gait with dynamic elastic response prosthetic feet: A pilot study, *J Rehabil Res Dev*, 27(4), 369, 1990.
73. Casillas, J., et al., Bioenergetic comparison of a new energy-storing foot and SACH foot in traumatic below-knee vascular amputations, *Arch Phys Med Rehabil*, 76, 39, 1995.
74. Lehmann, J., et al., Comprehensive analysis of energy storing prosthetic feet: Flex Foot and Seattle Foot versus Standard SACH foot, *Arch Phys Med Rehabil*, 74, 853, 1993.
75. Prince, F., et al., Mechanical efficiency during gait of adults with transtibial amputation: A pilot study comparing the SACH, Seattle, and Golden-Ankle prosthetic feet, *J Rehabil Res Dev*, 35(2), 177, 1998.
76. Cavagna, G., Willems, P., and Heglund, N., The role of gravity in human walking: Pendular energy exchange, external work and optimal speed, *J Physiol*, 528 (part 3), 657, 2000.
77. Cavagna, G., Thys, H., and Zamboni, A., The sources of external work in level walking and running, *J Physiol*, 262(3), 639, 1976.
78. Heglund, N., et al., Energy-saving gait mechanics with head-supported loads, *Nature*, 4375(6526), 52, 1995.
79. Gitter, A., Czerniecki, J., and Meinders, M., Effect of prosthetic mass on swing phase work during above-knee amputee ambulation, *Am J Phys Med Rehabil*, 76, 114, 1995.
80. Cunha-Filho, I., et al., Differential responses to measures of gait performance among healthy and neurologically impaired individuals, *Arch Phys Med Rehabil*, 84, 1774, 2003.
81. Detrembleur, C., et al., Energy cost, mechanical work, and efficiency of hemiparetic walking, *Gait Posture*, 18, 47, 2003.
82. Bhambhani, Y., Rowland, G., and Farag, M., Reliability of peak cardiorespiratory responses in patients with moderate to severe traumatic brain injury, *Arch Phys Med Rehabil*, 84(11), 1629, 2003.
83. MacKay-Lyons, M. J. and Makrides, L., Exercise capacity early after stroke, *Arch Phys Med Rehabil*, 83(12), 1697, 2002.

84. McCrory, M., et al., Energy expenditure, physical activity, and body composition of ambulatory adults with hereditary neuromuscular disease, *Am J Clin Nutr*, 67, 1162, 1998.

85. Ng, A. and Kent-Braun, J., Quantitation of lower physical activity in persons with multiple sclerosis, *Med Sci Sports Exerc*, 29(4), 517, 1997.

86. Pearson, O., et al., Quantification of walking mobility in neurological disorders, *Q J Med*, 97, 463, 2004.

87. American Heart Association, *Heart Disease and Stroke Statistics—2003 Update*, American Heart Association, Dallas, TX, 2002.

88. Bard, G., Energy expenditure of hemiplegic subjects during walking, *Arch Phys Med Rehabil*, 44, 368, 1963.

89. Hash, D., Energetics of wheelchair propulsion and walking in stroke patients, *Orthop Clin North Am*, 9, 372, 1978.

90. Stoquart, G., et al., Efficiency of work production by spastic muscles, *Gait Posture*, 22, 331, 2005.

91. Kelly, J. O., et al., Cardiorespiratory fitness and walking ability in subacute stroke patients, *Arch Phys Med Rehabil*, 84, 1780, 2003.

92. Franceschini, M., et al., Effects of an ankle-foot orthosis on spatiotemporal parameters and energy cost of hemiparetic gait, *Clin Rehabil*, 17, 368, 2003.

93. Danielsson, A. and Sunnerhagen, K., Energy expenditure in stroke subjects walking with a carbon composite ankle foot orthosis, *J Rehabil Med*, 36, 165, 2004.

94. David, D., et al., Oxygen consumption during machine-assisted and unassisted walking: A pilot study in hemiplegic and healthy humans, *Arch Phys Med Rehabil*, 87(4), 482, 2006.

95. Danielsson, A. and Sunnerhagen, K., Oxygen consumption during treadmill walking with and without body weight support in patients with hemiparesis after stroke and in healthy subjects, *Arch Phys Med Rehabil*, 81(7), 953, 2000.

96. Cunha, I., et al., Gait outcomes after acute stroke rehabilitation with supported treadmill ambulation training: A randomized controlled pilot study, *Arch Phys Med Rehabil*, 83, 1258, 2002.

97. Macko, R., et al., Treadmill aerobic exercise training reduces the energy expenditure and cardiovascular demands of hemiparetic gait in chronic stroke patients: A preliminary report, *Stroke*, 28(2), 326, 1997.

98. Macko, R., Ivey, F., and Forrester, L., Task-oriented aerobic exercise in chronic hemiparetic stroke: Training protocols and treatment effects, *Top Stroke Rehabil*, 12(1), 45, 2005.

99. Gordon, N. F., et al., Physical activity and exercise recommendations for stroke survivors, *Stroke*, 35, 1229, 2004.

100. American Spinal Injury Association, *Standards for Neurological Classification of Spinal Injury Patients*, American Spinal Injury Association, Chicago, IL, 1992.

101. Kawashima, N., et al., Effect of lesion level on the orthotic gait performance in individuals with complete paraplegia, *Spinal Cord*, 44, 487, 2006.

102. Bernard, P., et al., Influence of lesion level on the cardiorespiratory adaptations in paraplegic wheelchair athletes during muscular exercise, *Spinal Cord*, 38, 16, 2000.

103. Maynard, F., et al., International standards for neurological and functional classification of spinal cord injury, *Spinal Cord*, 35, 266, 1997.

104. Buchholz, A. and Pencharz, P., Energy expenditure in chronic spinal cord injury, *Curr Opin Clin Nutr Metab Care*, 7, 635, 2004.

105. IJzerman, M. J., et al., Validity and reproducibility of crutch force and heart rate measurements to assess energy expenditure of paraplegic gait, *Arch Phys Med Rehabil*, 80, 1017, 1999.

106. Miller, N., et al., Paraplegic energy expenditure during negotiation of architectural barriers, *Arch Phys Med Rehabil*, 65, 778, 1984.

107. Waters, R., et al., Prediction of ambulatory performance based on motor scores derived from standards of the American Spinal Injury Association, *Arch Phys Med Rehabil*, 75, 756, 1994.
108. Jacobs, P., et al., Relationships of oxygen uptake, heart rate, and ratings of perceived exertion in persons with paraplegia during functional neuromuscular stimulation assisted ambulation, *Spinal Cord*, 35, 292, 1997.
109. Barstow, T., et al., Peak and kinetic cardiorespiratory responses during arm and leg exercise in patients with spinal cord injury, *Spinal Cord*, 38, 340, 2000.
110. Kawashima, N., et al., Energy expenditure during walking with weight-bearing control (WBC) orthosis in thoracic level of paraplegic patients, *Spinal Cord*, 41, 506, 2003.
111. Bernardi, M., et al., The efficiency of walking of paraplegic patients using a reciprocating gait orthosis, *Paraplegia*, 33, 409, 1995.
112. Nene, A. and Patrick, J., Energy cost of paraplegic locomotion using the parawalker—Electrical stimulation "hybrid" orthosis, *Arch Phys Med Rehabil*, 71, 116, 1990.
113. Hirokawa, S., et al., Energy consumption in paraplegic ambulation using the reciprocating gait orthosis and electric stimulation of the thigh muscles, *Arch Phys Med Rehabil*, 71, 687, 1990.
114. Minetti, A., et al., Effects of stride frequency on mechanical power and energy expenditure of walking, *Med Sci Sports Exerc*, 27, 1194, 1995.
115. Moore, C., et al., Energy cost of walking in low lumbar myelomeningocele, *J Ped Orthop*, 21(3), 388, 2001.
116. Zamparo, P. and Pagliaro, P., The energy cost of level walking before and after hydrokinesi therapy in patients with spastic paresis, *Scan J Med Sci Sports*, 8, 222, 1998.
117. Williams, L., et al., Energy cost of walking and of wheelchair propulsion by children with myelodysplasia, *Dev Med Child Neurol*, 25, 617, 1983.
118. Waters, R., et al., Determinants of gait performance following spinal cord injury, *Arch Phys Med Rehabil*, 70(12), 811, 1989.
119. Thomas, J., et al., Changes in physical strain and physical capacity in men with spinal cord injuries, *Med Sci Sports Exerc*, 28(5), 551, 1996.
120. Odding, E., Roebroeck, M., and Stam, H. J., The epidemiology of cerebral palsy: Incidence, impairments and risk factors, *Disabil Rehabil*, 28(4), 183, 2006.
121. Johnston, T. E., et al., Energy cost of walking in children with cerebral palsy: Relation to the Gross Motor Functional Classification System, *Dev Med Child Neurol*, 46, 34, 2004.
122. Jones, J. and McLaughlin, J., Mechanical efficiency of children with spastic cerebral palsy, *Dev Med Child Neurol*, 35, 614, 1993.
123. Unnithan, V. B., Clifford, C., and Bar-Or, O., Evaluation by exercise testing of the child with cerebral palsy, *Sports Med*, 26(4), 239, 1998.
124. Campbell, J. and Ball, J., Energetics of walking in cerebral palsy, in energetics: Application to the study and management of locomotor disabilities, *Orthop Clin North Am*, 9, 374, 1978.
125. Keefer, D., et al., Interrelationships among thigh muscle co-contraction, quadriceps muscle strength and the aerobic demand of walking in children with cerebral palsy, *Electromyogr Clin Neurophysiol*, 44, 103, 2004.
126. Bowen, T., et al., Variability of energy-consumption measures in children with cerebral palsy, *J Ped Orthop*, 18, 738, 1998.
127. Rose, J., et al., Energy expenditure index of walking for normal children and for children with cerebral palsy, *Dev Med Child Neurol*, 32, 333, 1990.
128. Unnithan, V., et al., Role of cocontraction in the O_2 cost of walking in children with cerebral palsy, *Med Sci Sports Exerc*, 28, 1498, 1996.
129. Damiano, D. L., et al., Muscle force production and functional performance in spastic cerebral palsy: Relationship of cocontraction, *Arch Phys Med Rehabil*, 81, 895, 2000.

130. Rose, J., et al., Muscle pathology and clinical measures of disability in children with cerebral palsy, *J Orthop Res*, 12(6), 758, 1994.
131. Palisano, R., et al., Development and reliability of a system to classify gross motor function in children with cerebral palsy, *Dev Med Child Neurol*, 39, 214, 1997.
132. Palisano, R., et al., Validation of a model of gross motor function for children with cerebral palsy, *Phys Ther*, 89, 974, 2000.
133. Jeng, S., et al., Self-optimization of walking in nondisabled children and children with spastic hemiplegic cerebral palsy, *J Mot Behav*, 28(1), 15, 1996.
134. Smiley, S., et al., A comparison of the effects of solid, articulated, and posterior leaf-spring ankle-foot orthoses and shoes alone on gait and energy expenditure in children with spastic diplegic cerebral palsy, *Orthopedics*, 25(4), 411, 2002.
135. Park, E., Park, C., and Kim, J., Comparison of anterior and posterior walkers with respect to gait parameters and energy expenditure of children with spastic diplegic cerebral palsy, *Yonsi Med J*, 42(2), 180, 2001.
136. Duffy, C., Hill, A., and Graham, H., The influence of flexed-knee gait on the energy cost of walking in children, *Dev Med Child Neurol*, 39, 234, 1997.
137. Perry, J., Antonelli, D., and Ford, W., Analysis of knee-joint forces during flexed-knee stance, *J Bone Joint Surg*, 57A, 961, 1975.
138. Hsu, A. T., et al., Quadriceps force and myoelectric activity during flexed knee stance, *Clin Orthop Rel Res*, 288, 254, 1993.
139. Fernandez, J., Pitetti, K., and Betzen, M., Physiological capacities of individuals with cerebral palsy, *Hum Factors*, 32(4), 457, 1990.
140. Rose, J., et al., Energy cost of walking in normal children and in those with cerebral palsy: Comparison of heart rate and oxygen consumption, *J Ped Orthop*, 204, 276, 1989.
141. Correy, I. S., et al., Measurement of oxygen consumption in disabled children by the Cosmed K2 portable telemetry system, *Dev Med Child Neurol*, 38, 585, 1996.
142. Keefer, D. J., et al., Within- and between-day stability of treadmill walking VO_2 in children with hemiplegic cerebral palsy, *Gait Posture*, 22, 177, 2005.
143. Rose, J., Haskell, W., and Gamble, J., A comparison of oxygen pulse and respiratory exchange ratio in cerebral palsied and non-disabled children, *Arch Phys Med Rehabil*, 74, 702, 1993.
144. Dresen, M., et al., Aerobic energy expenditure of handicapped children after training, *Arch Phys Med Rehabil*, 66, 302, 1985.
145. Olgiati, R., Burgunder, J. -M., and Mumenthaler, M., Increased energy cost of walking in multiple sclerosis: Effect of spasticity, ataxia, and weakness, *Arch Phys Med Rehabil*, 69, 846, 1988.
146. Olgiati, R., Jacquet, J., and Di Prampero, P., Energy cost of walking and exertional dyspnea in multiple sclerosis, *Am Rev Respir Dis*, 124, 1005, 1986.
147. Koseoglu, B. F., et al., Cardiopulmonary and metabolic functions, aerobic capacity, fatigue and quality of life in patients with multiple sclerosis, *Acta Neurol Scand*, 114, 261, 2006.
148. Markus, H., Cox, M., and Tomkins, A., Raised resting energy expenditure in Parkinson's disease and its relationship to muscle rigidity, *Clin Sci*, 83, 199, 1992.
149. Ghosh, A., Ganguli, S., and Bose, K., Metabolic energy demand and optimal walking speed in post-polio subjects with lower limb afflictions, *Appl Ergon*, 13(4), 259, 1982.
150. Brehm, M.-A., Nollet, F., and Harlaar, J., Energy demands of walking in persons with postpoliomyelitis syndrome: Relationship with muscle strength and reproducibility, *Arch Phys Med Rehabil*, 87, 136, 2006.
151. Menard-Rothe, K., et al., Self-selected walking velocity for functional ambulation in patients with end-stage emphysema, *J Cardiopulm Rehabil*, 17(2), 85, 1997.
152. Richards, M., Davies, P., and Bell, S., Energy cost of physical activity in cystic fibrosis, *Eur J Clin Nutr*, 55, 690, 2001.

153. Skemp, K., et al., Measured energy expenditure during activities of daily living in pacemaker patients, *Clin Exerc Physiol*, 3(4), 213, 2001.
154. Marconi, C., et al., Energetics of walking in patients with peripheral arterial disease: A proposed functional evaluation protocol, *Clin Sci*, 105, 105, 2003.
155. Wilke, N. A., et al., Energy expenditure during household tasks in women with coronary artery disease, *Am J Cardiol*, 75, 670, 1995.
156. Perrault, H., Efficiency of movement in health and chronic disease, *Clin Invest Med*, 29(2), 117, 2006.
157. Velloso, M. and Jardim, J. R., Study of energy expenditure during activities of daily living using and not using body position recommended by energy conservation techniques in patients with COPD, *Chest*, 130(1), 126, 2006.
158. Jones, A., Dean, E., and Chow, C., Comparison of the oxygen cost of breathing exercises and spontaneous breathing in patients with stable chronic obstructive pulmonary disease, *Phys Ther*, 83(5), 424, 2003.
159. Holder, C., Haskvitz, E., and Weltman, A., The effects of assistive devices on the oxygen cost, cardiovascular stress, and perception of nonweight-bearing ambulation, *J Orthop Sports Phys Ther*, 18, 537, 1993.
160. Bateni, H. and Maki, B. E., Assistive devices for balance and mobility: Benefits, demands, and adverse consequences, *Arch Phys Med Rehabil*, 86, 134, 2005.
161. Waters, R. L., Energy expenditure. *Gait Analysis: Normal and Pathological Function*, Perry, J. (Ed.), Slack Inc., Thorofare, NJ, 1992, p. 443.
162. Imms, F. J., MacDonald, C., and Prestidge, S. P., Energy expenditure during walking in patients recovering from fractures of the leg, *Scan J Rehabil Med*, 8, 1, 1976.
163. Hamzeh, M., Bowker, P., and Sayegh, A., The energy costs of ambulation using two types of walkers, *Clin Rehabil*, 2, 119, 1988.
164. McBeath, A. A., Bahrke, M., and Balke, B., Efficiency of assisted ambulation determined by oxygen consumption measurement, *J Bone Joint Surg Am*, 56, 994, 1974.
165. Brattgard, S. -O., et al., Energy expenditure and heart rate in driving a wheel-chair ergometer, *Scan J Rehabil Med*, 2, 143, 1970.
166. Wells, C. L., Physiological response to upper extremity exercise and the clinical implications, *Cardiopulm Phys Ther J*, 9(4), 7, 1998.
167. Wolfe, G. A., Waters, R., and Hislop, H. J., Influence of floor surface on the energy cost of wheelchair propulsion, *Phys Ther*, 57(9), 1022, 1977.
168. Mukherjee, G., Bhowik, P., and Samanta, A., Energy cost of manual wheelchair propulsion at different speeds, *Int J Rehabil Res*, 25, 71, 2002.
169. Mukherjee, G. and Samanta, A., Arm-crank propelled three-wheeled chair: Physiological evaluation of the propulsion using one arm and both arm patterns, *Int J Rehabil Res*, 27, 321, 2004.
170. Snow, L., Aging with a physical disability: Is it safe to exercise? *Orthop Phys Ther Clin North Am*, 10(2), 251, 2001.
171. Brondel, L., et al., Energy cost and cardiorespiratory adaptation in the "Get-Up-and-Go" test in frail elderly women with postural abnormalities and in controls, *J Geront*, 60A(1), 98, 2005.
172. Tang, N., et al., Total daily energy expenditure in wasted chronic obstructive pulmonary disease patients, *Eur J Clin Nutr*, 56, 282, 2002.
173. Toth, M. J. and Poehlman, E. T., Energetic adaptation to chronic disease in the elderly, *Nutr Rev*, 58(3), 61, 2000.
174. Liou, T. -H., Pi-Sunyer, X., and Laferrére, B., Physical disability and obesity, *Nutr Rev*, 63(10), 321, 2005.

3 Pain

G. Lorimer Moseley and Lester Jones

CONTENTS

3.1   INTRODUCTION

A few years ago, Marras (2000) described the need for those working in occupational health to adopt and integrate the "state of the science" into the approach to low back disorders (p. 899). This included consideration of the multidimensional factors that can lead to an increased risk of developing an occupational disorder. No longer was occupational low back disorder to be seen as something that could be explained simply by biomechanical dysfunction or failure. And, no longer could a person in the workplace be assessed simply for their anthropometric dimensions and physical capabilities.

Such a need is not simply about back pain, but about occupational disorders. Marras' timely recommendation mirrored rapid increases in our understanding of pain and pain mechanisms, our knowledge of which has expanded exponentially since the landmark gate control theory of Melzack and Wall (1965). Pain is no longer exclusively attributed to pathology in the tissues, but is considered a complex human experience that depends on many factors from across physical, psychological, and social domains. As is always the case, the more we know, the more we realize we do not know. This chapter will present a broad overview of what we know of the biology of pain, its assessment and management, all within the context of ergonomics and occupational disorders.

3.1.1   DEFINITION OF PAIN

The International Association for the Study of Pain (IASP) defines pain as "… an unpleasant, sensory and emotional experience associated with actual or potential tissue damage, or described in terms of such damage" (Merskey and Bogduk, 1994). This definition remains broadly consistent with current concepts of pain. For example, pain is a result of complex cortical processing; pain depends on evaluations of threat to, and vulnerability of, the body; the nociceptive system is dynamic; pain is not a measure of the condition of the tissues. We think that understanding these key concepts is key to understanding the biology of pain.

3.2 CURRENT CONCEPTS OF PAIN

3.2.1 PAIN IS A RESULT OF COMPLEX CORTICAL PROCESSING

Once the notion of specific neural pathways for specific stimuli was proposed (the "specificity theories" of the 1600s), pain was considered a reliable and accurate indicator of the state of the tissues. The specificity theories held that the intensity of pain related to the extent of tissue damage, that pain receptors passed pain messages through pain pathways to pain centers in the brain. Nowadays, one might call this a structural-pathology model of pain.

The idea of pain receptors might be intuitively sensible, but it is nonsense. This can be demonstrated by considering what receptors actually do. Heat receptors detect a change in heat. Chemoreceptors detect a change in chemicals. Mechanoreceptors detect mechanical deformation. In each case, a property of the stimulus is detected by receptors that are specifically sensitive to that property, or a change in that property. However, pain is not a property that can be possessed by a stimulus. For example, a very hot iron does not possess the property of pain, nor does a very sharp knife. Granted, if one puts the very hot iron on their skin, one usually experiences pain, but that is different. Pain does not exist in the iron, nor in the knife. Rather, pain is an emergent property that exists only in our consciousness. The same argument applies to pain pathways—there is no pain message to transmit so the existence of pain pathways is also nonsense.

Anecdotal and experimental evidence demonstrates that pain is an output of the central nervous system. Pain can be evoked by many types of sensory inputs, and it is influenced by many conscious and nonconscious factors. So, how do we categorize the system that normally evokes pain, if to talk of pain receptors, pain messages and pain pathways is nonsense? We categorize it according to its very important role in alerting the brain to danger. We do have receptors that seem specifically suited to respond to dangerous changes in the tissues. The receptors and nerves that carry these danger messages constitute the nociceptive system.

The nociceptive system is complex. It includes

- High threshold and low threshold primary nociceptors: These neurons are small diameter myelinated (type Aδ) and unmyelinated (type C) fibers. They lie in the tissues of the body and are activated by dangerous and nondangerous stimuli. High threshold nociceptors are thought to be most important in evoking pain. For a review of peripheral mechanisms of nociception, see Myers et al. (2006).
- Second-order neurones that project from the dorsal horn of the spinal cord and ascend to the thalamus and brain via several different tracts.
- Cortical and subcortical neurones that respond to input from the above tracts and are modified by other sensory and brain inputs. Currently, it is not possible to determine which brain areas are involved in nociception and which are involved in pain. For a review of spinal and cortical mechanisms of nociception and pain, see Petrovic and Ingvar (2002), Gracely et al. (2004), Jones (2005), Ohara et al. (2005), Godinho et al. (2006), and Seminowicz and Davis (2006). The brain then "filters, selects, and modulates" these inputs (Melzack, 1999, p. S121).

3.2.1.1 Neuromatrix Theory

It is known that the brain produces pain. It is also known that many factors from across domains contribute to the brain's production of pain. However, we do not know how the brain produces pain. Melzack's body-self neuromatrix model (Melzack, 1990) for application to management of chronic pain disorders (see Moseley, 2003a) is useful for integrating what is currently known about pain within a clinically useful paradigm.

The neuromatrix theory considers that nociceptive (somatosensory) inputs, evaluative inputs, emotional influences, autonomic, immune, and neuroendocrine inputs all contribute to pain (see Janig et al., 2006 for an updated review of autonomic and endocrine system influences). That many systems respond to impending danger implies that pain can be considered the conscious component of a multisystemic response to protect the tissues from danger (Moseley, 2007). The interaction between the systems is complex and is only beginning to be understood. For example, the endocrine and autonomic nervous systems produce the protective stress response and interact directly with the nociceptive system; the immune system activates proinflammatory cytokines, which tackle the danger and interact directly with the nociceptive system (see Sommer et al., 2006 for detailed discussion), the motor system braces, moves, or protects the affected area, and interacts directly with the nociceptive system. Evidence that these systems are activated together with pain is readily available: raised blood concentration of immune mediators (Watkins and Maier, 2000), altered voluntary and postural muscle activity (Hodges et al., 2003), expressions of distress and fear (Vlaeyen and Linton, 2000), and symptoms of anxiety (Main, 1983).

In summary then, the neuromatrix theory describes pain as multidimensional, and therefore modifiable by, sensory experiences, evaluations based on prior learning, emotional contexts and experiences, behavior, and health status. It conceptualizes pain as one output of the central nervous system that occurs when the central nervous system perceives tissues to be under threat.

3.2.1.2 Cognitive-Emotional Modulation of Pain

Recognizing that pain is not just associated with emotions but is in part emotional is an important step in understanding human pain. Experimental evidence of this is well established and viable neurobiological mechanisms have been proposed. Cognitive modulation is also critical and is encapsulated by the context of the pain (e.g., its predictability, its timing, its meaning, its impact, its location, and its associated sensory cues). Experimental manipulation of the context of pain can have profound effects on pain intensity and unpleasantness (e.g., see Moseley and Arntz, 2007). Contextual factors also influence clinical (or nonexperimental) pain. In a broader sense, those factors constitute thoughts, feelings, and behaviors. Within an occupational setting, those thoughts, feelings, and behaviors might relate specifically to social and physical aspects of the work environment and the patient's place within it.

3.2.2 Thoughts, Feelings, and Behaviors

According to cognitive-behavioral principles, thoughts, feelings, and behaviors are all implicit in the course of recovery, or lack of recovery, after an initial injury or pain episode. Often, fear of pain, movement, and reinjury is key. The role of fear

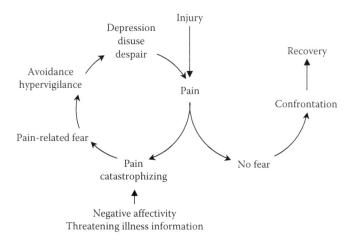

FIGURE 3.1   The fear avoidance model. (From Vlaeyen, J.W. and Linton, S.J., *Pain*, 85, 317, 2000. With permission.)

in recovery is well modeled by the fear avoidance model (Figure 3.1). In short, the model proposes that fear leads people to avoid, which confirms their rationale for avoiding it in the first place (by confirming the cognition that "to not move is to not provoke pain" they by implication confirm the cognition that "to move is to provoke pain"). The alternative path is to confront (more accurately, to "test out") movements and activities, rather than avoid them. This is about behavior, but behavior is fundamentally dependent on thoughts and feelings. For example, misinterpretations of bodily sensations and prediction of extreme negative consequences (i.e., catastrophizing), underpins fear, which causes avoidance. Participation in the activities (or adoption of the posture), allows the person to refresh their beliefs and maintain a more realistic self-efficacy for successful participation.

Self-efficacy, which has been shown to be an important predictor of behavior in people with pain, is also affected by misinterpretation of symptoms and catastrophizing. Someone believing pain to accurately indicate the state of the tissues will be likely to have low self-efficacy for participating in tasks that may cause harm, and logically so. A person who attributes pain to normal healing processes (as opposed to risk of more damage) or nervous system sensitization is likely to have high self-efficacy and is likely to persist at difficult tasks for longer (Asghari and Nicholas, 2001; Nicholas, 2007) (see Box 3.1). Self-efficacy can be directly assessed and targeted in cognitive-behavioral management. Self-efficacy is sensitive to treatment and is closely related

BOX 3.1   SELF-EFFICACY

Self-efficacy, a construct from Social Learning Theory (Bandura), is the belief a person has about his/her ability to perform a task. As such, it involves assessing the demands of a task and identifying the personal resources available to overcome these. Therefore, misinterpretation of sensations and overestimation of negative consequences would lower a person's self-efficacy.

to function (Nicholas et al., 1991). For more information on self-efficacy as it relates to pain assessment and management, see Nicholas et al. (2002).

Research has also raised concerns about the thoughts and beliefs of clinicians, and the impact of their beliefs on the outcome of treatment. There is strong evidence that the clinician's beliefs directly impact on patient's immediate response to treatment. For example, in an elegant placebo-controlled, double blind study of fentanyl (a powerful analgesic) during wisdom teeth removal (Gracely et al., 1985), the researchers manipulated the information given to dentists who were administering the injection. Dentists were incorrectly told that some patients had no chance of receiving fentanyl when in fact all patients had a 50% chance of receiving fentanyl. When the dentist correctly thought that the patient had a 50% chance of receiving fentanyl, pain dropped 2 points on a 10-point scale after the placebo injection pain. When the dentist incorrectly thought that the patient could not get fentanyl, pain increased by 5 points after the placebo injection. Other studies showed that rheumatologists' own beliefs about fear avoidance affected the decisions they made in relation to patients' management (Coudeyre et al., 2006) and that patients tended to hold similar pain-related beliefs to their primary treating practitioner (Poiraudeau et al., 2006).

3.2.3 ATTENTION AND EXPECTATION

Attention and expectation are both thought to influence pain, although the nature of the effect varies. It would seem intuitively sensible to allocate attentional resources to a potentially dangerous situation, or a potentially vulnerable body part. Thus, it would seem intuitively sensible to expect the threat of pain to cause a bias in attentional resources toward the source of that threat. However, experimental data are not so clear and extensive research attempting to define the role attention plays in pain perception remains inconclusive (Matthews et al., 1980; Eccleston, 1994; Crombez et al., 1996, 1997, 1998, 1999; Asmundson et al., 1997; Duckworth et al., 1997; Eccleston et al., 1997; McCracken, 1997; Eccleston and Crombez, 1999; Peters et al., 2000; Naveteur et al., 2005; Moseley and Arntz, 2007). The intuitive result, that paying attention to pain enhances the experience and attending to another stimulus nullifies pain, is supported by some data. However, there are also data to support the opposite responses, i.e., attending to pain reduces the experience and attending away from it increases the experience. Contextual and situational factors, and the individual's response to these, most likely moderate the relationship between pain and attention. For example, those who are catastrophic about pain and injury tend to attend to cues of impending pain and tend to report more pain. For a review of this topic, see Crombez et al. (2005).

Research into the expectation of pain also seems to demonstrate variable effects on pain. The key to the effect on pain seems to be the nature of the expectation. That is, if one expects the pain to be intense, it will probably be more intense than if one expects it to be mild. If the cue relates to how damaging the stimulus might be, it is likely to evoke more pain (Arntz and Claassens, 2004; Moseley and Arntz, 2007). This type of effect has been demonstrated in many studies using a variety of paradigms (Chua et al., 1999; Ploghaus et al., 1999; Sawamoto et al., 2000; Keltner et al., 2006; Moseley and Arntz, 2007) and the same principle applies to the expected effect of treatment. That is, if one expects a treatment to reduce pain, it will reduce pain more than the same treatment expected not to (Pollo et al., 2001; Benedetti et al., 2003). The literature on the influence of expectation on pain has been presented in two informative reviews (Wager, 2005).

3.2.4 ANXIETY

Linton (2005) identifies distress and catastrophizing about pain as strong predictors for the onset of back pain and that anxiety is the mediating factor. Again, this is not counterintuitive, but nor is it established to be true. The recent literature discussing the relationship between anxiety and pain provides no consensus. Increased levels of anxiety have been associated with increased pain both in experimentally induced pain (Tang and Gibson, 2005) and during clinical procedures (Gore et al., 2005; Pud and Amit, 2005; Schupp et al., 2005; Klages et al., 2006). However, it has also been reported that anxiety levels have no effect on pain (Arntz et al., 1990, 1994). The influence of anxiety on pain, to a large degree, appears to depend on attention (Arntz et al., 1994; Ploghaus et al., 2003), which brings us back to a recurring principle that modulation of pain by attention, anxiety, expectation, thoughts, feelings, and behaviors depends on the context of the pain. Ultimately, modulation seems to depend on the influence of the modulating factor on the implicitly perceived degree of danger to body tissues.

3.2.4.1 Social Influences

Social factors have been shown to modulate pain and health in general. Although a simplistic approach, we will group social influences as: "occupational," "sex and gender," and "ethnicity and culture." Separating social influences from psychological influences, in the real world, is probably impossible.

3.2.4.2 Occupational Influences

Proposals of a role for work organization and work stress, in contributing to work-related musculoskeletal disorders (Carayon et al., 1999), have gained increasing support. A recent review highlighted the importance of high work demands and low perceived control at work, in contributing to neck and upper limb symptoms in workers (Bongers et al., 2006). One possible explanation for such a link is that people are more likely to report symptoms in these conditions. Another is that stress alters motor performance—there is a large amount of evidence to suggest that to be the case. That psychological stress disrupts normal motor and postural performance has been established (Marras et al., 2000; Moseley et al., 2004b,c). There have also been developments in the understanding of how beliefs, moods, immune system, and nervous system interact (so-called psychoneuroimmunology). The demonstrated effect of cytokines on nociceptor activity is one example, but there are many others (see Butler, 2000). Although it is clear that issues such as psychosocial stress can influence recovery and the development of chronic problems once an initial episode has occurred (Bigos et al., 1991; Feuerstein et al., 2006), there are no strong data on whether psychosocial stress increases the likelihood of an initial episode (Van Nieuwenhuyse et al., 2006).

3.2.5 Sex and Gender

There seems to be both biological and psychosocial differences in the pain experience between women and men. Women generally are considered to have lower pain thresholds, at least for experimental pain (Soetanto et al., 2006), with evidence of a relationship between pain threshold and the phases of the menstrual cycle (Unruh, 1996). Socialization of pain responses may also be different in men and women (Myers et al., 2006), with some authors proposing that women are more likely to attribute negative emotion with threatening stimuli (Rhudy and Williams, 2005). We should remember, however, that most pain experiments have been undertaken by male researchers, which probably incurs a further systematic effect on data.

3.2.6 Ethnicity and Culture

Members from the same ethnic group are likely to share cultural values and traditions. Culture affects how people define and respond to illness and pain, and the language they use to articulate its intensity and quality. At the same time, there appears to be little physiological variation between ethnic groups. However, there are often variations in the treatment that different cultural groups receive, which could imply cultural insensitivity or prejudice on the part of caregivers, or expectations on the part of patients (see Lasch, 2002; Morris, 2001 for review).

Obviously there are many challenges to the clinician who aims to be culturally competent. Immigrants of an ethnic or cultural group will vary in how much they identify with their group. This might be due to factors such as age, education, ties to their birth country, and level of integration to a new community (Lasch, 2002; Morris, 2001). Furthermore, language translations may not be sensitive to important semantic differences describing the quality of pain (Fabrega and Tyma, 1976). Therefore, we contend that it is essential that a person-centered approach is adopted at all times, and that communication strategies are optimized.

3.2.6.1 Nociceptive System

For simplicity, the nociceptive system can be described as the initiator and transmitter of neural messages in response to noxious stimulation from the periphery to the brain. It involves multiple nerve pathways, and information is filtered and modulated at the spinal cord prior to processing by the brain. Nociception forms one aspect of the evaluation of threat and vulnerability, which will be discussed in this section.

3.2.7 Peripheral Mechanisms

Myelinated Aδ fibers and unmyelinated C fibers are probably the most important peripheral neurones contributing to nociception and are conventionally called nociceptors. However, many types of neurones in the periphery are thought to contribute to nociception (Meyer et al., 2006) and many Aδ and C fibers also respond to non-noxious stimulation (Craig, 2002). As per current convention, we will classify Aδ and C fibers as primary nociceptors.

Primary nociceptors respond to dangerous mechanical, chemical, and thermal stimuli, and are widely distributed throughout the internal tissues and external surfaces of the body. In healthy pain-free individuals, these neurones generate and transmit a nerve impulse in response to mechanical pressures or rapid changes in tissue temperature, or in response to the presence of provocative substances (including endogenous) at suprathreshold concentrations.

3.2.8 SPINAL MECHANISMS

As with other afferent fibers, the majority of primary nociceptors terminate in the dorsal horn of the spinal cord. The dorsal horn consists of numerous layers, which are defined according to the projections, and structural and functional properties, of their neurones. The termination sites for nociceptors, for the most part, are laminae I, II, and V. Most Aδ fibers terminate in lamina I, but some also terminate with Aβ fibers—as well as some C fibers—in lamina V. Most C fibers terminate in lamina II. Important features of lamina II neurones are that they project to other laminae, and they can be inhibitory or excitatory in their projections. This means that they potentially have a filtering or modulatory role on peripheral inputs. The neurones that project from lamina I are synapsing mainly with primary nociceptors and so are called nociceptive-specific second-order neurones. Second-order neurones projecting from lamina V respond to the different peripheral inputs terminating there (i.e., Aδ, C, and Aβ fibers). As they have to respond to a wide range of stimulus inputs, they are called wide-dynamic range neurones.

3.2.9 TRANSMISSION FROM THE DORSAL HORN TO THE BRAIN

Five ascending pathways transmit nociceptive information up the spinal cord. The spinothalamic tract is the largest and includes neurones that originate in laminae I and V of the dorsal horn. The spinoreticular, spinomesencephalic, cervicothalamic, and spinohypothalamic tracts also transmit ascending nociceptive information. Significantly, there is not a single pathway responsible for nociception. From an evolutionary perspective, multiple ascending pathways would seem more robust in the event of disease or injury. There are also many sites within the brain where nociceptive information is processed. Again, this may avoid the harmful consequences of a single "pain center" being damaged or becoming dysfunctional.

Importantly, the fact that multiple brain regions are active with pain indicates that there is a range of inputs available for sampling by the brain. According to neuromatrix theory, a specific and individual pattern of neural activity in these central nervous system structures will lead the brain to produce pain. The pattern of neural activity has been referred to as the pain neurosignature (Melzack, 1996) or pain neurotag (Butler and Moseley, 2003).

Once nociceptive information reaches the brain, there are several important principles that seem to govern how it is processed, and how, and if, pain is produced.

1. *Parallel processing*: Many brain areas are involved in pain. Most often, the thalamus, insula, primary (S1) and secondary (S2) somatosensory, and prefrontal cortices are activated when someone is in pain. These areas are called the pain matrix (Apkarian et al., 2005) (Figure 3.2). However, these areas are never the only areas involved and they are not always all involved—the pattern of brain activation varies greatly between and within individuals.

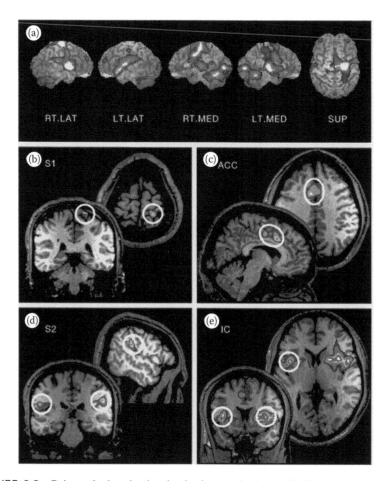

FIGURE 3.2 Pain-evoked activation in the human brain. (a) Surface-rendered subtraction images of activation patterns obtained with positron emission tomography (PET) scans, showing right lateral (RT.LAT), left lateral (LT.LAT), right medial (RT.MED), left medial (LT.MED), and superior (SUP) views. Activation observed during repetitive innocuous warm stimuli (40°C) is subtracted from that observed during repetitive painful heat stimulation (50°C). The scans began 40 s after the onset of the painful heat stimulation and reveal responses bilaterally in the anterior cingulate cortex (ACC), insular cortex (IC), thalamus, cerebellum, and sensorimotor cortex. (b–e) Functional and anatomical MRI of four subjects exposed to repetitive 9 s noxious heat stimuli on the leg (46°C) compared to repetitive warm stimuli (36°C). The circled areas represent regions showing a significantly greater activation during the noxious heat than during the warm stimuli. These areas include primary and secondary somatosensory cortices (SI, SII), ACC, and IC. For all images the right hemisphere is shown as right. Responses with a statistical significance of P 0.05 are shown superimposed in stereotactic coordinates on an MRI. (From McMahon, S.B. and Koltzenburg, M., *Wall & Melzack's Textbook of Pain*, Elsevier, London. With permission.)

2. *Different aspects of pain seem to involve different brain areas*: Some authors advocate the notion of two nociceptive/pain "systems"—the medial system and the lateral system (Jones, 2005). The medial nociceptive system includes the medial thalamic nuclei, and anterior cingulated and dorsolateral prefrontal cortices. It is described as slow and only broadly somatotopic, which means it does not have the capacity to code in detail the location in the body at which the stimulus occurred. Activity in this system has been proposed to subserve the affective-emotional qualities of pain (broadly speaking, the unpleasantness of pain rather than the intensity and quality of pain).

The lateral nociceptive system includes the lateral thalamic nuclei and the primary (S1) and secondary (S2) somatosensory cortices. It is described as fast and is highly somatotopic, which means it is able to code, in great detail, the tissue location at which the stimulus occurred. Activity in this system is proposed to subserve the sensory-discriminative qualities of pain (the intensity of the pain and the sensory characteristics of the stimulus (e.g., warm, sharp, deep, superficial). The intensity and unpleasantness of pain can be independently manipulated (e.g., Moseley and Arntz, 2007).

3.2.9.1   Consequences of Complex Processing

Pain is the consequence of complex cortical processing. One consequence of this complexity is that the response to any given noxious stimulus varies between, and within, individuals. A stimulus that is painful for one person may not be painful for another. Similarly, a stimulus that is painful for a given subject on one day may not be painful the next day.

Pain's complexity is one reason that diagnostic tests for the "cause" of pain are notoriously problematic. A series of imaging studies undertaken since the mid-1990s have demonstrated this. One study used magnetic resonance imaging (MRI) to identify the structure of intervertebral disks in people without back pain (Jensen, 1994). The majority had scans that were positive for disk lesions, several were positive for disk protrusions, and one for a disk extrusion. Yet they were all pain-free. While there was no follow up to see if these subjects developed pain later, the study demonstrated that evidence of tissue pathology should not be considered as evidence of pain.

Another similar study found similar structural changes in asymptomatic subjects (Boos et al., 1995). That study did undertake long-term follow up (5 years) and found that psychological and work-related factors at inception were better predictors of medical consultation than MRI findings were. A more recent study demonstrated that there was poor correlation between vertebral stress fracture as identified using computed tomography (CT) scan and pain or return to sport (Millson et al., 2004). The authors concluded that the findings on tissue structure provided by the CT scan, was not valuable objective information for clinical decision making.

There is also evidence of pain without identifiable tissue damage. This leads some to try harder and harder to identify tissue lesions, which, on the basis of the previous paragraph is fundamentally problematic unless double-blind diagnostic provocation tests are undertaken (Schwarzer et al., 1994). However, exhaustive tests still fail to find a "nociceptive driver" in most cases of low back pain, complex regional pain syndrome, fibromyalgia, and chronic fatigue syndrome. We contend that it is biologically corrupt to conclude that patients who fit the diagnostic criteria for these disorders are not genuinely suffering.

One example of pain in the absence of frank tissue trauma was particularly relevant to occupational medicine: repetitive strain injury (RSI). It was speculated that high-demand repetitious keyboarding caused microtrauma and inflammation, but the existence of such microtrauma is not supported by the literature, as no inflammatory component has been identified (for reviews see Awerbuch, 2004; Helliwell, 2004). One hypothesis is that workers in an environment that promotes anxiety, including where other workers are reporting injury (see Godinho et al., 2006), may be predisposed to feel pain (Keltner et al., 2006), and this may be especially the case with women (Rhudy and Williams, 2005).

It remains possible that further tissue pathology will be identified in such patients, but it should be reiterated that evidence of tissue pathology does not constitute evidence for the cause of pain. In summary, the body of evidence clearly demonstrates that nociception is neither sufficient, nor necessary, for pain.

The next sections will further explore why pain occurs, and argue that in persistent pain, central mechanisms are likely to be the most important influences.

3.2.10 PAIN DEPENDS ON EVALUATIONS OF THREAT AND VULNERABILITY

According to neuromatrix theory, pain is conceptualized as an output of the central nervous system, which occurs in response to perceived danger to body tissues. Key to this then is (1) the appraisal of the threat (e.g., noxious stimulation) and (2) the perceived vulnerability of the tissues to that threat. We conceptualize it like this: together, these tissues inform the brain at an unconscious level about the answer to this question: "How dangerous is this really?" There are many studies that have investigated this issue (see Butler and Moseley (2003) for a review of these studies) and it is beyond the scope of this chapter to list or discuss them all. However, the principle of these studies is relevant for our discussion. The principle is that anything that would lead the brain to conclude that the threat to tissues has increased should increase pain. Conversely, anything that would lead the brain to conclude that the threat to tissues has decreased should decrease pain. This gives the clinician the clinical reasoning capacity to predict what effect different issues from across the sensory, psychological, and social domains may have on a patient's pain.

Let us consider the keyboard operator who develops low level forearm pain and compare that person to one who has several colleagues who have lost their jobs because of chronic forearm pain. Intuitively, the perceived threat to the forearms should be greater in the second person, which implies that their pain should also be greater. This general principle is now widely regarded to be important in the phenomenon of RSI that swept Australia in the 1980s (Lucire, 2003).

Let us now consider the education component of a rehabilitation program for patients with chronic low back pain. What is the likely effect, on perceived vulnerability of the back, of focussing on disk pressures, disk herniations, postures that "protect" the back and movements that are "dangerous"? This is obviously a rhetorical question—it has been shown that conventional back school education programs actually heighten catastrophic interpretations of back pain, increase fear of reinjury, and perceived vulnerability of the back (Moseley, 2004a; Moseley et al., 2004a). This evaluation of perceived threat to tissues is important in descending facilitation and inhibition of the spinal cord means that, as the nociceptive system becomes more sensitive, "explanatory model" becomes more important.

3.2.11   ROLE OF SENSITIVITY OF THE NOCICEPTIVE SYSTEM IN PERSISTENT PAIN

Pain that persists beyond the time of the inflammatory-induced sensitivity associated with healing is considered to have a different mechanism than the acute postinjury process (Watkins and Maier, 2005; Banks and Watkins, 2006). We will consider both here, but emphasize the mechanisms of persistent pain, where attempts at treatment of a peripheral target tissue may not only be ineffective, but detrimental.

3.2.11.1   Sensitization of the Nociception/Pain System

Hyperalgesia (when noxious stimulation hurts more) and allodynia (when nonnoxious stimulation hurts) can be expected after tissue injury. It is appropriate that after recent damage to tissue, tenderness of the injured area and surrounding tissue makes the individual avoid provocation of the injury. In extreme cases of allodynia, however, light touch (especially by others) and the sensation of clothes rubbing on the skin can evoke severe pain. It is well acknowledged now that this type of sensitivity of the nervous system can produce disproportional pain responses to completely innocuous stimuli.

3.2.11.2   Peripheral Mechanisms

When pain is evoked by noxious stimuli, peripheral mechanisms can enhance sensitivity of the nociceptive system. These mechanisms include the presence of inflammatory mediators, decreased circulation (which increases the local concentration of H^+ ions), the presence of immune mediators, and activation of certain genes (see Figure 3.3 and Meyer et al. (2006) for an exhaustive review of peripheral mechanisms of modulation). Inflammatory mediators are released by tissue damage and by activation of nociceptors (neurogenic inflammation). The result of these sensitizing peripheral mechanisms is called peripheral sensitization, and it will commonly resolve as the inflammation response resolves.

3.2.11.3   Spinal Cord Mechanisms

A much studied receptor is the N-methyl-D-aspartate (NMDA) receptor. Located on the second-order nociceptors in the dorsal horn, the NMDA receptor responds to persistent or intense stimulation by allowing greater postsynaptic activity. An increase in the number of open channels on the postsynaptic membrane means that the second-order nociceptors will show an increased activation rate even though the peripheral input remains unchanged. Therefore, more messages relating to body tissue danger will be sent to the brain for processing. This is an upregulation of the (protective) nociceptive system.

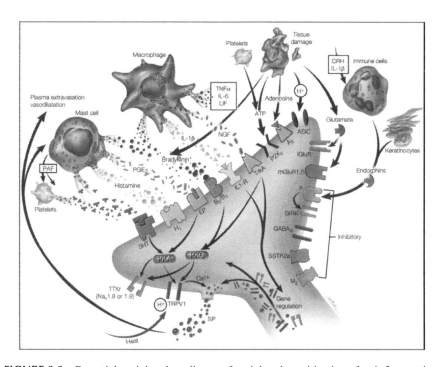

FIGURE 3.3   Potential peripheral mediators of peripheral sensitization after inflammation. Inflammation leads to the release of numerous chemicals from mast cells, macrophages, immune cells, and injured cells that may act directly or indirectly to alter the sensitivity of peripheral nerve terminals. ASIC, acid-sensing ion channel; CRH, corticotrophin-releasing hormone; GIRK, G-protein-coupled inward rectifying potassium channel; iGluR, ionotropic glutamate receptor; IL-1β, interleukin-1β; IL-6, interleukin-6; mGluR, metabotropic glutamate receptor; NGF, nerve growth factor; PAF, platelet-activating factor; PGE2, prostaglandin E2; PKA, protein kinase A; PKC, protein kinase C; SSTR2A, somatostatin receptor 2A; TNF-α, tumour necrosis factor-α; TrkA, tyrosine kinase receptor A; TTXr, tetrodotoxin-resistant sodium channel; μ, mu-opioid receptor; M2 muscarinic receptor; 5HT, serotonin; LIF, leukemia inhibitory factor. (From McMahon, S.B. and Koltzenburg, M., *Wall & Melzack's Textbook of Pain*, Elsevier, London. With permission.)

The interaction of nociception and other sensory information can also lead to enhanced sensitivity of the nociceptive system. Again this occurs in the dorsal horn, where wide-dynamic-range neurones in the laminae provide an interaction of at least three fiber types (i.e., Aδ, C, and Aβ fibers). This interaction appears to be important in the quality of pain, i.e., how people describe their pain. In the case of peripheral nerve damage or disease, the potential for enhancing sensitivity is magnified via the forming of new synapses between a wide-dynamic-range neurone and a sensitized neurone. This would allow direct communication between low threshold peripheral afferents (i.e., Aβ) and the nociceptive system and may explain painful responses to normally nonpainful stimuli, such as touch. Peripheral neural damage can also evoke axonal sprouting, which involves the extension of the nerve cell into an adjacent dorsal horn laminae, where it could form new synapses with the interneurones

(Woolf and Salter, 2000). For a reasonable detailed but accessible discussion of these processes, see Butler and Moseley (2003).

3.2.11.4 Neuropathic Pain

The pain associated with nerve damage is known as "neuropathic pain." Of course, as with nociception, it is only a contributor to whether the person feels pain. The use of the term "pain" to describe it is an inappropriate assumption that is carried with a lot of the nomenclature in pain literature. Neuropathic pain is commonly associated with what could be interpreted as bizarre symptoms such as feelings of "burning" or "electric shock," or even "insects crawling on skin" or "water running along a limb."

The neural tissue damage associated with stroke or other central nervous system trauma can alter the activity of inhibitory neurons, therefore enhancing pain sensitivity. In the peripheral nervous system, damage to neural structures, can result in ectopic impulse generation from the damaged structure or from the dorsal root ganglion (DRG). This type of response to nerve damage commonly results in mechanosensitivity, which is sometimes an indicator of neuropathic pain (Cousins and I. 1999, LaJoie et al., 2005; Box 3.2). When neurones are damaged their genetic expression can alter (Butler, 2000). One outcome of this is the upregulation of certain chemoreceptors. With this increased production of receptors, is an increase in sensitivity to the chemical that binds to the receptor. Adrenalin provides a good example, as neural firing will increase when adrenoreceptors are upregulated and blood concentration of adrenaline is increased or the sympathetic nervous system is activated.

The mechanisms of sensitization that have been most widely studied in models of neural injury remind us of the role of the nociceptive system as part of a greater body protection system. It is now acknowledged that interactions between the immune system, endocrine system and autonomic nervous system are important in all types of pain, including neuropathic pain (Watkins and Maier, 2005; Campbell and Meyer, 2006). Furthermore, management of patients with pain should consider tissues from across these systems.

These and other spinal and supraspinal influences on sensitivity are broadly considered central sensitization. In effect, it means that neurones that send a nociceptive message to the brain become more easily activated. It is widely thought, although not yet proven in human studies, that descending facilitation is sufficient to drive spinal nociceptive neurones once they are in a state of advanced sensitization.

BOX 3.2 NEUROPATHIC PAIN AND NEUROGENIC PAIN

Terminology: The terms neuropathic pain and neurogenic pain are commonly used in physiotherapy. Neuropathic pain refers to pain associated with pathology of neural tissue. Neurogenic pain refers to pain that is associated with sensitized neural tissue.

3.2.12 Cortical Reorganization and Sensitivity

Each of the mechanisms by which nociceptive transmission in the spinal cord becomes sensitized is also thought to occur in the brain. The ramifications of this will be wider than those of spinal changes because there are many more inputs here, from across all possible domains. Suffice to say that the principle is again important. That principle is that the pain neurosignature becomes more sensitive. Evidence of this has been obtained in patients with complex regional pain syndrome for whom imagined movements, in the absence of detectable muscle activity, increases pain and swelling (Moseley, 2004b) and visual input in the absence of somatic input also produces pain (Acerra and Moseley, 2005).

The other change that occurs in the brain in conjunction with persistent pain occurs within the cortical maps of the body. The most studied cortical map, or virtual body, is held in primary sensory cortex (S1). S1 changes have been reported in several patient groups. Two types of changes have been reported. First, the representation of the affected limb in patients with phantom limb pain and complex regional pain syndrome is smaller than the unaffected side (Flor et al., 1995; Pleger et al., 2006). Second, the representation of the affected area in patients with chronic back pain becomes bigger than in healthy controls and shifts toward the midline (Flor et al., 1997). In each case, the extent of the shift from normal relates to the intensity of pain. The importance of cortical reorganization in chronic pain states has not been established, but it is possible that it will offer a range of new treatment opportunities (see Acerra et al., 2007 for a review).

3.3 ASSESSMENT OF PAIN

3.3.1 Pain and its Meaning

When clinicians and researchers attempt to assess pain, they often attempt to measure it. However, pain is a subjective experience resistant to objective measurement and so many pain measurement tools rely on assumptions, including that people are willing and able to report their experience accurately.

Nevertheless we will highlight some of the tools commonly used in pain assessment (for a more extensive review see *Handbook of Pain Assessment* (Turk and Melzack, 2001)). First, we will highlight the importance of the clinical interview in an attempt to understand the individual's beliefs about their pain and the contribution of biological and cognitive-emotional factors to their pain, and in turn to the impact of their pain on their function.

3.3.2 Clinical Interview

Clinical interviews have conventionally focussed on symptoms: location, intensity, quality and temporal patterns, and signs. However, this information focuses very much on information relating to tissues and does not address the things the person's functional abilities, nor the psychosocial factors that are important in pain and its impact. The interview should identify factors that activate or sensitize the nociceptive system as well as elucidate factors that may preclude full recovery (see "Yellow Flags" later) (Table 3.1).

TABLE 3.1

Structured Interview for Biopsychosocial Assessment

Area of Examination	Information Gained
Orientation	Nature and location of symptoms; patient's story from onset to present, expectations of physiotherapy, questions and concerns about problem
Previous intervention	Investigations and understanding, treatment effects, advice received, causal beliefs
Medical history	Comorbidity and effect on function, special questions (red flag screening), medication
Effects on function and participation	Current social and employment situation, typical day, effects on work, restrictions on activity, assistance required, aids and adaptations, downtime, sleep
Coping strategies	Current coping strategies: active and passive, perceived consequences of change (e.g., increasing activity, exercise, pacing)
Socioeconomic	Effect on finances, benefits, medicolegal
Effect on family	Beliefs, responses, nature of support provided
Emotion	Nature and extent, effect on motivation
Preexamination	Body chart, behavior of symptoms

Source: Goldingay, S., *Topical Issues in Pain 5*, CNS Press, Falmouth, 2006. With permission.

3.3.3 MEASURES AND SCALES

Measures and scales can be valuable adjuncts to the interview and assist in broadening the assessment across the biopsychosocial domains.

3.3.3.1 Self-Report Measures

Given the subjectivity of pain, self-report measures are considered the gold standard in pain assessment. Common formats for measuring pain intensity are the visual analog scale (VAS) and the numerical rating scale (NRS). A VAS is usually a horizontal line 100 mm long. At each end is an anchor. The left anchor is usually "no pain" and the right anchor is usually "worst pain" or "worst pain imaginable." The patient marks a point on the line in answer to a specific question about their pain. The nature of the question determines the nature of the answer. For example, a clinician may want to know how much a certain activity hurts. If so, the question would need to refer to that activity. Alternatively, if the clinician wants to get an idea of the average pain they might ask "What is your average pain level over the last two days?" The distance from the mark to the left anchor is used as a measure of their pain (examples, in different languages, can be downloaded from British Pain Society Web site: www.britishpainsociety.org).

An NRS uses numbers instead of a line, such that 0 = "no pain" and 10 = "worst pain." The VAS is probably more sensitive to change, more difficult to measure, and less vulnerable to perseveration (perseveration refers to remembering what you said last time and responding the same way). The NRS is easier in a clinical setting because it is quick. It is probably sufficiently sensitive to detect clinically meaningful changes (a clinically meaningful or important change is usually considered to be about 2 points on a 10-point NRS scale (McQuay et al., 1997)).

The most widely used tool to assess the quality of pain is the short form of the McGill Pain Questionnaire (MPQ; Melzack, 1975). As per the neuromatrix model, the MPQ divides pain up into three dimensions and lists a variety of words for each. For example, words such as "sharp," "burning," and "intense" are listed to describe the sensory-discriminative aspect of pain (e.g., sharp, burning, intense), "punishing" is an example of the affective-motivational aspect of pain, and "annoying" an example of its cognitive-evaluative context. There are many other measures that emphasize different aspects of pain. Box 3.3 describes the MPQ and two other common measures (Jones and Moseley, 2008).

3.3.3.2 Behavioral Measures

Additional information can be gained by adopting behavioral measurement strategies. These strategies include the use of performance measures, such as repetitions, time and load, or observation of behaviors that might indicate distress, which may be indicative of pain. These may be most useful in situations where communication is a problem, in which case the uncertain relationship between behavior and pain must be acknowledged. Full review of behavioral measures is beyond the scope of this chapter, but the interested reader is referred to the *Handbook of Pain Assessment* (Turk and Melzack, 2001) and *Manage Your Pain* (Nicholas et al., 2002) for examples.

3.3.3.3 Measures of the Impact of Pain

The factors involved in the modulation of pain and the behavioral response to pain may be established during the clinical interview. It may be valuable to quantify those findings by using one of the many measures designed and tested for this purpose. The following is a brief account of the most widely used and documented.

3.3.3.4 Measuring Potential Impact of Beliefs and Thoughts

The fear avoidance beliefs questionnaire (FABQ) (Waddell et al., 1993) and the TAMPA scale of kinesiphobia (kinesiphobia means "fear of movement") (Miller et al., 1991) are designed to measure beliefs and behaviors relating to fear of movement, physical activity, and work. They have been used extensively and data are available from a range of patient and nonpatient populations. The pain catastrophizing scale (Sullivan et al., 1995) for measurement of catastrophic thinking about pain also has a large amount of data available. Three psychometrically robust measures, which are more commonly used in research than clinical settings, include the survey of pain attitudes (Jensen et al., 1987), the pain beliefs and perceptions inventory (Williams et al., 1994), and the pain anxiety symptoms scale (McCracken et al., 1992).

BOX 3.3   NOTES ON PAIN SCALES

McGill Pain Questionnaire (Melzack, 1975)
    Attempts to measure pain as a multidimensional experience

- Twenty categories of adjectives
- Four subclasses—sensory/affective/evaluative/miscellaneous
- Patients select adjectives that best describe pain experience
- Adjectives are weighted and a score—the pain rating index—for each subclass, is calculated
- Valid and reliable in range of contexts
- Takes a long time to fill out (a short version is also available)
- Patients may prefer to use other words to describe the quality of pain

Brief Pain Inventory (Keller et al., 2004)

- Patients self-categorize social status and current work situation
- Boxes are checked to indicate pain history
- Pain location is marked on a body chart
- Pain intensity and quality are determined by ratings on 0–10 scales or yes/no responses
- Seven questions are specific to the impact of pain: function, mood, life enjoyment
- Easily administered

Chronic Pain Index (Von Korff et al., 1994)

- Patients respond to eight questions about pain intensity and interference in life activities
- Pain intensity and interference of activity are seen as a single dimension reflecting severity
- Scoring method and grading system completed by assessor
- Presumes that dimension of severity includes biopsychosocial influences

3.3.3.4.1   *Red, Yellow, Blue, and Black Flags*

Common to the pain assessment process is a collection of signs, symptoms, and situations that act as indicators of special circumstances that need attention. The so-called "red flags" are signs and symptoms indicative of a serious pathology that requires, sometimes urgent, specialist care (e.g., cauda equina compression) (Greenhalgh and Selfe, 2006).

"Yellow flags" relate to signs and symptoms, including beliefs and attitudes, that are believed to increase the risk of reduced participation in a person's regular life situations. Although this approach was developed with guidelines for managing recent-onset (acute) low back pain, it is increasingly being used with people who have pain at other anatomical sites. Effectively, "yellow flags" are indicative of unrealistic and unhelpful beliefs about pain (Kendall et al., 1997). Assessment for these beliefs can be formalized using a standardized questionnaire, or alternatively, carefully selected questions can be incorporated into the clinical interview (Watson and Kendall, 2000).

In recognition of the importance of occupational factors in affecting return to work and healthcare visits, occupational specific factors have been grouped into "blue flags" and "black flags." Factors that would be identified as "blue flags" are those that relate just to that particular worker. For example, consider an individual who has work-related concerns about the attitudes of their line manager to them and their injury or rehabilitation. It is possible that the line manager's attitude, or the worker's perception of their manager's attitude, might impede return to work. "Black flags" indicate attention is needed to manage a workplace process or policy, i.e., something that has influence on all workers. For example, consider a workplace where there is no clear return to process or policy to support injured workers return to work (see Sowden, 2006).

In response to the negative focus of yellow, blue, and black flags Gifford (2006) proposed the introduction of another group of assessment findings: the "pink flags." These are indicative of a positive outcome to treatment. Examples might include realistic and helpful attitudes to pain and movement, evidence that a person has returned to regular activities (Box 3.4). While pink flags are in part a facetious addition to the flag battalion, they convey an important message to clinicians—that we should foster these things and reinforce them when they present.

3.3.3.4.2 Measures of Functional Limitation and Disability

There are a large number of self-report tools that aim to measure the functional impact of a person's pain. A large proportion of those tools concern back pain (e.g., the Roland Morris disability questionnaire (Roland and Morris, 1983) and the Oswestry questionnaire (Fisher and Johnston, 1997)) or neck pain (e.g., neck disability index; Vernon and Mior, 1991). These tools are widely used and a large amount of data from patient and nonpatient populations exists. There are also disability questionnaires

---

BOX 3.4   CLINICAL TIP—YELLOW FLAGS

Psychological Risk Factors
A high stress level
Distress and/or anxiety, depression
Passive coping strategies
Worry about the cause of pain, catastrophizing
Fear avoidance behavior and beliefs

Social Risk Factors
Poor relationships at work
Low job satisfaction
(Overmeer)

that are not anatomically focussed, for example the task-specific tools, whereby the patient selects a task or activity that they are unable to perform because of pain, and rates their ability to perform that task over the course of treatment. An advantage of such a tool is that it can be used with different populations. A disadvantage is that it makes it difficult to compare between treatments or between patients.

3.3.4 NOCICEPTIVE TRIGGERS

Investigations of structures and movements may be helpful in identifying noxious stimuli. Evidence of mechanical forces, pressure, and distention during aggravating postures (static and dynamic) should be sought. Areas of chemically mediated nociception, in association with the inflammatory mediators of peripheral sensitization, might be suspected at points of tenderness identified by palpation. However, consideration of peripheral noxious stimulation should always consider the profound effects of spinal and supraspinal mechanisms on pain sensitivity.

3.4 MANAGEMENT OF PAIN

3.4.1 EDUCATION

We believe that an essential component of the management of pain is intensive education about the biology of pain. Obviously this requires the educator to have appropriate knowledge, but also skills in facilitating effective learning. The benefits of an effective and detailed explanation of pain biology include changing beliefs and attitudes about pain, movement and activity (Moseley et al., 2004a), and increasing pain threshold during relevant tasks (Moseley, 2004a). When combining education with movement-based physiotherapy, pain is decreased and disability in the long term is reduced (Moseley, 2002, 2003b).

Effective education enables changed thinking from a new perspective. Unhelpful cognitions about pain, injury, and activity can be challenged and replaced. Unhelpful concepts of pain relating to tissue vulnerability can be replaced by new concepts that include neural sensitivity and central processing. Such a reconceptualization is likely to be a complex process requiring more than simply giving information, however, an example of the material used to explain pain biology is presented in *Explain Pain* (Butler and Moseley, 2003).

3.4.2 REDUCE AND MODIFY NOCICEPTION

3.4.2.1 Deactivating Peripheral Mechanisms of Nociception

Due to its sensitizing influence on nociceptors, the inflammatory response presents as the main target for deactivating peripheral mechanisms of nociception. It is worth remembering, however, that inflammation is a necessary and self-limiting process following injury. As such, the body has its own processes for deactivating the inflammatory response and the peripheral sensitization that it facilitates. This is achieved by the combined involvement of motor, immune, and vascular responses, effectively dissipating the substances that stimulate nociceptors and the chemical mediators responsible for peripheral sensitization.

Commonly, the clinician also intervenes by modifying the inflammation process. Such strategies are not thought to impede normal tissue healing, but by reducing pain and swelling, they aim to get people moving more quickly than they otherwise would. Conventional first aid to tissue trauma involves cooling and elevation of the injured part, firm bandaging, and reduced activity (rest, ice, compression, and elevation) with the intent of reducing blood flow and protecting injured tissue.

Pharmacological agents are also employed to reduce inflammation. Such agents are commonly designed to target the mechanisms involved in the production of prostaglandins. Use of these "anti-inflammatories" should be managed cautiously due to the importance of the inflammation process in tissue healing and the drastic side effects (including gastric ulceration) associated with prolonged or inappropriate use. Notably, the administration of anti-inflammatories is commonly systemic (e.g., orally or by injection), so the drug effects will extend beyond the target tissue. Even in local application of topical agents, there is a risk the active agent will be transported remotely in the circulation. Only those with appropriate expertise and medicolegal authority should be involved in giving advice and prescribing such medications.

Decisions about the introduction of movement and eventual return to activity are made with regard to the state (i.e., vulnerability) of the tissues, not simply with regard to pain. This is an important point. We have outlined why pain is not an accurate measure of the state of the tissues, and herein lies the implication of that assessment. If pain is not an accurate guide to the state of the tissues, then, taking a purely tissue-focused perspective, pain is not an appropriate marker for the reintroduction of activity. Indeed, movement may be another feature that assists in the dissipation of sensitizing substances through its promotion of blood flow, oxygen supply, waste product removal, and appropriate forces to guide healing. Therefore, delaying the reintroduction of movement because of pain may prolong pain. The clinician needs to have sound knowledge of the processes of healing and nociception to make this judgment. That is, the clinician must have both comprehensive biological knowledge and sound clinical reasoning. Finally, the clinician needs to manage the patient's concern about moving despite pain because it is these concerns determine both how, and how much, the patient will move.

3.4.2.2 Deactivating Spinal Mechanisms of Nociception

The desensitization of second-order neurones is influenced by two mechanisms, one involving peripheral stimulation and the other involving descending supraspinal influences. Novel peripheral input, such as transcutaneous electrical nerve stimulation (TENS), activates Aβ neurones. This nonnoxious stimulation "competes" with incoming nociceptive stimulation and can become the more prominent sensation. Descending modulation of spinal activity can be facilitatory or inhibitory. Inhibitory effects seem to be linked to positive emotional states and direct links to the spinal neurones from the emotional areas of the brain have been identified. The "gate control theory," now more than 40 years old, postulated that lamina II of the dorsal horn of the spine was the site of this inhibition of the nociceptive system (Melzack and Wall, 1965). Pain neuroscience has grown from this theory, and despite great advances in the understanding of pain, there is still strong support for this modulatory function of the dorsal horn. Intriguingly, there is good evidence that TENS is effective in pain of recent onset, presumably with recent trauma, and not effective in persistent pain states (McQuay et al., 1997). This may be a consequence of the greater role of sensitivity in persistent pain states we have described previously. There is a good argument that stimulation of Aβ neurones actually facilitates dorsal horn sensitization once sensitization is underway, because spinal nociceptive neurones can become sensitive to Aβ input.

3.4.2.3 Targeting Cortical Representations of the Body

An effect associated with persistent pain states is the alteration of the representation of the painful part in the primary sensory cortex (S1) (see Flor et al., 2006 and Moseley, 2006 for review). The plastic nature of the cortex means these changes may be due to altered neural input. That is, a change of normal tissue activity and stimulation, the so-called use it or lose it principle. However, a more specific mechanism, involving the inhibition of nonnoxious stimuli at the thalamus, has also been proposed (Rommel et al., 1999), although it is yet to be substantiated.

In any case, rehabilitation of people with persistent pain states may benefit from attempts to normalize the S1 representation (Flor, 2003, Maihofner et al., 2004, Pleger et al., 2005). Training the nervous system to be more discriminating to sensory stimuli appears to be beneficial in reducing pain for some patient groups (e.g., phantom limb pain (Flor et al., 2001) and complex regional pain syndrome (Moseley et al., 2008)). This reflects findings that tactile acuity is related to pain and changes to the S1 representation (Flor, 2003). While these findings may lead to the assumption that changes to the S1 representation cause pain (Harris, 1999), this is yet to be established (Moseley and Gandevia, 2005).

3.4.2.4 Reduce and Modify Psychological and Social Demands

As described earlier, it would seem that negative effects (e.g., distress, anxiety), cognitions (e.g., catastrophizing, expectations), and social factors (e.g., workplace demands) influence pain and the disability associated with pain. Not surprisingly then, cognitive-behavioral therapy (CBT) has emerged as a popular intervention. While there are different approaches to CBT, the literature tends not to distinguish between these approaches. Therefore, in this section, we will outline the use of cognitive-behavioral principles rather than theory, per se. The application of cognitive-behavioral principles, in a CBT framework or otherwise, aims to enhance coping skills and reduce psychopathology and disability. Techniques, such as goal setting, problem solving, cognitive restructuring, attention diversion, communication skills, and assertiveness training, are commonly employed. To reduce pain is not a target of CBT, but it is an effect (Morley et al., 1999).

3.4.2.5 Deactivating Brain Mechanisms of Nociception and Pain

We suggested earlier that pain is dependent on an evaluation by the central nervous system, of threat to body tissue. It follows then that any input that changes that evaluation will also change pain. The mechanisms for this have been suggested, but are not well defined. Probably, there is involvement of mechanisms that modulate descending inhibitory and excitatory influences on the dorsal horn neurones as well as suppression of activity in cortical structures (see Petrovic and Ingvar, 2002). However, again, the principle that pain is the conscious correlate of the implicit perception of threat to body tissues is able to inform the clinical implication of these mechanisms (see Moseley, 2007 for review).

3.4.2.6 Cognitive-Behavioral Principles

The basic premise underlying the use of cognitive-behavioral principles is that an individual's thoughts influence and interact with their emotions, beliefs, and behavior. Therefore, by challenging unhelpful thoughts and replacing them with more accurate and appropriate ones, improved mood and behavior can occur. With persistence, this may even lead to a reconceptualization of existing beliefs. Modifying behavior, for example participating rather than avoiding, allows for further challenging of preexisting thoughts and beliefs, and is also likely to positively affect mood.

3.4.2.7 Relaxation

There are many strategies, and personal preferences, for achieving a relaxed state. However, not all strategies enable relaxation during participation in necessary or desired activity. As well it would seem appropriate to be able to initiate a relaxation response, at a time when the pain is still controllable, but might be worsening. A recognized approach to relaxation that satisfies these requirements combines meditative, physiological, and psychological elements. It features a mantra, a visual imagery and attention to inhalation, expiration, and the tension in muscles. Through frequent training sessions, a relaxed state is linked to the mantra, the image, and the exhalation, allowing it to be initiated opportunistically. The benefits of relaxation in a person with pain include reducing negative emotional response to pain or the expectation of pain, reducing unnecessary muscle activity prior to movement, allowing more effective cognitive function and response. Compared to many other strategies, this strategy can be implemented without interruption to current activities, and hopefully allows the person to perform better and for longer periods of time.

3.4.2.8 Pacing

An identified cycle of activity in many people with persistent pain involves high level of activity—usually when symptoms are low—followed by very low levels of activity, in response to elevation of symptom intensity. It is sometimes called the "boom or bust cycle," and is problematic when the periods of very low activity interfere with things a person wants or needs to do (e.g., work). Pacing aims to change this pattern of activity by avoiding the two extreme levels. The person will instead function at a level that can be consistently reproduced day after day. This allows for more confident predictions of future performance and is more appropriate for regular participation in home, work, and social settings. Initially, the identified level of activity that can be performed regularly may still be too low for participation in the person's preferred lifestyle. However, by applying strategies, such as thought-challenging and relaxation, the individual may be able to do more despite pain.

As well, the person should be encouraged to use quotas to guide activity level, rather than pain being the guide. Quotas (e.g., repetitions of exercise, time spent on an activity) identify the level of activity to be performed regardless of the pain on the day. They should be set by the person in response to previous successful experiences. The person must resist responding to low levels of pain by increasing activity beyond the set quota and should endeavor to reach the quota even when pain is interfering. This should be done, with the knowledge from previous experience, that the task is achievable by challenging any unhelpful thoughts and using relaxation strategies during the task. A gradual increase in quotas allows activity to be paced up and should be achievable as the person becomes more competent in the use of cognitive strategies and used to the level of activity.

The rehabilitation professional should be able to facilitate this process of pacing up activity. Importantly, this requires effective education, the opportunity for the person with pain to experience successful performances, and the development of effective cognitive-behavioral strategies for self-management. Optimum levels of activity will most likely be achieved when the combined skills of thought challenging, relaxation, and pacing are well developed and consistently applied (see Nicholas and Tonkin, 2004 for more specific detail on goal setting, pacing, and quotas).

3.4.2.9   Graded Exposure

The use of a graded exercise program is common in the rehabilitation of people with persistent pain. This has many potential benefits including physical improvements such as strength, range of movement, and coordination, and psychological benefits such as improved self-efficacy and improved mood. There is also the possibility that there is a reduction in pain-related fear, as a person is able to confront fearful activities or situations in the safety of the rehabilitation setting.

Graded exposure to fearful activities is a much more formalized approach to this, and arguably more effective (Vlaeyen and Linton, 2000). With fear as the target of the intervention, a hierarchy of situations or events is constructed ranging from a situation of no fear (i.e., baseline) to one that provokes intense fear. Treatment using graded exposure involves presenting the fear-inducing stimuli in order of the hierarchy, progressing toward the most intense. This technique has been used successful in people with persistent pain including nonspecific low back pain (Vlaeyen et al., 2002) and complex regional pain syndrome (de Jong et al., 2005).

Notably, the application of these cognitive-behavioral principles forms just one aspect of the rehabilitation process, along with interdisciplinary interventions that tackle physical fitness, ergonomic factors, and work practices.

3.5   LIMITATIONS, OPPORTUNITIES, AND CONCLUSION

This chapter attempted to provide the reader with a broad overview of pain biology, assessment, and management. The complexity of the human experience, which is exemplified in the human experience of pain, means that this chapter can only provide a snapshot of the body of literature that is available. One objective that we considered to be particularly important was that the reader has sufficient material to understand how to think about pain. That is why we have reiterated the key principle—that pain can be conceptualized as conscious correlate of the brain's implicit perception of threat to body tissue. There are several other key "take-home messages:"

1. Pain depends on the brain's implicit appraisal of threat to body tissue. Nociception is very important, but it is neither sufficient nor necessary for pain.
2. Many factors from sensory, psychological, and occupation (social) domains modulate pain.
3. Pain treatment can target the underpinning mechanisms in pain. That is, anti-inflammatory strategies, including postural correction and appropriate work-related pacing to reduce peripheral sensitization, cognitive-behavioral strategies to promote descending inhibition, and provision of accurate information ("explaining pain") to modify the meaning of pain.
4. This chapter is a starting place. We have tried to reference the key paper or source where the reader would benefit greatly from further reading.

ACKNOWLEDGMENTS

G.L.M. is supported by the Nuffield Dominions Trust. L.J. is an honorary senior lecturer in pain sciences at the University of Sydney, Australia.

REFERENCES

Acerra N and Moseley GL 2005: Dysynchiria: Watching the mirror image of the unaffected limb elicits pain on the affected side. *Neurology* 65: 751–753.
Acerra N, Souvlis T, and Moseley G 2007: Stroke, complex regional pain syndrome and phantom limb pain: Can commonalities direct future management? *J Rehabil Med* 39: 109–114.
Apkarian AV, Bushnell MC, Treede R-D, and Zubieta J-K 2005: Human brain mechanisms of pain perception and regulation in health and disease. *Eur J Pain* 9: 463–484.
Arntz A and Claassens L 2004: The meaning of pain influences its experienced intensity. *Pain* 109: 20–25.
Arntz A, Dreessen L, and De Jong P 1994: The influence of anxiety on pain: Attentional and attributional mediators. *Pain* 56: 307–314.
Arntz A, Vaneck M, and Heijmans M 1990: Predictions of dental pain—The fear of any expected evil, is worse than the evil itself. *Behav Res Ther* 28: 29–41.
Asghari A, Nicholas MK 2001: Pain self-efficacy beliefs and pain behaviour. A prospective study. *Pain* 94: 85–100.
Asmundson GJ, Kuperos JL, and Norton GR 1997: Do patients with chronic pain selectively attend to pain-related information? Preliminary evidence for the mediating role of fear. *Pain* 72: 27–32.
Awerbuch M. 2004: Repetitive strain injuries: Has the Australian epidemic burnt out? *Intern Med J* 34(7): 416–419.
Banks WA and Watkins LR 2006: Mediation of chronic pain: Not by neurons alone. *Pain* 124: 1–2.
Benedetti F, Pollo A, Lopiano L, Lanotte M, Vighetti S, and Rainero I 2003: Conscious expectation and unconscious conditioning in analgesic, motor, and hormonal placebo/nocebo responses. *J Neurosci* 23: 4315–4323.

Bigos SJ, Battie MC, Spengler DM, Fisher LD, Fordyce WE, Hansson TH, Nachemson AL, and Wortley MD 1991: A prospective study of work perceptions and psychosocial factors affecting the report of back injury [published erratum appears in spine 1991 jun;16(6):688]. *Spine* 16: 1–6.

Bongers PM, Ijmker S, van den Heuvel S, and Blatter BM 2006: Epidemiology of work related neck and upper limb problems: Psychosocial and personal risk factors (part i) and effective interventions from a biobehavioural perspective (part ii). *J Occup Rehabil* 16: 279–302.

Boos N, Rieder R, Schade V, Spratt KF, Semmer N, and Aebi M 1995: 1995 Volvo Award in Clinical Sciences. The diagnostic accuracy of magnetic resonance imaging, work perception, and psychosocial factors in identifying symptomatic disc herniations. *Spine* 20: 2613–2625.

Butler D 2000: *The Sensitive Nervous System*. Adelaide: NOI Publications, 431 pp.

Butler D and Moseley GL 2003: *Explain Pain*. Adelaide: NOI Group Publishing, 114 pp.

Campbell JN and Meyer RA 2006: Mechanisms of neuropathic pain. *Neuron* 52: 77–92.

Carayon P, Smith MJ, and Haims MC 1999: Work organization, job stress, and work-related musculoskeletal disorders. *Hum Factors* 41: 644–663.

Chua P, Krams M, Toni I, Passingham R, and Dolan R 1999: A functional anatomy of anticipatory anxiety. *Neuroimage* 9: 563–571.

Coudeyre E, Rannou F, Tubach F, Baron G, Coriat F, Brin S, Revel M, and Poiraudeau S 2006: General practitioners' fear-avoidance beliefs influence their management of patients with low back pain. *Pain* 124: 330–337.

Cousins MC, I. P 1999: Acute and postoperative pain. In Wall PD and Melzack R (Eds.): *Textbook of Pain* (4th edn.). London: Churchill Livingstone, pp. 447–492.

Craig A 2002: How do you feel? Interoception: The sense of the physiological condition of the body. *Nature Rev Neurosci* 3: 655–666.

Crombez G, Eccleston C, Baeyens F, and Eelen P 1996: The disruptive nature of pain: An experimental investigation. *Behav Res Ther* 34: 911–918.

Crombez G, Eccleston C, Baeyens F, and Eelen P 1997: Habituation and the interference of pain with task performance. *Pain* 70: 149–154.

Crombez G, Eccleston C, Baeyens F, and Eelen P 1998: Attentional disruption is enhanced by the threat of pain. *Behav Res Ther* 36: 195–204.

Crombez G, Eccleston C, Baeyens F, van Houdenhove B, and van den Broeck A 1999: Attention to chronic pain is dependent upon pain-related fear. *J Psychosom Res* 47: 403–410.

Crombez G, Van Damme S, and Eccleston C 2005: Hypervigilance to pain: An experimental and clinical analysis. *Pain* 116: 4–7.

de Jong JR, Vlaeyen JWS, Onghena P, Cuypers C, Hollander MD, and Ruijgrok J 2005: Reduction of pain-related fear in complex regional pain syndrome type i: The application of graded exposure in vivo. *Pain* 116: 264–275.

Duckworth MP, Iezzi A, Adams HE, and Hale D 1997: Information processing in chronic pain disorder: A preliminary analysis. *J Psychopathol Behav Assess* 19: 239–255.

Eccleston C 1994: Chronic pain and attention: A cognitive approach. *Br J Clin Psychol* 33: 535–547.

Eccleston C and Crombez G 1999: Pain demands attention: A cognitive-affective model of the interruptive function of pain. *Psychol Bull* 125: 356–366.

Eccleston C, Crombez G, Aldrich S, and Stannard C 1997: Attention and somatic awareness in chronic pain. *Pain* 72: 209–215.

Fabrega H and Tyma S 1976: Language and cultural influences in description of pain. *Br J Med Psychol* 49: 349–371.

Feuerstein M, Harrington CB, Lopez M, and Haufler A 2006: How do job stress and ergonomic factors impact clinic visits in acute low back pain? A prospective study. *J Occup Environ Med* 48: 607–614.

Fisher K and Johnston M 1997: Validation of the oswestry low back pain disability questionnaire, its sensitivity as a measure of change following treatment and its relationship with other aspects of the chronic pain experience. *Physiother Theory Pract* 13: 67–80.

Flor H 2003: Cortical reorganisation and chronic pain: Implications for rehabilitation. *J Rehabil Med* 35: 66–72.

Flor H, Braun C, Elbert T, and Birbaumer N 1997: Extensive reorganization of primary somatosensory cortex in chronic back pain patients. *Neurosci Lett* 224: 5–8.

Flor H, Denke C, Schaefer M, and Grusser S 2001: Effect of sensory discrimination training on cortical reorganisation and phantom limb pain. *Lancet* 357: 1763–1764.

Flor H, Elbert T, Knecht S, Wienbruch C, Pantev C, Birbaumer N, Larbig W, and Taub E 1995: Phantom-limb pain as a perceptual correlate of cortical reorganization following arm amputation. *Nature* 375: 482–484.

Flor H, Nikolajsen L, and Jensen TS 2006: Phantom limb pain: A case of maladaptive CNS plasticity? *Nat Rev Neurosci* 7: 873–881.

Gifford L: Red and yellow flags and improving patient outcomes. *OCPPP Annual Congress 2006*, Nottingham, U.K.

Godinho F, Magnin M, Frot M, Perchet C, and Garcia-Larrea L 2006: Emotional modulation of pain: Is it the sensation or what we recall? *J Neurosci* 26: 11454–11461.

Gore M, Brandenburg NA, Dukes E, Hoffman DL, Tai KS, and Stacey B 2005: Pain severity in diabetic peripheral neuropathy is associated with patient functioning, symptom levels of anxiety and depression, and sleep. *J Pain Symptom Manage* 30: 374–385.

Gracely RH, Dubner R, Deeter WR, and Wolskee PJ 1985: Clinicians' expectations influence placebo analgesia. *Lancet* 1: 43.

Gracely RH, Geisser ME, Giesecke T, Grant MAB, Petzke F, Williams DA, and Clauw DJ 2004: Pain catastrophizing and neural responses to pain among persons with fibromyalgia. *Brain* 127: 835–843.

Greenhalgh S and Selfe J 2006: *Red flags. A Guide to Identifying Serious Pathology of the Spine.* Oxford: Churchill Livingstone Elsevier, 214 pp.

Harris AJ 1999: Cortical origin of pathological pain. *Lancet* 354: 1464–1466.

Helliwell PS and Taylor WJ. 2004: Repetitive strain injury. *Postgrad Med J* 80(946): 438–443.

Hodges PW, Moseley GL, Gabrielsson A, and Gandevia SC 2003: Experimental muscle pain changes feedforward postural responses of the trunk muscles. *Exp Brain Res* 151: 262–271.

Janig W, Chapman CR, and Green P 2006: Pain and body protection: sensory, autonomic, neuroendocrine and behavioural mechanisms in the control of inflammation and hyperalgesia. In: Flor H, Kalso E, and Dostrovsky J (Eds.): *11th World Congress of Pain*, Sydney: IASP Press.

Jensen M 1994: Magnetic resonance imaging of the lumbar spine in people without low back pain. *N Engl J Med* 331(2): 69–73.

Jensen MP, Karoly P, and Huger R 1987: The development and preliminary validation of an instrument to assess patients' attitudes toward pain. *J Psychosom Res* 31: 393–400.

Jones AKP 2005: The role of the cerebral cortex in pain perception. In Justins DM (Ed.): *Pain 2005—An Update Review*, Seattle, WA: IASP Press, pp. 59–68.

Jones L and Moseley GL 2008: Pain. In Porter S (Ed.): *Tidy's Physiotherapy* (14th edn.). Oxford: Elsevier, pp. 485–502.

Keller, S., Bann, C.M., Dodd, S.L., Schein, J., Mendoza, T.R., and Cleeland, C. 2004: Validity of the brief pain inventory for use in documenting the outcomes of patients with noncancer pain. *Clin J Pain*, 20(50): 309–318.

Keltner JR, Furst A, Fan C, Redfern R, Inglis B, and Fields HL 2006: Isolating the modulatory effect of expectation on pain transmission: A functional magnetic resonance imaging study. *J Neurosci* 26: 4437–4443.

Kendall NAS, Linton SJ, and Main CJ 1997. Guide to assessing psychosocial yellow flags in acute low back pain: Risk factors in long-term disability and work loss. Accident Rehabilitation and Compensation Insurance Corporation of New Zealand, and the National Health Committee Ministry of Health. Wellington, New Zealand, 1997.

Klages U, Kianifard S, Ulusoy O, and Wehrbein H 2006: Anxiety sensitivity as predictor of pain in patients undergoing restorative dental procedures. *Community Dent Oral Epidemiol* 34: 139–145.

LaJoie AS, McCabe SJ, Thomas B, and Edgell SE 2005: Determining the sensitivity and specificity of common diagnostic tests for carpal tunnel syndrome using latent class analysis. *Plast Reconstr Surg* 116: 502–507.

Lasch KE 2002: Culture and pain. Pain Clinical Updates, Accessed on 12 December 2008 from http://www.iasp-pain.org/AM/AMTemplate.cfm?Section=Home&TEMPLATE=/CM/ContentDisplay.cfm&CONTENTID=7578

Linton SJ 2005: Do psychological factors increase the risk for back pain in the general population in both a cross-sectional and prospective analysis. *Eur J Pain*, 9(4): 354–361.

Lucire Y 2003: *Constructing RSI: Belief and Desire.* Sydney, Australia: UNSW Press, 216 pp.

Maihofner C, Handwerker HO, Neundorfer B, and Birklein F 2004: Cortical reorganization during recovery from complex regional pain syndrome. *Neurology* 63: 693–701.

Main CJ 1983: The modified somatic perception questionnaire (mspq). *J Psychosom Res* 27: 503–514.

Marras WS 2000: Occupational low back disorder causation and control. *Ergonomics* 43: 880–902.

Marras WS, Davis KG, Heaney CA, Maronitis AB, and Allread WG 2000: The influence of psychosocial stress, gender, and personality on mechanical loading of the lumbar spine. *Spine* 25: 3045–3054.

Matthews KA, Schier MF, Brunson BI, and Carducci B 1980: Attention, unpredictability, and reports of physical symptoms eliminating the benefits of predictability. *J Personal Soc Psychol* 38: 525–537.

McCracken LM 1997: "Attention" to pain in persons with chronic pain: A behavioral approach. *Behav Ther* 28: 271–284.

McCracken LM, Zayfert C, and Gross RT 1992: The pain anxiety symptoms scale: Development and validation of a scale to measure fear of pain. *Pain* 50: 67–73.

McQuay HJ, Moore RA, Eccleston C, Morley S, and Williams AC 1997: Systematic review of outpatient services for chronic pain control. *Health Technol Assess* 1: i–iv, 1–135.

Melzack R 1975: The Mcgill pain questionnaire: Major properties and scoring methods. *Pain* 1: 277–299.

Melzack R 1990: Phantom limbs and the concept of a neuromatrix. *Trends Neurosci* 13: 88–92.

Melzack R 1996: Gate control theory. On the evolution of pain concepts. *Pain Forum* 5: 128–138.

Melzack R 1999: From the gate to the neuromatrix. *Pain* 6(Suppl.): S121–S126.

Melzack R and Wall PD 1965: Pain mechanisms: A new theory. *Science* 150: 971–979.

Merskey H and Bogduk N 1994: *Classification of Chronic Pain* (2nd edn.). Seattle, WA: IASP Press, 210 pp.

Meyer R, Ringkamp M, Campbell JN, and Raja SN 2006: Peripheral mechanisms of cutaneous nociception. In McMahon SB and Koltzenburg M (Eds.): *Textbook of Pain* (5th edn.). London: Elsevier, pp. 3–35.

Miller R, Kori S, and Todd D. The tampa scale for kinesiphobia. Unpublished report. Tampa, FL, 1991.

Millson HB, Gray J, Stretch RA, and Lambert MI 2004: Dissociation between back pain and bone stress reaction as measured by CT scan in young cricket fast bowlers. *Br J Sports Med* 38: 586–591.

Morley S, Eccleston C, and Williams A 1999: Systematic review and meta-analysis of randomized controlled trials of cognitive behaviour therapy and behaviour therapy for chronic pain in adults, excluding headache. *Pain* 80: 1–13.

Morris DB 2001: Narrative, ethics, and pain: Thinking with stories. *Narrative* 9(1): 55–77.

Moseley GL 2002: Combined physiotherapy and education is effective for chronic low back pain. A randomised controlled trial. *Aust J Physiother* 48: 297–302.

Moseley GL 2003a: A pain neuromatrix approach to patients with chronic pain. *Man Ther* 8: 130–140.

Moseley GL 2003b: Joining forces—Combining cognition-targeted motor control training with group or individual pain physiology education: A successful treatment for chronic low back pain. *J Man Manip Ther* 11: 88–94.

Moseley GL 2004a: Evidence for a direct relationship between cognitive and physical change during an education intervention in people with chronic low back pain. *Eur J Pain* 8: 39–45.

Moseley GL 2004b: Imagined movements cause pain and swelling in a patient with complex regional pain syndrome. *Neurology* 62: 1644.

Moseley GL 2006: Making sense of s1 mania—Are things really that simple? In Gifford L (Ed.): *Topical Issues in Pain,* Vol. 5. Falmouth: CNS Press, pp. 321–340.

Moseley GL 2007: Reconceptualising pain according to its underlying biology. *Phys Ther Rev* 12:169–178.

Moseley GL and Arntz A 2007: The context of a noxious stimulus affects the pain it evokes. *Pain* 133:64–71.

Moseley GL and Gandevia SC 2005: Sensory-motor incongruence and reports of "pain". *Rheumatology* 44: 1083–1085.

Moseley GL, Nicholas MK, and Hodges PW 2004a: A randomized controlled trial of intensive neurophysiology education in chronic low back pain. *Clin J Pain* 20: 324–330.

Moseley GL, Nicholas MK, and Hodges PW 2004b: Does anticipation of back pain predispose to back trouble? *Brain* 127: 2339–2347.

Moseley GL, Nicholas MK, and Hodges PW 2004c: Pain differs from non-painful attention-demanding or stressful tasks in its effect on postural control patterns of trunk muscles. *Exp Brain Res* 156: 64–71.

Moseley GL, Zalucki NM, and Wiech K 2008: Tactile discrimination, but not tactile stimulation alone, reduces chronic limb pain. *Pain* 137(3):600–608.

Myers CD, Tsao JCI, Glover DA, Kim SC, Turk N, and Zeltzer LK 2006: Sex, gender, and age: Contributions to laboratory pain responding in children and adolescents. *J Pain* 7: 556–564.

Naveteur J, Mars F, and Crombez G 2005: The effect of eye orientation on slowly increasing pain. *Eur J Pain* 9: 79–85.

Nicholas MK 2007: The pain self-efficacy questionnaire: Taking pain into account. *Eur J Pain* 11: 153–163.

Nicholas MK 2010: Cognitive behavioural pain management. In Moseley GL (Ed.): *Pain. Do You Get It?* Oxford: Elsevier.

Nicholas MK, Siddal P, Tonkin L, and Beeston L 2002: *Manage Your Pain.* Sydney: ABC Books.

Nicholas MK and Tonkin L 2004: Application of cognitive-behavioural principles to activity-based pain management programs. In Refshauge K and Gaff E (Eds.): *Musculoskeletal Physiotherapy: Clinical Science and Evidence Based Practice.* Oxford: Elsevier, pp. 277–293.

Nicholas MK, Wilson PH, and Goyen J 1991: Operant-behavioural and cognitive-behavioural treatment for chronic low back pain. *Behav Res Ther* 29: 225–238.

Ohara PT, Vit JP, and Jasmin L 2005: Cortical modulation of pain. *Cell Mol Life Sci* 62: 44–52.

Peters ML, Vlaeyen JW, and van Drunen C 2000: Do fibromyalgia patients display hypervigilance for innocuous somatosensory stimuli? Application of a body scanning reaction time paradigm. *Pain* 86: 283–292.

Petrovic P and Ingvar M 2002: Imaging cognitive modulation of pain processing. *Pain* 95: 1–5.

Pleger B, Ragert P, Schwenkreis P, Forster AF, Wilimzig C, Dinse H, Nicolas V, Maier C, and Tegenthoff M 2006: Patterns of cortical reorganization parallel impaired tactile discrimination and pain intensity in complex regional pain syndrome. *Neuroimage* 32: 503–510.

Pleger B, Tegenthoff M, Ragert P, Forster AF, Dinse HR, Schwenkreis P, Nicolas V, and Maier C 2005: Sensorimotor returning in complex regional pain syndrome parallels pain reduction. *Ann Neurol* 57: 425–429.

Ploghaus A, Becerra L, Borras C, and Borsook D 2003: Neural circuitry underlying pain modulation: Expectation, hypnosis, placebo. *Trends Cogn Sci* 7: 197–200.

Ploghaus A, Tracey I, Gati JS, Clare S, Menon RS, Matthews PM, and Rawlins JN 1999: Dissociating pain from its anticipation in the human brain. *Science* 284: 1979–1981.

Poiraudeau S, Rannou F, Baron G, Henanff AL, Coudeyre E, Rozenberg S, Huas D, Martineau C, Jolivet-Landreau I, and Garcia-Mace J 2006: Fear-avoidance beliefs about back pain in patients with subacute low back pain. *Pain* 124: 305–311.

Pollo A, Amanzio M, Arslanian A, Casadio C, Maggi G, and Benedetti F 2001: Response expectancies in placebo analgesia and their clinical relevance. *Pain* 93: 77–84.

Pud D and Amit A 2005: Anxiety as a predictor of pain magnitude following termination of first-trimester pregnancy. *Pain Med* 6: 143–148.

Rhudy JL and Williams AE 2005: Gender differences in pain: Do emotions play a role? *Gender Med* 2: 208–226.

Roland M and Morris R 1983: A study of the natural history of back pain. Part 1: Development of a reliable and sensitive measure of disability in low-back pain. *Spine* 8: 141–144.

Rommel O, Gehling M, Dertwinkel R, Witscher K, Zenz M, Malin JP, and Janig W 1999: Hemisensory impairment in patients with complex regional pain syndrome. *Pain* 80: 95–101.

Sawamoto N, Honda M, Okada T, Hanakawa T, Kanda M, Fukuyama H, Konishi J, and Shibasaki H 2000: Expectation of pain enhances responses to nonpainful somatosensory stimulation in the anterior cingulate cortex and parietal operculum/posterior insula: An event-related functional magnetic resonance imaging study. *J Neurosci* 20: 7438–7445.

Schupp CJ, Berbaum K, Berbaum M, and Lang EV 2005: Pain and anxiety during interventional radiologic procedures: Effect of patients' state anxiety at baseline and modulation by nonpharmacologic analgesia adjuncts. *J Vasc Interv Radiol* 16: 1585–1592.

Schwarzer AC, Aprill CN, Derby R, Fortin J, Kine G, and Bogduk N 1994: The false-positive rate of uncontrolled diagnostic blocks of the lumbar zygapophysial joints. *Pain* 58: 195–200.

Seminowicz DA and Davis KD 2006: Cortical responses to pain in healthy individuals depends on pain catastrophizing. *Pain* 120: 297–306.

Sommer C, Sorkin L, and Kress M 2006: Cytokine-induced pain: From molecular mechanisms to human pain states. In: Flor H, Kalso E, and Dostrovsky J (Eds.): *11th World Congress on Pain*, Sydney, Australia: IASP Press.

Soetanto AL, Chung JW, and Wong TK 2006: Are there gender differences in pain perception? *J Neurosci Nurs* 38: 172–176.

Sowden G 2006: Vocational rehabilitation. In Gifford L (Ed.): *Topical Issues in Pain 5*. Falmouth: CNS Press, pp. 149–66.

Sullivan MJL, Bishop SR, and Pivik J 1995: The pain catastrophizing scale: Development and validation. *Psychol Assessment* 7: 524–532.

Tang J and Gibson SJ 2005: A psychophysical evaluation of the relationship between trait anxiety, pain perception, and induced state anxiety. *J Pain* 6: 612–619.

Turk DC and Melzack R (Eds.). *Handbook of Pain Assessment* (2nd edn.) New York: Guildford Press, 2001.

Unruh AM 1996: Gender variations in clinical pain experience. *Pain* 65: 123–167.

Van Nieuwenhuyse A, Somville PR, Crombez G, Burdorf A, Verbeke G, Johannik K, Van den Bergh O, Masschelein R, Mairiaux P, and Moens GF 2006: The role of physical workload and pain related fear in the development of low back pain in young workers: Evidence from the belcoback study; results after one year of follow up. *Occup Environ Med* 63: 45–52.

Vernon H and Mior S 1991: The neck disability index: A study of reliability and validity. *J Manip Physiol Ther* 14: 409–415.

Vlaeyen JW and Linton SJ 2000: Fear-avoidance and its consequences in chronic musculoskeletal pain: A state of the art. *Pain* 85: 317–332.

Vlaeyen JWS, de Jong J, Geilen M, Heuts P, and van Breukelen G 2002: The treatment of fear of movement/(re)injury in chronic low back pain: Further evidence on the effectiveness of exposure in vivo. *Clin J Pain* 18: 251–261.

Von Korff M 1994: Studying the natural history of back pain. *Spine* 19(18 Suppl): 2041S–2046S.

Waddell G, Newton M, Henderson I, Somerville D, and Main CJ 1993: A fear-avoidance beliefs questionnaire (fabq) and the role of fear-avoidance beliefs in chronic low back pain and disability. *Pain* 52: 157–168.

Wager TD 2005: Expectations and anxiety as mediators of placebo effects in pain. *Pain* 115: 225–226.

Watkins L and Maier S 2000: The pain of being sick: Implications of immune-to-brain communication for understanding pain. *Ann Rev Psychol* 51: 29–57.

Watkins LR and Maier SF 2005: Immune regulation of central nervous system functions: From sickness responses to pathological pain. *J Intern Med* 257: 139–155.

Watson P and Kendall NAS 2000: Assessing psychosocial yellow flags. In Gifford L (Ed.): *Topical Issues in Pain*. Falmouth: CNS Press.

Williams DA, Robinson ME, and Geisser ME 1994: Pain beliefs: Assessment and utility. *Pain* 59: 71–78.

Woolf CJ and Salter MW 2000: Neuroscience—Neuronal plasticity: Increasing the gain in pain. *Science* 288: 1765–1768.

4 Aging and Ergonomics

Lili Liu and Robert Lederer

CONTENTS

4.1 INTRODUCTION

This chapter provides an overview of the demographics of aging and provides a revised definition of "old." The changing demographics have implications for current and future roles of rehabilitation professionals. In the past, rehabilitation focused on addressing the needs of populations with disabilities. With the aging of the baby-boomer population, most of whom will remain in the community, the focus of rehabilitation will shift from disability to the needs of older people who may or may not have a combination of disabilities. Concurrently, there is a movement focusing on environmental design as an approach to facilitating function in seniors who may or may not yet have limitations. In other words, given the right environment, product, or even service design, some disabilities would no longer be issues.

Ergonomics and human factors are examined from the perspective of age-related changes in physical, sensory, and cognitive functions. These changes are reviewed and some design recommendations for addressing these are provided. Next, we discuss the emerging role of rehabilitation professionals in design for aging and provide four examples of products designed by students in Occupational Therapy and Physical Therapy in collaboration with students in Industrial Design at the University of Alberta. These teams also included older adults in the design process. These award-winning designs emphasize the necessity of teamwork and interdisciplinary collaboration. We conclude with an example of the role of a rehabilitation professional as a leader in the conceptualization, design, usability testing, and clinical trial for a commercial version of an e-health wireless sensor technology. Throughout the design phase, ergonomic and human factors were considered in the context of usability of this technology for older adults living in the community.

4.2 DEMOGRAPHICS AND THE DEFINITION OF "OLD"

In Canada, close to 19% of the population will be 65 years or older by 2021, up from 12.3% in 1998.[1] The proportion of seniors in Canada will be four times as high as it was a century before.[1] The first of the baby-boomer generation, those born between 1947 and 1966 (or from 1946 to 1964 in the United States), will reach 65 years in 2012 (2011 in the United States). This group forms 32.4% or the largest proportion of the Canadian population.[2] In the United States, close to 36 million, or 12% of Americans, are aged 65 years or older. This is projected to increase to 72 million, or 20% of the U.S. population in 2030.[3] Globally, there are over 600 million people aged 60 years and older[4] (WHO, 2002). This will increase to 1.2 billion by 2025 and 2 billion by 2050.

It has been argued there is a need to revise our definition of "old." Based on computations using life tables over four decades, Denton and Spencer[5] demonstrate that if 65 years of age was accepted as old in 1951 for males, the definition should be revised to be about 68.5 years of age in 1991. If 65 years was viewed as a male-oriented definition of old in 1951, the corresponding definition for females should be 67.5 years of age in 1951, and 73 or 73.5 years of age in 1991.[5] Given the longer life span of both men and women over the last four decades, and the aging of populations globally, there will likely be an increasing number of older adults staying healthy and working beyond the age of 65 years.

4.3 ERGONOMICS AND OCCUPATIONAL PERFORMANCE

This shift in demographics requires a shift in environmental and product designs. The discipline of ergonomics has traditionally examined the fit of the workplace environment and the ability of human beings to perform safely and productively within that environment.[6] This focus of ergonomics excludes most older adults who are going through the transition from work to retirement, or who have retired but are still engaging in a productive role. They also form a large segment of the consumer population that demands well-designed products. Work or productivity is more appropriately considered in the context of "occupational performance," defined as an individual's experience of being engaged in self-care, productivity, and leisure,[7] or consisting of activities of daily living, instrumental activities of daily living, education, work, play, leisure, and social participation.[8] Although older adults may engage in work beyond 65 years, occupational performance within an older population encompasses activities beyond paid employment. These activities may be productive work performed on a part-time or volunteer basis, or they may be leisure and social activities. Older adults may choose or find themselves in caregiving roles for young children, or other older adults such as spouses, neighbors, and friends.

4.4 MOST OLDER ADULTS LIVE IN THE COMMUNITY

The majority of seniors live at home. In 2001, only about 9% of older women and 5% of older men in Canada lived in institutions and these proportions have declined since 1981.[9] Successful programs and designs meet the needs of seniors who form a major consumer base and address their quality of life in the community. There is great variability between seniors in terms of their levels of occupational performance. While one cannot always assume that a senior experiences challenges, it is prudent to consider the needs of as many clients or users as possible so that the process of aging and "future needs" are considered. This approach has been referred to as a "transgenerational" or "universal design" approach.

- *Consumer base*: The boomers, because of their sheer number, have had a large impact on sale of products, and their needs and lifestyle will continue to drive retail product sales. As the boomers age, they will encounter age-related physical, sensory, and cognitive conditions, as their parents are experiencing today. This experience in caring for their parents is having an impact on their expectations for their own "golden years."
- *Quality of life*: Tomorrow's seniors will be different from today's seniors. It is predicted that, as a whole, the boomers will have more discretionary funds, be more comfortable, and have better access to technologies, and the gender gap will not be as wide as today. There will also be various retirement schemes available to tomorrow's seniors. All of these factors contribute to a cohort of seniors who will have more control over their quality of life compared to today's seniors.
- *Transgenerational approach and universal design*: If we design our products and environments for older adults, we also design for our future selves and multiple generations benefit. A universal design approach also takes into consideration interactions between seniors and younger children, as well as seniors and their care providers who also have ergonomic needs.

4.5 AGE-RELATED CHANGES IN PHYSICAL, SENSORY, AND COGNITIVE FUNCTIONS

Rehabilitation professionals understand the physical, sensory and perceptual, and cognitive changes associated with aging. This aspect of their education and training makes them ideal members of a design team. Rehabilitation professionals, such as occupational and physical therapists, can serve as team members or consultants in opportunities such as home renovations for seniors, design, and postoccupancy assessments of residential care facilities. Health professionals who work with older adults routinely consider ergonomic factors when they perform assessments and provide interventions for this population. However, few therapists participate in the design of products and environments used by older adults. By using their gerontology expertise to inform builders, architects, designers, and policy makers, rehabilitation professionals can help ensure that designs meet ergonomic requirements of seniors. As the baby-boomer population begins to reach the age of 65 years in the next 5 years, there will be an increase in demand for rehabilitation professionals to provide services in the community for this population. It is anticipated that rehabilitation professionals will play a more important role in providing guidance to their clients on decisions regarding home modifications and other strategies to allow seniors to age-in-place. Common age-related changes are now discussed with design implications.

4.5.1 Physical Changes

There is heterogeneity among older adults with regard to physical function. Extrinsic and intrinsic factors contribute to the effects of aging on a person's physical abilities. Extrinsic factors include exercise, nutrition, physical injuries; intrinsic factors include one's genetic makeup and susceptibility to diseases. Typically, aging is associated with a change in muscle strength, endurance, flexibility, posture, and gait.

Lower extremity muscle strength can decline by up to 40% between 30 and 80 years of age.[10] In one study based on 275 participants ranging in age from 30 to 86 years, researchers found that quadriceps muscle strength declined with age and that forward shift of the center of pressure also decreased.[11] This is believed to be the reason that some older adults experience difficulty with sit-to-stand movements from a chair. This movement may be easier with quadriceps strengthening and education on how to get up from a chair. However, it is also important to address environmental factors. For example, clients should use chairs that are the right size for their height and chairs should have armrests, which can be used by the client to push up when doing a sit-to-stand movement. Indeed, it has been found that the timed "Up and Go" test is dependent on chair type and that chairs with armrests and seating heights of 44–47 cm are recommended.[12]

Endurance, or the capacity of muscle to contract continuously at submaximal levels, declines with age.[10] This can affect rehabilitation assessment outcomes. For example, if a client is required to perform maximally during an assessment, the outcome may not reflect the client's actual functional ability during the remainder of the day when energy level or endurance has declined. In a study on the necessity of three trials for the Functional Reach Test, researchers concluded that scores based on one trial, two trials, or the average of two trials for a Functional Reach Test Score were not significantly different from the scores obtained from standard three-trial averages.[13] Therefore, fewer trials during this type of assessment may adequately reflect a client's performance.

Reduced flexibility can occur as a result of biology, hypokinesis (inactivity), or disease, such as arthritis.[14] A decline in strength and spinal flexibility result in

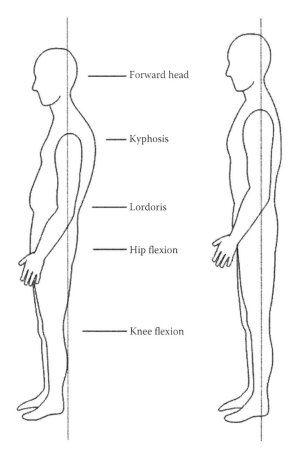

FIGURE 4.1 Posture changes with age. (Illustration with permission from Chris Maley was adapted from Bernstein, C. in *Posture Changes with Age*, F.A. Davis, Philadelphia, PA, 2002.)

postural changes in older adults[10,14] (Figure 4.1). The forward posture of the head and kyphosis reduce the range of upward gaze in older adults. Kinematic data has shown that aging is associated with diminished ankle range of motion or reduced plantar flexion excursion during push-off, and reduced knee extension at the end of swing.[15] In a study on kinematics of stair decent using a three-step stair, researchers reported that stair decent was significantly slower in older subjects compared to younger subjects.[16] Other age-related differences were a reduced peak knee flexion in the sagittal plane, and increased hip and pelvic motion in the frontal and transverse planes, i.e., motion outside the plane of progression. These age-related differences did not change after exercise training three times a week for 12 months.[16]

4.5.1.1 Upper Extremity Coordination

Reaching movements such as repetitive tapping tasks can slow down by 30%–90% with aging according to different studies.[17] This can be attributed to various factors including visual motor processing, central motor processing, and attention. Declining upper extremity strength and endurance may also be factors. Manual dexterity is also affected by aging and the effects can be seen in tasks such as tying shoelaces and fastening buttons.[17] While these age-related changes are observable under experimental conditions, especially when time is used as a variable, they typically do not affect healthy older adults in their daily functional activities.

Design considerations for age-related physical changes:

- Provide benches at regular distances in public spaces to allow older adults to rest.
- Entrance to public washrooms could be designed to allow a variety of mobility aids. Automatic sliding doors and entrances with no door (Figure 4.2) are common in airports. These accommodate the needs of older adults with mobility aids as well as travelers and their luggage.
- In homes, a space under the kitchen sink allows an older adult to work at the sink in a seated position (Figure 4.3). This design also works for wheelchair users.
- Evaluations and assessment batteries used with older adults should cause minimal burden on the client being assessed. If protocol allows, evaluation sessions may be divided to be conducted over two or more sessions.
- User-interface of electronic equipment, such as telephones and household appliances, should be user-friendly and logical to older adults.
- Location and height of signage should take into consideration lower upward gaze due to postural changes.

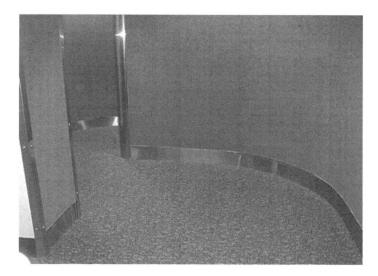

FIGURE 4.2   Door-free entrance to washroom facilitates use by people who have mobility aids and travelers with luggage. (Photo taken by Liu, L., 2004.)

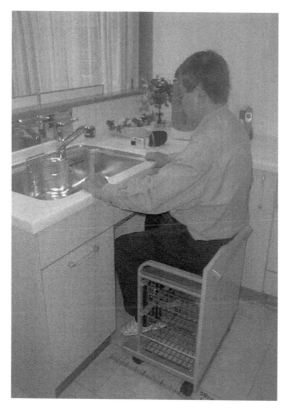

FIGURE 4.3 Junichi Hashimoto, an Edmonton architect, demonstrates use of roll-in seat at kitchen sink located in Hokkaido's Asai Gakuen University Universal Design Show Home. (Photo taken by Liu, L., 2004.)

4.5.2 SENSORY AND PERCEPTUAL CHANGES

4.5.2.1 Vision

In 2003, approximately 3 million Canadian seniors, or 82% of individuals 65 years or older, reported having vision problems.[18] Under normal lighting conditions, twice as much light is required at age 40 years as at age 20 years and three times as much at age 60 years.[19] Aging is associated with reduced visual field size, visual acuity, contrast sensitivity, increased sensitivity to glare and poorer color discrimination.[20] Cloudier lenses, smaller pupils, and fewer rods in the aged eye result in reduced amount of light reaching the retina. Changes in color perception are more evident after the age of 60 years.[21] The reception of short wavelengths (blue) are affected first, then gradually the rest of the spectrum, but the reception of long wavelengths (red) remain relatively unaffected.[21] Yellowing lenses cause seniors to experience difficulty discriminating between color combinations of yellow/white, blue/green, dark blue/black, and purple/dark red.[22] Older adults require more time than younger adults to adapt to darkness.[23] For example, for older adults in their seventies, the point at which rods take over is delayed by 2.5 min compared to adults in their twenties.[23] The time it takes 70-year-olds to reach baseline light sensitivity is over 10 min longer than for 20-year-olds.[23] Driving at night becomes difficult for seniors because of the need to adjust to oncoming headlights and poorly lit streets and signage. Even in the absence of eye disease, decline in visual functions such as delayed dark adaptation restrict older adults' performance in visual tasks that rely on time-critical decisions such as driving, wayfinding in a dark theater, finding one's way to a toilet, or performing work-related tasks.

Cataracts are a leading cause of vision impairment among seniors. In 2003, 20% of Canadians had cataracts.[18] Individuals with cataracts are sensitive to glare, have blurred vision, and difficulty reading in dim light. There is also reduced depth perception at edges of stairs and curbs. Cataract is typically corrected with surgery but can result in loss of vision if left untreated.

A second major cause of vision decline in older adults is macular degeneration, which affects central vision and occurs in 13%–16% of Canadians.[24] Glaucoma affects nearly 7% of Canadians[24] and results in progressive peripheral field loss, reduced contrast sensitivity, and poor night vision.[20] Macular degeneration results in a loss of ability to distinguish facial features, colors, and reduced depth perception. Some seniors have a combination of both.

For age-related changes in vision, design the following considerations:

- Increase size of print including pictures and signage.
- Locate signage at eye level, which may be lower for older adults who use mobility devices such as canes, walkers, or wheelchairs.
- Increase contrast of print; black print on white background is best for most people. In a dimly lit room, white on black is better. However, for people with cataracts, it is necessary to reduce the amount of scatter light surrounding the task, i.e., white letters on black background is easier to read.[20]
- Increase luminance contrast, for example, between floors and walls, door frames and walls, or toilet seat and toilet, can help people with blurry vision to orient themselves in space. Limit the contrast to relevant objects or environmental cues as too many contrasts can make cues difficult to interpret.
- Use color to differentiate between tasks, particularly when luminance contrast is low. Use colors such as orange or red.
- Illuminance preferences differ widely between young and older adults. In fact, older adults prefer lower lighting than younger adults, possibly because of the amount of scattered light produced in the older eyes.[20,25] Therefore, provide options of levels of lighting for older adults to choose from.
- Prevent glare on flooring and other surfaces by choosing material that is not glossy. If carpeting makes mobility difficult, nonglare flooring, such as Marmoleum, other types of nonslip flooring, and tiles are available in the market. Indirect lighting reduces glare. Window coverings can be used to reduce or eliminate glare during part of the day.
- Keep flooring simple; complex patterns (Figure 4.4) can be misinterpreted as "holes" by people with partial vision.

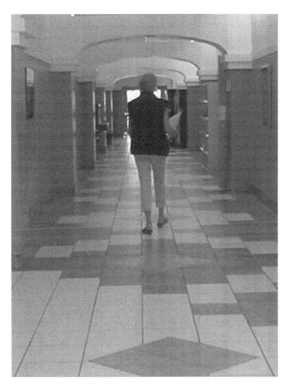

FIGURE 4.4 Complex floor patterns can confuse older adults with low vision. (Photo taken by Liu, L., 2005.)

- Avoid "dangerous edges" (Figure 4.5a) by using high contrast between wall and flooring (Figure 4.5b). Complex visual cues on stairs can be confusing (Figure 4.6a), keep cues simple by contrasting the tread from the riser and nosing of each step (Figure 4.6b).

4.5.2.2 Hearing, Taste, Smell, and Touch

Approximately one-third of older adults between 65 and 74 years, and 50% of those between 75 and 79 years experience hearing loss.[26] Hearing loss can be conductive, sensorineural, or mixed type. Causes of hearing loss include noise exposure, tumors, and diseases. The most common type of hearing loss is "presbycusis," which refers to "sensorineural hearing loss that is associated with aging"[26] (p. 1315). An older adult tends to have difficulty discerning high-frequency sounds such as higher-pitched voices of women or children. Older adults can have difficulty understanding speech when conversing in a crowd or when there is background noise.

Our sense of smell and fine taste begins to decline in the sixth decade.[26] Olfactory function declines by 40% with aging[27] and can affect one's ability to detect unpleasant odors. By age 50 years, adults can lose up to 50% of their taste buds at the front of the tongue.[27] As sweet and salty taste buds atrophy first, older adults may

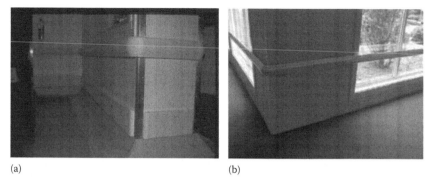

(a)   (b)

FIGURE 4.5 (a) Dangerous edge. (Photo taken by Liu, L., 2002.) (b) High contrast between wall and floor facilitates wayfinding for people with low vision, or for cognitively impaired older adults. (Photo taken by Liu, L., 2004.)

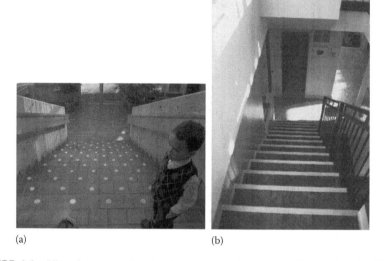

(a)   (b)

FIGURE 4.6 View from top of stairs: (a) complex visual cues. (Photo taken by Liu, L., 2003); and (b) simple, effective visual cues. (Photo taken by Wickman, R., 2006.)

think that their food taste bitter or sour. These sensory changes frequently result in lowered appetites and a declined interest in meals.

Touch sensitivity varies widely among older adults, but touch thresholds among older adults have been shown to be significantly higher than in younger adults.[28] Thermal sensitivity in the extremities declines with age, particularly in the foot.[29]

Designing considerations for age-related changes in hearing, taste, smell, and touch:

- Approach all older clients with the assumption that there is some degree of hearing loss. This prepares the professional to use approaches that help ensure a client fully participates in the communication process.

- The environment for interview and intervention should facilitate communication through senses other than hearing, such as vision and touch. Communication should occur with eye contact, with minimal or no competing background noise.
- Auditory signals from telephone and smoke detector may not be detectable by older adults who are hard of hearing. Redundancies such as a visual signal can be installed. Remote monitoring of frail older adults living alone is a possibility. This can be done through the use of webcams, provided issues of privacy and security are carefully addressed.
- Demonstrate to clients and family caregivers strategies to deal with declining smell. For example, refrigerated foods can be labeled with an expiry date so that older adults do not have to rely on smell to detect when food is no longer fit for eating. Seniors may not detect leaking gas through smell, therefore, an auditory gas detector can be installed in homes. As taste is affected by aging, older adults who cook for others can rely on measuring utensils and avoid cooking to their taste.
- A decrease in tactile sensitivity stimuli can mean that older clients apply firmer pressure on buttons that operate devices. They are adversely affected by thermal extremes; therefore, provide living spaces where they can control the thermostat or room temperature.

4.5.3 COGNITIVE CHANGES

Longitudinal studies show that in normal aging, crystallized intelligence, or cumulative information and knowledge, can increase up to the seventh decade and may not decrease until late old age.[30] However, cognitive speed and memory show a linear decline from early adulthood and the decline may accelerate in late old age.[30] Evidence suggests that cognitive speed can decline by 20% at age 40 years and by 40%–60% at age 80 years.[30] With respect to memory, aging is associated with a decline in episodic memory, or memory for events,[31] for example, where we put our keys or parked the car, where we had met someone, and when we had an appointment. Semantic memory associated with highly practiced skills, such as playing the piano and typing, remains constant with aging. However, semantic memory for new information and skills is subjected to age-related declines in performance.[31]

Working memory, or the temporary storage of information, is affected by aging. The multicomponent model of working memory first introduced by Baddeley and Hitch[32] described working memory as consisting of a central executive system, which manipulates information within working memory and controls two storage systems: the phonological loop (auditory information) and the visuospatial scratchpad (visual and spatial information). Recently, based on evidence that not all information can be categorized as auditory or visuospatial alone, a fourth system has been added to the model—the episodic buffer.[33] It is postulated that the episodic buffer holds information from other systems and long-term memory and integrates them into scenes or episodes.[34]

Working memory has been demonstrated to decline with age. For example, in one study, subjects aged 20 to more than 75 years were divided into four groups and given memory updating tasks.[35] The tasks required them to remember the smallest items in each list and to update each piece of information by minimizing irrelevant information or intrusions from items on the previous lists. Researchers reported that the oldest old group, or those older than 75 years, performed worse in memory updating, had the most intrusion errors, and demonstrated the most difficulty with increased task demand.[35] Similar findings have been reported in experimental tasks that simulate everyday activities. In a study that examined age-related cognitive changes, subjects were asked to use a touch screen to follow a series of 14 event-based shopping errand instructions using a virtual street scene on a computer.[36] Older subjects aged 61–80 years and younger university student subjects participated in the study. Researchers concluded that older subjects were less likely than the younger subjects to remember the correct action (e.g., buy a map) associated with a location cue (e.g., Barnes and Noble). Further, older subjects performed significantly worse when they had only one trial, as opposed to three trials, to learn the association between the cue and action.[36]

Design considerations for age-related changes in memory:

- Create environments that are familiar to older adults. This is particularly important in a residential care facility that targets residents from a specific culture, such as Chinese elders, or a specific cohort, such as veterans. Familiarity facilitates a sense of "homelikeness" and allows learning through integration of new information with long-term memory.
- Instructions for therapeutic intervention or operation of equipment and devices should be restricted to a minimal number of steps. If learning of more complex steps is involved, adequate time, education, and follow-up should be designed into the training process.
- Redundant cues, e.g., visual and auditory, would facilitate registration of information. For example, when giving verbal instructions, also provide visual demonstration or illustration. Therapeutic tasks should be meaningful to older users to draw on semantic memory.

4.6 AGING AND UNIVERSAL DESIGN

Rehabilitation professionals have an understanding of the aging process and ergonomics. They strive to enable older adults to function and remain within their homes or chosen environments. Rehabilitation professionals are often the first service providers to encounter a need for a home or workplace to be adapted for a client who has experienced a temporary, chronic, or permanent disability. In this way, rehabilitation professionals are consultants to the process of environmental, product, or task modification for a client. As the aging demographic continues to grow, more of the "young-old," or the preretirement cohort, are planning for their future. When there is an opportunity for home renovation or for building a new home, some individuals seek advice on how to "age-proof" or "future-proof" their homes. Rehabilitation professionals who provide consultations in these situations take on a proactive role that will benefit current and future generations. The concept of universal design focuses on the creation of environments and products that meet the needs of older adults. This is a different perspective from the traditional rehabilitation approach of improving an individual's function so that the individual may adapt to the environment.

While the concept of universal design is too broad of a concept for some, and may not seem possible to mandate or legislate, the concept of "visitability" is practical. Visitability can be viewed as a subset of universal design. Visitability is a movement begun by Eleanor Smith of Concrete Change[37] to "change construction practices so that virtually all new homes—not merely those custom-built for occupants who currently have disabilities—offer a few specific features that make the home easier for people who develop a mobility impairment to live in and visit." A visitable home must possess at least the following three features:

- Wide passage doors
- At least a half bath/powder room on the main floor
- At least one zero-step entrance approached by an accessible route on a firm surface no steeper than 1:12, proceeding from a driveway or public sidewalk (Figure 4.7)

Bolingbrook, Illinois passed legislation in 2004 for all homebuilders and developers to adhere to a "Visitability Ordinance." An updated list of visitability initiatives across the United States is available at the Centre for Inclusive Design and Environment's Web site.[38] In Canada, a visitability initiative has begun under the leadership of Laurie Ringaert and in partnership with the Canadian Centre on Disability Studies. More information can be found on their Web site.[39]

Accessibility as a movement was precursor to the current trend of designing for aging. The Americans with Disability Act (ADA) of 1990[40,41] has been the driving force behind barrier-free design in the United States. The Act specifies that

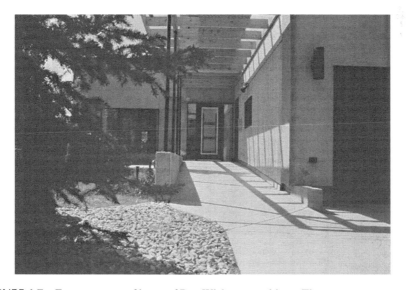

FIGURE 4.7 Front entrance of home of Ron Wickman, architect. The entrance was created to make R. Wickman's home visitable for his father, Percy Wickman, who used a wheelchair. Percy Wickman served as a politician and was an advocate for persons with disabilities. (Photo taken by Wickman, R., 2006.)

persons with disabilities cannot be discriminated against with respect to employment, transportation, public accommodations, and telecommunications. Although Canada does not have legislation like the ADA, standards do exist for accessible design. For example, the Canadian Standards Association (CSA) International has several National Standard of Canada reports including Accessible Design for the Built Environment,[42] which describes how to make buildings accessible for people with physical or sensory disabilities; and barrier-free design for automated banking machines (ATM),[43] which describes requirements for designing and manufacturing accessible wall-mounted and stand alone, but excluding drive through, ATMs.

More recently, aging is becoming a driving force behind universal or inclusive design. Inclusion of older people and people with disabilities in the mainstream of design does not guarantee the design to be usable by all individuals.[44] However, consideration of design needs from the perspective of older adults can help ensure that a designer considers multiple disabilities (physical, sensory, and cognitive) that challenge older adults. The CSA standards for Inclusive Design for an Aging Population[45] provide core principles, guiding concepts and tools for the design, and provision of products, services, and environments for seniors and those with age-related disabilities. It is important to note that in these guidelines, design of services is included with the design of products and environments. This is in recognition of the importance of good service to address needs that cannot be addressed through good physical design, as well, user satisfaction of a product or environment depends on the associated service and support.

As the proportion of seniors increases globally, the trend is to go beyond designing for people with disabilities or age-related ailments, and to adopt a more inclusive attitude, with attention to esthetics as well as aging-in-place. "Universal design is the design of products, buildings, and exterior spaces to be usable by all people to the greatest extent possible without the need for adaptation or specialized design."[46,47] Proponents of universal design do not negate the need for customized and accessible design altogether. Instead, they are striving to remove boundaries between designs for mainstream and designs for some special populations. For example, environmental control units were originally designed as assistive devices for people with disabilities. Now, variations of these, such as the television remote control, are used by everyone. Indeed, the concept of "smart houses" relies on electronic control of the living environment, remotely or preprogrammed to meet the needs of the resident. When a product or environment benefits the mainstream population, there is a reduction in stigma faced by people regardless of their disability or age. As well, it accommodates people who are "temporarily" handicapped.

The seven principles of universal design were created by a group of 10 experts in 1997 at the Centre for Universal Design, North Carolina State University.[48] Each principle is accompanied by four or five guidelines. The principles are

1. *Equitable use*: The design is useful and marketable to people with diverse abilities.
2. *Flexibility in use*: The design accommodates a wide range of individual preferences and abilities.

3. *Simple and intuitive use*: Use of the design is easy to understand, regardless of the user's experience, knowledge, language skills, or current concentration level.

4. *Perceptible information*: The design communicates necessary information effectively to the user, regardless of ambient conditions or the user's sensory abilities.

5. *Tolerance for error*: The design minimizes hazards and the adverse consequences of accidental or unintended actions.

6. *Low physical effort*: The design can be used efficiently and comfortably, and with a minimum of fatigue.

7. *Size and space for approach and use*: Appropriate size and space is provided for approach, reach, manipulation, and use, regardless of the user's body size, posture, or mobility.

Table 4.1 provides a Product Evaluation Countdown (CUD, 2002), a scale that can be used by consumers to evaluate the usability of a product.[49] A survey of items related to the principles of universal design has been developed by Story and colleagues[50,51] and tested in a controlled usability tests of products.[52]

4.7 DESIGN FOR AGING—STUDENTS IN REHABILITATION LEARN A RELEVANT ROLE

Aging populations can benefit from designs that accommodate a wide range of functional needs, yet are esthetically acceptable and not stigmatizing. One strategy is to provide learning content on assistive technology and devices in the context of universal design. Another strategy is to promote interdisciplinary collaboration between students in rehabilitation and students in design. Some examples of the outcomes of such collaboration are now presented. One purpose is to provide the reader with illustrations of how ergonomics and human factor can be applied to the design of products that enable daily function in older adults, yet the products are inclusive, not segregating. Another purpose is to highlight the benefits of interdisciplinary collaboration between rehabilitation professionals and designers. Of course, successful design must also be informed by the users—older adults themselves.

Since 1997, the Faculty of Rehabilitation Medicine and the Faculty of Arts have collaborated in providing students with opportunities to apply universal design principles to product designs for seniors.* Students in Rehabilitation Medicine† and Industrial Design are familiarized with the following concepts:

---

* Rehabilitation course instructor: Lili Liu; industrial design course instructors: Peter Galonski (from 1997 to 1999) and Robert Lederer (from 1999 to present).
† Rehabilitation medicine students were in either the fourth year of the BSc occupational therapy, or the third year of the BSc physical therapy program.

TABLE 4.1
Universal Design: Product Evaluation Countdown

Have you ever regretted buying a product because it turned out to be difficult to use? Maybe the package was hard for you to open, the instructions were hard to understand, or the controls were hard to operate.

Each of us is unique in our abilities to think, see, hear, handle things, and move around. Products that are easy to use for one person may not be easy for another, whether because of the user's personal abilities or their environment. Everyone has different personal preferences too.

Each of us must consider our own abilities and preferences, and sometimes also the abilities and preferences of other people in our household, when we select products.

Universal design is an approach to make products and environments as usable as possible for people of all ages and abilities.

The checklist on the following pages is based on the seven Principles of Universal Design. This list can help you think about your own needs and those of other potential users when selecting products.

When you use this checklist to count down your evaluation of a product, you will agree with some statements more than others. The more statements you agree with, the more likely it is that the product will be easy to use, for you and the other people who might use it—and the less likely you will regret buying it.

This work was supported by a grant from the National Institute on Disability and Rehabilitation Research, U.S. Dept. of Education. The opinions contained in this publication are those of the grantee and do not necessarily reflect those of the sponsor.

© 2002 The Center for Universal Design, N.C. State University Campus Box 8613, Raleigh, NC 27695-8613

1-800-647-6777; cud@ncsu.edu

http://www.design.ncsu.edu/cud

PRINCIPLE 7. Size and Space for Approach and Use

7A.	It's easy for me to see all the important elements of this product from any position (such as standing or seated). *Comments:*	Not Important	Strongly Disagree	Disagree	Neutral	Agree	Strongly Agree
7B.	It's easy for me to reach all the important elements of this product from any position (such as standing or seated). *Comments:*	Not Important	Strongly Disagree	Disagree	Neutral	Agree	Strongly Agree

	Not Important	Strongly Disagree	Disagree	Neutral	Agree	Strongly Agree
7C. This product fits my hand size. *Comments:*	Not Important	Strongly Disagree	Disagree	Neutral	Agree	Strongly Agree
7D. There is enough space for me to use this product with the devices or assistance that I need. *Comments:*	Not Important	Strongly Disagree	Disagree	Neutral	Agree	Strongly Agree

PRINCIPLE 6. Low Physical Effort

	Not Important	Strongly Disagree	Disagree	Neutral	Agree	Strongly Agree
6A. I can use this product comfortably—without awkward movements or uncomfortable postures. *Comments:*	Not Important	Strongly Disagree	Disagree	Neutral	Agree	Strongly Agree
6B. I can use this product without overexerting myself. *Comments:*	Not Important	Strongly Disagree	Disagree	Neutral	Agree	Strongly Agree
6C. I can use this product without having to repeat any motion enough to cause fatigue or pain. *Comments:*	Not Important	Strongly Disagree	Disagree	Neutral	Agree	Strongly Agree
6D. I don't have to rest after using this product. *Comments:*	Not Important	Strongly Disagree	Disagree	Neutral	Agree	Strongly Agree

PRINCIPLE 5. Tolerance for Error

	Not Important	Strongly Disagree	Disagree	Neutral	Agree	Strongly Agree
5A. The product features I use most are the easiest to reach. *Comments:*	Not Important	Strongly Disagree	Disagree	Neutral	Agree	Strongly Agree
5B. This product protects me from potential hazards. *Comments:*	Not Important	Strongly Disagree	Disagree	Neutral	Agree	Strongly Agree
5C. If I make a mistake, it won't cause damage or hurt me. *Comments:*	Not Important	Strongly Disagree	Disagree	Neutral	Agree	Strongly Agree
5D. This product forces me to pay attention during critical tasks. *Comments:*	Not Important	Strongly Disagree	Disagree	Neutral	Agree	Strongly Agree

(continued)

TABLE 4.1 (continued)
Universal Design: Product Evaluation Countdown

PRINCIPLE 4.   Perceptible Information

		Not Important	Strongly Disagree	Disagree	Neutral	Agree	Strongly Agree
4A.	I can use this product without hearing.	Not Important	Strongly Disagree	Disagree	Neutral	Agree	Strongly Agree
	Comments:						
4B.	I can use this product without vision.	Not Important	Strongly Disagree	Disagree	Neutral	Agree	Strongly Agree
	Comments:						
4C.	I can easily identify the features of this product in order to use instruction manuals or telephone help lines.	Not Important	Strongly Disagree	Disagree	Neutral	Agree	Strongly Agree
	Comments:						
4D.	I can use this product with the aids, devices, or techniques that I use.	Not Important	Strongly Disagree	Disagree	Neutral	Agree	Strongly Agree
	Comments:						

PRINCIPLE 3.   Simple and Intuitive Use

		Not Important	Strongly Disagree	Disagree	Neutral	Agree	Strongly Agree
3A.	This product is as simple and straightforward as it can be.	Not Important	Strongly Disagree	Disagree	Neutral	Agree	Strongly Agree
	Comments:						
3B.	This product works just like I expect it to work.	Not Important	Strongly Disagree	Disagree	Neutral	Agree	Strongly Agree
	Comments:						
3C.	I understand the language used in this product.	Not Important	Strongly Disagree	Disagree	Neutral	Agree	Strongly Agree
	Comments:						
3D.	The most important features of this product are the most obvious.	Not Important	Strongly Disagree	Disagree	Neutral	Agree	Strongly Agree
	Comments:						
3E.	This product lets me know that I'm using it the right way.	Not Important	Strongly Disagree	Disagree	Neutral	Agree	Strongly Agree
	Comments:						

PRINCIPLE 2. Flexibility in Use

2A.	I can use this product in whatever way is effective for me.	Not Important	Strongly Disagree	Disagree	Neutral	Agree	Strongly Agree
	Comments:						
2B.	I can use this product with either my right or left side (hand or foot) alone.	Not Important	Strongly Disagree	Disagree	Neutral	Agree	Strongly Agree
	Comments:						
2C.	I can use this product precisely and accurately.	Not Important	Strongly Disagree	Disagree	Neutral	Agree	Strongly Agree
	Comments:						
2D.	I can use this product at whatever pace I want (quickly or slowly).	Not Important	Strongly Disagree	Disagree	Neutral	Agree	Strongly Agree
	Comments:						

PRINCIPLE 1. Equitable Use

1A.	This product is as usable for me as it is for anyone else.	Not Important	Strongly Disagree	Disagree	Neutral	Agree	Strongly Agree
	Comments:						
1B.	Using this product doesn't make me feel segregated or stigmatized.	Not Important	Strongly Disagree	Disagree	Neutral	Agree	Strongly Agree
	Comments:						
1C.	This product gives me needed privacy, security, and safety.	Not Important	Strongly Disagree	Disagree	Neutral	Agree	Strongly Agree
	Comments:						
1D.	The design of this product appeals to me.	Not Important	Strongly Disagree	Disagree	Neutral	Agree	Strongly Agree
	Comments:						

Source: CUD, *Universal Design: Product Evaluation Countdown,* Centre for Universal Design, NCSU, 2002. With permission.

- *Partnerships and team work*
  - ○ Students learn about each discipline's areas of expertise, develop group norms, and establish team expectations. Students learn about patents and intellectual property.
- *Research*
  - ○ Market—demographics, functional needs of older people, who is the buyer and who is the end user, pros and cons of existing products, history of the product and future trends, levels of consumer awareness. Development of a persona (case study) helps teams focus on their goals.
  - ○ Function—what does the product do, how is it used, what are the mechanisms, how many tasks must it be capable of, will it do these with the least aggravation to the user, adaptability or additions. Students begin to apply principles of universal design.
  - ○ Ergonomics—activity analysis, what are the user-interface concerns, how is the product handled and used, how does the individual directly engage with it, how easy is it to use, what are the safety concerns, and willingness of user to use it. Students often engage older adults at this stage, if not earlier, to validate their ideas.
  - ○ Engineering—structure considerations, material choices, manufacturing options, recycling issues, mechanics, standards, codes.
  - ○ Economics—do the numbers of users warrant mass production versus batch production, long-term production investment or short-term investment, affordability, stages in production, or a range of products.
  - ○ Ideation—act of generating an innovative approach to address and solve the problem or need. Through brainstorming, lateral thinking, and thinking out of the box, the rehabilitation students and industrial design students bring as many options and ideas as possible to address the components of the design problem. To avoid committing to a quick solution, design teams will consider a broad range of options as they fill the idea funnel (create as many options as possible, eliminate options and develop ideas, and refine and select options). Considerations during ideation state include: form follows function, form follows content, product identity, symbolism, communication, visual language, cultural issues, trends, retro, materials, color, perception. The presentation to the client is in the form of sketches or quick form studies. From this presentation, choices, selections, and composites are made, which are then developed and put back into the design funnel.
  - ○ Concept development—Still a number of options are on the table, and teams go through eliminations. Evaluations during the concept development stage include
    - ■ Functional concerns (will it do what is expected).
    - ■ Scale, proportion, composition (do these work).
    - ■ Perception (does its appearance reflect its value or added value or what it does, is it appropriate).
    - ■ Does the form show the user how it works or its orientation.
    - ■ Two or three renderings or accurate models of the concept are presented. Selections are made and the project moves into further design refinement and drawings for mold making. Technical problems are addressed.

- Teams may stop at this stage to make an actual full-scale model or prototype to test the product.
- Students verify they have addressed the relevant principles of universal design. Students also verify they have addressed relevant human factors and ergonomics of the targeted users. These factors include cognitive abilities (memory, speed of processing), perceptual abilities (vision, hearing, touch), physical abilities (strength, endurance, balance, coordination), and behavior (wandering, social interaction).

The following student designs illustrate how aging and ergonomics are considered in the context of universal design. The high success rate of this collaborative initiative, as demonstrated by the number of award-winning designs, highlights the importance of interdisciplinary collaboration.

4.7.1 EXAMPLE 1

The Tee Planter (Figure 4.8a) was designed by industrial design students Darren Tonn and Reza Bacchus, and rehabilitation students Paul Laliberte and D'Arcy Gainor. It received a Bronze Medal in the 2000 American Society on Aging Universal Design Competition.

This universal design is appealing to golfers of all ages. The students used a persona of a 68-year-old male who had osteoarthritis, a right hip replacement, and chronic low back pain. The objective was to create a design that would eliminate repetitive bending and squatting (Figure 4.8b) so that individuals can play an entire game of golf without having to bend over. Such a device would be useful for individuals with restricted range of motion in the hip, knee, and ankle joints, lower extremity amputees, paraplegics, individuals who need to conserve energy, hypertension, balance deficits, arthritis, or golfers who love gadgets.

An elbow-shaped device is placed at the end of a golf club (Figure 4.8c). When a golf and tee are placed inside the device, high-density foam keeps them in place (Figure 4.8d through f). When pressure is applied on the ball and tee as it is being planted into the ground, a space is created between the foam and the ball (Figure 4.8g), allowing the device to be removed leaving the ball and tee in place (Figure 4.8h). The device can be used to scoop the ball out of the hole (Figure 4.8i), it can also be pulled off the end of the club so it could be fitted onto the end of any club handle, or it can be clipped to the belt or bag, making it versatile and portable.

The simple solution has no moving parts. Its organic shape imitates the hand motion of planting the ball and tee into the ground. It does not stigmatize and could be used by all golfers to consistently plant the tee and ball.

4.7.2 EXAMPLE 2

The Aurora Universal Iron was designed by industrial design students Heather Eadie and Helen Gregson, and rehabilitation students Jocelyn Cromwell and Cindy Holmes. The students wanted to address the common conditions in older populations: reduced vision, decreased stamina, decreased strength, arthritis, weakness due to stroke, and paralysis, as well as other chronic conditions such as multiple sclerosis. The design of most irons do not take into consideration these obstacles faced by

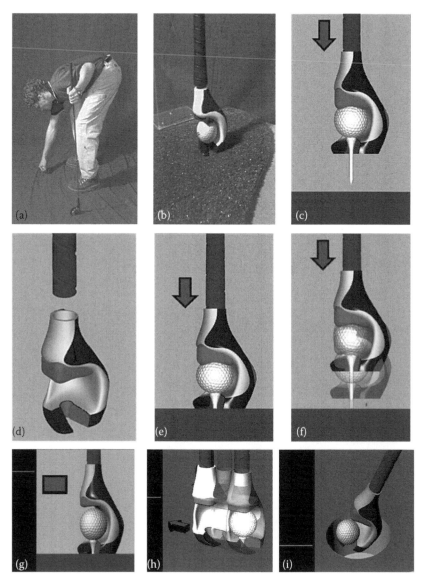

FIGURE 4.8   (a–i) The "Tee Planter." (Photos and images by Darren Tonn, Reza Bacchus, Paul Laliberte, and D'Arcy Gainor, 1999.)

older adults. Iron handles are not ergonomically designed and cause improper positioning of wrist and hand (Figure 4.9a). Dials and controls are difficult to read and use (Figure 4.9b). Cords can be difficult to manage.

The shape and position of the handle are redesigned. Two handles allow for several possible hand positions depending on user needs and increases the number of people who can use the iron (Figure 4.9c and d). The cylindrical handle is angled at 60° to encourage correct positioning of the wrist. The handle tapers

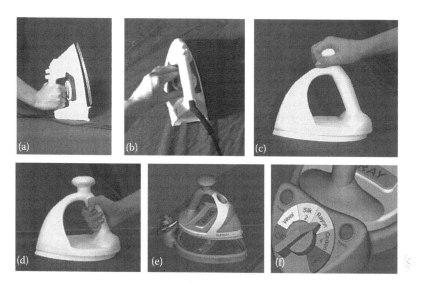

FIGURE 4.9   (a–f) The "Aurora." (Photos and images by Heather Eadie, Helen Gregson, Jocelyn Cromwell, and Cindy Holmes, 1999.)

from 3.5 cm diameter at the top to 3 cm diameter at the bottom. This allows for a comfortable hand position for any size of hand and creates a power grip, thereby increasing control of the iron. There is ample space around the handle to accommodate larger hands and knuckles. The round, knob-type handle at the top of the iron is 6 cm in diameter and fits comfortably in the palm of most hands. This handle can be used by people with decreased dexterity and poor mobility of the hand. Both handles provide comfortable hand positioning while the user is sitting or standing. The handles have comfortable rubber foam grips to provide tactile input and to facilitate control.

The Aurora is cordless (Figure 4.9e). The iron has a lighter weight than existing designs because the mechanics are located in the charger unit. It allows greater freedom of movement because there is no cord to get in the way. Larger, easier to use controls are located on the charger unit rather than on the iron itself. The large temperature controls are easy to read and dials or buttons click into place (Figure 4.9f). The need to lift the iron and rest it on its end is eliminated. The soleplate is Teflon-coated to ease gliding. The teardrop shape allows for greater efficiency of movement because it has no straight edges and can be moved in any direction. The clear water tank, with large opening, is easy to fill. Safety features include a bumper around the soleplate, automatic shutoff, and easy cord management.

Ideally, the Aurora would be used as part of an improved system of ironing. The act of ironing itself can be quite tiring as it involves standing for a prolonged period of time and a lot of bending and twisting to move garments. The ironing board and seat should be adjustable. An attached clothing basket and hanging rack should be used to minimize energy expenditure through reduced movement. Rounded, wider boards provide more work area within easy reach. Clothing is also less prone to fall off a wider board.

4.7.3 EXAMPLE 3

The Real Chair (Figure 4.10a) was designed by industrial design students Trish Bell and Chet Domanski, and rehabilitation students Jen Dong and Donna Scovil. It received a Silver Medal in the 2000 American Society on Aging Universal Design Competition. The purpose of the design was to address the issue of "geri-chairs" used in nursing homes with residents. Current chairs are institutional in appearance, large, and can be heavy, making residents dependent on help from staff. The students wanted to present a rolling seat that was more esthetically acceptable. Staff can assist a resident to sit or transfer into the chair, then roll the resident comfortably to the edge of the table. When a resident has completed his or her meal, the resident can push away from the table instead of waiting for assistance from staff. A braking mechanism is activated when pressure is placed on the armrest, thereby allowing the user to safely stand up or transfer to a wheelchair (Figure 4.10b).

Specifications include lumbar support 8 in. above the seat. Padding toward the front of the armrest indicate where to place hands when standing or sitting. Polyurethane castors can be used on both linoleum and carpet and do not mark surfaces. Crypton fabric is suggested as it is resistant to spills, stains, and bacteria.

4.7.4 EXAMPLE 4

The Simplicity Range was designed by industrial design students Cam Frith and Zsolt Kovacs, and rehabilitation students Sophie Wilderdijk and Mary Ellen Lamont. This design won the Gold Medal in the 2000 American Society on Aging competition. This design addressed the functional limitations experienced by many older adults in performing instrumental activities of daily living such as meal preparation. An analysis of the task of using a conventional showed that users are required to bend down to open the oven door, reach into the oven or move a rack out of the oven, and lift meals from the oven onto the counter. These movements require adequate

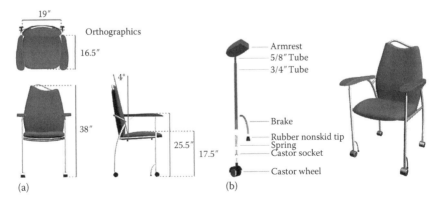

FIGURE 4.10 (a,b) The "Real Chair." (Images by Trish Bel, Chet Domanski, Jen Dong, and Donna Scovil, 1999.)

range of motion and strength in the upper extremities, back and lower extremities, power grip, visual acuity, depth perception, and good balance. Leg weakness can prevent someone from using proper body mechanics such as bending the knees. Ovens with side-hinged doors do not address the problem of lifting heavy items with arms extended into the hot oven. Bottom-hindged wall ovens require users to lift items from countertop and the door can impede reach into the oven. One German (AEG) design uses a sliding door, but the rack is fixed. Commonly, it is not intuitive for users to know which knobs operate which burners. Digital controls require dexterity and displays may be difficult for older adults to read due to lack of contrast and small print.

The Simplicity Range has the following features that make it ergonomically suitable for the older individual to use. Large control knobs with 180° turning range reduces hand and wrist motion (Figure 4.11a). The high contrast visual scale and incremental steps facilitates accurate and intuitive operation. The oven door pulls straight out, and the rack is affixed to the door rather than the interior of the oven. The oven door can be opened with minimal joint range demands in the hands, wrists, hips, and knees, assisting individuals with osteoporosis, total hip replacement, disk degeneration, and arthritis (Figure 4.11b). The self-raising rack eliminates need for reaching in or lifting the item (Figure 4.11c).

The induction stovetop is common in the market. As a feature of the Simplicity Range, the stovetop can be used to temporarily hold the meal after it comes out of the oven, thereby eliminating the need to life the meal. Advantages of an induction stovetop include easier cleanup of spills, no flames or hot-elements, which can ignite fabric.

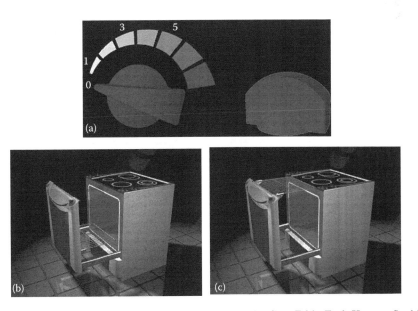

FIGURE 4.11 (a–c) The "Simplicity Range." (Images by Cam Frith, Zsolt Kovacs, Sophie Wilderdijk, and Mary Ellen Lamont, 1999.)

4.8 ROLE OF REHABILITATION IN CONCEPTUALIZATION, DESIGN, CLINICAL TRIAL, USABILITY TESTING, AND COMMERCIALIZATION

"Usability" or "user friendliness" and "ease of use[53]" refer to a set of characteristics of a product or environment from the perspective of users. Usability testing relates to the concept of iterative design where a design in an early stage is presented to users who provide data on aspects of the design that work and other aspects that cause frustration. If warranted, the product is redesigned and retested.[53] Rehabilitation professionals can undertake or participate in usability testing of products by applying their knowledge base of aging, function, and ergonomics. This knowledge should increase the chances that a product meets the needs of older adult users. In environmental design, rehabilitation professionals can provide consultation at the design phase and conduct or participate in postoccupancy evaluations, which will inform future designs. Rehabilitation researchers can apply quantitative and qualitative research approaches that correspond to their research objectives and respondent characteristics.

4.9 REHABILITATION AS A LEADER IN DESIGN FOR AGING

Nichols et al.[54] describe a hypothetical case study of a home telemedicine system for older adults to illustrate task analysis and age-related changes that need to be considered in designs for aging. The hypothetical case involved a system that required clients to measure their blood glucose level and then to transmit the data into a computer each evening using USB. This section describes the realization of this hypothetical case study through wireless technology that does not even require home care clients to use a computer.

Telehealth is the delivery of health services at a distance, in real time or asynchronously. These health services include assessments, interventions, follow-up, consultations with specialists, and supervision of support personnel or helping and supporting informal caregivers in the delivery of rehabilitation interventions. Telehealth encompasses telerehabilitation, teledermatology, telepsychiatry, etc. Telehealth may also be used interchangeably with telemedicine. In 2002, Dr. Masako Miyazaki (Figure 4.12), an occupational therapist and researcher at the University of Alberta, conceptualized the application of Bluetooth technology for wireless monitoring of physiological readings of home care clients. The wireless wearable physiological monitor (WWPM) was designed and developed by a team of engineers, computing scientists, health professionals, and other scientists from Canada and Japan. The system is depicted in Figure 4.13. Pulse data are collected continuously by the wearable pulse sensor (WPS) (Figure 4.14a) and the data are picked up by the wireless system (WS) (Figure 4.14b), which are sent to a central server. A glucose meter can be used to collect blood and send glucose level readings to the server via the WS. A client's health professional can use a password to sign onto a Web site to read the client's physiological data. The client and the health professional can use the WS to program regular reminders such as take medications, blood sugar readings, or to call the health professional. Clients can also contact the health professional by pushing the "Call" button.

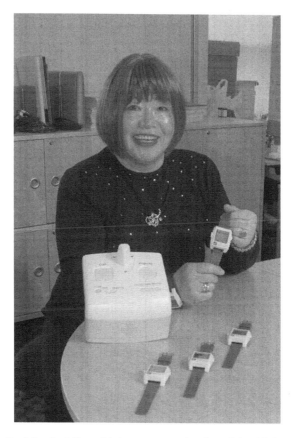

FIGURE 4.12   Dr. Masako Miyazaki demonstrates the size of the WPS which is worn on the wrist like a watch, and the WS, which uses Bluetooth to transmit data to a central server. (Photo by Bourque, T., *Edmontonians*, March 2006.)

The features of the watch and WS were originally designed with a focus on elderly clients as the target users. This elderly population would be receiving home care services and be monitored by a health care team for chronic conditions such as diabetes and heart disease. In addition, these individuals would be experiencing common age-related conditions such as functional limitations in vision, hearing, mobility, balance, coordination, and finger dexterity. Therefore, careful consideration of these factors, in addition to the technological requirements of Bluetooth, resulted in the designs depicted in Figure 4.14a and b. Visual displays, labels, and buttons on the WPS are large. Buttons and labels on the WS are readable with good contrast (black on white). An instruction manual used 16 points Arial font, actual photos of the technologies, and training was provided to clients and their informal caregivers.

Once the WWPM system and devices were designed and developed, they were tested in a trial consisting of 98 home care clients with chronic conditions, 25 community-residing frail seniors, and 26 healthy older adults. The trial examined the feasibility, validity, and usability of the WWPM. All older adult participants and

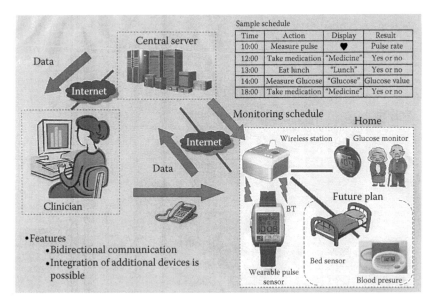

FIGURE 4.13   Wireless wearable physiological monitor. (Image by Miyazaki, M., 2005.)

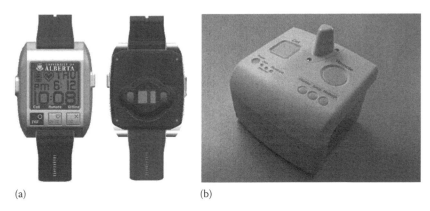

(a)   (b)

FIGURE 4.14   (a) WPS. (Image by Miyazaki, M., 2005.) (b) Wireless system. (Photo taken by Miyazaki, M., 2007.)

health professionals involved completed questionnaires or interviews to provide feedback based on their experiences. The data included the usability of the WPS, glucose meter, and the WS from the perspectives of clients and health professionals. The trial proved to be a constructive and valuable phase in the further development of the WWPM. However, as considerations for age-related functional challenges were addressed at the beginning, recommendations for modifications after the trial were not considered to be major. The trial also informed developers and health professionals about strategies for using the WPS with clients who experienced mild cognitive impairment. Despite the clarity of the user-interface, clients with impaired executive function were using the Call buttons when they did not need to call a health professional. In these cases, where a family caregiver was with the client, an effective strategy was to hide the WS under a cloth or cover so that the client could not see the system.

4.10 SUMMARY

As older adults form an increasing client base for rehabilitation professionals, the focus of health services need to be directed to the community where older adults prefer to live. In order to enhance their quality of life and promote aging-in-place, more attention needs to be directed to the design of products, environments, and services. Rehabilitation professionals have expertise in ergonomics and human factors as they relate to age-related changes. In collaboration with members of the design disciplines, rehabilitation professionals can make a noticeable impact on older adults as a population.

REFERENCES

1. Statistics Canada, *A Portrait of Seniors in Canada*, Catalogue number 89-519-XPE, Statistics Canada, Ottawa, 1997.
2. Foot, D., *Boom, Bust & Echo 2000—Profiting from the Demographic Shift in the 21st Century*, Stoddart, Toronto, 2000.
3. Wan, H. et al., *U.S. Census Bureau, Current Population Reports, P23-209, 65+ in the United States*, U.S. Government Printing Office, Washington, DC, 2005.
4. WHO, *Ageing and Life Course*, http://www.who.int/ageing/en/ (accessed January 4, 2007).
5. Denton, F. T. and Spencer, B. G., How old is old? Revising the definition based on life table criteria, *Math. Popul. Stud.*, 7, 147–159, 1999.
6. Helander, M. G., The human factors profession, in: *Handbook of Human Factors and Ergonomics*, Salvendy, G. (Ed.), Wiley-Interscience, New York, 1997, pp. 3–16.
7. CAOT, *Enabling Occupation*, CAOT Publishing, Ottawa, 1997.
8. AOTA, Occupational therapy practice framework: Domain and process, AOTA, Bethesda, MD, 2002, 56, 609–639.
9. Statistics Canada, 2001 Census, Statistics Canada, Ottawa, 2006.
10. Shumway-Cook, A. and Woollacott, M. H. (Eds.), Aging and postural control, in: *Motor Control— Theory and Practical Applications*, Lippincott Williams & Wilkins, Baltimore, MD, 2001, pp. 222–247.
11. Miyoshi, K. et al., Effect of ageing on quadriceps muscle strength and on the forward shift of centre of pressure during sit-to-stand movement from a chair, *J. Phys. Ther. Sci.*, 17, 23–28, 2005.
12. Siggeirsdottir, K. et al., The timed 'Up & Go' is dependent on chair type, *Clin. Rehabil.*, 16, 609–616, 2002.
13. Billek-Sawhney, B. and Gay, J., The Functional Reach Test—are 3 trials necessary? *Top. Geriatr. Rehabil.*, 21, 144–148, 2005.
14. Lewis, C. B. and Kellems, S., Musculoskeletal changes with age: Clinical implications, in: *Aging the Health-Care Challenge*, Lewis, C.B. (Ed.), F.A. Davis, Philadelphia, PA, 2002, pp. 104–126.
15. Olney, S. J. and Culham, E. G., Changes in posture and gait, in: *Physiotherapy with Older People*, Pickles, B., Compton, A., Cott, C., Simpson, J., and Vandervoort, A. (Eds.), W.B. Saunders, London, 1995, pp. 81–94.

16. Mian, O. S. et al., Kinematics of stair decent in young and older adults and the impact of exercise training, *Gait Posture*, 25, 9–17, 2007.

17. Shumway-Cook, A. and Woollacott, M. H. (Eds.), Reach, grasp, and manipulation: Changes across the life span, in: *Motor Control—Theory and Practical Applications*, 2nd edn., Lippincott Williams & Wilkins, Baltimore, MD, 2001, Chapter 17.

18. Millar, W. J., *Vision Problems among Seniors*, Catalogue 82-003-XIE 16, Statistics Canada, Ottawa, 2004, 45–59.

19. Huppert, F., Designing for older users, in: *Inclusive Design—Design for the Whole Population*, Clarkson, R., Coleman, R., Keates, S., and Lebbon, C. (Eds.), Springer, London, 2003, pp. 31–49.

20. Boyce, P. R., Lighting for the elderly, *Technol. Disabil.*, 15, 165–180, 2003.

21. Cooper, B. A., Ward, M., Gowland, C. A., and McIntosh, J. M., *Journals of Gerontology, Series B, Psychological Sciences and Social Sciences*, 46, 320–324, 1991.

22. Ishihara, K. et al., Age-related decline in color perception and difficulties with daily activities-measurement, questionnaire, optical and computer-graphics simulation studies, *Int. J. Ind. Ergon.*, 28, 153–163, 2001.

23. Jackson, G. R., Owsley, C., and McGwin, G. Jr., Aging and dark adaptation, *Vision Res.*, 39, 3975–3982, 1999.

24. Maberley, D. A. L. et al., The prevalence of low vision and blindness in Canada, *Eye*, 20, 341–346, 2006.

25. Lindner, H. et al., Subjective lighting needs of the old and pathological eye, *Lighting Res. Technol.*, 21, 1–10, 1989.

26. Anonymous, Taste and smell disorders, in: *The Merck Manual of Geriatrics*, Abrams, W. B., Beers, M. H., and Berkow, R. (Eds.), Merck Research Laboratories, Whitehouse Station, NJ, 1995, p. 1345.

27. Carruthers, C. A. H. and Lane, J., Aging process, in: *Occupational Therapy with Elders—Strategies for the COTA*, Lohman, H., Padilla, R. L., and Byers-Connon, S. (Eds.), Mosby, St. Louis, MO, 1998, pp. 22–28.

28. Thornbury, J. M. and Mistretta, C. M., Tactile sensitivity as a function of age, *J. Gerontol.*, 36, 34–39, 1981.

29. Stevens, J. C. and Choo, K. K., Temperature sensitivity of the body surface over the lifespan, *Somatosens. Mot. Res.*, 15, 13–28, 1998.

30. Christensen, H., What cognitive changes can be expected with normal aging? *Aust. NZ J. Psychiatry*, 35, 768–775, 2001.

31. Burke, D. M. and MacKay, D. G., Memory, language, and ageing, *Phil. Trans. R. Soc. Lond. B*, 352, 1845–1856, 1997.

32. Baddeley, A. and Hitch, G., Working memory, in: *The Psychology of Learning and Motivation*, Vol. 8, Bower, G. A. (Ed.), Academic Press, New York, 1974.

33. Baddeley, B. A., The episodic buffer, *Trends Cog. Sci.*, 4, 417–423, 2000.

34. Repovs, G. and Baddeley, A., The multicomponent model of working memory: Exploration in experimental cognitive psychology, *Neuroscience*, 139, 5–21, 2006.

35. De Beni, R. and Palladino, P., Decline in working memory updating through ageing: Intrusion error analyses, *Memory*, 12, 75–89, 2004.

36. Farrimond, S., Knight, R. G., and Titov, N., The effects of aging on remembering intentions: Performance on a simulated shopping task, *Appl. Cognit. Psychol.*, 20, 533–555, 2006.

37. Smith, E., Visitability defined 2003, http://www.concretechange.org/Definition_of_Visitability.htm (accessed January 30, 2007).

38. Anonymous, Centre for Inclusive Design and Environmental Access, http://www.ap.buffalo.edu/idea/visitability (accessed January 30, 2007).

39. Canadian Centre on Disability Studies, Visitability, http://www.visitablehousing canada.com (accessed January 30, 2007).

40. Anonymous, American Disabilities Act, http://www.ada.gov/pubs/ada.htm (accessed January 30, 2007).
41. Rothstein, J. M., Roy, S. H., and Wolf, S. L., Americans with Disabilities Act and accessibility issues (including wheelchair information), in: *The Rehabilitation Specialist's Handbook*, F.A. Davis Company, Philadelphia, PA, 2005, pp. 1–51.
42. CSA International, Accessibility for the built environment, CAN/CSA-B651-04, Toronto, 2004.
43. CSA International, Barrier-free design for automated banking machines, CAN/CSA-B651.1-01, Toronto, 2001.
44. Vanderheiden, G. C., Design for people with functional limitations, in: *Handbook of Human Factors and Ergonomics*, Salvendy, G. (Ed.), John Wiley, Hoboken, NJ, 2006, pp. 1387–1417.
45. CSA International, Inclusive design for an aging population, CAN/CSA-5659-01, Toronto, 2007.
46. Mace, R. L., Hardie, G. J., and Place, J. P., Accessible environments: Toward universal design, http://www.design.ncsu.edu/cud/pubs_p/docs/ACC%20Environments.pdf (accessed January 30, 2007).
47. Mace, R., About universal design, http://www.design.ncsu.edu/cud/about_ud/about_ud.htm (accessed January 30, 2007).
48. Centre for Universal Design. *The Principles of Universal Design*, Version 2.0, North Carolina State University, Raleigh, NC, 1997.
49. Centre for Universal Design, Universal Design: Product Evaluation Countdown, http://www.design.ncsu.edu/cud/pubs_p/docs/UDPEC.pdf (accessed January 15, 2007).
50. Story, M. F., Meuller, J. L., and Montoya-Weiss, M., Progress in the development of universal design measures, in: *Proceedings of the RESNA Annual Conference*, Orlando, FL, 2000, pp. 132–134.
51. Story, M. F., Meuller, J. L., and Montoya-Weiss, M., Completion of the universal design performance measures, in: *Proceedings of the RESNA Annual Conference*, Reno, NV, June 22–26, 2001, pp. 109–111.
52. Beecher, V. and Paquet, V., Survey instrument for the universal design of consumer products, *Appl. Ergon.*, 36, 363–372, 2005.
53. Lewis, J. R., Usability testing, in: *Handbook of Human Factors and Ergonomics*, Salvendy, G. (Ed.), John Wiley, Hoboken, NJ, 2006, pp. 1275–1316.
54. Nicols, T. A., Rogers, W. A., and Fisk, A. D., Design for aging, in: *Handbook of Human Factors and Ergonomics*, Salvendy, G. (Ed.), John Wiley, Hoboken, NJ, 2006, pp. 1418–1445.

Section B

Disorders and Disabilities

5 Gait and Ergonomics: Normal and Pathological

Siobhan Strike

CONTENTS

This chapter reviews many of the publications related to gait and presents them in a way that is applicable to ergonomics for health professionals. This chapter initially introduces walking gait, the aim of walking, and overviews how this aim is achieved. The factors that result in pathological gait are outlined, and the implications on the achievement of the aim of walking are highlighted. Selected mechanical issues pertinent to understanding gait, loading, the anatomical implications of the link-chain system, and efficiency are detailed. The mechanics of gait, which gives an in-depth review of the outcome and process measures that cause and result in gait, are detailed. The effect pathologies have on these mechanics are illustrated. Finally, an analysis of how all these elements combine is given through a detailed description of transtibial amputee gait.

5.1   NATURE OF WALKING GAIT

There are many different definitions for walking or gait [1–4], but common to all is the statement that gait involves progression/locomotion and that support/stability is seen as key.

Walking is such an automatic response for most people that its complexity is often underestimated. We learn to walk without instruction and there is little deviation from the "norm," suggesting that walking is instinctive rather than cognitive. It is dependent upon the progressive maturation of the central nervous system (CNS) [5] and infants usually begin to walk at 9–18 months.

In order to ensure that progression with stability is achieved, each individual will develop a unique mechanical solution, a fact that is illustrated when we recognize a person simply from the way they walk. This individual solution is developed in response to individual anthropometrics (height and weight in particular), strength, flexibility, habit, and posture. The environment or the requirements of the task can further alter our gait. For instance, if the body is tired, injured, or as it ages, the way in which we walk can alter. These accommodations are due to organism constraints. We walk differently to accommodate different ground surfaces, inclines or to avoid obstacles, illustrating our adaptability toward environmental constraints. Depending on the nature of the task, we can alter our walking to carry a load or to achieve quicker or slower walking speeds, illustrating our ability to adapt to task constraints. Given that we can adapt in response to constraints, we can be identified as mechanically "dynamic" systems. Other factors, which influence our individual walking style, are clothing, footwear, and psychosocial status.

Given the flexibility of the locomotor system, factors which influence walking can result in new movement patterns. These patterns can be "internalized" over a period of time such that they become the automatic response. Thus interventions, such as orthoses or prosthetic setups, should be allowed to be learned before their true effect can be understood. If an intervention is temporary (i.e., a fracture cast) then when it is removed, the locomotor system will return to the "normal" walking gait.

5.2   INTRODUCTION TO THE BIOMECHANICS OF GAIT

The primary aim of walking is to progress the body safely from one place to another. Later sections will detail the mechanisms that cause walking. Here, a brief overview of the requirement to allow progression and support with efficiency is detailed.

5.2.1   PROGRESSION

Progression is achieved through the interplay between potential and kinetic energy. The center of mass (CoM) is raised over the stance limb and forward progress occurs when it moves forward and downward to the double support phase. From this depth, it must be moved forward and upward again over the contralateral limb. To achieve this movement of the CoM, the limbs provide the kinetic energy. The trail leg (i.e., the limb entering swing) pushes and the stance leg pulls the trunk from the low point of double support to the high point of midstance [6]. This mechanism is one of the fundamental functions of the limb during stance—to extend in terminal stance in order to achieve this required push off. An inability to achieve this results in a pathological gait. Once the limb has achieved this push-off, it is swinging and it must be able to advance to a position where it can take over the supporting role [3]. Again, failure to advance will result in an inability to achieve progress and therefore pathological gait or an inability to achieve any gait will result.

5.2.2   STABILITY

Successful gait depends on each limb being able to support the body without collapsing and balance must be maintained in single stance [3]. The CoM is moved over a base of support that is constantly changing from stable (double support) to unstable (single support). Stability is challenged as the body is top heavy and the segments are continually moving so that the position of the CoM over the base of support is always altering. To ensure stability the stance foot must be stable on the floor, there must be adequate body balance, the lower extremity in stance must allow for the clear swing of the contralateral limb and the limb must resist collapse. In order to prevent collapse, there must be a net extensor moment at the three main joints, the hip, the knee, and the ankle. These large moments along with gravitational forces are being imposed on the system while it is being supported on one leg for 40% of the time. Inability to achieve stability in stance results in a pathological gait. Assistive devices (such as crutches, canes, orthoses) can be used to enhance stability. However, if these devices introduce excessive stability, then progress can be difficult.

In summary, normal gait is characterized by locomotion of the body from one place to another through bipedal action of the lower limbs. If the body cannot maintain balance and support, or if the trunk cannot advance and the limbs cannot progress then pathological gait occurs.

5.3   PATHOLOGICAL GAIT

In pathological gait, progress and support can be accomplished, but through an abnormal movement or by using some form of assistive device (cane, crutch, orthoses, prosthesis). Common causes of pathological gait are: deformity, muscle weakness, impaired control, and pain [2]. These can cause an abnormal mechanical response. Alternatively, the abnormal mechanical response could be a compensation at another joint.

Deformity results from insufficient passive mobility in the tissues to allow sufficient postures and joint ranges of motion to allow for a normal walking pattern to be achieved. Both progression and stability can be affected due to a deformity. Progression is affected through the lack of energy supply from the limbs to facilitate trunk advancement and, frequently, poor progression of the limb in swing. Support can be compromised through unstable postures while the limb is in support. Contracture and/or pain are common causes and a leg length discrepancy is a common outcome.

Muscle weakness can result from disuse atrophy and neurological impairments. Both progress and stability can be compromised from muscle weakness, and its effect is most often seen in the movement of the limb in swing. Insufficient strength in the hip flexors and ankle plantarflexors prior to swing will result in a weak push from the trail leg. The resulting reduced momentum, which helps to advance the trunk over the contralateral supporting limb, results in slower gait. It is reasonably easy to compensate for muscle weakness at other joints or through the use of assistive devices. For amputees, compensations as a result of weakness in the residual limb can be accommodated at other joints, notably the hip in late stance and the contralateral hip in early stance. As a result, the trunk can be raised to the high point of midstance.

Impaired control, including sensory loss, can affect the gait to such an extent that it is no longer possible. Proprioception informs the walker of the location of the limb and if this is impaired, then tripping or poor limb loading can result. Stability is compromised as a result. This can be seen in amputees who delay the loading of the prosthesis to ensure that it is safely placed on the floor. A CNS lesion (in cerebral palsy, cerebral vascular accident, spinal chord injury) will affect gait and the level/extent of the lesion can result in sufficient paralysis to prevent gait. Here both progression and stability are compromised. In some instances, through using assistive devices, including orthoses compensations for voluntary control can ensure gait can occur.

Pain can cause deviations to try to remove pain from the area. The loading on the system is therefore altered. Pain can lead to a deformity and/or weakness from disuse or inhibition. Pain can be alleviated with assistive devices, treatment or rehabilitation, as long as the reallocation of load does not lead to pain in another site.

Disabled individuals develop remaining capabilities in their adapted gait pattern to achieve the aim of locomotion. Any clinical intervention should be implemented with practitioners being aware that trying to "normalize" the gait pattern may be detrimental to the achievement of gait. Rehabilitation should be informed by an understanding of the capabilities of the anatomy of the individual and their dynamics and these should be maximized to enable the achievement of gait. For instance, Fonseca et al. [7] illustrate that the features of cerebral palsy result in a stiffer locomotor system that may store more elastic energy in the muscles. They follow that the raising the CoM higher than normal in midstance allows the body to fall further onto a plantarflexed foot, which increases the loading on the stiff plantarflexors. When the limb rebounds the elastic energy return is closer to that of running and so progress occurs. As such, the gait pattern adopted is not a limitation, but an adaptation to the changed body dynamics, which facilitates the achievement of gait.

After a stroke, many people are left with an altered gait pattern as a result of impaired control affecting balance and motor control and muscle weakness affecting progress and stability. The result is a slower, less efficient walking pattern. Olney and Richards [8] showed that hemiparetic gait could be classified as having (a) reduced hip joint angle amplitude in sagittal plane, caused by reduced hip flexion at heel strike and reduced extension at toe-off; (b) reduced knee flexion at toe-off and during swing, with increased knee extension at initial contact, and (c) increased plantarflexion at initial contact and in swing and decreased plantarflexion at toe-off. The ineffective ankle dorsiflexion during swing and failure to achieve heel strike at initial contact results in modified synergistic patterns and secondary compensations such as vaulting, circumduction or pelvic tilt to ensure swing-through (Section 5.9.8).

In rehabilitating stroke patients, there is controversy regarding the extent to which the normal mechanics are required for functional recovery. Similar to Fonseca et al. [7] for cerebral palsy, Huitema et al. [9] suggest that the adaptation of compensatory mechanisms may facilitate functional recovery [9]. Particularly, they found that the development of a stiff knee gait by stroke patients can be predicted by calculating the difference between the knee angle at midstance and midswing. If this value is below 10° in the first stages of recovered gait, then it will never reach a normal level and stiff-knee gait will result. If the stiff knee can be functional and recognized as such early in the rehabilitation process, they suggest that it may be useful to train the patient using the compensatory walking pattern, rather than trying to change the gait to normal. This idea needs further research to assess its efficacy as generally it is felt that early treatment to regain normal movements as much as possible and to avoid the development of compensatory mechanisms is the best rehabilitation.

5.4   MECHANICAL CONCEPTS PERTINENT TO UNDERSTANDING GAIT

Pathological gait results in progress with adequate support; however, the means by which these are achieved are altered. Before the mechanics of gait can be reviewed, the mechanical concepts of loading, the kinematic chain and efficiency are briefly outlined.

5.4.1   LOADING

Given the nature of walking, the body is loaded with each ground contact. The overall load on the body is reflected in the ground reaction force (GRF), which indicates the force on the CoM. The direction and magnitude of this force can be represented as a vector (Figure 5.1) known as the ground reaction vector (GRV), which has its origin at the center of pressure (CoP).

As the joints and tissues are loaded deformation results. The extent of the deformation is dependent on the properties under load, the size and shape of the tissue,

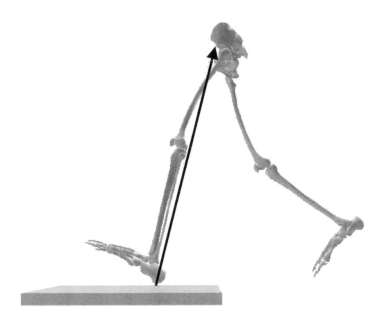

FIGURE 5.1 Skeleton at initial contact. The GRV is represented by an arrow. The GRV originates at the CoP and indicates the magnitude and direction of the overall force acting on the body. The force vector can cause, or tend to cause, flexion or extension at a joint depending on where it passes relative to the joint. An internal moment, caused by muscular contraction, will facilitate or counteract the tendency toward flexion or extension caused by the external force.

environmental factors and specific to the force—its magnitude, direction, point of application, duration, and frequency. The resultant load on the CoM in able-bodied walking is not particularly high, reaching no more than a little over one body weight in the loading and propulsion phases—up to nine times body weight have been recorded in some jumping activities. As such, the load on the joints and tissues is well within their mechanical limits and, under normal circumstances, tolerance is easily achieved. This may not be the case under extreme conditions. For instance, stress fractures are known to occur in the military as a result of walking long distances, carrying heavy loads and/or repeated marching. Army recruits have shown that the knee effects substantial compensations during backpack loaded marching. These high loads have been associated with shock attenuation or the reduction of excessive loads elsewhere. Interestingly, after marching for 40 min, the altered knee mechanics were not sustained, suggesting the fatigue may occur and the compensations could not be sustained [10]. Carrying a load on the back also has an effect on normal walking gait. Adolescent girls walked more slowly and with decreased pelvic motion with increased load. Hip flexion and extension increased as did the joint moments and power with increased mass [11]. Research indicates that backpack loading be limited to 10% body weight to avoid excessive loading on the musculoskeletal system. Lateral bending of the trunk to counteract the asymmetric placement of a load (e.g., a shoulder strap over one shoulder) has been suggested as a risk factor for a number of low-back disorders. Asymmetric loading has been shown to affect posture, with increased forward lean through thoracic adjustments and lateral bending through lumbar adjustments [12]. High heels distort the biomechanics of the foot and lower limbs to redirect the forces in unusual directions and may result in injury. Ankle plantarflexion, knee flexion, the timing of subtalar and knee joint action and the vertical and braking forces have been shown to be affected by increased heel height. Poor alignment may result in other complications. The resultant abnormal direction of the loading may be implicated in the development of secondary injuries or the inability to walk without aids, or not at all.

In pathological conditions, even though the loading may not be much higher than normal, the consequence of an altered magnitude (GRF) or direction of the load (GRV), or the anatomy experiencing the load may be more extreme. Stress fractures can be caused by the GRV with reference to the position of the body segments. For instance, if dealing with osteoporosis or osteoarthritis in the lower limb joints, the loading may result in joint pain or fractures. Postarthroplasty assistive devices such as canes are used in rehabilitation to reduce the force on the prosthetic device and on the incised muscles. The use of an assistive device such as a cane, held contralaterally for a hip arthroplasty, can also help in preventing a lurching gait by reducing weight-bearing pain and by assisting the weakened hip abductor muscles.

5.4.2 KINEMATIC CHAIN

Fundamental to understanding the biomechanics of gait, and specifically the compensatory mechanisms if a pathology is introduced, is the mechanical concept of the linked segment. The mechanical flexibility of the locomotor system is as a result of the fact that the human body is made of a system of levers, which do not act independently of one another. The linked segments form a kinematic chain, which can enhance the range of motion and the overall load-bearing capacity of the system.

In gait, when the limb is in stance, it is a closed chain as the distal segment (the foot) is fixed. In this situation, movement at one joint has an effect on the more proximal joints and this motion is relatively predictable. For instance, at initial contact, the foot strikes the floor and the kinematic chain becomes closed. If wearing high heels, the foot is plantarflexed and to achieve foot flat, the knee, hip or pelvis will have to compensate. In a novice high heel wearer, the compensation is typically achieved through increased knee flexion similar to crouched gait or through trunk lean. In more experienced heel wearers, hip abduction and pelvic rotation are the compensatory mechanisms. Specifically the increased knee moment compensations have been indicated as relevant in the development and/or progression of knee osteoarthritis [13].

Pathologically, if there is limited dorsiflexion, at midstance, the knee and hip will compensate. The hip may flex, externally rotate and abduct, the knee may flex or even hyperextend to facilitate foot-flat. In early hip osteoarthritis, reduced hip extension is associated with kinematic changes in the pelvis to maintain effective extension of the lower limb at push-off.

When the limb is in swing, it is an open chain and the joints have more freedom to move independent of each other, but can still compensate. For instance, with limited dorsiflexion, toe clearance at midswing can become an issue, but the knee or hip can flex or the pelvis can hike to ensure that the person does not trip. These modifications are detailed further in the description of walking below.

So, when one joint or a muscle/muscle group affecting a joint is not functioning correctly, compensations will be evident at adjacent joints in the kinematic chain, and depending on the extent of the problem at more than one joint. If trying to correct an abnormal mechanism at one joint, it is important to remember the effect this manipulation will have on the remaining joints.

5.4.3 EFFICIENCY

Walking gait should be efficient as walking usually needs to be sustained for a period of time. In many pathological conditions, if efficiency is not feasible then walking will not occur and wheelchair locomotion will be preferred.

Mann [14] states that the act of walking is a result of the blending and compromising of physical and biological forces in order to achieve maximum efficiency at minimum cost. For efficient progress to occur, energy must be conserved so that the act of walking can continue over a prolonged period of time in steady state. To increase efficiency, the body must (a) maximize the use of gravitational force, which it does through converting potential energy to kinetic energy, (b) minimize the excursion of the CoM and control momentum, and (c) minimize the use of muscles.

To minimize the excursion of the body's CoM, it travels in a three-dimensional sinusoidal pathway. As shown, the CoM is farthest to the right and high at right midstance, central and low at double support and farthest left and high at left midstance. It is useful to think of this pathway as a three-dimensional "~" with the highest and widest position at midstance and the lowest and most central position at double support. If this movement of the CoM is deviated from the "~" through deformity, pain or impaired control, or if the excursion is jagged as a result of muscle weakness, then this is energy expensive and therefore undesirable.

Momentum is used in such a way that for natural walking speed the least energy per meter traveled is expended through the conservation of momentum. At slow and fast speeds the energy expended increases [15]. Walking slowly requires that momentum is removed from the system by eccentric muscle contractions to maintain the slow pace. At fast speeds, momentum, through energy, must be continually added to the system through larger concentric muscle contractions to maintain the pace. Pathological gait is often slower as the mechanics required for efficient momentum use are disrupted through muscle weakness and impaired control. Deformity and pain can result in the ineffective raising and lowering of the trunk and the subsequent requirement for additional momentum to be added to the system.

Minimizing the use of muscles is achieved by taking advantage of the human body's ability to transfer energy passively from one segment to another. Winter [4] describes two major energy-saving mechanisms used by the body. One uses the passive flow of energy across a joint, obvious in the terminal swing phase of walking when the swinging foot and leg transfer energy through the thigh to the trunk. The trunk then conserves the potential energy and converts it to kinetic energy to accelerate the head, arms, and trunk (HAT) in the forward direction. During terminal stance, the power generated by the plantarflexor muscles also transfers through the knee to the thigh to help lift the stance limb into swing. In pathological gait, if the limb does not have sufficient energy, then the reduced energy flow will have to be supplied through active contraction, or the gait will be slower. In stroke or aged gait, the energy in the swinging limb is reduced due to reduced hip flexor and ankle plantarflexor activity. As a result the energy available to be transferred to the trunk is reduced and slower gait follows. The other mechanism involves the active energy transfer across muscles when the adjacent joints are rotating in the same direction. A further mechanism, which reduces energy expenditure, is to take advantage of the stretch-shortening cycle. Here, the muscles function such that they tend to stretch in gait and the "stretch energy" is returned without the need for active contraction. As detailed above, Fonseca et al. [7] illustrated that the altered mechanism evident in CP gait takes advantage of the stiff plantarflexors to store more stretch energy to compensate for the reduced capacity to actively contract these muscles, thereby taking advantage of this energy-saving mechanism to achieve progression.

It is through understanding the process by which we walk and the loading pattern of the movement that we can understand the adaptations and consequences of pathological walking. When these compensatory mechanisms are understood, it is generally easier to understand the role and development of devices or rehabilitation to functionally restore capacity.

5.5 FUNCTIONAL RESTORATION: DEVICES AND TRAINING

An important aspect of the understanding of gait is the ability to enhance the capacity of the body to improve functional mobility—that is to achieve stable progression. Understanding the mechanics of any disruption or the influence of assistive devices and rehabilitation enhances the capacity of the body to improve functional mobility.

The design of any assistive device, such as a prosthesis, orthosis, cane, crutch, etc., should begin with the identification of biomechanical prerequisites to ensure the success of the component. It should end with a comprehensive biomechanical analysis of the device's functional qualities. In developing devices, it is important to consider the mechanical character of the human-device system. The basic biomechanical patterns that are necessary to perform locomotor functions effectively must be identified and along with the patient's reserve capacities. The device should effectively make use of all force and energy resources (both internal and external) available to ensure safe loading, acceptable compensations, and efficient progress.

In order to maximize the mechanical character of the device to ensure that functional restoration can occur the device must take into account pressure-sensitive and pressure-tolerant areas of the body and ensure that high loads/pressure are directed to these areas [16]. The appropriate material characteristics (isotropic nature of the material, its viscoelasticity, hysteresis properties, the load/deformation and the stress/strain curves) of the device must also be taken into consideration when analyzing the type of loading (i.e., tension, compression, shear, torsion, and bending) on the device. As external devices need to interface at some point with the human, the neurovascular system must be able to withstand the pressure at the interface and so load distribution is important.

When an assistive device is used, the gait is known as partial weight-bearing (PWB) gait. Typically if the cane or crutch or walker is being used to give relief from pain by helping to unload the limb or it is used to compensate for muscle weakness, it is used contralaterally. As the aim of the device is to unload a limb, successful implementation of the device should be evidenced by a reduced GRF on the affected side. It can be difficult for a therapist to accurately determine the magnitude of the load that is placed on the loaded limb. Two common strategies used to estimate magnitude of the load the patient is applying to the limb are (a) to stand on the therapist's hand and for the therapist to estimate the load and (b) to stand on a bathroom scale and the patient loads the limb to the prescribed weight. Youdas et al. [17] have shown that it is possible to train healthy subjects using the bathroom scale to place 50% of body weight on a designated limb when walking with auxiliary crutches at self-selected level walking. Using forearm crutches was almost as successful, a mean vertical load of 56% was applied. The wheeled walker was not successful with a mean peak of 64% on the "affected" limb and a reduced loading of 85% on the "unaffected" limb—indicating the upper extremities were used to transmit the load to the wheeled walker even when the unaffected limb was in stance. A single point cane only reduced the load on the affected limb to 76%. Ajemian et al. [18] showed that after total hip arthroplasty the use of a cane, held in the contralateral hand, reduced the hip abduction moments on the operative side. The hip abduction moment on the nonoperative side increased and they warned that clinicians should be mindful of the effects of the cane as an assistive device on the contralateral hip. To assist with unstable gait, a cane is typically used ipsilaterally.

Exercise is fundamental to functional mobility, as all mobility requires the capacity to exercise the neuromuscular system. The level of exercise and the expectation for exercise participation varies with different groups. Exercise is also an integral part of rehabilitation. Generally, the purposes of exercise in rehabilitation includes: remediating or preventing impairments; enhancing function; reducing risk of injury; optimizing overall health, and enhancing fitness and well-being [19], increasing circulation, increasing strength, increasing ROM, preventing or correcting contractures, develop coordination, reduce edema and promote healing, promote mobility and self-care, and increase cardiorespiratory fitness [16]. Specific retraining of the motor system can improve muscle recruitment and timing, which can reduce the compensatory mechanisms. Through exercise, muscular strength is enhanced and the ability to absorb load through eccentric contractions developed. Proprioception and fine motor control can also be developed through the selection of the appropriate exercise program and the consequent ability to cope with unstable situations is developed. Exercise programs undertaken by the elderly have been shown to improve walking.

By understanding the limitations of the specific pathology, rehabilitation can be accurately directed with appropriate goals set to enhance gait.

5.6 GAIT AND SYMMETRY

Many pathological gait patterns, for example, bilateral amputee, hemiplegia, unilateral osteoarthritis, have asymmetry as a feature of the biomechanics. Often clinical and rehabilitation decisions are made on the basis of the results of the gait analysis that indicates where these asymmetries lie. In much of the earlier gait literature, which provides the normative data, there was the assumption of gait symmetry the right and left limbs operated in the same manner and the data for the limbs were often pooled. However, Sadeghi et al. [20] have indicated a functional gait asymmetry. They also showed that the left and right limbs have different roles to play in achieving gait [21]. The right limb acted as a mobilizer characterized by a strong hip power at push-off. They also found that there was a strong secondary support function at midstance. The left limb was associated with the function of stabilizing and the variables associated with stability were associated primarily with the knee and were evidenced throughout the gait cycle.

5.7 GAIT ANALYSIS—VARIABLES AND THEIR SELECTION

Gait analysis is the term used to describe and analyze the process of producing the biomechanics of the movement. There have been a number of comprehensive studies conducted on "normal" walking [1–4], which characterize their gait. These allow for a framework to help in the understanding of the impact of disorders on the system and can help in the development of rehabilitation programs or the development of new assistive devices. Further, any deviation from the norm can be illustrated and can therefore help in the interpretation of the data collected for those with some pathology. Generally, a biomechanical analysis of human movement investigates variables, which can be identified as outcome—is the result successful, i.e., is stable efficient progress achieved; and process—how does the body operate mechanically in order to achieve this outcome.

As outcome variables relate the success of the movement, they are often more easily measured. The complexity of the process variables can mean that sophisticated measuring tools are required. Over the past 30 years advances in technology have resulted in the widespread availability of measurement systems and as such the collection and analysis of biomechanical data in gait laboratories is reasonably commonplace. Nonetheless, the accurate collection and interpretation of this data reflects its complexity and requires specialist knowledge in the field.

5.7.1 OUTCOME VARIABLES

As the main aim of walking is to safely transport the body, these are the key outcome variables, which should initially be assessed. Linear displacement of the CoM is the first assessment of gait. Safety in transport is usually related to stability in stance, which requires a net extensor moment at the three lower limb joints.

Outcome measures that further elucidate the extent to which the displacement of the CoM was successfully achieved are often referred to as temporal and spatial measures (TS). These give more information on the components which make up the overall displacement of the CoM. TS variables are widely used to describe normal and pathological gait. The variables are well defined in the literature and are broadly accepted. Typical TS variables are velocity, cadence, step, and stride length. Others that are frequently reported are step and swing period, single and double support time, and percentage of stride. Stance and swing are initially defined; stance when in the limb is in support and swing with in the limb is in the air (Figure 5.2). Stance makes up about 60% of the gait cycle and the remaining 40% is in swing. In total,

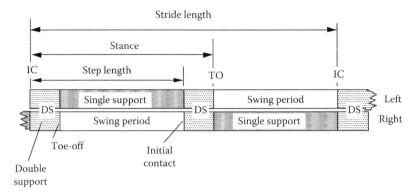

FIGURE 5.2   Timing of a single gait cycle. IC indicates initial contact, DS indicates double support, TO indicates toe-off.

double support is about 20% of the gait cycle, equally divided between initial double support and terminal double support. Single support is about 40% (the same duration as the contralateral swing). Subphases of stance and swing are also defined, though the phasing is somewhat more variable (Section 5.9).

5.7.2   TEMPOROSPATIAL VARIABLES

A stride is the distance (along the direction of progression) from the initial contact of one foot to the next initial contact of that (ipsilateral) foot. Initial contact is often heel strike, but for some pathological conditions, the heel does not necessarily contact the ground. Typically, normal stride length is about 1.46 m in men and 1.28 m in women [2]. Children have established an adult stride length by about 11 years [2]. Step length is the distance from initial contact of one foot to the initial contact of the other (contralateral) foot. Stride length, therefore, is the sum of the length of the two steps of which the stride is comprised. Stride length, when traveling in a straight line, is symmetrical. Step length need not necessarily be symmetrical, and in many pathological conditions, it is not symmetrical. Stride time is the interval between the foot contacts. Velocity of the CoM is often recorded and gives quality information regarding the displacement, i.e., it tells us how fast the person is walking. Normal walking velocity is approximately 1.3–1.6 m/s [1] with different age groups and pathologies achieving different velocities. Cadence refers to the number of steps or strides per minute or second and can reflect the capacity to walk of the participant. Normal walking cadence is about 110–115 steps/min. The speed of walking is equal to the cadence times the step length, if the steps are shorter the cadence increases at the same velocity. The temporal characteristics of gait vary with walking speed. When walking speed increases the stance phase and double support period gets shorter and the swing phase increases. Eventually, walking is no longer sustainable and running must occur. Running is defined by a period of flight/no support. When the cadence reaches about 180 steps/min then gait switches from walking to running.

Comfortable walking speed declines with advancing age and the decline begins in approximately the seventh decade of life. Kerrigan et al. [22] found that the natural velocity of elderly walkers was 1.19 m/s. Their cadence was 119 steps/min and stride length was 1.2 m. Younger walkers had the same cadence, but walking velocity was higher (1.37 m/s) due to a longer stride (1.38 m). Hyndman et al. [23] found that people with a stroke walked with a slower velocity and a shorter stride length than aged-matched controls.

Healthy individuals who are asked to walk with assistive devices and load a limb to 50%, evidence a slower walking speed (1.281 m/s slows to 0.563–0.761 m/s depending on the type of device). The slower walking is as a result of both reduced cadence 110.9 reduced to 69.4–75.5 steps/min and stride length 138.4 shortened to 112.9–124.3 cm. In early unilateral osteoarthritis, patients walked at a significantly slower speed (1.05 m/s) than an equivalent nonclinical group (1.18 m/s). The slower walking speed was as a result of both a significantly reduced stride length (1.16 against 1.24 m) and a significantly reduced cadence (108.62 against 114.27 steps/min). Total hip arthroplasty patients monitored preoperative and at 4 and 8 months postoperatively showed an increase in walking speed over time and a significant difference was found preoperatively (0.95 m/s) and at 8 months postoperation (1.08 m/s). When using a cane, the subjects walked 3% slower than when walking independently [18]. Table 5.1 indicates the mean velocity, cadence, and stride length for different groups. All data are presented in the same units, so some calculations have been made to facilitate comparisons.

Table 5.1 illustrates the wide range of values for different populations. The TS variables of gait can change depending on the environment, size of the room, and even if the data are collected inside or outside. As a result many studies complete their own control trials in order to understand the normal range of the group if an

TABLE 5.1
Temporospatial Characteristics for a Normal and Nonpathological Populations

	Velocity (m/s)	Cadence (step/min)	Stride Length (m)
Men [1]	1.3–1.6	110–115	1.4–1.6
Women [1]	1.2–1.5	115–120	1.3–1.5
Elderly [22]	1.19	119	1.2
Adult [22]	1.37	119	1.38
Poststroke [8]	0.23–0.73		
Poststroke hemiparetic [24]	0.346	83.4	0.52
Early OA [25]	1.05	108.62	1.16
Elderly fallers [26]	0.89	107	138
Elderly nonfallers [26]	1.21	120	1.22
TTA SACH foot [27]	1.32	118	1.36
Hip arthroplasty before surgery [18]	0.95		
Hip arthroplasty after surgery [18]	1.08		

alteration is being made to that group, or if comparing disability to nondisability. Control groups should be age and activity level matched as much as possible. When it is not possible to height match patients, it may be more appropriate to try to normalize the data. The most appropriate way is to convert the variables to dimensionless quantities (e.g., Ref. [1]).

When assessing the process by which the TS variables have been affected, i.e., how did the joint mechanics alter as a result of a pathology or of aging, it is important to ensure that the altered mechanics are not simply an effect of the slower walking, but as a result of the disability or aging. It is reasonably common to make allowances in interpreting pathological gait results in comparison to normal gait to account for the different walking speed. A relationship between many variables and speed has been established [28], which can be helpful in making diagnostic decisions. It can be useful to ask the controls to walk at the same speed as the disabled group (e.g., Ref. [24]).

Gait performance has been seen to deteriorate when participants carry out a secondary task. Tasks such as talking, carrying a tray/glass, stepping over obstacles, and responding verbally to sounds have been shown to slow gait. Hyndman et al. [23] introduced a cognitive task—remembering a seven-item shopping list—to the task of walking 5 m. Both stroke patients and control groups walked more slowly, with a shorter stride length. Further, stride length was reduced for fallers compared to nonfallers in the stroke group. Walking speed has been shown to be affected when the environment is changed such as walking in a mall. Lord et al. [29] showed that gait speed of stroke patients in the clinic was 0.68 m/s while this slowed to 0.60 m/s in a mall. This was related to the unpredictability of the constraints imposed by the environment. Step length and step frequency were not significantly different between the clinic and mall, but were much more stable in the clinic. This can have implications for rehabilitation, which is confined to the clinic as the skill may not be sufficiently malleable to cope with the unpredictability of natural environments.

5.7.3   TS Variables and Functional Mobility

In order to achieve community mobility, people need to be able to walk at a 1.22 m/s (in order to be able to cross a street controlled by a traffic light) for 332–360 m [30,31]. They also need to be able to negotiate a 17.8–20.3 cm curb, manage stairs, and a ramp. Older people with disabilities are more likely to take fewer trips and more likely to have more days in which no trips outside the house were taken compared to older people without disabilities [32]. On those trips, the people with a disability were not able to maintain the speed of those around them and they completed the trips accompanied by someone, while those without a disability were able to keep up with those around them and complete 95% of the trips unaccompanied.

5.8   PROCESS VARIABLES

Process variables indicate how the participant walked, i.e., the mechanics that produce the movement. To get accurate results, more sophisticated equipment is required and the more in-depth the variable, the more complex the technology.

In order to locomote, the leg acts as a system of rotating elements coupled in series, each storing and releasing energy through passive muscle absorption of strain energy or through active muscle activation. The net torque results in rotations of segments about the ankle, knee, and hip joints. If the rotations are constrained as a result of a disruption to the joints or muscles, which are involved in producing the movement, then the gait will be hampered. Locomotion will not be achieved or it may be achieved inefficiently (compared to normal gait) or not safely.

Movement is caused (or tends to be caused) by the application of a force. The forces which we analyze in human walking are due to muscle activation or gravity. Ligament and tendon forces are often included with muscle forces as analyzing them separately is not feasible using most biomechanical equipment. Bone forces are also difficult to quantify but are sometimes calculated, particularly for the assessment of joint replacements. Centrifugal forces, arising from rotations of the body segments, act to decrease the vertical GRF but only by minor amounts [33] and are often not analyzed. The friction force is only considered in certain circumstances (e.g., slipping, surface assessment) and the fluid force as a result of air resistance is not considered of sufficient magnitude to be included in an analysis. If possible, the body will make use of gravity and momentum to try to reduce the involvement of the muscles as they are "free" energy as distinct from "costly energy" required when a muscle contracts.

Analyzing muscle activation and how the body maximizes the gravitational force are key to an effective biomechanical analysis of walking. Through a method known as "inverse dynamics" the joint moments and powers required to produce the movement can be calculated. For an in-depth description of how these variables are calculated, see Refs. [1,4]. The variable analyzed to assess the effectiveness of the muscle activation is power. A power generation (positive) result indicates that the joint muscles are involved in a concentric contraction. Power absorption (negative result) indicates muscles are contracting through an eccentric contraction to take energy out of the segment. Power relates to a net result at the joint therefore it cannot indicate the specific muscles involved in the contraction. Cocontractions are also not indicated through this result, which can result in poor interpretation for pathological gait. It is often useful to include an electromyographic (EMG) analysis to indicate which muscles are contracting, for how long at what percentage maximum voluntary contraction (%MVC). Increasingly, simplified dynamic models and more sophisticated muscle-actuated simulations are being used to investigate the effects of various gait features and muscle roles on the production of movement [33,34].

In gait, muscle roles are often associated with propulsion and/or support as these are the key elements in successful gait. Different muscles can have different roles during different phases of the gait cycle, and in some instances, different muscles acting about the same joint can have different roles. For example, there has been much controversy surrounding the role of the ankle plantarflexors during late stance. Three main theories have been proposed regarding this muscle group. They are that the ankle plantarflexors (a) provide controlled roll-off and do not actively contribute to progression but help in the controlled fall of the trunk [2], (b) actively contribute to forward progression through a push-off at terminal stance and the energy generated at the plantarflexors is transferred to the trunk to provide both support and forward progression [35], and (c) accelerate the limb into swing and forward progression is provided through the angular momentum of the swing limb, which is transferred to the trunk [36]. Neptune et al. [34], using muscle-actuated simulations, have indicated that in fact these theories are not mutually exclusive and that the role of the plantar-flexors needs to be described in terms of the particular muscles, which conduct different roles. In single-leg stance, both the soleus and gastrocnemius provide vertical support, in mid-single-leg stance, the soleus decelerates the forward rotation of the tibia so that the knee extends and the trunk is allowed to pass over the supporting foot. The gastrocnemius acts to flex the knee at this time. If the soleus is impaired, a compensation would be necessary to prevent the knee collapsing during the middle of single-leg stance. In late single-leg stance and early propulsion, both the soleus and gastrocnemius accelerate the trunk forward, with the soleus providing 60% and the gastrocnemius providing 25% of the trunk forward acceleration.

5.9   PHASES OF THE GAIT CYCLE

To examine the process variables, it is common to break the movement into smaller phases and to identify the aim of each subphase. This allows the mechanics associated with achieving that aim to be more easily identified and interpreted.

There are a number of systems of subphasing the gait cycle. Perry [2] indicates weight acceptance, single limb support, and limb advancement as the key tasks to be achieved in the gait cycle. She divided the stance phase into five distinct subphases to reflect these tasks. The system used is a common phasing system: initial contact, load response, midstance, terminal stance, and preswing. Swing is divided into three phases: initial swing, midswing, and terminal swing. Sutherland [5] described three phases of stance: initial double support, single limb support, second double support, followed by the three swing phases outlined above, Winter [37] developed a slightly more functional gait cycle with the three stance phases coinciding with Sutherland [5], though the names are more descriptive of the function of the phase: weight acceptance; midstance; push-off, and he divides swing into two phases: lift-off and reach. Kirtley [1] adapts this further to identify the fundamental functions outlined by Perry [2] in the phasing: loading; support/progression; and propulsion and swing. Figure 5.3 illustrates the start and end of the three stance phases.

The following sections detailing the biomechanics, or process, by which gait is achieved will follow the phasing outlined by Kirtley [1], though swing is detailed as a separate phase here. Detailed data for normal gait are available from a number of sources [1–4,6] and the reader is referred to them if a more comprehensive understanding is required.

In studying the biomechanics of walking, it is reasonably common to divide the body into the mechanical "locomotor" system, consisting of the lower limbs and pelvis and the "passenger" system comprising the HAT. This is for the ease of mechanical interpretation and to simplify the model and complexity of the data. There is growing evidence that muscle slings link the lower and upper body and that the opposing movement of the arms and limbs with the gluteus muscles and the latissimus dorsi working together contributes to movement. Further research is required in this field to develop this theory.

Figures in the following sections are illustrated for a male walking at 1.68 m/s with a stride length of 1.55 m. Three-dimensional gait analysis was conducted using

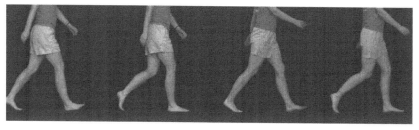

Loading   Support/progression   Propulsion

FIGURE 5.3 Photographs of normal gait indicating start and end of right limb stance phases. The phase is the interval between these images. Loading is the period between image 1 and image 2, weight is borne, the foot is lowered to the floor and the contralateral limb is in propulsion. Support/progression is the period between image 2 and image 3, the trunk passes over the supporting limb and the contralateral limb is in swing. Propulsion is the period between image 3 and image 4, the limb is propelled into swing and contralateral stance loading occurs.

a seven-camera, VICON 512 (Oxford Metrics, UK) motion analysis system (120 Hz) synchronized with a single Kistler force plate set at a sampling frequency of 600 Hz. Fifteen retroreflective markers were attached to anatomical landmarks in accordance with Davis et al. [38]. The three-dimensional maker trajectory data was filtered using Woltring's cross-validated quintic spline routine as incorporated in "Plug-In Gait." The data was then processed creating a three-dimensional link segment model. Kinematic and kinetic data were derived using the built-in facilities of VICON's "Plug-in Gait" software and was used for calculating the three-dimensional kinematics and kinetics (through inverse dynamics).

5.9.1   LOADING: 0%–10% CYCLE

Aims of this phase: Safe contact with the floor; ensure stable limb and absorb force/shock; smooth transfer of body weight from trailing limb; active bearing of weight.

Overall, the role of the foot is to absorb impact and adjust to surface irregularities. This is achieved by absorbing shock in the heel pad, eccentrically contracting the dorsiflexors, and pronating the subtalar joint to make the foot compliant and flexible [1]. The support of the trunk is primarily provided by the ankle dorsiflexors [33].

The role of the knee is to absorb shock by the eccentric contraction of the knee extensors, which also maintains weight-bearing stability at the knee [2]. The role of the hip, through an eccentric contraction of the hip abductors and the activation of the core muscles, is to maintain stability of the pelvis and to ensure that an erect posture of the trunk is preserved. A concentric contraction of the hip extensors (H1S) helps to pull the trunk over the supporting limb.

As load is transferred to the stance limb, compression begins and deformation occurs. Under normal conditions, this deformation is well within the critical limits of the whole body and the individual joints and tissues. Weight is taken on the new stance limb, though at the early stage (0%–2%) in the cycle the muscles have not "taken control" of the movement and there can be a peak in the Fz, often known at the impact peak. It is a matter of debate as to whether this shock does any harm [3,39].

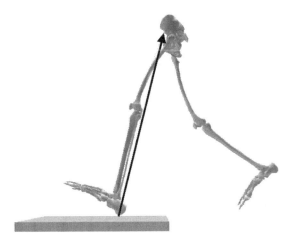

FIGURE 5.4 External GRV causes an external plantarflexor, knee flexor, and hip flexor moment. This is counteracted by an internal dorsiflexor, which controls the lowering of the foot to the floor, and a knee extensor and hip extensor moment, which stops the limb from collapsing as it is loaded.

In the sagittal plane, the GRV is directed behind the ankle and knee and in front of the hip (Figure 5.4). This causes an external plantarflexor moment at the ankle and flexor moment at the knee and at the hip. The ankle dorsiflexors contract eccentrically to control the lowering of the foot to foot-flat and providing smooth transition to stance. The knee extensors activate to control knee flexion allowing up to 20° of flexion (K1S). This movement helps to control the downward acceleration of the CoM. A hip extensor moment helps to control hip flexion and maintains 30° of flexion. Once the hip is stabilized, it moves from flexion to extension through a concentric contraction of the hip extensors (H1S) (Figure 5.4).

In the frontal plane, the GRV is directed medially and a strong adduction moment is exerted at the hip and knee that follows the rapid transfer of body weight onto the limb (Figure 5.5). The contralateral pelvis drops as the limb is being unloaded is limited to 5° by this strong hip abductor moment, which generates power through a concentric contraction (H1F). The external adductor moment that acts on the knee is largely controlled by the iliotibial band. The vector causes subtalar valgus, which is restrained by the tibialis anterior and posterior.

In the transverse plane, the subtalar valgus causes internal rotation at the talus and the accompanying rotation of the tibia results in an internal torque at the knee. The external rotators of the hip prevent the femur from internally rotating and this prevents excessive internal rotation at the knee. The limited internal rotation, which occurs at the hip, assists advancement of the contralateral limb in progression phase.

5.9.2 EFFECTS OF JOINT PATHOLOGIES

Due to the kinematic chain, if a pathology exists at one joint, it can effect other joints in the chain and compensations can also occur at different points in the chain.

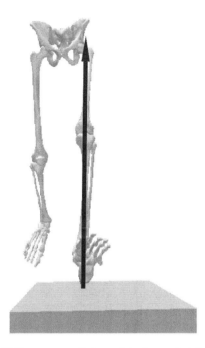

FIGURE 5.5 External GRV passes medially and the internal abductor hip moment, caused by an eccentric contraction of the muscles, controls the drop of the pelvis.

A common pathology evidenced in this phase is that initial contact is made with the forefoot. Pathologies at the foot, knee, and hip can cause and effect this condition. With the foot in equinus forefoot initial contact occurs and the GRV passes anterior rather than posterior to the ankle. Due to the location of the CoP a large external dorsiflexor moment occurs. The cause of the equinus could be an ankle plantarflexor contracture. Poor alignment of a prosthesis can also result in a similar plantarflexor position. To resolve the forefoot strike, if the person tries to contact in footflat then the compensation may be knee hyperextension and possibly increased foot (if present) pronation. Pseudoequinus can occur if the knee is excessively flexed at initial contact. Here, the ankle is normal, but the flexed knee enforces forefoot contact. Higher up the chain, if there are flexor hip contractures present, the implications for this phase of the gait cycle mean that the pelvis tilts anteriorly and the knee can be excessively flexed to ensure the heel contact the ground. This requires increased quadricep activity and results in crouched gait. For all these conditions, the initial contact is poorly aligned to absorb the subsequent load, which cannot be easily accommodated by the eccentric contraction at the hip and knee. Further, H1S is inhibited and so raising the trunk to the high point of midstance is difficult. As a result, anterior trunk lean can compensate to move the CoM forward. Reduced step length is evident with hip and knee flexor contractures.

At the ankle, loss of dorsiflexor function results in uncontrolled plantarflexion and footslap occurs. If the knee at the end of the previous swing phase cannot absorb the momentum of the swinging limb prior to initial contact, then the force experienced at initial contact may be high, and the orientation of the limb may cause higher loads. If the knee extensors are weak, excessive knee flexion can be seen, though more often the knee will remain fully extended throughout early stance and the gait will be abrupt in this phase.

In pathologies where the ankle and knee mechanisms do not work effectively, an excessive vertical displacement of the CoM can result, which is energy expensive. This is often seen in TT amputees and those with a peronial nerve disorder.

If the knees are in valgus or varus, the GRV may pass inside or outside the knee joint and if the knee abductor or adductor muscles are insufficiently strong to balance the load then the knee may collapse. A leg length discrepancy results in an asymmetrical pelvis and asymmetrical loading on the limbs.

Wearing high heels results in a larger plantarflexor moment as a result of the increased moment arm. The pretibial muscles have to generate a larger eccentric contraction to control the lowering of the foot to foot flat.

5.9.3 Support/Progression: 10%–50% Cycle

Aims of this phase: Stable base over which the trunk can travel to progress; support and balance without collapsing; facilitate swing of contralateral limb. Single support means that the load is taken solely by the stance limb.

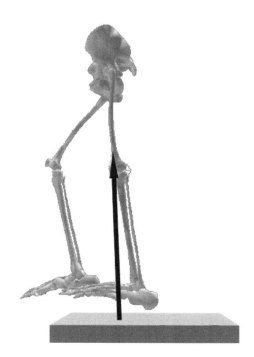

FIGURE 5.6 GRV passes anterior to the knee and hip keeping them extended. This extension by the external moment means that the muscles do not have to contract to maintain an extended limb in this phase. The eccentric contraction of the ankle plantarflexors restrains the passage of the trunk over the foot and helps to ensure stability and effective progression.

Overall, the role of the foot is to provide a flat stable base over which the body can progress, i.e., the trunk can be raised to the high point of midstance. The ankle must restrain the shank. The knee must extend to increase the weight-bearing capacity of the joint and to facilitate the raising of the trunk. The hip must provide stability, and support through a contraction of the gluteus medius and minimus with gravity assisting significantly [33], which also facilitates an upright alignment of the trunk.

In the sagittal plane, the ankle, knee, and hip work together to ensure that progress occurs with minimal overall energy cost. The ankle plantarflexors generate a large plantarflexor moment with an eccentric contraction at the soleus in which the muscle does negative work (A1S) [6]. That keeps the GRV vector passing anterior to the knee joint and behind the hip to stabilize these joints (Figure 5.6). This external extensor moment around the knee keeps the knee stable without the use of the knee extensors. Knee hyperextension is prevented by the posterior capsule ligaments and the gastrocnemius muscle and the result is an internal flexor moment.

In the frontal plane the hip stabilizes the pelvis with abductor muscle action to maintain it in a level posture as the contralateral limb swings through (Figure 5.7).

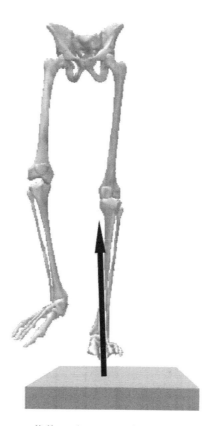

FIGURE 5.7   GRV passes medially and an eccentric contraction by the hip abductors keeps stops the pelvis from dropping more than about 5°. Maintaining a balanced pelvis ensures that there is sufficient clearance for the contralateral swinging limb to clear the floor.

5.9.4 PATHOLOGIES

The large plantarflexor moment, which restrains the shank and keeps the GRV anterior to the knee is a major mechanism for support in this phase [33,35]. Weakness of the plantarflexors allows the GRV to pass behind the knee and tends to cause collapse at this joint, with repercussions at the ankle and hip in the kinematic chain. This collapse is evident in "crouch gait."

Crouch gait (seen in diplegic cerebral palsy) is a multilevel pathology affecting the ankle, knee, and hip. There is often spacisticity of the hamstrings and iliopsoas. Due to the weak plantarflexors, the GRV passes posterior to the knee and so a flexor moment results in collapse of the joint and a consequent collapse at the hip. A common compensation for the unstable knee is anterior lean of the trunk shifting the GRV anterior to the knee again. To improve stability a KAFO, which ensures that hyperextension is prevented, can be prescribed. These devices have been developed to allow for flexion of the knee in swing while providing full stability in stance by automatically locking on loading in the stance phase. Both mechanical and electronic locking mechanisms are available. While the magnitude of the knee flexion in swing may not be as great as those in normal gait using the orthosis [40], it is sufficient to eliminate the need for vaulting.

Knee valgus/varus can result in the GRF vector passing medial or lateral to the knee in this phase. This increased moment can result in the increased stress on the collateral ligaments at the knee (or lax ligaments could cause the instability with results in valgus/varus) or increased load in the medial or lateral compartments of the joint. This may be a precursor to degenerative osteoarthritis. Lateral trunk lean may help to unload the medial compartment. Orthoses can also help to counteract these moments.

Contralateral swing through occurs in this phase. Any issues related to ensuring toe clearance can affect ipsilateral stance. For instance, if the contralateral swinging limb is long, then toe clearance can be ensured by trunk lean or pelvis hiking. However, these compensations can move the GRVr more medially on the supporting limb and increase loading on it. Further, the loading on the ipsilateral hip abductors is energy demanding and can effect stability in stance. An alternative method of clearing the long limb is through circumduction, which, again, can affect stance stability. Vaulting, through active ankle plantarflexion, on the stance limb is sometimes evident. This is energy expensive and increases lack of stability.

If the stance limb has weak hip abductors, the pelvis on the swinging side is more likely to drop and swing clearance needs to be ensured by the knee and ankle on the swinging side (Section 5.9.7). This gait is known as Trendelenburg gait and an obvious compensation is to lean the trunk toward the weak side, thus reducing the required hip abductor moment. This gait gives the appearance of waddling.

In patients with OA, Trendelenburg gait compensation is related to a painful hip. The load on the hip is reduced by decreasing gluteus medius activity, increasing pelvic tilt, and inclining the trunk on the side of the supporting limb. This is done to ensure that the moment arm between the hip and the CoM of the upper body is reduced in the frontal plane. The effect on the lumbar spine is not fully understood.

To try to reduce the loading on the hip in the support phase after a total hip arthroplasty, a cane is often recommended. Mechanically, contralateral use helps to reduce the loading on the affected hip primarily by decreasing the hip abductor muscle force required to balance the pelvis during single support. Ajemian et al. [18] found that the hip abductor moment on the affected hip decreased by 26%. However, the contralateral hip force increased by 28%. They concluded that this could hasten degeneration of an asytomatic joint and that sustained use of a cane after adequate healing should be monitored to avoid overloading the joint. Toward the end of support, if the ankle plantarflexors are weak or missing, then the foot rocker is missing and there is a loss of heel-off.

If there is posterior trunk lean in this phase (as a result of hip extensor weakness), then the GRV will pass further behind the hip and a larger extensor moment is evident. The resulting increased stability needs to be overcome to ensure progress.

In the transverse plane, toeing in can result in femoral anteversion. To bring the foot straight and avoid large torsion moments on the supporting limb, the hip externally rotates.

5.9.5 PROPULSION: 50%–60% CYCLE

Aims: Facilitate initial contact of contralateral limb; initiation of limb advancement into swing, which influences the subsequent raising of the trunk in contralateral loading and support.

This is the second double support of stance limb, ipsilaterally active ankle plantarflexion push-off (Figure 5.8) and hip flexion pull-off (Figure 5.9) propel the limb into swing. The angular momentum of the limb in swing is crucial for forward progression and it is determined at this stage. If the ankle plantarflexors or hip flexors do not contribute effectively to this phase then the contralateral stance is effected. Knee flexion, controlled by a knee power absorption (K3) is required to unload and shorten the limb and flexion velocity is crucial to successful swing. Females have indicated a greater knee flexion moment and a greater power absorption than males.

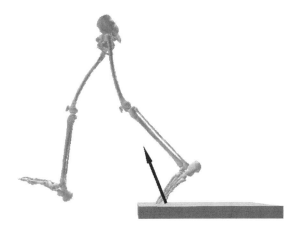

FIGURE 5.8 GRV at A2. The ankle push-off as a result of a powerful plantarflexor concentric contraction helps to propel the limb into swing. The energy produced in this phase is crucial to progress the trunk through contralateral stance. K3, the eccentric muscular contraction to control knee flexion also occurs now.

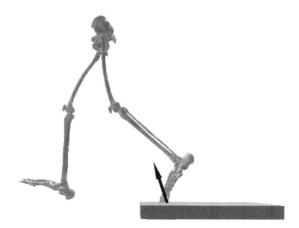

FIGURE 5.9 Just after A2, the hip pull-off power (H3) occurs. This hip power as a result of the concentric contraction of the hip flexors helps to propel the limb into swing. The distal to proximal pattern indicates a powerful coordination to increase the velocity of the limb at toe-off. The energy produced in this phase is crucial to progress the trunk through contralateral stance.

In order to propel the limb into swing, two key power bursts occur as a result of a concentric contraction. The ankle push-off power (A2S) is crucial with the gastrocnemius being the key muscle involved [34]. The hip, which was extended, often up to $10°$ of hyperextension at late support now actively flexes with a concentric contraction (H3S), which contributes to pulling the limb into swing. The plantarflexors generate almost all the support of the whole body in this phase [33].

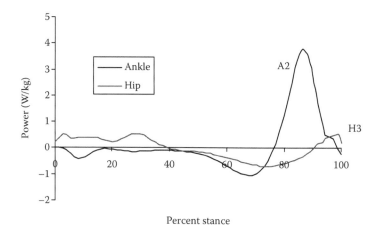

5.9.6 PATHOLOGIES

Walkers who do not have the active plantarflexion on the affected side, compensate, if possible, with the hip flexors. These produce more power than for the able-bodied. The contralateral hip, which is in loading, also compensates with an increased H1S.

When wearing high heels, the ankle plantarflexors cannot produce the A2S power as effectively and again, the compensation of increased hip pull-off assists the limb to advance. Hip flexion contractures can result in reduced step length, and the resulting knee flexion can result in "drop-off."

For the elderly, reduced gait velocity appears to be due to a reduced hip extension and to reduced peak power generation and reduced peak ankle plantarflexion [22]. A consequence of the reduced hip extension appears to be an increased anterior pelvic tilt to try to maintain a reasonable step length [22]. They suggest that the reduced range and power at the ankle could be due to reduced strength or could be a strategy to preserve balance during walking, to maintain greater foot–floor contact.

If the hip medial/lateral rotators are too tight, the resulting reduced pelvic rotation can result in a reduced step length and pronation or supination at the foot. Conversely, if there are pronation or supination deviations, then torsion at the knee and hip can occur and again due to the lack of rotation, the step length is reduced.

5.9.7 SWING: 60%–100% CYCLE

Aim: To advance the limb to a position to take over support in the next stance phase.

Loading from the ground is absent and only gravity, muscle and centrifugal forces are active. Once the limb is in swing, it swings much like a pendulum, though, the limb is shortened by knee flexion, which is required to ensure toe clearance. Muscle actions are necessary to check the large knee flexion velocity and the rectus femoris plays an important role in regulating the knee flexion. Knee flexion velocity at toe-off is highly correlated with the knee flexion in this phase [41]. This knee flexion velocity is in turn highly related to the ankle push-off at propulsion [6]. As the foot clears the ground by approximately 5 cm, the foot can be in danger of tripping as a result of, for instance, an uneven surface. Excessive knee flexion and ankle dorsiflexion can occur, or the pelvis can be raised. There are consequences for the stance limb in midstance (Section 5.9.4).

To prepare for the following stance, angular momentum must be removed from the swinging limb to ensure that it is safely placed on the floor for the next stance phase. Hip extensors eccentrically contact to control the swinging limb. The knee flexors eccentrically contract (K4S) to control the knee extension, which occurs as the foot swings forward to complete the stride. Rotational kinetic energy from the swinging limb is returned to the trunk through the hip joint and helps in forward progression by helping to raise the trunk through loading into single support [6]. Females demonstrated greater hip flexion and less extension before initial contact.

5.9.8 PATHOLOGIES

Pathologies, which can influence foot clearance, include foot-drop as a consequence of a lower-motor neuron lesion, dynamic or fixed equinus. In these cases, there are four options to ensure ground clearance (a) hip hiking; (b) circumduction; (c) vaulting; and (d) high-stepping. Often all the four are used to some extent. Other pathologies can affect the contralateral limb in stance (Section 5.9.4).

5.9.9 Detailed Description of Gait for Transtibial Amputees

For the transtibial amputee (TAA), the lower limb and ankle joint is missing. The disruption to the distal end of the kinematic chain means that the amputee can achieve a stable walking pattern through compensations at the remaining joints. As the amputation moves higher, or as it affects the contralateral limb, the extent of the compensations increases and the deviation from normal gait increases.

For a unilateral TTA, the aims of walking, to progress, in a stable and efficient manner can be achieved. The type of prosthesis, the alignment of the prosthesis, the length of the stump, the time since amputation, type of socket, liner, etc., can all have an affect on the gait of the amputee.

To ensure progression, the amputee must effectively initiate swing and then, once the limb is swinging, must ensure the prosthesis is swinging sufficiently fast so that the limb may be placed safely on the ground for the subsequent stance phase. Stability is somewhat compromised and the energy cost of walking is increased.

The key issue for the TTA is compensating for the loss of the ankle. As the ankle plays a key role at different parts of the gait cycle, the mechanical limitations of the prosthesis result in limited adaptability of the prosthesis. Different prostheses have been developed to try to enhance their mechanical characteristics to improve the walking pattern and reduce the compensatory mechanisms. The prostheses fall into two main categories, inert prostheses (typically SACH foot or uniaxial foot) and dynamic prostheses (typically flex-foot, mercury, seattle). The dynamic feet are often known as dynamic elastic response (DER) prostheses. The primary difference between these two prostheses is the "liveliness" of the pylon/foot. They are unresponsive in the inert foot—aside from the cushion heel of the SACH foot or the plantar/dorsiflexor bumpers on the uniaxial foot. For the dynamic feet, elements of the prosthesis have been designed to store energy in a spring mechanism early in stance and to return this energy in late stance, thus mimicking the A1S absorption of the normal ankle in midstance and A2S generation of power at terminal stance. These prostheses have had mixed success in enhancing TTA gait.

Perry and Shanfield [42] noted a difference in the forefoot area of the various designs, which allowed for different rates of progress for the CoP along the base of the foot. The FF had a more rapid progression of the trunk over the prosthesis during prosthetic support. The rate of progress of the CoP may be related to stability and those with a fast progress can be perceived as unstable by some amputees. In spite of the increased dorsiflexion at the ankle and the increased dorsiflexor moment in late stance for the FF, there was no corresponding increased velocity for the amputee nor a reduction of the energy expended by the amputee. This may have been as a result of any increased mobility being absorbed by the FF shank and not translating to the knee or hip [43].

An oft-reported aspect of the performance of DER prostheses is the "net efficiency" of the prosthesis. This relates to the ratio of the energy returned relative the energy absorbed, with a high net efficiency being rated as good. However, the net efficiency of the prostheses is not a suitable performance characteristic as it does not take into account the timing of energy storage and recovery and the effects that this timing will have on the gait of the amputee.

TABLE 5.2

Temporal Characteristics of TT Amputees Using Different Prostheses

	Velocity (m/s)	Cadence (step/min)	Stride Length (m)	Prosthetic Stance (% cycle)
Winter and Sienko [44]	0.97	92	1.27	—
SACH [45]	1.04	—	1.23	47.8
Seattle [45]	1.1	—	1.28	47.98
SACH [27]	1.32	118	1.36	43.8
CCII [27]	1.342	118.4	1.38	43.8

— Indicates no data reported.

5.9.10 OUTCOME MEASURES

Generally, the outcome measures for TTA indicate that the gait is not as successful as for the able-bodied. Velocity is reduced, stride length is shorter, step length and swing timing are asymmetric, and results vary for different prostheses. General temporal characteristics for transtibial amputees include decreased speed, shorter stride length and asymmetric step, and swing timings between the intact and prosthetic limbs, which vary for different prostheses. Table 5.2 summarizes some of the temporal characteristics reported in the literature.

Some of the data in Table 5.2 has been modified so that it could be reported in a comparative format. Due to different protocols and the different prostheses comparisons can only be made between prostheses in studies by the same researchers. Colborne et al. [45] reports strides/min rather than steps/min as 50.8 (±5.49) for the SACH and 52.4 (±10.6) for the Seattle prostheses. Anzel et al. [46] found that the speed of the amputee using the FF was 84 m/min, which was significantly faster than the 75.4 m/min when using the SACH foot. Using the Seattle, CCII, and Quantum, the speed was 79–81 m/min.

In the following section, the figures are based on a transtibial male walking at 1.42 m/s with a stride length of 1.46 m and a cadence of 117 steps/min. Data were collected and processed as for the participant above, but the markers were placed on the prostheses in anatomically matched positions. The amputee was wearing a patellar tendon bearing socket with an endolite limb, a teletorsion pylon, and a multiflex ankle. Process variables are discussed with the prosthesis as the focus limb.

5.9.11 LOADING

At initial contact, the prosthesis must safely take the load. Poor alignment can result in excessive knee extension, or flexion with consequent implications for the hip. Depending on the type of prosthesis, dorsiflexion is reduced or increased. If the alignment is such that the knee extends excessively, then the shock absorption capacity of the limb is reduced and the hip has to compensate (Figure 5.10). Alternatively, if there is too much flexion, then the movement of the CoM can be disrupted and the tibia can advance too quickly for the heel rocker to be effective. In order to compensate, the hip extensors will compensate to raise the body up to midstance. The trunk may also lean forward.

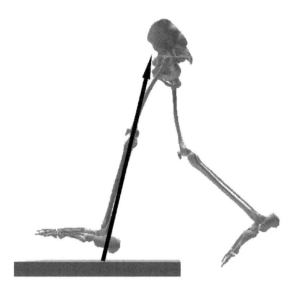

FIGURE 5.10 Direction of the GRV is altered due to the poor positioning of the limb at initial contact. It passes through the ankle and the knee and anterior to the hip. The ankle and knee remain stable and as the phase progresses the knee extension is maintained. The result is a stiff-kneed gait and is a common consequence of the abnormal ankle motion as a result of the passive prosthesis. More hip flexion than normal is a common consequence as a result of the kinematic chain.

During loading, the prosthesis is compressed. There is some deformation of the "cushion heel" of the SACH foot. The uniaxial prosthesis allows limited plantar-flexion due to the moment caused by the GRV passing behind the joint at the ankle. It is controlled by the rear rubber bumper. In the more dynamic prostheses, the dynamic element deforms to store elastic energy in the material of the prosthesis. This deformation simulates to a lesser degree than normal the plantarflexion of the foot. The absence of controlled plantarflexion results in footflat being delayed due to the length of time it takes for the amputee's leg to rotate forward until the foot is flat [44].

Saunderson and Martin [47] found that when using the FF there was a prolonged flexor moment at the knee in the first half of stance. They attributed the high extensor moment at the hip to the need to compensate for the knee flexor moment in the first half of stance, and that this was important to maintain the leg in extension and to move the body over the stance leg. The magnitude of H1S was more than twice that of normal and was maintained for longer than normal actually lasting for more than the first half of stance. This is attributed to the hip assisting in the control of knee flexion and in aiding to pull the trunk over the stance foot (Figure 5.10). This use of hip extensor power is known to increase as speed increases. In the frontal plane, the biomechanics are almost normal, though the loading may be more lateral to ensure stability (Figure 5.11).

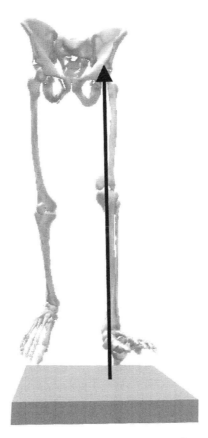

FIGURE 5.11 GRV passes medially, though often less than for nonpathological gait. The more lateral loading is to ensure a safe contact and stability in loading in the absence of adequate proprioception. An internal abductor hip moment, caused by an eccentric contraction of the muscles, controls the drop of the pelvis.

5.9.12 SUPPORT/PROGRESSION

Here, the ankle rocker is disrupted and the tibial restraint can be difficult to time. As a result the knee remains in flexion and the thigh does not move forward in a smooth manner (Figure 5.12).

As the forefoot bends over the keel, reduced dorsiflexion occurs. This limited motion prevents the amputee from taking longer steps due to the limited lean allowed by the body [48].

For the uniaxial prosthesis, in the transition to midstance the GRV passes rapidly along the plantar surface of the foot. As the rear bumper unloads and the front bumper is loaded, the foot begins to dorsiflex. This limited motion could also be a reason for increased energy expenditure due to the resulting elevation of the CoM.

Generally, the knee remains partly flexed throughout stance. The normal power burst at midstance (K2S) used to extend the knee and raise the CoM of the body is

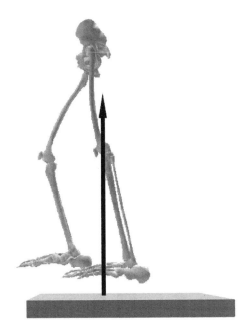

FIGURE 5.12   Lack of the eccentric contraction by the plantarflexors means that the GRV passes along the plantar surface of the foot faster than normal. As a result the knee remains flexed to compensate. The hips produce a larger than normal extensor moment to ensure the limb remains extended.

missing. Colborne et al. [45] noted the strong hip extensor moment throughout most of stance and the tendency for the knee to collapse is prevented by the hip. In the frontal plane the biomechanics are close to normal (Figure 5.13).

5.9.13   PROPULSION

At terminal stance, the lack of the ankle plantarflexors results in a reduced A2S and there is little power to begin to supply momentum to the limb for swing. The hips compensate and the H3S is larger than normal. In inert prostheses, the limb is lifted into swing from the more proximal joints, rather than pushed from the more distal joints. For the more dynamic prostheses, there is evidence that the A2S exists, but the timing and magnitude is not as effective as for a normal ankle and the hip continues to compensate (Figures 5.14 and 5.15).

The knee absorption power at toe-off quite normal.

5.9.14   SWING

Amputees must have both the strength to swing the limb and the ability to control the position of the limb when it is being loaded. For swing, there may be some knee or hip flexion to ensure toe clearance in midswing. The limb does not swing as quickly and knee power absorption at the end of swing (K4) is lower than normal as minimal power is needed to slow the slowly swinging prosthesis [44].

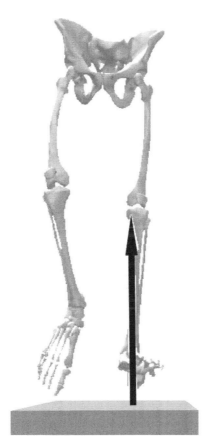

FIGURE 5.13   GRV passes medially and an eccentric contraction by the hip abductors keeps stops the pelvis from dropping more than about 5°. Maintaining a balanced pelvis ensures that there is sufficient clearance for the contralateral swinging limb to clear the floor. There is little difference between amputee and normal gait in this frontal plane in this phase.

A small extensor moment at the hip to stop the thigh rotating in preparation for heelstrike is evident.

The intact limb as the focus limb requires the key compensation during loading. Even when using dynamic prostheses contralaterally, the mean power pattern shows a large power burst at H1 when the hip extensors are shortened under tension to propel the body forward and thus compensate for the lack of energy generation by the missing contralateral ankle plantarflexors in contralateral propulsion.

5.9.15   BIOMECHANICALLY BASED SPECIFIC NEEDS OF THE TTA

To enhance progression and to facilitate stability, the following features of the pathological gait need to be addressed—"deformity" in the prosthesis, which results in a lack of ankle motion and inhibits knee motion as a result of the amputation, "development

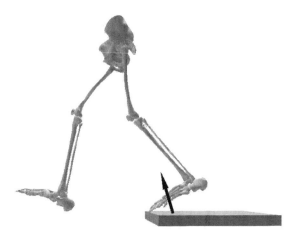

FIGURE 5.14 GRV at A2. The ankle push-off as a result of a powerful plantarflexor concentric contraction is missing in inert limbs and is reduced compared to normal in dynamic limbs. The reduced power results in reduced energy produced in this phase. In order to progress the trunk through contralateral stance the hip at H3 and contralaterally at H1 compensates. K3, the eccentric muscular contraction to control knee flexion is normal.

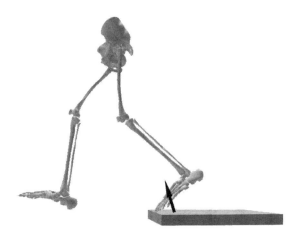

FIGURE 5.15 Just after A2, the hip pull-off power (H3) occurs. This hip power as a result of the concentric contraction of the hip flexors is larger than normal to compensate for the reduced power at the ankle. The energy produced in this phase is insufficient to fully compensate for the lacking ankle plantarflexors and progression is slower than normal, a result of the reduced stride length.

of muscle strength" on the muscles of the knee and hip on the amputated side, and the development of the prosthesis to replicate the action of the ankle dorsiflexors at loading, the plantarflexors eccentric contraction in support and plantarflexors concentric contraction in progression, "enhanced proprioception" especially at loading and propulsion and reduction of "pain" in the stump. Through rehabilitation, exercise and prosthetic development many of these areas can be addressed such that the TTA evidences little compensations to achieve gait.

5.10   CONCLUSION

Human walking gait is a complex movement, which, if successful, results in progression and support. Efficiency is required to sustain the walking mechanics over a distance. The biomechanics are the result of the individual's accommodation of imposed constraints. Walking is achieved through an interplay of internal and external forces. When pathological gait is being assessed, it is important to fully understand normal gait in order to be able to understand the adopted compensations. These compensations should not be viewed in isolation, and should not necessarily be "fixed" as the compensation is, in itself, a valid solution. Functional devices can be used to enhance gait, that is, to facilitate a more mechanically efficient or effective progression of a safely supported system.

REFERENCES

1. Kirtley, C., *Clinical Gait Analysis: Theory and Practice*. 2006, Edinburgh: Churchill Livingstone.
2. Perry, J., *Gait Analysis: Normal and Pathological Function*. 1992, Thorofare, NJ: Slack Incorporated.
3. Whittle, M., *Gait Analysis: An Introduction*. 3rd ed. 2002, Oxford: Butterworth-Heinemann.
4. Winter, D., *Biomechanics and Motor Control of Human Gait*. 1987, Waterloo: University of Waterloo Press.
5. Sutherland, D.H., R.A. Olshen, E.N. Biden, and M.P. Wyatt, *The Development of Mature Walking*. 1988, Philadelphia, PA: JB Lippincott.
6. Gage, J., *Gait Analysis and Cerebral Palsy*. 1991, Oxford: Blackwell Scientific Publications.
7. Fonseca, S.T., et al., A dynamical model of locomotion in spastic hemiplegic cerebral palsy: Influence of walking speed. *Clinical Biomechanics*, 2001. **16**(9): 793–805.
8. Olney, S.J. and C. Richards, Hemiparetic gait following stroke. Part I: Characteristics. *Gait & Posture*, 1996. **4**(2): 136–148.
9. Huitema, R.B., et al., Functional recovery of gait and joint kinematics after right hemispheric stroke. *Archives of Physical Medicine and Rehabilitation*, 2004. **85**(12): 1982–1988.
10. Quesada, P.M., L.J. Mengelkock, R.C. Hale, and S.R. Simon, Biomechanical and metabolic effects of varying backpack loading on simulated marching. *Ergonomics*, 2000. **43**(3): 293–309.
11. Chow, D.H., et al., The effect of backpack load on the gait of normal adolescent girls. *Ergonomics*, 2005. **48**(6): 642–656.
12. Fowler, N.E., A.L.F. Rodacki, and C.D. Rodacki, Changes in stature and spine kinematics during a loaded walking task. *Gait & Posture*, 2006. **23**(2): 133–141.
13. Kerrigan, D.C., et al., Moderate-heeled shoes and knee joint torques relevant to the development and progression of knee osteoarthritis. *Archives of Physical Medicine and Rehabilitation*, 2005. **86**(5): 871–875.
14. Mann, R., Biomechanics of the foot and ankle, in *Surgery of the Foot*, R. Mann, Ed. 1986, St. Louis, MO: Mosby.
15. Perry, J., Normal and pathological gait, in *Atlas of Orthotics*, American Association of Orthopaedic Surgeons, 1985, St. Louis, MO: Mosby. 76–111.
16. Miller, S., Biomechanical Implications of Prosthetics and Orthotics, in *Prosthetics and Orthotics: Lower Limb and Spinal*, R. Seymour, Editor. 2002, Baltimore, MD: Lippincott Williams and Wilkins.

17. Youdas, J.W., et al., Partial weight-bearing gait using conventional assistive devices. *Archives of Physical Medicine and Rehabilitation*, 2005. **86**(3): 394–398.
18. Ajemian, S., et al., Cane-assisted gait biomechanics and electromyography after total hip arthroplasty. *Archives of Physical Medicine and Rehabilitation*, 2004. **85**(12): 1966–1971.
19. American Physical Therapy Association, *A Guide to Physical Therapist Practice*. 2nd ed. 2001.
20. Sadeghi, H., et al., Symmetry and limb dominance in able-bodied gait: A review. *Gait & Posture*, 2000. **12**(1): 34–45.
21. Sadeghi, H., Local or global asymmetry in gait of people without impairments. *Gait & Posture*, 2003. **17**(3): 197–204.
22. Kerrigan, D.C., et al., Biomechanical gait alterations independent of speed in the healthy elderly: Evidence for specific limiting impairments, *Archives of Physical Medicine and Rehabilitation*, 1998. **79**(3): 317–322.
23. Hyndman, D., et al., Interference between balance, gait and cognitive task performance among people with stroke living in the community. *Disability and Rehabilitation*, 2006. **28**(13–14): 849–56.
24. Chen, G., et al., Gait differences between individuals with post-stroke hemiparesis and non-disabled controls at matched speeds. *Gait & Posture*, 2005. **22**(1): 51–56.
25. Watelain, E., et al., Pelvic and lower limb compensatory actions of subjects in an early stage of hip osteoarthritis. *Archives of Physical Medicine and Rehabilitation*, 2001. **82**(12): 1705–1711.
26. Kerrigan, D.C., et al., Kinetic alterations independent of walking speed in elderly fallers. *Archives of Physical Medicine and Rehabilitation*, 2000. **81**(6): 730–735.
27. Barr, A., et al., Biomechanical comparison of the energy-storing capabilities of SACH and Carbon Copy II prosthetic feet during the stance phase of gait in a person with below-knee amputation. *Physical Therapy*, 1992. **72**(5): 344–354.
28. Lelas, J.L., et al., Predicting peak kinematic and kinetic parameters from gait speed. *Gait & Posture*, 2003. **17**(2): 106–112.
29. Lord, S.E., et al., The effect of environment and task on Gait parameters after stroke: A randomized comparison of measurement conditions. *Archives of Physical Medicine and Rehabilitation*, 2006. **87**(7): 967–973.
30. Lerner-Frankiel, M.B., S. Varga, M.B. Brown, et al., Functional community ambulation: What are your criteria? *Clinical Management in Physical Therapy*, 1986. **6**(2): 12–15.
31. Cohen, J.J., J.D. Sveen, J.M. Walker, and K. Brummel-Smith, Establishing criteria for community ambulation. *Topics in Geriatric Rehabilitation*, 1987. **3**(1): 71–77.
32. Shumway-Cook, A., et al., Environmental demands associated with community mobility in older adults with and without mobility disabilities. *Physical Therapy*, 2002. **82**(7): 670–681.
33. Anderson, F.C. and M.G. Pandy, Individual muscle contributions to support in normal walking. *Gait & Posture*, 2003. **17**(2): 159–169.
34. Neptune, R.R., S.A. Kautz, and F.E. Zajac, Contributions of the individual ankle plantar flexors to support, forward progression and swing initiation during walking. *Journal of Biomechanics*, 2001. **34**(11): 1387–1398.
35. Kepple, T.M., K.L. Siegel, and S.J. Stanhope, Relative contributions of the lower extremity joint moments to forward progression and support during gait. *Gait & Posture*, 1997. **6**(1): 1–8.
36. Mienders, M., A. Gitter, and J.M. Czerniecki, The role of the ankle plantar flexor muscle work during walking. *Scandinavian Journal of Rehabilitation Medicine*, 1998. **30**(1): 39–46.
37. Winter, D.A., Concerning the scientific basis for the diagnosis of pathological gait for rehabilitation protocols. *Physiotherapy Canada*, 1985. **37**(4): 245–252.

38. Davis, I. and B. Roy, et al., A gait analysis data collection and reduction technique. *Human Movement Science*, 1991. **10**(5): 575–587.

39. Radin, E., R. Martin, D. Burr, B. Caterson, and R. Boyd, Mechanical factors influencing cartilage damage, in *Osteoarthritis, Current Clinical and Fundamental Problems*, J. Peyron, Ed. 1985, CIBA-Geigy: Basel, Switzerland. pp. 90–99.

40. Hebert, J.S. and A.B. Liggins, Gait evaluation of an automatic stance-control knee orthosis in a patient with postpoliomyelitis. *Archives of Physical Medicine and Rehabilitation*, 2005. **86**(8): 1676–1680.

41. Piazza, S.J. and S.L. Delp, The influence of muscles on knee flexion during the swing phase of gait. *Journal of Biomechanics*, 1996. **29**(6): 723–733.

42. Perry, J. and S. Shanfield, Efficiency of dynamic elastic response prosthetic feet. *Journal and Rehabilitation Research and Development*, 1993. **30**: 137–143.

43. Torburn, L., C.M. Powers, R. Guiterrez, and J. Perry, Energy expenditure during ambulation in dysvascular and traumatic below-knee amputees: A comparison with five prosthetic feet. *Journal and Rehabilitation Research and Development*, 1995. **32**: 111–119.

44. Winter, D.A. and S.E. Sienko, Biomechanics of below-knee amputee gait. *Journal of Biomechanics*, 1988. **21**(5): 361–367.

45. Colborne, G.R., et al., Analysis of mechanical and metabolic factors in the Gait of congenital below knee amputees: A comparison of the SACH and seattle feet. *American Journal of Physical Medicine and Rehabilitation*, 1992. **71**: 272–278.

46. Anzel, S., J. Perry, E. Ayyappa, L. Torburn, and C.M. Powers, Efficiency of dynamic Elastic Response Feet. *Rehabilitation R&D Progress Reports*, 1991. **29**: 32–33.

47. Saunderson, D.J. and P.E. Martin. *Joint Kinetics in Unilateral Below Knee Amputees During Walking*. in *NACOB*. 1992. Chicago, IL.

48. Wagner, J., et al., Motion analysis of SACH versus flex-foot in moderately active below-knee amputees. *Clinical Prosthetics and Orthotics*, 1987. **11**: 55–62.

6 Wheelchair Ambulation: Biomechanics and Ergonomic Considerations*

Lucas H. V. van der Woude, Sonja de Groot, Dirkjan H. E. J. Veeger, Stefan van Drongelen, and Thomas W. J. Janssen

CONTENTS

6.1 INTRODUCTION

Wheeled mobility is a necessity in daily ambulation for a growing number of people. In the Netherlands the number of wheelchair users is estimated to be around 150,000 [180]. Based on this estimate, the figure for the United

---

* Based on a position stand presented at the Meeting "Health, Sports and Innovations," Session "Sports and Disability," Brussels, Belgium, 27–28 May 2005 and published in adapted form in *Science et Sports* 21, 226–235, 2006 and *Medical Engineering & Physics* 28, 905–915, 2005.

States and Europe may be extrapolated to, respectively, a rough 2.6 and 3.9 million—on average elderly—people. The majority of these people will use a self-or assistant-propelled manual wheelchair. This chapter will focus on the self-propelled wheelchair. By nature, the use of the upper-body and arms, a limited (age-related) fitness, and the impairment itself, a wheelchair-confined lifestyle will hamper individual mobility and participation. Simmons et al. [152] conclude their study "Wheelchairs as mobility restraints..." with: "Improving wheelchair skills with targeted intervention programs, along with making wheelchairs more 'user friendly' ... could result in more wheelchair propulsion with resultant improvements in the resident's independence, freedom of movement and quality of life."

This statement, evidently coming from the heart, seemingly sets the scene for a straightforward research agenda. However, this puts the complexity of wheeled mobility into a somewhat too simplified perspective. Wheeled mobility is indeed a complex issue both in theory and practice and its study requires a systematic approach that can do well with a clear conceptual framework.

Although mobility is an essential element in daily life, its importance is usually only then recognized when it is for some reason (temporarily) limited, as is the case in those who are wheelchair dependent. Mobility is a multilayered concept. One can speak of joint mobility, but also of mobility as an element of daily activities and of course within the context of participation we use the term mobility (social range of action, freedom of movement). All three mentioned connotations of mobility substantiate the main objectives of an integral (often lifelong) rehabilitation process. As such, mobility can be positioned at each of the three domains of functioning within the International Classification of Functioning, Disability, and Health (ICF) model [198]. This model is exemplified for (the rehabilitation of) persons with a spinal cord injury (SCI) in Figure 6.1. It is in many ways the conceptual starting point of the different aspects

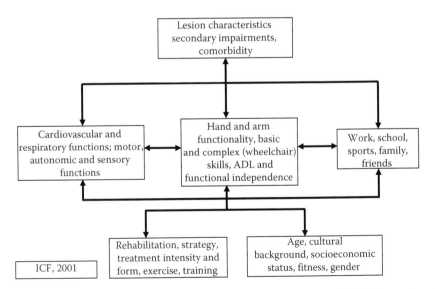

FIGURE 6.1 ICF model, as applied to persons with a SCI. (From WHO, *International Classification of Functioning, Disability and Health*, Geneva, World Health Organisation, 2001. With permission.)

of (biomechanics and ergonomics) research in rehabilitation and in the related issues of restoration of (wheeled) mobility, activities of daily living, and sports for those with a disability.

Within the context of a chronic impairment, rehabilitation focuses on restoration of mobility in its widest sense. Continuing to be a mobile individual and having an optimal social and physical range of action are key objectives in rehabilitation of those with lower-limb impairments. In today's rehabilitation field, this goes beyond the mere restoration, compensation, and (technology-based) adaptation of sensomotor function, functional capacity, activities of daily living (ADL), functional capacity, and independence. A physically active lifestyle, including sports, during and after rehabilitation is becoming an increasingly important issue on the rehabilitation research agenda [37,58,65,138]. Understanding the underlying mechanisms and processes of adaptation and/or the compensation of function and functioning, with or without the use of optimal assistive technology, is the core of biomechanics and ergonomics-based rehabilitation research and knowledge. The underlying multicausal and multilayered rehabilitation paradigm is "To restore function and functionality, and to stimulate optimal activity and participation."

Wheelchairs are assistive devices crucial for daily functioning of those with lower-limb impairments. The interaction between assistive technology and the (disabled) human system is complex by definition and requires a detailed research approach from a combined ergonomics and biophysical rehabilitation perspective.

As an example, the long-term use of assistive technology* and its consequences on the musculoskeletal system have become an important issue in manual wheelchair research, where the continued imbalance between the task stresses, physical strain, and overall mechanical and physiological work capacity leads to overuse injuries in the upper extremities [13]. In general when assistive technology for (wheeled) mobility and the biological system do not optimally match and function, a debilitative cycle may start that can lead to an inactive lifestyle [88,98], leading to disuse and even nonuse of assistive technology, and consequently to an increased risk for secondary health complications. This stresses the important preventive role of an integrative ergonomics approach within the field of rehabilitation and assistive technology, as is clearly exemplified in the Human-Activity-Assistive-Technology (HAAT) model of Cook and Hussey [32] (Figure 6.2). This model emphasized the, not too often explicitly recognized in the scientific literature [25,103,111,116,151,155,201], ergonomics basis of assistive and rehabilitation technology, and of the rehabilitation approach in a broader context [92,111,121].

Optimal functioning of the human movement system in the context of (wheeled) mobility restoration can be conceptualized as a continued effort of the biological system to maintain a proper balance between external stresses, internal strain, and the (physical) work capacity. As such, the stress–strain–work capacity model of

---

* For example, "…a broad range of devices, services, strategies and practices that are conceived and applied to ameliorate the problems faced by individuals who have disabilities…"

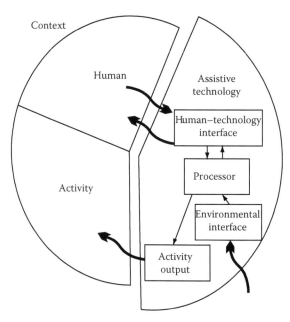

FIGURE 6.2   The HAAT model. (From Cook, A. and Hussey, S., *Assistive Technologies: Principles and Practice*, Mosby Year Book Inc., St Louis, MO, 2002. With permission.)

van Dijk et al. [57] expresses the interdependency of these domains in a flow diagram (Figure 6.3), applicable also in rehabilitation and indeed useful in the context of assistive technology research and practice. "Overall work capacity" must be interpreted here as the total sum of maximum physical, cognitive, mental, and social aspects of the human capacity in every day functioning.

Although the individual is by definition viewed as a biopsychosocial entity, the issues addressed in the following will primarily have a biophysical perspective.

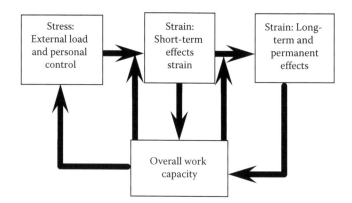

FIGURE 6.3   The stress–strain–work capacity model of van Dijk et al. (From van Dijk et al., *TSG*, 68, 3, 1990. With permission.)

From an ergonomics perspective, the external stresses in the context of wheeled mobility for instance are a consequence of (1) the combined effect of mechanical wheelchair characteristics and environmental conditions and (2) from the fine-tuning of the wheelchair–user interface [6,112,120,160,175]. Beyond that, (3) physical work capacity is defined by the overall functional capacity of the cardiovascular, respiratory, and the neuromuscular systems, and clearly is dependent on such individual characteristics as impairment, age, gender, training status, genetics, and expertise. In manual wheelchair use, the optimal level of, and interplay among, these three different domains are crucial for a maximum range of mobility, as it would be for any other assistive devices for ambulation, as indeed can be represented with Cook and Hussey's "ergonomics" model for assistive technology [31] (Figure 6.2).

Having the different conceptual models at the background of our mind, the current chapter will address important practical and research issues of a mobile and physically active lifestyle for those in rehabilitation, especially in those who are wheelchair dependent. In addition, it will provide a framework of biophysical and ergonomics considerations for manual wheelchair practice and research.

6.2 WHEELING AND (IN-)ACTIVITY

The importance of a physically active lifestyle was recognized for the general population in research [21,80,81] and by influential (political) bodies such as the American College of Sports Medicine,[*] Centers for Disease Control,[†] and the World Health Organization.[‡] Recently, it became even more evident, that (restoration of) an active lifestyle is highly more important for those with a chronic disease or those involved in (clinical) rehabilitation [37,58,65,138,163].

The focus onto the health-related mobility problem of a wheelchair-confined life in individuals with a SCI was already recognized by Clarke [28] in 1966 and later stressed by Voigt and Bahn [195], Hjeltnes and Vokac [88], Dallmeijer et al. [43], and Janssen et al. [43,98,99]. Sports have played a major role in an active lifestyle over the years. Today, being active in daily life is considered essential for general health. More and more, the risks of a sedentary lifestyle have become apparent in international literature as being one of the keystones to the prevention of many chronic diseases such as diabetes type II, the metabolic syndrome, forms of cancer, and cardiovascular disease [37,58,65,138,163]. The prominent role of an active lifestyle in the prevention of long-term health problems has become a specific issue that must be on the rehabilitation and sports-research agenda [58,65,138,163], especially in those who are limited in their mobility, such as people who are wheelchair-dependent. Sports and an active lifestyle have been shown to have a marked effect on life satisfaction [158], quality of life, and participation [79,128,129]. The risk of an inactive life, the problem of inefficiency of the manual wheeling task in general, and the subsequent risks of mechanical overload has boosted the research activity

---

[*] www.acsm.org

[†] www.cdc.gov/nccdphp/dnpa/surveill.htm

[‡] www.who.int/hpr/physactiv/health.benefits.shtml

over the years and has changed wheelchair design from the chromium-plated sling seat format in the early years toward a much more specialized and often individually fine-tuned assistive device today.

6.3   WHEELING AND UPPER-BODY OVERUSE

Wheelchair arm work is physically straining, and this is even more so for individuals who are not well trained. Next to the cardiovascular risk of an inactive lifestyle, an important other long-term secondary health problem in wheelchair-confined individuals is upper-body musculoskeletal overuse [15,40,59,66,106,145,181]. Overuse—especially in the shoulders and wrists, but also neck and low back—are seen in both sedentary as well as highly active wheelchair users. In various studies, a direct link has been made between this overuse problem and the repetitious and daily use of the hand rim wheelchair [140] in combination with other daily activities such as weight-relief lifts and body transfers [62,67,68,132,182]. Especially the latter have been suggested to generate local peak strains on the upper body. Internal joint forces have been described to exceed forces equal to body weight [184–186]. Wheelchair propulsion itself is in that sense a relatively low intensity, but highly frequent stress [190]. Based on the work of Veeger et al. [190] and van Drongelen et al. [185,186] (Figure 6.4), it can be suggested that an estimated minimum daily period of 1 h hand rim propulsion would lead to some 1800 bimanual pushes. Using biomechanical modeling, each push generates an unilateral reaction or compression force in the shoulder joint of some 40 kg (390 N). In that same day a wheelchair user will make some 15 lifts and or transfers. Each lift leads to a joint compression or contact force of 110 kg (1080 N), which has been shown to be even higher (+55 kg (540 N)) in those with trunk and arm impairments, such as tetraplegia. The combination of high-repetition–low-intensity wheeling with the relatively low number but highly intense daily transfers, lifts, and other activities—in association with the lack of recovery time of the upper extremities in individuals in a wheelchair during a day—seem to explain the high prevalence (50%–70% of the population is at risk [59,126,145]) of upper-extremity complaints after 10–15 years of wheelchair use.

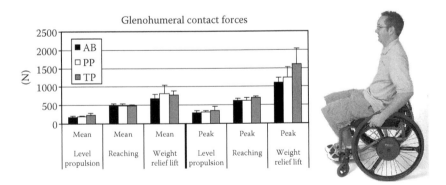

FIGURE 6.4   Model outcome: mean and peak GH contact forces in three ADL tasks for five able-bodied subjects (AB), eight persons with paraplegia (PP), and four with tetraplegia (TP) [184–186].

It is expected that next to impairment (i.e., high/low lesion), technique and boundary conditions (i.e., wheelchair fit, physical environment), balanced upper-body physical conditioning [66,181] may influence the risk of these activities for overuse problems [40]. Prevention of overuse, such as through improved (hand rim) wheelchair design [135], must directly impact the balance of stress–strain and capacity of wheeling and daily wheelchair use, especially with respect to muscle force/power and the balance of muscle capacity around complex joints, such as the shoulder and the wrist. Practical consequences are the need for ergonomic optimization of both wheelchair technology and the built environment [108]. The latter should limit too high physical exertions due to, for example, negotiation of (side) slopes, curbs, and floor surface characteristics. In addition, other techniques of transfers and the use of appropriate transfer-assist devices [30,73] must be trained in early rehabilitation. Finally, a well-trained upper-body musculature must help prevent an imbalance among muscle groups and the disturbance of the mechanical balance around the highly flexible, but complex structures of the shoulder and wrist joints [40,66].

To develop an understanding of dose–response relationships, research should study the longitudinal development of overuse problems in combination with mechanical strain in association to specifics of daily activities, wheelchair design, and that of the built environment and individual physical capacity (e.g., muscle strength), both in sedentary persons and athletes. In addition, intervention studies [40] should be further elaborated on. With regards to the underlying mechanisms of tissue damage, effects of both incidental peak stresses as well as highly repetitive but submaximal stresses should be studied with different laboratory techniques. Eventually, this may lead to more evidence-based guidelines for the prevention of upper extremity overuse in those with a SCI [16], as well as other groups of wheelchair users.

A BRIEF HISTORICAL SIDESTEP (1)

The presence of wheelchairs for ambulation dates back to ancient times.* In 1655 Stephen Farfler, a paraplegic watchmaker, built his own—mainly wooden self-propelled three-wheeled arm crank wheelchair—in many ways much a physical archetype of today's hand cycle. Yet, serious wheelchair research was only to start in the late 1960s, initially from a mechanical point of view. Focus was made on materials, durability, safety, and vehicle mechanics [22,64,131,156]. Despite a start in the late 1960s [17,20] at a much later stage interest in manual wheelchair propulsion was directed toward the physiological and health-related consequences. Even more recently, attention was more consistently also geared toward the biomechanical aspects of wheelchair propulsion [18,33–35,91,139,143,161,188]. A detailed engineering perspective of different aspects of wheeled mobility is given by Cooper [36].

Initially, biomechanics and physiology focused on performance-related issues with relatively simple technology and methodology. Despite the major improvement in technology, propulsion technique is still not very well understood. More recently, biomechanics research has been geared toward the musculoskeletal problems of long-term wheelchair use and sports. Today, within the framework of active wheelchair

---

* www.wheelchairnet.org/WCN_WCU/SlideLectures/Sawatzky/WC_history.html

use, a number of relevant research questions can be categorized and receive increasing attention in international literature. There are a number of performance associated issues: propulsion technique, (peak) power production, short-term peak power or anaerobic power production. But also disability-related issues must be raised, for instance with respect to questions directly associated with the human stress–strain–capacity problem, all in relation to the ergonomics of wheelchair design and fitting.

Obviously, a wide variety of hand-propelled wheelchairs is available on the market today. One cannot speak of the wheelchair, even when we isolate the hand rim-propelled wheelchair that is predominantly used in daily life and sports. Indeed, just small variations in wheelchair configuration may lead to differences in the human–machine interaction and in vehicle mechanics. This will subsequently influence physiological and biomechanical measures of performance.

6.4   RESEARCH TECHNOLOGY AND WHEELCHAIR PROPULSION

To study the physiological and mechanical strain of manual wheelchair propulsion and wheelchair sports performance in rehabilitation today, specific technologies (often limited to laboratory settings) are required to measure with detail and accuracy. The development of computer technology, human movement sciences, biology, engineering, and electronics into the interdisciplinary field of biomechatronics over the past decades has driven the design and availability of precise and fast measurement technology, such as motion sensors, in- and outside the rehabilitation research laboratory.

Primarily for its complexity, few studies have evaluated the more overall functional use of (sports) wheelchairs [49]. Functional evaluation of wheelchairs is often conducted in standardized laboratory experiments on treadmills or ergometers [175], allowing detailed physiology and biomechanics (using simulation devices such as treadmills or ergometers; Figure 6.5.), but with limited face validity. These set-ups allow repeated and specific physiological steady-state or peak exercise testing in sedentary and expert wheelchair users, as well as evaluation of propulsion technique and mechanical strain. Small numbers of subjects are generally used in these

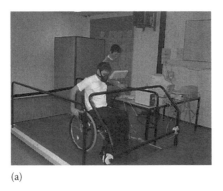
(a)

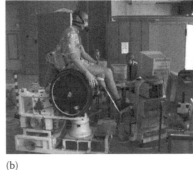
(b)

FIGURE 6.5   (a) Exercise testing on a motor-driven treadmill and (b) on a computer-controlled wheelchair ergometer.

studies. This research effort has led to the start of the development of more or less evidence-based guidelines for exercise prescription in rehabilitation [58,65].

Measurement outside the laboratory and on the track has become more feasible due to the further development and miniaturization of monitoring devices, portable metabolic analyzers, and motion sensor technology. Especially in wheelchair sports, but also in rehabilitation, this opens up new avenues for performance-related (longitudinal) research.

The study of daily physical activity and associated health issues require large subject numbers. Apart from heart rate monitoring [43,89,98] and the common use of questionnaires for (in-)activity and lifestyle research, the use of small computer-based activity sensors has recently entered research into activity monitoring, also in the field of rehabilitation and sports [76,157]. Accelerometer monitoring of home- and community-based ambulatory activity during and after rehabilitation allow to study quantity of movement [26,130,133,153,162], thus opening ways to stimulate and advise on activity and lifestyle. Only few physical activity questionnaires are available for specific use in rehabilitation populations [163], while the sensor-based techniques require elaborate validation and reliability research for different subpopulations in rehabilitation. However, it is important to stimulate this type of research. Some of these more complex sensor techniques not only allow to observe the quantity but also the quality of ambulation in real life over a longer period of time [26], even in hand rim wheelchair propulsion [133].

To study the force impact of wheeling and other ADL on the musculoskeletal system requires not only detailed biomechanical modeling [182,190], but also the accurate measurement of 3D forces and moments of the hands on the propulsion mechanism. 3D force measurement is available in some ergometers [191] (Figure 6.5b), but today also in instrumented wheels [5,41,144,186,190,202]. A six degrees of freedom force measuring hand rim wheel (Figure 6.6) is currently

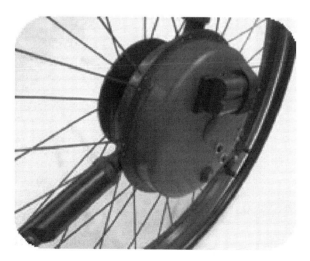

FIGURE 6.6   The Smartwheel, a six degrees of freedom force-sensing measurement hand rim wheel.

available commercially.* Obviously, detailed propulsion technique and power output can be studied with these (expensive) devices in sports and rehabilitation practice, but interpretation is not self-evident.

Less expensive tools for ambulant power output measurement—outdoors during rehabilitation, sports, and recreation, or in daily wheelchair use—for hand rim wheelchairs may become available in the near future, based on bicycle measurement technology such as the Power Tap[+] and SRM[‡] [9], which is currently being applied in hand cycle systems. Power output in wheelchair ambulation is an important performance indicator—next to the traditional peak oxygen uptake—being specific, sensitive and reliable, and closely linked to daily wheelchair activity [44,105,175,187].

6.5 MANUAL WHEELCHAIRS

Obviously, manual wheelchair technology has dramatically improved over the last decades, although the central concept of the most frequently employed hand-propelled wheelchair in the western world, the hand rim wheelchair, has not clearly changed. The transfer of the sling-seat chromium-plated wheelchair of the 1950s toward the function-specific (all lightweight and high-tech material, solid frame wheelchairs; and e.g., in track wheelchairs: speed and endurance-oriented design, aerodynamic low bucket seat, large wheels, smaller hand rims; or: basketball wheelchairs: highly maneuverable and acceleration-oriented design, large camber angle and small castors, normal sized rim diameter; Figure 6.7) and modern looking design of today took place in different phases, initiated primarily through wheelchair sports developments. Research clearly contributed, but many innovations originated initially from sports practice. In the context of mobility, the hand rim wheelchair has become a task-specific, versatile, and functional device.

THEORETICAL SIDESTEP (2): A BIOMECHANICAL RESEARCH STRATEGY

Cyclic movement

Manual wheelchair propulsion is frequently studied as a cyclic movement pattern [171] a given propelling motion is repeated over time at a given frequency (f), generally to maintain a certain stationary velocity (v). This implies that in each stroke or push of the wheel the athlete produces a more or less equal amount of work (A). The advantage of this approach is that physiological measures (i.e., energy cost, physical strain) can elegantly be linked to biomechanical measures (i.e., power output, work, force, and torque production). The product of push frequency (f) and work (A) gives the average external power output (P_o), according to

$$P_o = fA \, (\mathrm{W}) \tag{6.1}$$

---

* www.3rivers.com
[+] www.analyticcycling.com
[‡] www.srm.de

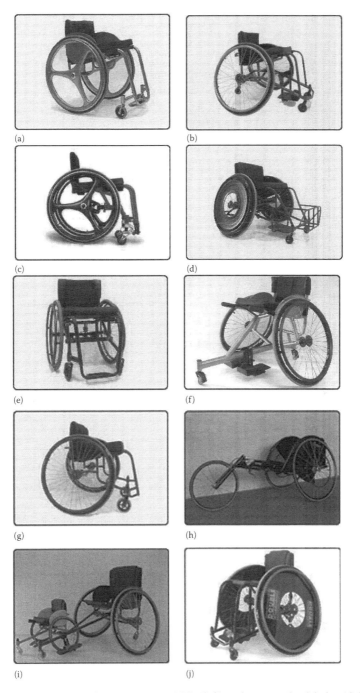

FIGURE 6.7 A sample of contemporary ADL (left) and sports wheelchairs (right, top to bottom basketball, rugby, tennis, wheeling, and hockey).*

---

* www.doubleperformance.nl

The work produced in each push constitutes the integral of the momentary torque (M) applied by the hands to the hand rim over a more or less fixed angular displacement (Q). In hand rim propulsion, the push is discontinuous, under steady-state conditions highly reproducible, and generally is limited to an angle of 70°–80° [7,168], given the constraints of the sitting posture, functional anatomy of the upper-body, and the spatial orientation of the rim. Equation 6.1 can be rewritten as

$$P_o = f\Sigma M dQ \ (\text{W}) \tag{6.2}$$

where torque is the product of the bimanual tangential force, that is applied on the hand rim, and the radius of the hand rim.

Measurement of angular displacement and the torque around the wheel-axle requires specialized experimental techniques for motion analysis and force measurement, which are not widely available. Therefore a different approach to determine P_o is frequently employed. Here the forces resisting the wheelchair–user combination are taken as the starting point for the calculation of power output. The wheelchair–user combination is approached as a free body that moves at a given speed (v) and encounters the following (drag) forces; rolling friction (F_{roll}), air resistance (F_{air}), gravitational effects when going up/down a slope ($mg \cdot \sin \alpha$), and internal friction (F_{int}). Details of these forces will be discussed below. The product of the sum of these drag forces (F_{drag}) and the linear velocity of the free body equals the power output that must be produced to maintain that velocity, according to

$$P_o = F_{drag}v \ (\text{W}) \tag{6.3}$$

The drag force can fairly easily be determined through a drag test [149,150].

Arm work and gross mechanical efficiency

Power production during hand rim wheelchair propulsion is achieved by upper-body work, primarily the arms. The relatively small muscle mass of the upper extremities and increased tendency for local fatigue leads to a much lower maximal work capacity in comparison to legwork. Peak upper-body oxygen uptake is usually 60%–85% of that in leg work [175]. Measurement of power output in wheelchair exercise testing, in combination with physiological measurements of the cardiorespiratory strain, gives additional information on the physical capacity of the person, and is also required for the calculation of the efficiency of the wheelchair–user system. The gross mechanical efficiency (ME) is defined as the ratio between externally produced energy (power out) and internally liberated energy (E_n: i.e., oxygen cost under submaximal, physiological steady-state conditions), according to

$$\text{ME} = (P_o E_n^{-1}) \times 100 \ (\%) \tag{6.4}$$

6.5.1 Vehicle Mechanics

Overall, innovation in vehicle mechanics has changed the specifics of the daily use and sports wheelchair dramatically in the light of load reduction, stability, and endurance. As is indicated in Table 6.1, various aspects of wheelchair design

TABLE 6.1
Mechanical Factors and Their Way in Which They Influence Rolling Resistance of Hand Rim Wheelchairs

Factors	Rolling Resistance
Body mass ↑	↑
Wheelchair mass ↑	↑
Tire pressure ↓	↑
Wheel size ↑	↓
Hardness floor ↓	↑
Camber angle ↑	?
Toe-in/out ↑	↑↑
Castor shimmy ↑	↑
For-aft position center of mass closer to large rear wheels	↓
Folding frame (versus box frame)	↑
Maintenance ↓	↑

Source: van der Woude, L.H., et al., *Med. Eng. Phys.*, 23, 713, 2001. With permission.

and technology have a major impact on rolling resistance [108] and thus on the mechanical and metabolic strain of the user [170].

The rolling resistance is the major opposing force in daily life and is heavily influenced by relatively straightforward aspects of "bicycle technology," such as wheel and tire characteristics, frame design, overall weight, etc. From a practical perspective, much profit can relatively easily be gained from proper and regular maintenance and from the choice of material, especially critical in the light of prevention of mechanical overuse and physical inactivity. Many different wheel and tire characteristics have been studied in fair detail [93,147,168] for that purpose.

THEORETICAL SIDESTEP (3): VEHICLE MECHANICS

The mechanical performance of a wheelchair is subject to rolling friction, air drag, and internal friction of the wheelchair. Task load can be expressed as external power, or the energy per unit time that is required to maintain the speed of the wheelchair–user combination. With the help of a so-called "power balance," the forces and energy sources responsible can be systematically evaluated [170]. The power balance for wheelchair propulsion can be expressed in the following equation:

$$P_o = (F_{roll} + F_{air} + F_{int} + mg \sin \alpha + ma) \cdot v \ (W) \tag{6.5}$$

where
   P_o is the external power output
   a is the acceleration of the system
   m is the mass of the wheelchair + user
   α is the angle of slope or inclination

If a wheelchair is kept at a constant speed, the athlete has to produce a certain amount of energy per unit time, or power. This is called external power (P_o). This external power is produced by the user and requires a much higher amount of internal power. The external power output is necessary to overcome energy losses in the system. The wheelchair–user combination will lose energy in the form of rolling resistance, air resistance, and internal resistance in the mechanical structures of the chair. When more external power is produced than is needed to overcome these losses, the chair will accelerate. The magnitude of acceleration will be dependent on the weight of the chair (ma). Also, the surplus of external power can be used to overcome a slope ($mg \sin \lambda$). On the other hand, negotiating a slope will, at a given external power output, lead to slowing down of the system. The terms ma and $mg \sin \lambda$ should not be considered as straight losses since they will work both ways. Energy, invested in acceleration or climbing, will be "harvested" when coasting or descending. In the following, we will briefly discuss the sources of energy losses; rolling resistance, air resistance, and internal friction.

Rolling resistance

In daily use conditions, rolling resistance generally is the major resisting force. Below relative head wind conditions of 2 m s^{-1}, air drag is still negligible. Rolling resistance can be determined in different manners. A coast-down technique is frequently used to determine rolling friction characteristic of the wheelchair in combination with different floor surfaces, or the effect of combined air and rolling resistance. A second method is the drag test. Also, rolling resistance can be measured by measuring the push force as is exerted by a wheelchair attendant to evaluate different floor surfaces [99,102] (Figure 6.8). This may lead to considerably high resisting forces and as a consequence to high start-up and push forces, as described by Koontz et al. [108].

   Apart from floor surface, rolling friction is essentially dependent on the characteristics of the wheels and tires; rolling resistance is lower for wheels with a larger radius and for harder tires. Rolling resistance can be expressed as the following equation:

$$F_{roll} = \eta_1 (N_1 R_1^{-1}) + \eta_2 (N_2 R_2^{-1}) \, (N) \qquad (6.6)$$

where
   R_1 and R_2 are the radii of the front and rear wheels
   N_1 and N_2 indicate the relative weight on those wheels
   η_1, η_2 are the friction coefficients

The magnitude of the friction coefficients is related to the amount of deformation of tire and floor surface. This deformation dissipates energy [189]. Deformation is dependent on tire pressure, tread and profile, or wheel diameter, but also on wheel alignment (Table 6). Wheel toe-in or toe-out has a considerable effect on rolling resistance.

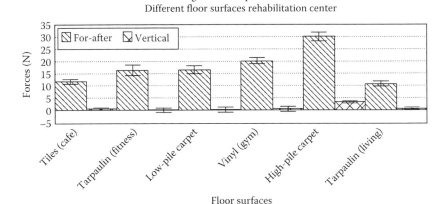

FIGURE 6.8 Effects of different floor surfaces on the horizontal (for-after) push force (measured with an experimental push wheelchair with two degrees of freedom force transducer). (From van der Woude, L.H., et al., *Med. Eng. Phys.*, 23, 713, 2001. With permission.)

For camber this is not so clear. It appears that, according to experimental results of Veeger et al. [196], camber of the rear wheels has no negative effect on rolling friction. However, Weege [23,196] advocates the opposite on the basis of theoretical considerations.

A special—frequently encountered problem in daily wheelchair use and racing— is the effect of a side slope [64]. The wheelchair generally will have the tendency to coast down a slope, which makes the steering of the wheelchair complicated and increases rolling resistance due to the effect on the alignment of the front casters. For that purpose track and racing wheelchairs are equipped with steering mechanisms that fixes the direction of the front wheel in a preset direction.

Air resistance

The second important factor in the power balance equation (Equation 6.6) is air resistance. In wheelchair racing this factor is by far the most important source of energy losses. Air resistance is dependent on the drag coefficient (C_d), frontal plane area (A), air density (∂), and velocity of the air flow relative to the object (v):

$$F_{air} = \frac{1}{2}\partial A C_d v^2 \text{ (N)} \tag{6.7}$$

As mentioned earlier, air resistance will be of minor importance at low speeds, but at high speeds and/or wind velocities air resistance will be the most important source of resistance. Following Abel and Frank [29] at slow speed (1 m s^{-1}) air drag will be below 1 N, while at 5 m s^{-1} the drag force due to air resistance is ±14 N, which implies an average power output of (5 × 14=) 70 W for wind resistance only at that wheelchair speed. It is obvious that the frontal plane area is dependent on the posture of the athlete. Although a wind tunnel experiment has been performed [64] as well as empirical measurements, no recent figures on air resistance have been published in association with contemporary wheelchair sitting posture and propulsion technique. However, from cycling or speed skating many new developments were transferred to wheelchair racing. Next to frontal plane area reduction, adaptation of the seat position and orientation of the segments of the body, and the application of skin suits will influence the drag coefficient. Especially in hand cycling both optimization of aerodynamics and the power producing muscle mass of arms and trunk has led to higher speeds and endurance.

Internal friction

Energy losses within the wheelchair are caused by bearing friction around the wheel axles and in the wheel suspension of the castor wheels and possibly by the deformation of the frame in folding wheelchairs during the force exertion in the push phase. Bearing friction generally is very small, and given that the hubs have annular bearings and are well maintained and lubricated, this friction coefficient will not exceed 0.001 [32]. However, the losses in ill-maintained bearings can be considerable. An experimental comparison of one subject with a worn out castor wheel bearing in his racing wheelchair with seven companion racers in a similar design wheelchair showed that the mean values for power output of the seven subjects (with a higher overall mean body weight) was 20 W lower at a velocity of 3.3 m s^{-1}, which implies—at a theoretical gross ME of 8%—an increase in oxygen consumption of 0.75 L min^{-1} for the subject in the wheelchair with the worn-out castor. This occurred despite the fact that this subject had a lower body weight than the other seven subjects.

An unknown aspect of internal energy dissipation is the loss of propulsion energy due to deformation of the frame elements. This will clearly be possible in folding wheelchairs, but has not been addressed empirically. The use of levers and cranks does introduce a chain, chain wheel and gearbox-related friction.

The change in frame construction material from the original steel into other materials (aluminum, titanium, and carbon fiber-reinforced materials, chrome alloy) has had a strong impact on the design, mass, stability, strength, and endurance of the wheelchair today [175]. Over the years, the folding mechanism has been replaced by the box frame design in many hand rim wheelchair models, thus reducing the potential internal loss of energy of propulsion into nonstiff joints, nuts, and bolts.

Depending on the conditions of use, tires and wheels can be changed or are wheelchair task-specific, e.g., tennis, basketball, wheelchair rugby, track wheelchairs. These are all different and highly task-specific in design. The choice of tires and castor wheels will not only depend on rolling characteristics and conditions of use but also on riding comfort. "No-more flats" have a reduced spring characteristic and a higher rolling resistance compared to pneumatic tires [38,56,200], but no risk of a puncture. Above that, "no-more flats" have a worse shock absorbance quality. Comfort is not the only reason to seek for shock absorption and reduction of vibration in hand rim wheelchairs. Vibration and shocks may impact the condition of the spinal column and produce low back pain [64,72,102]; prevention may be relevant in those sensitive to spinal or low back pain. Pneumatic tires have good spring and shock reducing characteristics, but may require more power to propel on certain materials in comparison to harder wheel/tire materials [90]. The "Spinergy"™*

---

* www.spinergy.com

PBO fiber spokes (and hubs and rims) that are seen today, are ultralightweight, are stronger, and suggested to be better on shock absorption than the traditional wheel technology. In addition to shock absorption of the usual pneumatic tires, some wheelchairs are equipped with suspension in the castors or at the rear. This may indeed be comfortable, but leads to increased energy consumption [170].

Vehicle mechanical aspects that further impact wheelchair stability, versatility, and energy cost of wheeling are camber of the rear wheels and the for-aft position. The optimum must be strived for within the individual demands of the user. All in all, construction and mass of the wheelchair are pivotal to performance. The body mass of the person in the chair is often of greater importance than wheelchair mass, however. Body weight management is an important aspect in both rehabilitation and sports practice that should not be underestimated. In addition, environmental characteristics are of crucial importance [44,87,119,154,168,199], but are difficult to influence.

6.5.2 PHYSICAL WORK CAPACITY

Apart from age, gender, and genetics, upper-body exercise capacity and ME are dependent on training status, expertise, impairment, and the mode of exercise. Hand rim wheelchair propulsion shows lower efficiency and peak power output values, when compared to arm crank exercise or hand cycling [78], as is for instance summarized in data from Haisma et al. [45] and Dallmeijer et al. [78] (Figure 6.9).

In individuals with a SCI, work capacity is generally associated with lesion level. Haisma et al. [77,78] showed that in the initial rehabilitation (T1) the physical work

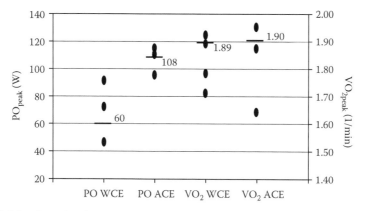

FIGURE 6.9 Overview from literature (each dot represents the mean outcome of a separate study; the dash indicates the weighted mean of the different studies) of peak performance (power output, PO; peak oxygen uptake, VO_2) levels in persons with SCI during hand rim propulsion wheel chair exercise (WCE) and arm crank exercise (ACE). (From Haisma, J.A. et al., *Spinal Cord.*, 44, 642, 2006. With permission.)

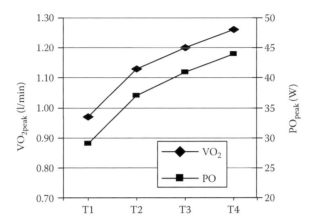

FIGURE 6.10 Model outcomes of peak hand rim wheelchair performance on a motor-driven treadmill (PO, peak power output; VO₂, peak oxygen uptake) in persons with SCI during (T1–T3) and one year after conclusion of clinical rehabilitation (T4), based on multilevel regression analysis. (From Haisma, J.A., et al., *Arch. Phys. Med. Rehabil.*, 87, 741–748, 2006. With permission.)

capacity generally improved from a generally extremely low value, just after the lesion, to values almost double that value one year after conclusion of rehabilitation at T4, however consistently being lower for those with a cervical spinal cord lesion when compared to those with paraplegia (Figure 6.10).

A critical review of literature shows many other sources of variation in exercise testing modes and protocols, which will influence the outcome and comparability of results. The bottom line, however, is that hand rim arm work is limited but can be very well trained [164,167]. It is also evident that people with lower-limb disabilities have a lower work capacity than able-bodied individuals performing leg exercise. Despite that, people with lower-limb disabilities will improve performance due to training and exercise. Athletes overall exhibit higher levels of performance than nonathletes and especially sedentary individuals [94,97,164], as exemplified in Tables 6.2 and 6.3. Anaerobic or sprint work capacity has been studied less frequently in wheelchair users [46,77,97,167], but is probably equally important as aerobic capacity or body muscle strength during daily functioning. In addition, there appear to be strong associations among anaerobic, aerobic, and upper-body strength outcome measures for wheelchair users [42,88,98]. Physical strain of standardized daily wheelchair arm work (expressed as percentage heart rate reserve) is inversely associated to work capacity [98,105], even in a longitudinal context and during rehabilitation [10].

6.5.3 WHEELCHAIR–USER INTERFACE

Of utmost importance for performance in sports is the individual tuning of wheelchair–user interface, where the wheelchair is fully fitted to the individual functional characteristics. Over the years, the importance of fine-tuning the wheelchair–user

TABLE 6.2

Aerobic Capacity in Male Wheelchair Athletes and Sedentary Subjects of Some Selected Arm Crank and Wheelchair Ergometry Studies

Authors	Mode	N	ISMGF	Disability	VO$_2$ (L/min)	VO$_2$ (ml/kg/min)	Heart Rate (b/min)	Power output (W)
Gass and Camp (1979)	MDT	8		T4–L3		40.6		
Wicks et al. (1983)	MDT	40	Ic–V	C7–S1	2.23	32.9	175	81.1
Davis and Shephard (1988)	ACE	15	III–V	T6–L5	2.24		182	97
Veeger et al. (1991a)	MDT	9		T4–T6	1.72		177	
		1	Ic	C7–C8	1.64	27.3	150	
		6	II	T1–T5	1.84	23.0	170	66
		10	III	T6–T10	1.97	26.8	175	80
		13	IV	T11–L3	2.42	36.9	182	85
		7	V	L4–S1	2.38	40.6	182	79
		3	Other	POL	2.94	39.4	160	93
Gass et al. (1995)	MDT	10			1.94	27.1	181	
Vinet et al. (1997)	WCE	8	III–IV	T8–L3	2.67	40.6	174	
Pare and Simard (1993)	WCE	35	II–V	<T1	1.63	23.9	187	39
Sedentary								
Huonker et al. (1998)	WCE	29		T1-S2	1.76	34.59	183	89
Athletes								
Sedentary	WCE	20		SB, T2–T12	1.14	23.9	162	50
Keyser et al. (1999)	WCE	15		a.o. SB, T2–T12	1.14	14.6	146	
Woude et al. (2002)	WCE	3	T1	C5/6–C7	0.67		110	22
		4	T2	C7	1.30		133	51
		8	T3	T5–L1	2.04		183	86
		23	T4	T6–S1 POL, SB	2.29		187	106

Source: van der Woude, L.H., et al., *Med. Eng. Phys.* 23, 713, 2001. With permission.

ACE, arm crank exercise; MDT, motor-driven treadmill; WCE, wheelchair ergometry; T1 t/m T4, ISMGF functional classification; AMP, amputees; CP, cerebral palsy; HEM, hemiplegia; KA, knee artrodesis; POL, polio; SB, spina bifida; SCI, spinal cord injury; F, female.

TABLE 6.3

Wheelchair Sprint Power Production in Wheelchair Athletes and Sedentary Subjects (Men and Women) for a Number of Wheelchair and Armcrank Studies

Authors	Modus	N	ISMGF	Disability	Peak Sprint P_o (W)	Peak Sprint P_o (W/kg)
Coutts and	WCE	2	Ia, Ib	C6–C7	46	0.77
Stogryn		3	III–V	T9–T12, POL	143	2.02
(1987)		1 (F)	IV	T10	85	1.73
Lees and Arthur (1988)	WCE	6	II–V	T1–L5	102–149[a]	
Janssen et al. (1993)	WCE	9	I		41.4	0.51
Sedentary		6	II		70.4	0.85
		15	III		95.9	1.22
		12	IV		114.4	1.45
		2	V		100.5	1.47
Woude et al.	WCE	3	T1	C5/6–C7	23	0.36
(1997)		4	T2	C7	68	1.03
		8	T3	T5–L1	100	1.65
		23	T4	T6–S1 POL, SB	138	2.36
		6 (1F)		CP	35	0.51
		6 (1F)		AMP, KA, HEM	121	1.85
		4 (F)	T2	C5–C7, POL	38	0.83
		3 (F)	T3	T8, SB	77	1.47
		3 (F)	T4	T12–S1, SB, POL	76	1.51
Hutzler	ACE	13	II	T1–T5	280	
et al. (1998)		15	III–VI	T6–S5	336	
		10	AMP	AMP	443	
		12	POL	POL	394	
		40	All		341	

Source: van der Woude, L.H., et al., *Med. Eng. Phys.*, 23, 713, 2001. With permission.

ACE, armcrank ergometry; WCE, wheelchair ergometry; T1 t/m T4, ISMGF functional classification; AMP, amputees; CP, cerebral palsy; HEM, hemiplegia; KA, knee artrodesis; POL, polio; SB, spina bifida; F, female.

[a] Values in dependence of different workloads.

interface to the individual has gradually reached daily practice in rehabilitation [10,113,120,159]. Geometry of the interface—e.g., propulsion mechanism, seat inclination and height, for-aft position, rim form, size and surface, camber angle— markedly affects propulsion technique, efficiency, and thus energy cost and probably mechanical loading [12,75,109,122,136,146,174,197]. First and foremost is the role of the propulsion mechanism itself, which will be discussed in the next paragraph. Since hand rim propulsion is common in western countries, some of these will be discussed below.

Seat or rear wheel axle position and height has been studied by different groups and was shown to affect efficiency as well as different indices of propulsion technique in experimentation or through modeling [173,174]. Especially, the different segment orientation of the arms and trunk will affect the force–length characteristics at which the muscles operate. The different study outcomes on seat height are however not very well comparable.

Unpublished results in a group of individuals with a SCI (Figure 6.11) show a tendency toward an optimum seat height in the range of 110°–130° elbow angle (which is defined according to a standardized seating posture, hands at top-dead-center, shoulders over the wheel axis; full extension = 180°). A similar study in able-bodied subjects suggests an optimum seat height at 100°–110° [75,109,122,146,197]. The for-aft axle position has been evaluated [74,122], and may be indeed individually optimized, but is more complex, since in practice it will influence both task load (rolling resistance) as well as the wheelchair–user interfacing characteristics.

Individual fine-tuning of the wheelchair–user interface is all in all an important prerequisite for long-term healthy wheeling in daily life and in sports. Available guidelines, based on common practice, are limited and still lacking a sufficient evidence base.

THEORETICAL SIDESTEP (4): RIM RADIUS, GEAR RATIO, AND CAMBER

The use of a different hand rim diameter size—essentially using a different gear setting—is often seen in wheelchair racing (often a much smaller rim size) or rehabilitation (in unilateral use of two differently sized rims simultaneously on one side); obviously rim size is limited by the wheel size. The hand rim radius is in fact a gearing level. Smaller hand rims—often seen in racing—will result in a larger force and smaller hand velocity at a given traveling speed. It is logical that different task conditions will require different hand rim diameters or gearing levels: groups of well-trained subjects may want a gearing, which enables them to compete at high velocities, whereas

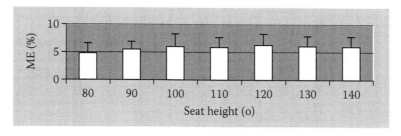

FIGURE 6.11   Effect of seat height (expressed in degrees elbow angle (full extension = 180°) on gross ME (mean ± SD); ME (%)) in $N = 12$ subjects with a SCI.

a steep incline for physically less able subjects will demand a low gear. The relevance of different gear ratios in hand rim wheelchairs is stressed by the results of different experimental studies [193].

Veeger et al. [177] showed that at equal submaximal power output, a higher mechanical advantage (0.43–0.87) i.e., a higher hand velocity—and simultaneously a lower mean resisting force—led to a higher cardiorespiratory response. Simultaneously, the increase in linear hand velocity during the push phase led to a decrease in effective force, which decreased from 71% to 58%. In addition, the amount of negative work at the beginning and end of the push increased with a higher mechanical advantage. Application of a variable gearing in hand rim wheelchairs is worth considering, but complicated, technically speaking. But different rim diameters are more common, especially in track wheelchairs. In wheelchair sports athletes tend to individualize their choice of hand rim size, tube diameter, and profile. To study the physiological effects of rim size, Woude et al. [137] conducted an experiment with a racing wheelchair and five different rim diameters in which track athletes participated at speeds up to 4.2 m s^{-1}. Rim diameter varied from 0.30 to 0.56 m. Results showed that the largest rim led to the highest physiological strain and lowest efficiency levels. Heart rate showed a mean difference of 20% (10–20 b min^{-1}) between the smallest and the largest rim size. Again the linear speed of the hand rim limited performance: five out of eight athletes were unable to perform at a velocity of 4.2 m s^{-1} (power output did not exceed 50 W!). The full advantage of variable gearing, however, is met in hand cycles and lever systems. However, the appropriate choice of ratio will be power and velocity dependent.

Richter and Axelson studied the possible role of compliance of the hand rim, in the reduction of mechanical impact on the hand, and showed positive effects of a specific compliant hand rim design on impact force [169]. Results suggest the possible preventive role of such material on wrist and shoulder overuse. Results of van der Woude and de Groot [189] evaluating different hand rim profiles and surface material did not show significant results on efficiency or force production, but showed subjective preference among the nonwheelchair users for a round foam rubber (7.5 ± 0.53 cm) coated hand rim.

Camber

The majority of sports wheelchairs are equipped with cambered rear wheels. There appears to be a biomechanical rationale for the suggested better performance with cambered wheels: with the top of the wheels as near as possible to the trunk the rims are in a plane more or less passing through the shoulder joint. This would prevent the upper arms to abduct in the frontal plane, thus reducing static effort of the shoulder muscles. The effective force vector can also be directed as closely as possible to the shoulder joint. Whether these assumptions were valid, was studied by Veeger et al. [141] for basketball wheelchair use during propulsion at speeds of 0.56 to 1.39 m s^{-1} on a motor-driven treadmill ($N = 8$ nonwheelchair users). During four subsequent exercise tests the camber angle varied randomly from 0° to 3°, 6°, and 9°. The cardiorespiratory parameters indicated no positive or negative effect of camber angle in this wheelchair model. Similar findings were seen for the kinematics: no change in abduction angle was evident with camber angle. The electromyography signal even showed an absence of activity of the major shoulder abductor (m.deltoideus pars medialis) during the push phase. The authors explained this phenomenon by stating that the abduction, that occurs during the push phase, is not an active process, but a side effect of the action of the major shoulder muscles (mm.pectoralis major and the deltoideus pars anterior). Their activity would lead both to anteflexion as well as abduction and endorotation, because of the closed kinetic chain that exists between the hand and the shoulder in the push phase. It thus appears that camber does not affect the functional load. However, also the positive effect of camber on stability is relevant, as well as the fact that the hands are protected when passing along objects.

An estimated 90% of all wheelchairs is hand rim-propelled [191,192]. Although hand rim wheelchair propulsion has been described as a physically straining form of ambulation, this propulsion mode has been on the market for over 60 years and will remain to do so, despite its disadvantages of a low efficiency and high mechanical load. The hand rim is the propulsion mechanism that evidently interacts the closest with the human system as possible: each stroke of the hands propels, brakes, or turns the wheelchair with direct visual, proprioceptive, and kinesthetic feedback to the user, directly expressing information about position, speed, and spatial orientation of the body. Also, the wheelchair is relatively small and maneuverable in small spaces and transportable.

THEORETICAL SIDESTEP (5): HAND RIM WHEELCHAIR PROPULSION TECHNIQUE

Propulsion forces

Hand rim wheelchair propulsion comprises a pushing phase and a recovery phase. During the pushing phase, the hands make contact with the rims and force is applied by the athlete to the rims. Since the hands hold the rims and therefore automatically follow the circular movement of those rims, the movement of the hands and arms can be characterized as a guided movement. In guided movements the forces that are applied by the hands do not directly influence the trajectory of the hands. As a consequence, it is possible to apply force that is not tangential to the hand rims. Any force that has a tangential force component will contribute to propulsion. The propulsive force can, but does not have to be applied tangential to the hand rims.

Experimental results have shown that propulsion forces are indeed not tangentially directed (Figure 6.12). Veeger et al. [202] introduced the term fraction effective force (FEF) as a measure for the effectiveness of force application. The FEF is defined as

$$FEF = F_m * |F_{tot}|^{-1} \times 100 \; (\%) \qquad (6.8)$$

where
F_m is the tangential force component
$|F_{tot}|$ is the magnitude of the propulsion force (Figure 6.12)

FEF and ME

In general the FEF was below 80%. Wu et al. [14] reported values of 47%–49% for riding at a self-selected pace on level ground and average FEF values of 63%–74% for riding on a ramp of 2.9°–7.1°. Boninger et al. [193] found values of 52%–54% for the force ratio F_m^2/F_{tot}^2, which is a slightly different definition for the FEF than is used here. Apart from an effect of speed or gear ratio on FEF [50,110], FEF seems to be a stable attribute of the human system in hand rim propulsion. Effects of learning [47], training [169], or hand rim profile [52] were negligible. A feedback-based learning process to maximize FEF was successful on FEF, but had a negative effect on gross ME, indicating a nonnatural

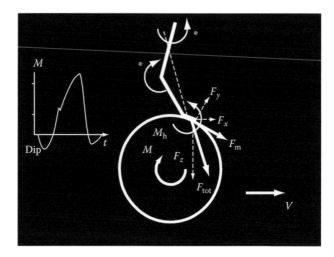

FIGURE 6.12 A typical description of characteristics of a hand rim wheelchair push (propelling from left to right at speed V): the effective tangential force component (F_m) and torque (M), the net torque around elbow and shoulder (*), the three orthogonal constituents (F_x, F_y, F_z) of the total force vector (F_{tot}), the hand torque (M_h), and the typical negative force values (dip) at the start and end of the push phase in the description of M over time (t).

adaptation of the human system [52,109]. FEF and force production appear inherently associated to the functional anatomy of the human system and the geometry of the task. Optimization on the mere mechanics of manual force and force effectiveness (e.g., a maximal tangential force component) thus is not necessarily consistent with optimization of energy cost and gross ME [142,144,183]. Much work has to be done in that realm, preferably using modeling techniques [47,50,190].

Timing

As in other cyclic tasks, proficiency of performance is first and foremost expressed in changes in the timing of the motion pattern. A reduction of the cycle frequency (and by definition an increase in the amount of work per cycle) is typical in the initial phase of learning and training hand rim wheelchair propulsion [53]. Although different hand trajectories in hand rim propulsion have been described, it remains unclear which would be the optimum pattern in terms of mechanical efficiency [176]. Woude et al. [71] and Goosey et al. [6,60,86] have shown that both experienced and inexperienced wheelchair users have a preferred push frequency, which shows the lowest energy cost and highest efficiency values, compared to lower or higher paced frequencies. It is difficult to suggest any clear guidelines for technique from these timing data, other than accepting that human system seeks for energetically optimum performance forms and conditions in cyclic wheelchair arm work.

Motor learning and training

Rehabilitation in lower-limb-disabled individuals is basically a continuous process of training and (motor) learning. Hand rim wheelchair training has been evaluated in very few studies [47,172]. Even less is known of motor learning underlying practice and training. Little is known of these processes. De Groot et al. [50–54] showed in her studies that apart from shifts in energy cost and gross ME as a consequence of motor learning, timing show typical changes toward a lower cycle frequency and thus a longer stroke time and recovery cycle. Changes in the force pattern and FEF are not that obvious. Changes in muscle activation patterns are also much more difficult to detect.

6.6   ALTERNATIVE PROPULSION MECHANISMS

Given the very limited work capacity of wheelchair users in general, stresses of hand rim mobility results in fatigue and local discomfort of the upper extremity with the described risk of repetitive strain injuries. The natural solution could be the provision of electric wheelchairs, but the already existing health-threatening inactivity cycle will not be stopped in this way. For this purpose, alternative wheelchair propulsion mechanisms (especially levers and cranks) have been the subject of study since the late 1960s [178].

The use of an alternative propulsion mechanism has evidently been studied as a solution to the drawbacks of hand rim wheelchair use (Figure 6.13).* A review of Woude et al. [19,179] substantiates the benefits of other than hand rim-propelled wheelchairs in terms of energy cost and physical strain (Table 6.4). However, little to nothing is known in literature about the biomechanical and physiological mechanisms that may explain the beneficial performance, especially of hand cycling [178].

Different experiments on lever and crank-propelled wheelchairs have shown that these propulsion mechanisms indeed are less straining and more efficient than hand rims in general [123–125]. Lever, and especially, crank-propelled tricycle wheelchairs prove their important role in more extreme environmental conditions in many nonwestern countries [178]. They allow higher velocities over a longer duration at the same or even a lower physical strain due to the following factors: a natural grip of the hands to a well-formed handle bar, with the arms moving within the visual field, mostly making a fully circular motion, not needing the coupling–uncoupling actions in hand rim propulsion. In addition, cranks and levers allow the use of all flexor and extensor muscles around the arm–shoulder joints to actively contribute to external work over the full motion cycle; the latter in contrast to hand

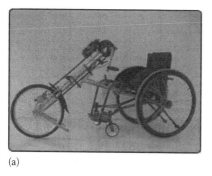 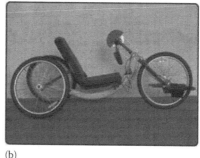

(a)   (b)

FIGURE 6.13   Two examples of contemporary hand cycles. (a) A tracker or attach-unit hand cycle and (b) a fixed frame race hand cycle.

---

* www.doubleperformance.nl

TABLE 6.4

Characteristics of Different Propulsion Mechanisms, Partly Based on Experimental Data

	Hand Rim		Hand Cycle			
	Basket	Racing	Fixed	Attach-unit	Lever	Hub
Max ME (%)	<10	<8	>13	>13	>13	>12
Strain CVS	High	High	Low	Low	Low	Low?
Strain MSS	High	High	Low	Low	Low	Low?
Risk RSI	High	High	Low?	Low?	Low?	Low?
Top speed (km h⁻¹)	15	30	>30	30	30	30
Mass (kg)	<10	<8	10–15	15	10–15	<10
Coupling hand	–	–	++	++	++	+
Force direction	–	–	+	+	++	+
Bi-modal	–	+	+	+	+	+
Continuous work production	–	+	+	+	+	+
Outdoor use	+	++	+++	+++	++	+
Maneuverability	++	±	–	–	–	–
Indoor use	++	±	–	±	–	–
Steering	++	±	±	±	±	–
Brake	±	–	+	+	+	–
Transportation	++	++	–	+	–	±
Maintenance	+	+	±	±	±	+

Source: van der Woude, L.H., et al., *Med. Eng. Phys.*, 23, 713, 2001. With permission.

Note: CVS, cardiovascular system; MMS, musculoskeletal system; RSI, repetitive strain injury; ME, mechanical efficiency. Lever propulsion is a cyclic arm movement with an almost horizontal push (and pull) action in front of the body. The hub crank is a small crank fixed to the hub of the wheel that allows a full 360° circular motion in racing wheelchairs. –: negative; +: positive aspect.

rim propulsion where the discontinuous motion allows active work only during 30%–40% of the cycle [1,45,48,194].

The use of modern technology and lightweight materials has led to the reintroduc-tion of the synchronous hand cycle for outdoor use [2,48,61,96,107,118,179]. Disadvantages of the early hand cycles—such as weight, size, and limited maneuverability—have partly been overcome. The contemporary lightweight well-looking tricycles have multiple gears, as well as good braking and steering qualities. Even those individuals with high level spinal cord lesions can in- and egress and can couple to the pedals with special gloves. Using a synchronous arm mode, both arms move in the same angular pattern, thus preventing a conflict with the simultaneous steering task [45,165,179], and a higher efficiency and power output can be obtained [3,4,39,114,115]. The use of tracker or attach-unit system (an add-on front wheel crank unit, which is combined with the daily hand rim wheelchair) has made the crank propulsion mechanism more practical in daily life outdoors for both transportation as well as recreation, but the hand rim-propelled wheelchair remains crucial indoors.

The current booming development of crank-propelled tricycles in the industrialized countries serves not only the young and active wheelchair user, but also the less well-trained individual or those with more extensive limitations. In the end, the frequent active use of other than hand rim-propelled wheelchairs may help prevent some of the secondary complications among the wheelchair user population today.

6.6.1 POWER SUPPORT

Recent developments in both measurement technology as well as the electronic motors allow the use of wheel-hub-mounted power support motor technology (Figure 6.14) in, for instance, hand rim wheelchairs [39,114,115], as well as hand cycles. Depending on the individual tuning, and based on the manual force input of the wheelchair user into the propulsion mechanism, the motor will or will not support the user in overcoming an obstacle, a ramp, or rough terrain, albeit ordinary daily wheeling. As a consequence, cardiorespiratory strain and most likely mechanical strain will be reduced under these wheeling conditions [27,55,83–85]. Especially in those persons who are temporarily injured to the upper extremity or very frail subjects, this type of power support will be relevant. For the latter group, the power support system may help to extend the use transition to an electrical wheelchair. Less

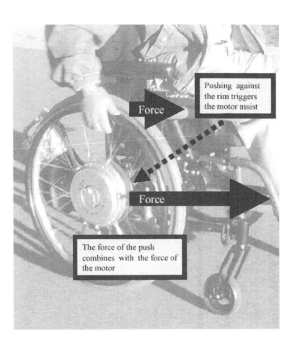

FIGURE 6.14   A wheel-hub mounted power support system for a hand rim wheelchair.

positive aspects of such a system are its additional mass and the limited control and delay that may be present in the power support regulation.

6.7 OTHER ASSISTIVE TECHNOLOGY FOR AN ACTIVE LIFESTYLE

Within the broader context of an active lifestyle and restoration of mobility in SCI and individuals with other lower-limb impairments, biotechnical research over the past decades not only evolved in the field of wheeled mobility, but also with respect to walking and lower-limb functioning. Body weight-supported treadmill walking [117] and the use of gait-assisting robotics have an impact on therapeutic exercise training in SCI and stroke rehabilitation. Also, robotics in ADL and upper-extremity support [24,104,203] and the upper-extremity neuroprostheses based upon (implemented) electrical stimulation (ES) for those with tetraplegia [11,27,84,85] are examples of specific assistive technology that supports restoration of function and functionality in among others persons with SCI, but seem to warrant a lifelong rehabilitation commitment.

Neuromuscular and functional ES does not limit itself to upper-body exercise, as can be seen from the different applications over the past. ES (treadmill) walking [82,95,134] and cycling have been in the field for more than four decades and have shown its possible clinical benefits in scientific research to a large extent [8,63,70,82,134]. The therapeutic use of stationary recumbent ES bicycles in SCI has become a common therapeutic element in various western countries, especially for those with SCI, and has stimulated the development of technology for ES

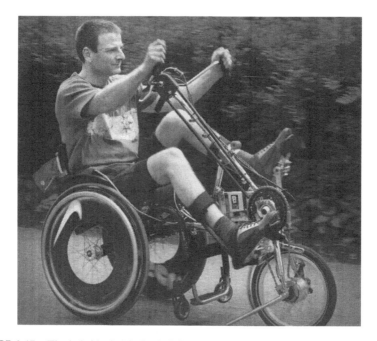

FIGURE 6.15 The hybrid tricycle Berkelbike in use.

recumbent cycling in real life [82], allowing a more active lifestyle even in high-lesion SCI. These hybrid devices use simultaneously voluntary upper-body arm work and ES leg work in subjects with SCI or stroke. An example is the Berkelbike [8,82], shown in Figure 6.15.* These new devices will require an additional ergonomics-oriented research input to reach an optimal long-term functioning of the "assistive technology–user combination."

Eventually, this will determine the quality and usability of assistive technology in daily life and directly impact on nonuse. Population surveys among wheelchair users, although complex, must provide a better understanding of user demands, functional and technical requirements of assistive technology, and thus functionality and durability in the context of its economic value [141].

6.8   ERGONOMIC GUIDELINES

A recent comprehensive analysis of international literature by a distinguished group of experts in the Consortium for Spinal Cord Medicine [16] has provided a first set of useful ergonomic guidelines for individuals with a SCI who use a hand rim wheelchair. A summary of these guidelines is given in Table 6.5. As is recognized by the authors, the real scientific evidence-base of the formulated guidelines is very limited and is in itself a strong stimulus for continued research and (international) collaboration in order to improve our understanding of the issues at hand and to provide additional evidence for certain guidelines and new perspectives.

6.9   CONCLUSIONS

Systematic biomechanics and ergonomics research has contributed to the evolution of wheeled mobility technology in rehabilitation and daily life, and in wheeled sports and subsequent rehabilitation technology. Innovations in assistive technology and the understanding of a wheelchair-confined lifestyle have led to improved but still highly limited evidence-based rehabilitation practice, and beyond that toward an increased freedom of mobility and quality of life of wheelchair-confined individuals. Understanding of the underlying causal and preventive mechanisms of (secondary) health issues, the role of an active lifestyle and fitness training and sports, will serve to further evolve rehabilitation guidelines and treatment, and the active daily functioning of individuals using manual wheelchairs. Much work has still to be done to further help improve the state of the art of mobility in both sedentary and athletic lower-limb-disabled individuals, as is indicated with the presented elements for a research agenda on rehabilitation technology and patient-related (experimental and prospective) research are suggested.

Apart from optimizing the wheelchair–user interface, one needs to carefully consider maximizing overall work capacity of users and further reduction of the vehicle mechanical losses to ensure a real optimum level of mobility.

Despite an increasingly strong research effort over the past decades, existing guidelines for wheelchair design and fitting as well as for the prevention of overuse problems in hand rim wheelchair use lack a sufficiently strong evidence-base.

---

* www.berkelbike.nl

TABLE 6.5
Summary of Recommendations from the Consortium
for Spinal Cord Medicine

Summary of Recommendations

Initial Assessment of Acute SCI

1. Educate health care providers and persons with SCI about the risk of upper limb pain and injury,the means of prevention, treatment options, and the need to maintain fitness.
2. Routinely assess the patient's function, ergonomics, equipment, and level of pain as part of a periodic health review. This review should include evaluation of
   - Transfer and wheelchair propulsion techniques.
   - Equipment (wheelchair and transfer device).
   - Current health status.

Ergonomics

3. Minimize the frequency of repetitive upper limb tasks.
4. Minimize the force required to complete upper limb tasks.
5. Minimize extreme or potentially injurious positions at all joints.
   - Avoid extreme positions of the wrist.
   - Avoid positioning the hand above the shoulder.
   - Avoid potentially injurious or extreme positions at the shoulder, including extreme internal rotation and abduction.

Equipment Selection, Training, and Environmental Adaptations

6. With high-risk patients, evaluate and discuss the pros and cons of changing to a power wheelchair system as a way to prevent repetitive injuries.
7. Provide manual wheelchair users with SCI a high-strength, fully customizable manual wheelchair made of the lightest possible material.
8. Adjust the rear axle as far forward as possible without compromising the stability of the user.
9. Position the rear axle so that when the hand is placed at the top dead-center position on the pushrim, the angle between the upper arm and forearm is between $100°$ and $120°$.
10. Educate the patient to
    - Use long, smooth strokes that limit high impacts on the pushrim.
    - Allow the hand to drift down naturally, keeping it below the pushrim when not in actual contact with that part of the wheelchair.
11. Promote an appropriate seated posture and stabilization relative to balance and stability needs.
12. For individuals with upper limb paralysis and/or pain, appropriately position the upper limb in bed and in a mobility device. The following principles should be followed:
    - Avoid direct pressure on the shoulder.
    - Provide support to the upper limb at all points.
    - When the individual is supine, position the upper limb in abduction and external rotation on a regular basis.
    - Avoid pulling on the arm when positioning individuals.
    - Remember that preventing pain is a primary goal of positioning.
13. Provide seat elevation or possibly a standing position to individuals with SCI who use power wheelchairs and have arm function.

TABLE 6.5 (continued)
Summary of Recommendations from the Consortium
for Spinal Cord Medicine

14. Complete a thorough assessment of the patient's environment, obtain the appropriate equipment, and complete modifications to the home, ideally to Americans with Disabilities Act (ADA) standards.
15. Instruct individuals with SCI who complete independent transfers to
    - Perform level transfers when possible.
    - Avoid positions of impingement when possible.
    - Avoid placing either hand on a flat surface when a handgrip is possible during transfers.
    - Vary the technique used and the arm that leads.
16. Consider the use of a transfer-assist device for all individuals with SCI. Strongly encourage individuals with arm pain and/or upper limb weakness to use a transfer-assist device.

Exercise

17. Incorporate flexibility exercises into an overall fitness program sufficient to maintain normal glenohumeral motion and pectoral muscle mobility.
18. Incorporate resistance training as an integral part of an adult fitness program. The training should be individualized and progressive, should be of sufficient intensity to enhance strength and muscular endurance, and should provide stimulus to exercise all the major muscle groups to pain-free fatigue.

Management of Acute and Subacute Upper Limb Injuries and Pain

19. In general, manage musculoskeletal upper limb injuries in the SCI population in a similar fashion as in the unimpaired population.
20. Plan and provide intervention for acute pain as early as possible in order to prevent the development of chronic pain.
21. Consider a medical and rehabilitative approach to initial treatment in most instances of nontraumatic upper limb injury among individuals with SCI.
22. Because relative rest of an injured or postsurgical upper limb in SCI is difficult to achieve, strongly consider the following measures:
    - Use of resting night splints in carpal tunnel syndrome.
    - Home modifications or additional assistance.
    - Admission to a medical facility if pain cannot be relieved or if complete rest is indicated.
23. Place special emphasis on maintaining optimal range of motion during rehabilitation from upper limb injury.
24. Consider alternative techniques for activities when upper limb pain or injury is present.
25. Emphasize that the patient's return to normal activity after an injury or surgery must occur gradually.
26. Closely monitor the results of treatment, and if the pain is not relieved, continued workups and treatment are appropriate.
27. Consider surgery if the patient has chronic neuromusculoskeletal pain and has failed to regain functional capacity with medical and rehabilitative treatment and if the likelihood of a successful surgical and functional outcome outweighs the likelihood of an unsuccessful procedure.

(continued)

TABLE 6.5 (continued)
Summary of Recommendations from the Consortium
for Spinal Cord Medicine

28. Operate on upper limb fractures if indicated and when medically feasible.
29. Be aware of and plan for the recovery time needed after surgical procedures.
30. Assess the patient's use of complementary and alternative medicine techniques and beware of possible negative interactions.

Treatment of Chronic Musculoskeletal Pain to Maintain Function

31. Because chronic pain related to musculoskeletal disorders is a complex, multidimensional clinical problem, consider the use of an interdisciplinary approach to assessment and treatment planning. Begin treatment with a careful assessment of the following:
   - Etiology
   - Pain intensity
   - Functional capacities
   - Psychosocial distress associated with the condition
32. Treat chronic pain and associated symptomatology in an interdisciplinary fashion and incorporate multiple modalities based on the constellation of symptoms revealed by the comprehensive assessment.
33. Monitor outcomes regularly to maximize the likelihood of providing effective treatment.
34. Encourage manual wheelchair users with chronic upper limb pain to seriously consider use of a power wheelchair.
35. Monitor psychosocial adjustment to secondary upper limb injuries and provide treatment if necessary.

Source: Boninger, M.L., et al. *Clinical Practice Guidelines: Spinal Cord Medicine*: *Paralyzed Veterans of America*, 2005, pp. 1–36. With permission.

REFERENCES

1. Abel, T., M. Kroner, S. Rojas Vega, C. Peters, C. Klose, and P. Platen. Energy expenditure in wheelchair racing and handbiking—a basis for prevention of cardiovascular diseases in those with disabilities. *Eur J Cardiovasc Prev Rehabil.* 10:371–376, 2003.
2. Abel, T., S. Schneider, P. Platen, and H. K. Struder. Performance diagnostics in handbiking during competition. *Spinal Cord.* 44:211–216, 2006.
3. Algood, S. D., R. A. Cooper, S. G. Fitzgerald, R. Cooper, and M. L. Boninger. Effect of a pushrim-activated power-assist wheelchair on the functional capabilities of persons with tetraplegia. *Arch Phys Med Rehabil.* 86:380–386, 2005.
4. Arva, J., S. G. Fitzgerald, R. A. Cooper, and M. L. Boninger. Mechanical efficiency and user power requirement with a pushrim activated power assisted wheelchair. *Med Eng Phys.* 23:699–705, 2001.
5. Asato, K. T., R. A. Cooper, R. N. Robertson, and J. F. Ster. SMARTwheel: Development abd testing of a system for measuring manual wheelchair propulsion dynamics. *IEEE Trans Biomed Eng.* 40:1320–1324, 1993.
6. Bennedik, K. and P. Engel. Technische und physiologische Aspekte bei Benutzung handbetriebener Krankenfahrstuhle. *Rehabilitation.* 11:94–108, 1972.
7. Bennedik, K., P. Engel, and G. Hildebrandt. *Der Rollstuhl.* Rheinstetten: Schindele Verlag, 1978.

8. Berkelmans, R., J. Duysens, and M. Arns. The development of a hybrid FES bike. *J Rehabil Res Dev.* 41:S54, 2004.
9. Bertucci, W., S. Duc, V. Villerius, J. N. Pernin, and F. Grappe. Validity and reliability of the PowerTap mobile cycling powermeter when compared with the SRM device. *Int J Sports Med.* 26:868–873, 2005.
10. Biemans, M. A., J. Dekker, and L. H. van der Woude. The internal consistency and validity of the self-assessment Parkinson's disease disability scale. *Clin Rehabil.* 15:221–228, 2001.
11. Bijak, M., M. Rakosm, C. Hofer, W. Mayer, M. Strohhofer, D. Rascka, and M. Kern. Clinical application of an eight channel stimulation system for mobilization of individuals with paraplegia. *Technol Disabil.* 17:85–92, 2005.
12. Boninger, M. L., M. Baldwin, R. A. Cooper, A. Koontz, and L. Chan. Manual wheelchair pushrim biomechanics and axle position. *Arch Phys Med Rehabil.* 81:608–613, 2000.
13. Boninger, M. L., R. A. Cooper, S. G. Fitzgerald, J. Lin, R. Cooper, B. Dicianno, and B. Liu. Investigating neck pain in wheelchair users. *Am J Phys Med Rehabil.* 82: 197–202, 2003.
14. Boninger, M. L., R. A. Cooper, R. N. Robertson, and S. D. Shimada. Three-dimensional pushrim forces during two speeds of wheelchair propulsion. *Am J Phys Med Rehabil.* 76:420–426, 1997.
15. Boninger, M. L., A. M. Koontz, S. A. Sisto, T. A. Dyson-Hudson, M. Chang, R. Price, and R. A. Cooper. Pushrim biomechanics and injury prevention in spinal cord injury: Recommendations based on CULP-SCI investigations. *J Rehabil Res Dev.* 42:9–20, 2005.
16. Boninger, M. L., R. L. Waters, T. Chase, M. P. J. M. Dijkers, H. Gellmann, R. J. Gironda, B. Goldstein, S. Johnson-Taylor, A. M. Koontz, and S. L. McDowell. *Clinical Practice Guidelines: Spinal Cord Medicine*: Paralyzed Veterans of America, 2005, pp. 1–36.
17. Brattgard, S. -O., G. Grimby, and O. Hook. Energy expenditure and heart rate in driving a wheelchair ergometer. *Scand. J. Rehab. Med.* 2:143–148, 1970.
18. Brauer, R. L. and B. A. Hertig. Torque generation on wheelchair handrims. *Proceedings of the 1981 Biomechanics Symposium; ASME/ASCE Mechanics Conference*, vol. 43, pp. 113–116, 1981.
19. Bressel, E., M. Bressel, M. Marquez, and G. D. Heise. The effect of handgrip position on upper extremity neuromuscular responses to arm cranking exercise. *J Electromyogr Kinesiol.* 11:291–298, 2001.
20. Brouha, L. and H. Krobath. Continuous recording of cardiac and respiratory functions in normal and handicapped people. *Human Factors.* 9:567–572, 1967.
21. Brown, D. R., R. R. Pate, M. Pratt, F. Wheeler, D. Buchner, B. Ainsworth, and C. Macera. Physical activity and public health: training courses for researchers and practitioners. *Public Health Rep.* 116:197–202, 2001.
22. Brubaker, C. E. and C. A. McLaurin. Ergonomics of wheelchair propulsion. In: *Wheelchair III; Report of a Wheelchair on Specially Adapted Wheelchairs and Sports Wheelchairs*, 1982, pp. 22–37.
23. Brubaker, C. E., C. A. McLaurin, and I. S. McClay. Effects of side slope on wheelchair performance. *J Rehabil Res Dev.* 23:55–58, 1986.
24. Bryden, A. M., K. S. Wuolle, P. K. Murray, and P. H. Peckham. Perceived outcomes and utilization of upper extremity surgical reconstruction in individuals with tetraplegia at model spinal cord injury systems. *Spinal Cord.* 42:169–176, 2004.
25. Buckle, P. and D. Stubbs. The contribution of ergonomics to the rehabilitation of back pain patients. *J Soc Occup Med.* 39:56–60, 1989.
26. Bussmann, H. B., P. J. Reuvekamp, P. H. Veltink, W. L. Martens, and H. J. Stam. Validity and reliability of measurements obtained with an "activity monitor" in people with and without a transtibial amputation. *Phys Ther.* 78:989–998, 1998.

27. Carvalho, D., M. de Cassia Zanchetta, J. Sereni, and A. Cliquet Jr. Metabolic and cardiorespiratory responses of tetraplegic subjects during treadmill walking using neuromuscular electrical stimulation and partial body weight support. *Spinal Cord.* 42:1–6, 2005.

28. Clarke, K. Caloric costs of activity in paraplegic persons. *Arch Phys Med Rehab.* 47:427–435, 1966.

29. Coe, P. L. Aerodynamic characteristics of wheelchairs. *NASA Technical Memorandum* 80191, 1979.

30. Coggrave, M. and L. Rose. A specialist seating assessment clinic: Changing pressure relief practice. *Spinal Cord.* 41:692–695, 2003.

31. Cook, A. and S. Hussey. *Assistive Technologies: Principles and Practice.* St Louis, MO: Mosby Year Book Inc., 2002.

32. Cooper, R. *Rehabilitation Engineering: Applied to Mobility and Manipulation.* Bristol: Institute of Physics Publishing, 1995.

33. Cooper, R. A. An exploratory study of racing wheelchair propulsion dynamics. *Adapted Physical Activity Quart.* 7:74–85, 1990.

34. Cooper, R. A. A force/energy optimization model for wheelchair athletics. *IIEE Trans Syst Man Cybernetics.* 20:444–449, 1990.

35. Cooper, R. A. Racing chair lingo. Sports 'n Spokes, March/April, 29–32 Or how to order a racing wheelchair: 29–32, 1988.

36. Cooper, R. A. *Rehabilitation Engineering: Applied to Mobility and Manipulation.* Bristol: Medical Science Series, 1995.

37. Cooper, R. A., L. A. Quatrano, P. W. Axelson, W. Harlan, M. Stineman, B. Franklin, J. S. Krause, J. Bach, H. Chambers, E. Y. Chao, M. Alexander, and P. Painter. Research on physical activity and health among people with disabilities: a consensus statement. *J Rehabil Res Dev.* 36:142–154, 1999.

38. Cooper, R. A., E. Wolf, S. G. Fitzgerald, M. L. Boninger, R. Ulerich, and W. A. Ammer. Seat and footrest shocks and vibrations in manual wheelchairs with and without suspension. *Arch Phys Med Rehabil.* 84:96–102, 2003.

39. Corfman, T. A., R. A. Cooper, M. L. Boninger, A. M. Koontz, and S. G. Fitzgerald. Range of motion and stroke frequency differences between manual wheelchair propulsion and pushrim-activated power-assisted wheelchair propulsion. *J Spinal Cord Med.* 26:135–140, 2003.

40. Curtis, K. A., T. M. Tyner, L. Zachary, G. Lentell, D. Brink, T. Didyk, K. Gean, J. Hall, M. Hooper, J. Klos, S. Lesina, and B. Pacillas. Effect of a standard exercise protocol on shoulder pain in long-term wheelchair users. *Spinal Cord.* 37:421–429, 1999.

41. Dabonneville, M., P. Kauffmann, P. Vaslin, N. de Saint Remy, and Y. Couetard. A self-contained wireless wheelchair ergometer designed for biomechanical measures in real life conditions. *Technol Disabil.* 17:63–76, 2005.

42. Dallmeijer, A. J., M. T. Hopman, H. H. van As, and L. H. van der Woude. Physical capacity and physical strain in persons with tetraplegia; the role of sport activity. *Spinal Cord.* 34:729–735, 1996.

43. Dallmeijer, A. J., M. T. Hopman, and L. H. van der Woude. Lipid, lipoprotein, and apolipoprotein profiles in active and sedentary men with tetraplegia. *Arch Phys Med Rehabil.* 78:1173–1176, 1997.

44. Dallmeijer, A. J., O. J. Kilkens, M. W. Post, S. de Groot, E. L. Angenot, F. W. van Asbeck, A. V. Nene, and L. H. van der Woude. Hand-rim wheelchair propulsion capacity during rehabilitation of persons with spinal cord injury. *J Rehabil Res Dev.* 42:55–64, 2005.

45. Dallmeijer, A. J., L. Ottjes, E. de Waardt, and L. H. van der Woude. A physiological comparison of synchronous and asynchronous hand cycling. *Int J Sports Med.* 25: 622–626, 2004.

46. Dallmeijer, A. J., L. H. van der Woude, A. P. Hollander, and H. H. van As. Physical performance during rehabilitation in persons with spinal cord injuries. *Med Sci Sports Exerc.* 31:1330–1335, 1999.

47. Dallmeijer, A. J., L. H. V. v. d. Woude, and C. S. Pathuis. Adaptations in wheelchair propulsion technique after training in able-bodied subjects. In: *Biomedical Aspects of Manual Wheelchair Propulsion. The State of the Art II.* L. H. V. v. d. Woude, M. T. E. Hopman, and C. H. Kemenade (Eds.) Amsterdam: IOS Press, 1999, pp. 224–226.

48. Dallmeijer, A. J., I. D. Zentgraaff, N. I. Zijp, and L. H. van der Woude. Submaximal physical strain and peak performance in handcycling versus handrim wheelchair propulsion. *Spinal Cord.* 42:91–98, 2004.

49. de Groot, S., P. Gervais, J. V. Coppoolse, K. Natho, Y. Bhambhani, R. Staedward, and G. Wheeler. Evaluation of a new basketball wheelchair design. *Technol Disabil.* 15:7–18, 2003.

50. De Groot, S., D. H. Veeger, A. P. Hollander, and L. H. van der Woude. Wheelchair propulsion technique and mechanical efficiency after 3 wk of practice. *Med Sci Sports Exerc.* 34:756–766, 2002.

51. de Groot, S., H. E. Veeger, A. P. Hollander, and L. H. van der Woude. Adaptations in physiology and propulsion techniques during the initial phase of learning manual wheelchair propulsion. *Am J Phys Med Rehabil.* 82:504–510, 2003.

52. de Groot, S., H. E. Veeger, A. P. Hollander, and L. H. van der Woude. Consequence of feedback-based learning of an effective hand rim wheelchair force production on mechanical efficiency. *Clin Biomech (Bristol, Avon).* 17:219–226, 2002.

53. de Groot, S., H. E. Veeger, A. P. Hollander, and L. H. van der Woude. Effect of wheelchair stroke pattern on mechanical efficiency. *Am J Phys Med Rehabil.* 83:640–649, 2004.

54. de Groot, S., H. E. Veeger, A. P. Hollander, and L. H. van der Woude. Short-term adaptations in co-ordination during the initial phase of learning manual wheelchair propulsion. *J Electromyogr Kinesiol.* 13:217–228, 2003.

55. Dietz, V. and G. Colombo. Recovery from spinal cord injury—underlying mechanisms and efficacy of rehabilitation. *Acta Neurochir Suppl.* 89:95–100, 2004.

56. DiGiovine, C. P., R. A. Cooper, E. Wolf, S. G. Fitzgerald, and M. L. Boninger. Analysis of whole-body vibration during manual wheelchair propulsion: A comparison of seat cushions and back supports for individuals without a disability. *Assist Technol.* 15: 129–144, 2003.

57. van Dijk, F., M. V. Dormolen, M. Kompier, and T. Meijman. Herwaardering model arbeidsbelastbaarheid (Dutch). *TSG.* 68:3–10, 1990.

58. Durstine, J. L. and G. E. Moore. *ACSM's Exercise Management for Persons with Chronic Diseases and Disabilities.* Champaign, IL: Human Kinetics, ACSM, 2003.

59. Dyson-Hudson, T. A. and S. C. Kirshblum. Shoulder pain in chronic spinal cord injury, Part I: Epidemiology, etiology, and pathomechanics. *J Spinal Cord Med.* 27:4–17, 2004.

60. Engel, P. and G. Hidebrandt. Zur Arbeitsphysiologischen Beurteilung verschiedener handbetriebener Krankenfahrstuhlemodelle. *Z Phys Med.* 2:95–102, 1971.

61. Faupin, A., P. Gorce, P. Campillo, A. Thevenon, and O. Remy-Neris. Kinematic analysis of handbike propulsion in various gear ratios: implications for joint pain. *Clin Biomech (Bristol, Avon).* 21:560–566, 2006.

62. Finley, M. A., K. J. McQuade, and M. M. Rodgers. Scapular kinematics during transfers in manual wheelchair users with and without shoulder impingement. *Clin Biomech (Bristol, Avon).* 20:32–40, 2005.

63. Formusek, C. and G. Davis. Technical design of a novel isokinetic FES exercise bicycle for spinal cord injured individuals. *J Rehabil Res Dev.* 41:S53, 2004.

64. Frank, T. G. and E. W. Abel. Measurement of the turning, rolling and obstacle resistance of wheelchair castor wheels. *J Biomed Eng.* 11:462–466, 1989.
65. Frontera, W. *Exercise in Rehabilitation Medicine.* Champaign: Human Kinetics, 1999.
66. Fullerton, H. D., J. J. Borckardt, and A. P. Alfano. Shoulder pain: A comparison of wheelchair athletes and nonathletic wheelchair users. *Med Sci Sports Exerc.* 35:1958–1961, 2003.
67. Gagnon, D., S. Nadeau, D. Gravel, L. Noreau, C. Lariviere, and D. Gagnon. Biomechanical analysis of a posterior transfer maneuver on a level surface in individuals with high and low-level spinal cord injuries. *Clin Biomech (Bristol, Avon).* 18:319–331, 2003.
68. Gagnon, D., S. Nadeau, D. Gravel, L. Noreau, C. Lariviere, and B. McFadyen. Movement patterns and muscular demands during posterior transfers toward an elevated surface in individuals with spinal cord injury. *Spinal Cord.* 43:74–84, 2005.
69. Gangelhoff, J., L. Cordain, A. Tucker, and J. Sockler. Metabolic and heart rate responses to submaximal arm lever and arm crank ergometry. *Arch Phys Med Rehabil.* 69:101–105, 1988.
70. Gfohler, M., M. Loicht, and P. Lugner. Exercise tricycle for paraplegics. *Med Biol Eng Comput.* 36:118–121, 1998.
71. Goosey, V. L., I. G. Campbell, and N. E. Fowler. Effect of push frequency on the economy of wheelchair racers. *Med Sci Sports Exerc.* 32:174–181, 2000.
72. Gordon, J., J. J. Kauzlarich, and J. G. Thacker. Tests of two new polyurethane foam wheelchair tires. *J Rehabil Res Dev.* 26:33–46, 1989.
73. Grevelding, P. and R. Bohannon. Reduced push forces accompany device use during sliding transfers of seated subjects. *J Reh Res Dev.* 38:135–139, 2001.
74. Guo, L. Y., F. C. Su, and K. N. An. Effect of handrim diameter on manual wheelchair propulsion: mechanical energy and power flow analysis. *Clin Biomech (Bristol, Avon).* 21:107–115, 2006.
75. Gutierrez, D. D., S. J. Mulroy, C. J. Newsam, J. K. Gronley, and J. Perry. Effect of fore-aft seat position on shoulder demands during wheelchair propulsion: Part 2. An electromyographic analysis. *J Spinal Cord Med.* 28:222–229, 2005.
76. Haeuber, E., M. Shaughnessey, L. Forrester, K. Coleman, and R. Macko. Accelerometer monitoring of home- and community based ambulatory activity after stroke. *Arch Phys Med Rehabil.* 85:1997–2001, 2004.
77. Haisma, J. A., J. B. Bussmann, H. J. Stam, T. A. Sluis, M. P. Bergen, A. J. Dallmeijer, S. de Groot, and L. H. van der Woude. Changes in physical capacity during and after inpatient rehabilitation in subjects with a spinal cord injury. *Arch Phys Med Rehabil.* 87:741–748, 2006.
78. Haisma, J. A., L. H. van der Woude, H. J. Stam, M. P. Bergen, T. A. Sluis, and J. B. Bussmann. Physical capacity in wheelchair-dependent persons with a spinal cord injury: A critical review of the literature. *Spinal Cord.* 44:642–652, 2006.
79. Hart, K. and H. Rintala. Long-term outcomes following spinal cord injury. *NeuroRehabilitation.* 5:57–73, 1995.
80. Haskell, W. L. and J. B. Wolffe Memorial Lecture. Health consequences of physical activity: Understanding and challenges regarding dose–response. *Med Sci Sports Exerc.* 26:649–660, 1994.
81. Haskell, W. L. Physical activity, sport, and health: Toward the next century. *Res Q Exerc Sport.* 67:S37–47, 1996.
82. Heesterbeek, P., H. Berkelsmans, D. Thijssen, H. van Kuppevelt, M. Hopman, and J. Duysens. Increased physical fitness after 4-week training on a new hybrid FES-cycle in persons. *Technol Disabil.* 17:103–110, 2005.
83. Herman, R., J. He, S. D'Luzansky, W. Willis, and S. Dilli. Spinal cord stimulation facilitates functional walking in a chronic, incomplete spinal cord injured. *Spinal Cord.* 40:65–68, 2002.

84. Hesse, S., C. Werner, and A. Barbelden. Electromechanical gait training with functional electrical stimulation: case studies in spinal cord injury. *Spinal Cord.* 42:346–352, 2005.

85. Hicks, A., M. Adams, K. Martin Ginnis, L. Giangregorio, A. Latimer, S. Phillips, and N. McCartney. Long-term body-weight-supported treadmill training and subsequent follow-up in persons with chronic SCI: Effects on functional walking ability and measures of subjective well-being. *Spinal Cord.* 43:291–298, 2005.

86. Hildebrandt, G., E. D. Voigt, D. Bahn, B. Berendes, and J. Kroger. Energy cost of propelling a wheelchair at various speeds: cardiac response and the affect of steering accuracy. *Arch Phys Med Rehabil.* 131–136, 1970.

87. Hintzy, F., N. Tordi, and S. Perrey. Muscular efficiency during arm cranking and wheelchair exercise: a comparison. *Int J Sports Med.* 23:408–414, 2002.

88. Hjeltnes. Circulatory strain in everyday life of paraplegics. *Scand J Rehabil Med.* 11:67–73, 1979.

89. Hjeltnes, N. and Z. Vokac. Circulatory strain in everyday life of paraplegics. *Scand J Rehabil Med.* 11:67–73, 1979.

90. Hughes, B., B. J. Sawatzky, and A. T. Hol. A comparison of spinergy versus standard steel-spoke wheelchair wheels. *Arch Phys Med Rehabil.* 86:596–601, 2005.

91. Hughes, C. J., W. H. Weimar, P. N. Sheth, and C. E. Brubaker. Biomechanics of wheelchair propulsion as a function of seat position and user-to-chair interface. *Arch Phys Med Rehabil.* 73:263–269, 1992.

92. Human, Factors, Special, and Issue. Assisting people with functional impairments. *Human Factors.* 32:379–502, 1990.

93. Ingen Schenau, G. J. v. Cycle power: A predictive model. *Endeavour* (*New Series*). 12(1), 44–47, 1988.

94. Jacobs, P. L., E. T. Mahoney, and B. Johnson. Reliability of arm Wingate Anaerobic Testing in persons with complete paraplegia. *J Spinal Cord Med.* 26:141–144, 2003.

95. Janssen, T., R. Glaser, and D. Schuster. Clinical efficacy of electrical stimulation exercise training: Effects on health, fitness, and function. *Top Spinal Cord Inj Rehabil.* 3:33–49, 1998.

96. Janssen, T. W., A. J. Dallmeijer, and L. H. van der Woude. Physical capacity and race performance of handcycle users. *J Rehabil Res Dev.* 38:33–40, 2001.

97. Janssen, T. W., C. A. van Oers, A. P. Hollander, H. E. Veeger, and L. H. van der Woude. Isometric strength, sprint power, and aerobic power in individuals with a spinal cord injury. *Med Sci Sports Exerc.* 25:863–870, 1993.

98. Janssen, T. W., C. A. van Oers, E. P. Rozendaal, E. M. Willemsen, A. P. Hollander, and L. H. van der Woude. Changes in physical strain and physical capacity in men with spinal cord injuries. *Med Sci Sports Exerc.* 28:551–559, 1996.

99. Janssen, T. W., C. A. van Oers, G. J. van Kamp, B. J. TenVoorde, L. H. van der Woude, and A. P. Hollander. Coronary heart disease risk indicators, aerobic power, and physical activity in men with spinal cord injuries. *Arch Phys Med Rehabil.* 78:697–705, 1997.

100. Kauzlarich, J. J. Wheelchair rolling resistance and tire design. In: *Biomedical Aspects of Manual Wheelchair Propulsion: State of the Art III.* L. H. V. v. d. Woude, M. T. E. Hopman, and C. H. v. Kemenade (Eds.). Amsterdam: IOS Press, 1999, pp. 158–172.

101. Kauzlarich, J. J., T. E. Bruning, 3rd, and J. G. Thacker. Wheelchair caster shimmy II: Damping. *J Rehabil Res Dev.* 37:305–313, 2000.

102. Kauzlarich, J. J. and J. G. Thacker. Wheelchair tire rolling resistance and fatigue. *J Rehabil Res Dev.* 22(2):25–41, 1985.

103. Khalaf, K. A., M. Parnianpour, P. J. Sparto, and S. R. Simon. Modeling of functional trunk muscle performance: Interfacing ergonomics and spine rehabilitation in response to the ADA. *J Rehabil Res Dev.* 34:459–469, 1997.

104. Kilgore, K. L., P. H. Peckham, M. W. Keith, F. W. Montague, R. L. Hart, M. M. Gazdik, A. M. Bryden, S. A. Snyder, and T. G. Stage. Durability of implanted electrodes and leads in an upper-limb neuroprosthesis. *J Rehabil Res Dev*. 40:457–468, 2003.

105. Kilkens, O. J., A. J. Dallmeijer, A. V. Nene, M. W. Post, and L. H. van der Woude. The longitudinal relation between physical capacity and wheelchair skill performance during inpatient rehabilitation of people with spinal cord injury. *Arch Phys Med Rehabil*. 86:1575–1581, 2005.

106. Kirby, R. L., C. L. Fahie, C. Smith, E. L. Chester, and D. A. Macleod. Neck discomfort of wheelchair users: Effect of neck position. *Disabil Rehabil*. 26:9–15, 2004.

107. Knechtle, B., G. Muller, and H. Knecht. Optimal exercise intensities for fat metabolism in handbike cycling and cycling. *Spinal Cord*. 42:564–572, 2004.

108. Koontz, A. M., R. A. Cooper, M. L. Boninger, Y. Yang, B. G. Impink, and L. H. van der Woude. A kinetic analysis of manual wheelchair propulsion during start-up on select indoor and outdoor surfaces. *J Rehabil Res Dev*. 42:447–458, 2005.

109. Kotajarvi, B., M. B. Sabick, K. N. An, K. D. Zhao, K. R. Kaufman, and J. R. Basford. The effect of seat position on wheelchair biomechanics. *J Reh Res Dev*. 41:403–414, 2004.

110. Kotajarvi, B. R., J. R. Basford, K. N. An, D. A. Morrow, and K. R. Kaufman. The effect of visual biofeedback on the propulsion effectiveness of experienced wheelchair users. *Arch Phys Med Rehabil*. 87:510–515, 2006.

111. Kumar, S. Ergonomics in rehabilitation. *Disabil Rehabil*. 18:113–114, 1996.

112. Lesser, W. Arbeitsphysiologische, biomechanische und anthropometrische Untersuchungen an Rollstuhlen. *3. Statuskoll.*, 1984.

113. Lesser, W. Arbeitsphysiologische Untersuchungen des Rollstuhls mit Greifreifenantrieb. *Med Orthop Techn*. 5:139–143, 1981.

114. Levy, C. E. and J. W. Chow. Pushrim-activated power-assist wheelchairs: Elegance in motion. *Am J Phys Med Rehabil*. 83:166–167, 2004.

115. Levy, C. E., J. W. Chow, M. D. Tillman, C. Hanson, T. Donohue, and W. C. Mann. Variable-ratio pushrim-activated power-assist wheelchair eases wheeling over a variety of terrains for elders. *Arch Phys Med Rehabil*. 85:104–112, 2004.

116. Loisel, P., L. Gosselin, P. Durand, J. Lemaire, S. Poitras, and L. Abenhaim. Implementation of a participatory ergonomics program in the rehabilitation of workers suffering from subacute back pain. *Appl Ergon*. 32:53–60, 2001.

117. Lum, P. S., C. G. Burgar, P. C. Shor, M. Majmundar, and M. van der Loos. Robot-assisted movement training compared with conventional therapy techniques for the rehabilitation of upper-limb motor function after stroke. *Arch Phys Med Rehabil*. 83:952–959, 2002.

118. Maki, K. C., W. E. Langbein, and C. Reid-Lokos. Energy cost and locomotive economy of handbike and rowcycle propulsion by persons with spinal cord injury. *J Rehabil Res Dev*. 32:170–178, 1995.

119. Martel, G., L. Noreau, and J. Jobin. Physiological responses to maximal exercise on arm cranking and wheelchair ergometer with paraplegics. *Paraplegia*. 29:447–456, 1991.

120. McLaurin, C. A. and C. E. Brubaker. Biomechanics and the wheelchair. *Prosthet Orthot Int*. 15:24–37, 1991.

121. Mital, A. and W. Karwowski. *Ergonomics in Rehabilitation*. London: Taylor & Francis, 1988.

122. Morrow, D. A., L. Y. Guo, K. D. Zhao, F. C. Su, and K. N. An. A 2-D model of wheelchair propulsion. *Disabil Rehabil*. 25:192–196, 2003.

123. Mukherjee, G., P. Bhowmik, and A. Samanta. Effect of chronic use of different propulsion systems in wheelchair design on the aerobic capacity of Indian users. *Indian J Med Res*. 121:747–758, 2005.

124. Mukherjee, G., P. Bhowmik, and A. Samanta. Physical fitness training for wheelchair ambulation by the arm crank propulsion technique. *Clin Rehabil*. 15:125–132, 2001.

125. Mukherjee, G. and A. Samanta. Arm-crank propelled three-wheeled chair: Physiological evaluation of the propulsion using one arm and both arm patterns. *Int J Rehabil Res.* 27:321–324, 2004.

126. Nichols, P. J., P. A. Norman, and J. R. Ennis. Wheelchair user's shoulder? Shoulder pain in patients with spinal cord lesions. *Scand J Rehabil Med.* 11:29–32, 1979.

127. Niesing, R., F. Eijskoot, R. Kranse, A. H. den Ouden, J. Storm, H. E. Veeger, L. H. van der Woude, and C. J. Snijders. Computer-controlled wheelchair ergometer. *Med Biol Eng Comput.* 28:329–338, 1990.

128. Noreau, L. and R. J. Shephard. Return to work after spinal cord injury: The potential contribution of physical fitness. *Paraplegia.* 30:563–572, 1992.

129. Noreau, L. and R. J. Shephard. Spinal cord injury, exercise and quality of life. *Sports Med.* 20:226–250, 1995.

130. Nunn, A., J. McLeod, I. Brown, A. Ting, P. Early, and R. Hawkins. Monitoring patients with SCI during activity using a datalogger. *J Rehabil Res Dev.* 41:47, 2004.

131. Peizer, E., D. Wright, and H. Freiberger. Bioengineering methods of wheelchair evaluation. *Bull Prosthetics Res.* 77–100, 1964.

132. Perry, J., J. K. Gronley, C. J. Newsam, M. L. Reyes, and S. J. Mulroy. Electromyographic analysis of the shoulder muscles during depression transfers in subjects with low-level paraplegia. *Arch Phys Med Rehabil.* 77:350–355, 1996.

133. Postma, K., H. J. van den Berg-Emons, J. B. Bussmann, T. A. Sluis, M. P. Bergen, and H. J. Stam. Validity of the detection of wheelchair propulsion as measured with an activity monitor in patients with spinal cord injury. *Spinal Cord.* 43:550–557, 2005.

134. Reichenfelser, W., M. Gfoehler, and T. Angeli. Design of a test and training tricycle for subjects with paraplegia. *Technol Disabil.* 17:93–101, 2005.

135. Richter, M. Low impact wheelchair propulsion: Achievable and acceptable. *J Rehabil Res Dev*, 42(3), Suppl.1:21–35, 2005.

136. Richter, W. M. The effect of seat position on manual wheelchair propulsion biomechanics: a quasi-static model-based approach. *Med Eng Phys.* 23:707–712, 2001.

137. Richter, W. M. and P. W. Axelson. Low-impact wheelchair propulsion: Achievable and acceptable. *J Rehabil Res Dev.* 42:21–34, 2005.

138. Rimmer, J. H. and D. Braddock. Health promotion for people with physical, cognitive and sensory disabilities: an emerging national priority. *Am J Health Promot.* 16:220–224, ii, 2002.

139. Rodgers, M. M., G. W. Gayle, S. F. Figoni, M. Kobayashi, J. Lieh, and R. M. Glaser. Biomechanics of wheelchair propulsion during fatigue. *Arch Phys Med Rehab.* 75: 85–93, 1994.

140. Rodgers, M. M., K. J. McQuade, E. K. Rasch, R. E. Keyser, and M. A. Finley. Upper-limb fatigue-related joint power shifts in experienced wheelchair users and nonwheelchair users. *J Rehabil Res Dev.* 40:27–37, 2003.

141. Roebroeck, M., R. Rozendal, and L. v. d. Woude. *Methodology of Consumer Evaluation of Hand Propelled Wheelchairs*: EEC, COMAC-BME, 1989.

142. Rozendaal, L. A. and D. E. Veeger. Force direction in manual wheel chair propulsion: Balance between effect and cost. *Clin Biomech (Bristol, Avon).* 15(Suppl 1):S39–S41, 2000.

143. Ruggles, D. L., T. Cahalan, and K. N. An. Biomechanics of wheelchair propulsion by able-bodied subjects. *Arch Phys Med Rehabil.* 75:540–544, 1994.

144. Sabick, M., B. Kotajarvi, and K. -A. An. A new method to quantify demand on the upper extremity during manual wheelchair propulsion. *Arch Phys Med Rehab.* 85:1151–1159, 2004.

145. Samuelsson, K. A., H. Tropp, and B. Gerdle. Shoulder pain and its consequences in paraplegic spinal cord-injured, wheelchair users. *Spinal Cord.* 42:41–46, 2004.

146. Samuelsson, K. A., H. Tropp, E. Nylander, and B. Gerdle. The effect of rear-wheel position on seating ergonomics and mobility efficiency in wheelchair users with spinal cord injuries: A pilot study. *J Rehabil Res Dev*. 41:65–74, 2004.
147. Sawatzky, B. J., W. O. Kim, and I. Denison. The ergonomics of different tyres and tyre pressure during wheelchair propulsion. *Ergonomics*. 47:1475–1483, 2004.
148. Sawatzky, B. J., W. C. Miller, and I. Denison. Measuring energy expenditure using heart rate to assess the effects of wheelchair tyre pressure. *Clin Rehabil*. 19:182–187, 2005.
149. Sawka, M. N. Physiology of upper body exercise. *Exerc Sport Sci*. 14:175–211, 1986.
150. Sawka, M. N., M. E. Foley, N. A. Pimental, and K. B. Pandolf. Physiological factors affecting upper-body aerobic exercise. *Ergonomics*. 26(7):639–646, 1983.
151. Schuldt, K. On neck muscle activity and load reduction in sitting postures. An electromyographic and biomechanical study with applications in ergonomics and rehabilitation. *Scand J Rehabil Med Suppl*. 19:1–49, 1988.
152. Simmons, S. F., J. F. Schnelle, P. G. MacRae, and J. G. Ouslander. Wheelchairs as mobility restraints: Predictors of wheelchair activity in nonambulatory nursing home residents. *J Am Geriatr Soc*. 43:384–388, 1995.
153. Smith, D. G., E. Domholdt, K. L. Coleman, M. A. Del Aguila, and D. A. Boone. Ambulatory activity in men with diabetes: Relationship between self-reported and real-world performance-based measures. *J Rehabil Res Dev*. 41:571–580, 2004.
154. Smith, P. A., R. M. Glaser, J. S. Petrofsky, P. D. Underwood, G. B. Smith, and J. J. Richard. Arm crank vs handrim wheelchair propulsion: metabolic and cardiopulmonary responses. *Arch Phys Med Rehabil*. 64:249–254, 1983.
155. Soede, M. Rehabilitation technology or the ergonomics of ergonomics. *Ergonomics*. 33:367–373, 1990.
156. Staros, A. Testing of manually-propelled wheelchairs. The need for international standards. *Prosthet Orthot Int*. 5:75–84, 1981.
157. Steele, B., B. Belza, K. Cain, C. Warms, J. Coopersmith, and J. Howard. Bodies in motion: Monitoring daily activity and exercise with motion sensors in people with chronic pulmonary disease. *J Reh Res Dev*. 40:45–58, 2003.
158. Tasiemski, T., P. Kennedy, B. P. Gardner, and N. Taylor. The association of sports and physical recreation with life satisfaction in a community sample of people with spinal cord injuries. *NeuroRehabilitation*. 20:253–265, 2005.
159. Traut, L. Gestaltung ergonomisch relevanter Konstruktionsparameter am Antriebsystem des Greifreifenrolstuhls -Teil 1. *Orthopadie Technik*. 7:394–399, 1989.
160. Traut, L. Gestaltung ergonomisch relevanter Konstruktionsparameter am Antriebsystem des Greifreifenrolstuhls -Teil 1-Teil II. *Orthopadie Technik*. 7;8:394–399;456–460, 1989.
161. Tupling, S. J., G. M. Davis, M. R. Pierrynowski, and R. J. Shephard. Arm strength and impulse generation: Initiation of wheelchair movement by the physically disabled. *Ergonomics*. 29(2):303–311, 1986.
162. van der Ploeg, H., K. Streppel, A. van der Beek, L. van der Woude, M. Vollenbroek-Hutten, and W. van Mechelen. The physical activity scale for individuals with physical disabilities: Test–retest reliability and comparison with two accelerometers. *J Phys Act Health*. 4(1): 96–100, 2007.
163. van der Ploeg, H. P., A. J. van der Beek, L. H. van der Woude, and W. van Mechelen. Physical activity for people with a disability: A conceptual model. *Sports Med*. 34:639–649, 2004.
164. van der Woude, L. H., W. H. Bakker, J. W. Elkhuizen, H. E. Veeger, and T. Gwinn. Anaerobic work capacity in elite wheelchair athletes. *Am J Phys Med Rehabil*. 76:355–365, 1997.
165. van der Woude, L. H., I. Bosmans, B. Bervoets, and H. E. Veeger. Handcycling: Different modes and gear ratios. *J Med Eng Technol*. 24:242–249, 2000.
166. van der Woude, L. H., E. Botden, I. Vriend, and D. Veeger. Mechanical advantage in wheelchair lever propulsion: Effect on physical strain and efficiency. *J Rehabil Res Dev*. 34:286–294, 1997.

167. van der Woude, L. H., C. Bouten, H. E. Veeger, and T. Gwinn. Aerobic work capacity in elite wheelchair athletes: A cross-sectional analysis. *Am J Phys Med Rehabil.* 81:261–271, 2002.

168. van der Woude, L. H., G. de Groot, A. P. Hollander, G. J. van Ingen Schenau, and R. H. Rozendal. Wheelchair ergonomics and physiological testing of prototypes. *Ergonomics.* 29:1561–1573, 1986.

169. van der Woude, L. H., M. Formanoy, and S. de Groot. Hand rim configuration: Effects on physical strain and technique in unimpaired subjects? *Med Eng Phys.* 25:765–774, 2003.

170. van der Woude, L. H., C. Geurts, H. Winkelman, and H. E. Veeger. Measurement of wheelchair rolling resistance with a handle bar push technique. *J Med Eng Technol.* 27:249–258, 2003.

171. van der Woude, L. H., K. M. Hendrich, H. E. Veeger, G. J. van Ingen Schenau, R. H. Rozendal, G. de Groot, and A. P. Hollander. Manual wheelchair propulsion: Effects of power output on physiology and technique. *Med Sci Sports Exerc.* 20:70–78, 1988.

172. van der Woude, L. H., J. J. van Croonenborg, I. Wolff, A. J. Dallmeijer, and A. P. Hollander. Physical work capacity after 7 wk of wheelchair training: Effect of intensity in able-bodied subjects. *Med Sci Sports Exerc.* 31:331–341, 1999.

173. van der Woude, L. H., D. J. Veeger, and R. H. Rozendal. Seat height in hand rim wheelchair propulsion: a follow-up study. *J Reh Sci.* 3:79–83, 1990.

174. van der Woude, L. H., D. J. Veeger, R. H. Rozendal, and T. J. Sargeant. Seat height in handrim wheelchair propulsion. *J Rehabil Res Dev.* 26:31–50, 1989.

175. van der Woude, L. H., H. E. Veeger, A. J. Dallmeijer, T. W. Janssen, and L. A. Rozendaal. Biomechanics and physiology in active manual wheelchair propulsion. *Med Eng Phys.* 23:713–733, 2001.

176. van der Woude, L. H., H. E. Veeger, R. H. Rozendal, and A. J. Sargeant. Optimum cycle frequencies in hand-rim wheelchair propulsion. Wheelchair propulsion technique. *Eur J Appl Physiol Occup Physiol.* 58:625–632, 1989.

177. van der Woude, L. H., H. E. Veeger, R. H. Rozendal, G. J. van Ingen Schenau, F. Rooth, and P. van Nierop. Wheelchair racing: Effects of rim diameter and speed on physiology and technique. *Med Sci Sports Exerc.* 20:492–500, 1988.

178. van der Woude, L. H. V., A. J. Dallmeijer, T. W. J. Janssen, and D. Veeger. Alternative modes of manual wheelchair ambulation—An overview. *Am J Phys Med Rehabil.* 80:765–777, 2001.

179. van der Woude, L. H. V., A. Horstman, P. Faas, S. Mechielsen, H. Abbasi Bafghi, and J. J. de Koning. Asynchronous versus asynchronous hand cycling. *Med Eng Phys.* 30(5):574–580, 2008.

180. van Drongelen, A., B. Roszek, E. Hilbers-Modderman, M. Kallewaard, and C. Wassenaar. *Wheelchair Incidents.* Bilthoven: RIVM, 2002.

181. van Drongelen, S., S. de Groot, H. E. Veeger, E. L. Angenot, A. J. Dallmeijer, M. W. Post, and L. H. van der Woude. Upper extremity musculoskeletal pain during and after rehabilitation in wheelchair-using persons with a spinal cord injury. *Spinal Cord*, 44(3):152–159, 2006.

182. van Drongelen, S., L. van der Woude, T. Janssen, E. Angenot, and H. Veeger. Glenohumeral contact forces and muscle forces in wheelchair-related activities of daily living in able-bodied, subjects versus subjects with paraplegia and tetraplegia. *Arch Phys Med Rehabil.* 86(7):1434–1440, 2005.

183. van Drongelen, S., L. van der Woude, T. Janssen, E. Angenot, and H. Veeger. Glenohumeral contact forces and muscle forces in wheelchair-related activities of daily living in able-bodied, subjects versus subjects with paraplegia and tetraplegia. *Arch Phys Med Rehabil.* 86:1434–1440, 2005.

184. van Drongelen, S., L. van der Woude, and H. Veeger. Load on the shoulder during weight-relief lifts in men with a spinal-cord injury. *JRRD.* 41:S18, 2004.

185. van Drongelen, S., L. H. van der Woude, T. W. Janssen, E. L. Angenot, E. K. Chadwick, and D. H. Veeger. Mechanical load on the upper extremity during wheelchair activities. *Arch Phys Med Rehabil.* 86:1214–1220, 2005.
186. van Drongelen, S., L. H. van der Woude, T. W. Janssen, E. L. Angenot, E. K. Chadwick, and H. E. Veeger. Glenohumeral joint loading in tetraplegia during weight relief lifting: A simulation study. *Clin Biomech (Bristol, Avon)*, 21(2):128–137, 2006.
187. van Ingen Schenau, G. J. Cycle power: a predictive model. *Endeavour.* 12:44–47, 1988.
188. Vanlandewijck, Y. C., A. J. Spaepen, and R. J. Lysens. Wheelchair propulsion: Functional ability dependent factors in wheelchair basketball players. *Scand J Rehabil Med.* 26:37–48, 1994.
189. Veeger, D., L. H. van der Woude, and R. H. Rozendal. The effect of rear wheel camber in manual wheelchair propulsion. *J Rehabil Res Dev.* 26:37–46, 1989.
190. Veeger, H. E., L. A. Rozendaal, and F. C. van der Helm. Load on the shoulder in low intensity wheelchair propulsion. *Clin Biomech (Bristol, Avon).* 17:211–218, 2002.
191. Veeger, H. E., L. H. van der Woude, and R. H. Rozendal. A computerized wheelchair ergometer. Results of a comparison study. *Scand J Rehabil Med.* 24:17–23, 1992.
192. Veeger, H. E., L. H. van der Woude, and R. H. Rozendal. A computerized wheelchair ergometer. Results of a comparison study. *Scand J Rehabil Med.* 24:17–23, 1992.
193. Veeger, H. E., L. H. van der Woude, and R. H. Rozendal. Effect of handrim velocity on mechanical efficiency in wheelchair propulsion. *Med Sci Sports Exerc.* 24: 100–107, 1992.
194. Verellen, J., D. Theisen, and Y. Vanlandewijck. Influence of crank rate in hand cycling. *Med Sci Sports Exerc.* 36:1826–1831, 2004.
195. Voigt, E. D. and D. Bahn. Metabolism and pulse rate in physically handicapped when propelling a wheel chair up and incline. *Scand J Rehabil Med.* 1:101–106, 1969.
196. Weege, R. D. V. Technische Voraussetzungen fur den Aktivsport im Rollstuhl. *Orthopaedie Technik.* 36(6):395–402, 1985.
197. Wei, S. H., S. Huang, C. J. Jiang, and J. C. Chiu. Wrist kinematic characterization of wheelchair propulsion in various seating positions: Implication to wrist pain. *Clin Biomech (Bristol, Avon).* 18:S46–52, 2003.
198. WHO. *International Classification of Functioning, Disability and Health.* Geneva: World Health Organisation, 2001.
199. Wicks, J. R., N. B. Oldridge, B. J. Cameron, and N. L. Jones. Arm cranking and wheelchair ergometry in elite spinal cord-injured athletes. *Med Sci Sports Exerc.* 15:224–231, 1983.
200. Wolf, E. J., M. S. Cooper, C. P. DiGiovine, M. L. Boninger, and S. Guo. Using the absorbed power method to evaluate effectiveness of vibration absorption of selected seat cushions during manual wheelchair propulsion. *Med Eng Phys.* 26:799–806, 2004.
201. Woolfrey, P. G. and R. L. Kirby. Ergonomics in rehabilitation: A comparison of two methods of moving an empty manual wheelchair short distances. *Arch Phys Med Rehabil.* 79:955–958, 1998.
202. Wu, H. W., L. J. Berglund, F. C. Su, B. Yu, A. Westreich, K. J. Kim, and K. N. An. An instrumented wheel for kinetic analysis of wheelchair propulsion. *J Biomech Eng.* 120:533–535, 1998.
203. Wuolle, K. S., A. M. Bryden, P. H. Peckham, P. K. Murray, and M. Keith. Satisfaction with upper-extremity surgery in individuals with tetraplegia. *Arch Phys Med Rehabil.* 84:1145–1149, 2003.

7 Seats, Seating, and Seat Selection: Implications for Pressure Ulcers

Leandro R. Solis and Vivian K. Mushahwar

CONTENTS

7.1   INTRODUCTION

A routine day in the life of most people involves spending a significant amount of time seated, whether it is in a classroom or at work, in a vehicle, or at home. The seat we use is often chosen by chance or availability (classroom, work). In other instances, a seat is chosen based on one's own personal preference (home). The process of picking the appropriate seat might seem trivial to most people, but when considering that one spends a significant part of the day seated, much thought should be given to the seat of choice in order to reduce the chances of medical complications associated with prolonged sitting. Several studies have shown that prolonged sitting can increase the risk of developing lower back pain, shoulder pain, and neck pain. These musculoskeletal disorders are frequent causes of sick leave that lead to the loss of millions of work days every year (Kvarnstrom, 1983; Johanning, 2000; Morken et al., 2003; Cagnie et al., 2007; Krismer et al., 2007).

Ariëns et al. (2001) reported that sitting at work for more than 95% of the working hours is a risk factor for developing neck pain. A study performed with European truck drivers found that 81% of the participants reported a musculoskeletal problem in at least one area of the body during the year prior to the study. Lower back pain had the highest incidence at 60%, followed by shoulder pain (39%), knee pain (36%), and neck pain (34%) (Robb and Mansfield, 2007). An increase in car driving time also leads to an increase in the number of absent days from work due to lower back pain (Porter and Gyi, 2002). Even among teenagers, prolonged periods of sitting are associated with a higher incidence of neck and shoulder pain (Auvinen et al., 2007). Moreover, sedentary activities, such as watching television and reading, were associated with neck pain in girls, while working or playing on a computer were associated with neck pain in boys.

While most able-bodied individuals can experience some type of posture-related pain at any time during their life due to prolonged sitting, postural disorders are not the only medical complication associated with prolonged sitting. A different disorder arises when the seated individual has reduced mobility and sensation, such as a person with a spinal cord injury (SCI) who is wheelchair dependent. While an able-bodied individual subconsciously moves periodically in his/her chair to relieve the discomfort of sitting, the same may not be possible for a person with SCI.

Approximately 75% of a person's body weight is supported by the buttocks and the ischial tuberosities when sitting upright. In this position, the soft tissue (skin, fat, fascia, muscle) between the seat surface and the ischial tuberosities is compressed, thereby reducing blood flow and generating mechanical stresses and strains in the tissue, especially in the muscles around the bony prominences. If this condition is maintained for an extended period of time, a pressure ulcer begins to develop in the affected tissue, in particular the muscle. The time required for an ulcer to begin developing can vary for each individual depending on the muscle mass and overall health of the person; however, a seat that distributes pressure around the buttocks poorly will lead to a reduction in the time required for an ulcer to begin forming.

7.1.1 INCIDENCE OF PRESSURE ULCERS

A pressure ulcer is defined by the National Pressure Ulcer Advisory Panel (NPUAP) in the United States, as a "localized injury to the skin and/or underlying tissue usually over a bony prominence, as a result of pressure in combination with shear and/or friction" (Black et al., 2007). Although the general layperson is usually unaware of the prevalence of pressure ulcers, ulcers are one of the main complications associated with immobilization and loss of sensation. Populations at risk of developing pressure ulcers include the elderly, residents of long-term care facilities and nursing homes, patients in acute and critical care units, patients who must undergo lengthy surgeries, as well as individuals who have suffered neurological insults such as SCI or stroke (Labbe et al., 1987; Conine et al., 1989; Woolsey and McGarry, 1991; Salzberg et al., 1996; Zanca et al., 2003; Edlich et al., 2004). A review of all published Medline articles during 1990–2000 conducted by the NPUAP indicated that clinical incidence rate of pressure ulcers is 7%–38% in acute care settings; 8%–40% in critical care settings; 4%–21% in the operating room; 7%–23% in long-term care; and 16%–17% in homecare settings (Panel, 2001). Variation in the incidence rates was reported to be due to variations in the definitions of an ulcer, formulas used to calculate incidence rates, mixed populations and sources of data, as well as random variation among the different studies.

Ulcers can develop within a few hours of immobilization. Aronovitch (2007) reported that among patients who developed a pressure ulcer intraoperatively, the median time of the surgery was 4.48 h. The estimated annual cost of treating hospital-acquired pressure ulcers alone in North America is in the range of $2.2 to $3.6 billion (Zanca et al., 2003) and $2.6 to $4.0 billion in the United Kingdom (Bennett et al., 2004). Although the risk and incidence of pressure ulcers increase with age, pressure ulcers can also develop in immobilized infants and children, where the incidence rates in pediatric intensive care units have been reported to be as high as 27% (Curley et al., 2003).

Individuals with SCI are especially at risk of developing ulcers due to their impaired sensation and atrophied muscles (Guthrie and Goulian, 1973; Thiyagarajan and Silver, 1984). More than 80% of individuals with SCI develop pressure ulcers (Salzberg et al., 1996), with incidence rates varying depending on the level and completeness of injury. Richardson and Meyer (1981) reported a 60% incidence rate in individuals with complete quadriplegia, 42% in incomplete quadriplegia, 52% in complete paraplegia, and 29% in incomplete paraplegia. Similarly, Young and Burns (1981) reported a 40%–45% incidence of pressure ulcers per year in all grades of sensory and motor quadriplegia. In a 3 year study focusing on veterans with SCI, Garber and Rintala (2003) showed that 39% of the participants were diagnosed with at least one pressure ulcer at any given time of the study and each experienced an average of four ulcers. Pressure ulcers on the pelvic area accounted for 67% of all ulcers and 76% of those required hospitalization. Originally, pressure ulcers were referred to as "bedsores" or "decubitus ulcers" due to the high incidence of this type of lesions in individuals confined to a bed; however, ulcers also develop in wheelchair users. The most susceptible location for pressure ulcers in wheelchair users is the tissue over the ischial tuberosities where muscle–bone interface forces are greatest (Ferguson-Pell, 1980; Drummond et al., 1982; Breuls et al., 2003b). Ischial ulcers represent 24% of the total incidence of pressure ulcers (Liu et al., 1999).

Severe ulcers require an average hospital stay of 2 months and cost $15,800–$72,680 to heal (Rischbieth et al., 1998). Given that 320,000 North Americans are currently living with SCI, the annual costs of treating pelvic ulcers in 39% of this population alone are $1.0–$4.6 billion. In addition to the financial consequences, pressure ulcers lead to further debilitation in individuals whose physical abilities are already compromised, further reduction in general independence and productivity, and lowering of self-esteem and self-worth (Krouskop et al., 1983). This results in a considerable decrease in the individual's overall quality of life.

The gravest risk associated with a developed pressure ulcer is the possibility of death from complications associated with an open infected wound, such as bacteremia (Galpin et al., 1976; Bryan et al., 1983; Wall et al., 2003). Higher mortality rates have been observed in individuals with pressure ulcers compared to age-matched subjects without ulcers, in particular among the elderly (Brandeis et al., 1990). In the United States between 1990 and 2001, pressure ulcers were reported as a cause of death for 114,380 persons (Redelings et al., 2005). A widely known case of death due to complications associated with a pressure ulcer was the tragic loss of the actor Christopher Reeve, who in 2004 died of cardiac complications caused by an infected pressure ulcer.

7.2 ETIOLOGY OF PRESSURE ULCERS

Pressure ulcers are a medical complication associated with immobilization, affecting bedridden individuals and wheelchair users. Pressure ulcers develop when soft tissue is compressed between a bony prominence and a surface for an extended period of time (Guthrie and Goulian, 1973; Fennegan, 1983; Swarts et al., 1988; Woolsey and McGarry, 1991; Salcido et al., 1995). The regions of the body commonly affected by pressure ulcers include the sacrum, ischium, heels, elbows, scapulae, trochanters, and the occiput (Figure 7.1). The main factors behind the formation of a pressure ulcer are the high mechanical stress and shear forces generated during the compression of the soft tissue. The prolonged exposure of the tissue to these excessive forces can directly

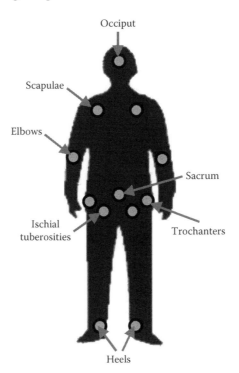

FIGURE 7.1   Regions at risk of developing pressure ulcers.

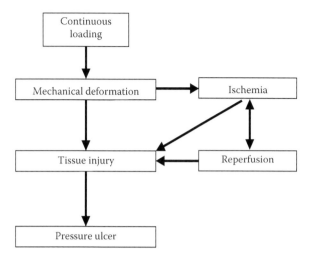

FIGURE 7.2   Pressure ulcer formation process.

lead to irreparable cell damage due to tissue deformation (Daniel et al., 1981; Bouten et al., 2003; Breuls et al., 2003b; Linder-Ganz and Gefen, 2004; Linder-Ganz et al., 2006, 2007; Stekelenburg et al., 2006b, 2007). In addition, extended loading of the tissue renders the tissue ischemic, limiting or eliminating the flow of oxygen and nutrients into the affected tissue and the removal of metabolic waste away from it. In the process of pressure ulcer development, ischemia is a major cause of injury to the tissue (Kosiak et al., 1958; Kosiak, 1959, 1961). Subsequent reperfusion of ischemic and already injured tissue can further increase the damage to the tissue (Grace, 1994; Gute et al., 1998; Peirce et al., 2000; Tsuji et al., 2005), initiating a negative cycle of metabolic changes in the tissue that lead to the formation of a pressure ulcer (Figure 7.2).

7.2.1   Effects of Ischemia and Reperfusion

Pressure in excess of that for capillary perfusion causes capillary occlusion, and interrupts the supply of oxygen and nutrients to the tissue and the removal of carbon dioxide and metabolic waste (Lyder, 2003). The lack of oxygen forces the cells to switch to anaerobic respiration, which in turn alters the concentration of energy metabolites important for cell function and homeostasis. The rate of adenosine triphosphate (ATP) production decreases and the levels of creatine phosphate (PCr) and glycogen decrease as they are used to produce new ATP. The levels of lactic acid and inorganic phosphate (Pi) increase, causing a decrease in pH, which in turn leads to clumping of nuclear chromatin and DNA inactivation (Grace, 1994; Tupling et al., 2001b). The duration of cell survival under anaerobic conditions depends on the type of the cell: skeletal muscles being highly sensitive to the lack of oxygen. Levels of ATP in the intracellular muscle space are reduced by 26% and 96% 30 min and 4 h after ischemia, while lactic acid is increased by 35% and 1000%, respectively (Tupling et al., 2001a,b; Kabaroudis et al., 2003). Levels of PCr and glycogen are reduced by 99.4% and 88% and Pi is increased by 400% 4 h after ischemia (Tupling et al., 2001a,b). Depletion of ATP also disrupts the Na^+K^+-ATPase pump, which maintains the balance of osmotic pressure between the intra- and extracellular environments. Upon failure of the pump, K^+ diffuses out of the cell while Na^+ accumulates inside accompanied by an accumulation of water, leading to cell swelling and eventual bursting of the membrane.

Under ischemic conditions, substrates for producing oxygen free radicals are formed. The enzyme xanthine dehydrogenase (XDH), which is found in the sarcolemma and mitochondria of aerobic muscle fibers and in the capillary endothelial cells of skeletal muscle, is converted to xanthine oxidase (XO). Moreover, ATP is broken down into hypoxanthine and xanthine, releasing iron in the process (Gute et al., 1998). As the duration of ischemia increases, the concentrations of XO, hypoxanthine, and xanthine increase.

Paradoxically, reperfusion of tissue following prolonged periods of ischemia can result in further injury even though restoration of blood flow is essential to maintain the living conditions of the cells (Grace, 1994). In the presence of oxygen, XO reacts with hypoxanthine to produce superoxide (O_2^-), and with xanthine to produce hydrogen peroxide (H_2O_2). Hydrogen peroxide in turn reacts with iron and produces hydroxyl radical (OH). Therefore, the sudden increase in available oxygen triggers a large production of H_2O_2 and free radicals that have three main harmful effects: (1) peroxidation of cell membranes; (2) oxidative modifications of proteins; and (3) lesions in DNA. These changes further damage the cell, leading it to necrosis (Labbe et al., 1987; Grace, 1994; Gute et al., 1998; Appell et al., 1999; Kabaroudis et al., 2003). Reperfusion also brings to the affected tissue large amounts of neutrophils whose increased infiltration has been associated with increased amounts of damage to the tissue (Grace, 1994; Gute et al., 1998). Leukocyte accumulation leads to an increase in tissue edema. Moreover, some leukocytes are believed to aggregate in the capillaries, occluding them, and partly contributing to the "no-reflow" effect, where tissue oxygenation is not restored even when there is normal blood flow in the arteries. This cascade of morphological, biochemical, and functional changes in the cell leads to its death (Finestone et al., 1991; Gilsdorf et al., 1991; Sagach et al., 1992; Grace, 1994; Tupling et al., 2001a,b).

7.2.2 Effects of Excessive Mechanical Compression

Excessive deformation of tissue, caused by the mechanical forces generated during loading, is recognized not only as the cause of ischemia in the tissue that leads to pressure ulcer formation, but also as a direct cause of tissue injury. These mechanical forces are (1) normal stress, (2) shear stress, and (3) friction. Normal stress is the distribution of force applied to a determined area of the tissue in a direction perpendicular to the support surface, as a result of the loading of the tissue. This type of stress is commonly referred to as "pressure," and causes the compression of the tissue between a bony prominence and the support surface. A study of the effects of pressure and its role in the etiology of pressure ulcers conducted by Kosiak identified an inverse relationship between the magnitude of pressure applied to the tissue, and the duration of the application (Kosiak, 1959). Higher levels of pressure applied for shorter periods of time were found to be as damaging to the tissue as lower levels of pressure applied for prolonged periods (Kosiak, 1959). Although traditionally high pressure levels were only considered the main cause for ischemia, which was in turn considered as the main cause for pressure ulcer formation, recent studies have shown that high pressure levels are capable of directly injuring the tissue. At the cellular level, in vitro studies have shown that the compression of single cells as well as that of engineered tissue causes deformation in the cell's membrane, which can be irreversible and lead to cell death (Bouten et al., 2001; Peeters et al., 2003; Breuls et al., 2003a). Animal experiments have also indicated that the combined effects of compressive loading and ischemia cause greater tissue injury than ischemia alone (Stekelenburg et al., 2007). Normal stress is the main cause for the formation of deep tissue injury (DTI) (see Section 7.4).

Shear stresses are forces distributed parallel to the support surface. In the etiology of pressure ulcers, they are usually accompanied by friction, which is the force that opposes the movement between two surfaces. These types of forces are generated by the degree of inclination of the upper body in an individual lying in bed or sitting in a wheelchair, or by the manner in which a person is repositioned. When inclined, the body tends to slide downward due to gravity, generating friction between the skin and the bed, which opposes the direction of movement. This generates shear stresses in the tissue, with the deep tissue pulling downward as the superficial tissue pulls upward. Similar forces are generated when a person is repositioned without being completely lifted. A study conducted by Goldstein and Sanders (1998) showed that shear forces injure superficial tissue layers, and the onset of injury becomes more rapid as the shear forces increase. Repeated exposure to friction causes tearing of the skin, and is considered a factor in the etiology of superficial pressure ulcers (Dinsdale, 1973; Dinsdale, 1974). Tissue could also be subjected to torsional stress, however, this specific type of stress is not considered a cause for tissue injury in the pressure ulcer formation process.

7.2.3 OTHER FACTORS

Several other factors have been associated with the formation of pressure ulcers, such as incontinence, poor nutritional status, cardiovascular diseases, atrophied muscles, and the presence of scar tissue from previous pressure ulcers. Although these factors on their own do not generate a pressure ulcer, a person afflicted by any of them is at a higher risk of developing a pressure ulcer.

Incontinence typically arises as a complication from a SCI or as a result of aging. When present, incontinence increases the amount of moisture in the skin. Prolonged exposure to moisture can lead to maceration and breakdown of the skin. Several studies have associated the presence of incontinence with a higher risk of pressure ulcer development (Brandeis et al., 1994; Schnelle et al., 1997; Benoit and Watts, 2007). Besides providing excessive moisture, incontinence can also lead to skin breakdown because of its contents. Urine contains several metabolic waste products, in particular urea, which can lead to skin irritation due to its acidic nature. In addition, once an ulcer has developed, incontinence increases the risk of infection of the wound.

A poor nutritional status can affect a person's health in many forms, in addition to the risk of development of pressure ulcers. Individuals with nutritional deficits are more likely to develop a pressure ulcer and have lower healing rates once an ulcer has developed (Thomas, 1997; Mathus-Vliegen, 2004). In particular, lower levels of serum albumin have been associated with higher risks of developing pressure ulcers (Gengenbacher et al., 2002; Reed et al., 2003).

One effect of immobilization, especially after a SCI is the lack of muscle tone and atrophy of the muscles below the lesion level. Loss of muscle mass in the gluteal region leads to higher interface pressure levels around the ischial tuberosities, the location most at risk of developing pressure ulcers in wheelchair users.

People who have had a pressure ulcer are also at higher risk of developing a recurring ulcer, primarily due to scar formation and compromised tissue integrity after the ulcer has healed (Woolsey and McGarry, 1991). Deep scars act as promoters for pressure ulcer development because of their mismatched mechanical properties with the surrounding muscle; this subjects the surrounding tissue to heightened interfacial stresses, increasing the likelihood of ischemia and excessive mechanical deformation.

7.3 CLASSIFICATION OF PRESSURE ULCERS

Traditionally, pressure ulcer development had been considered to initiate at the level of the skin and progress to encompass the underlying fat, muscle, and bone tissue. Based on the progression of the lesion, pressure ulcers are classified according to a scale set forth by the NPUAP (Black et al., 2007). This scale was originally defined in 1989 and has been updated over the years as knowledge related to pressure ulcers advanced. These are the four stages in the scale (Figure 7.3):

Stage I: Redness or discoloration of intact skin compared to surrounding areas, usually over bony prominences. Changes in skin temperature and consistency may also be present.

Stage II: Shallow wound that may appear as an open blister or abrasion. Damage to the tissue is limited to the dermis and/or epidermis.

Stage III: Full thickness tissue loss appearing as a deep crater wound. Damage to the tissue involves the skin and subcutaneous fat, but not the muscle or bone.

Stage IV: Full thickness tissue loss appearing as a deep crater wound. Extensive damage to the skin and all underlying tissues, including the fat, muscle, and bone may be present.

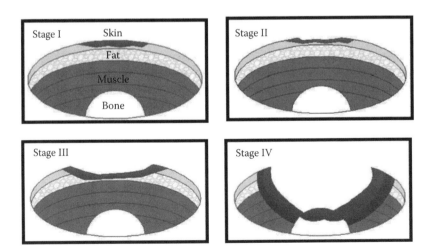

FIGURE 7.3 Classification of pressure ulcers.

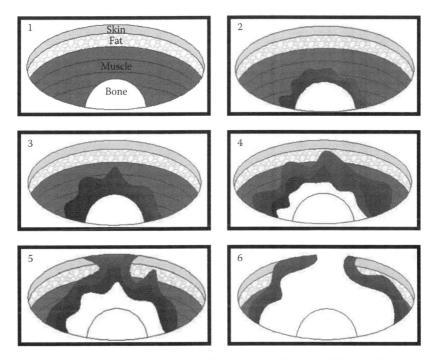

FIGURE 7.4   Progression of DTI from unaffected tissue (1) to stage IV ulcer (6).

Candidate factors for ulcers originating at the level of the skin are friction between skin and an external surface, tissue hygiene, moisture, increased temperature, circulatory integrity, and nutrition (Salcido et al., 1995).

The development of pressure ulcers can also initiate at deep bone–muscle interfaces, and progress toward the skin destroying the surrounding tissue (Daniel et al., 1981) (Figure 7.4). This type of ulcer would first appear as a bruise or purple lesion on the skin that would quickly deteriorate into a stage III or IV ulcer. Pressure ulcers with this etiology had not been formally considered as a type of pressure ulcer. It was not until 2001 when the NPUAP defined this type of pressure ulcer DTI, and created a task force to review the literature regarding this type of pressure ulcer etiology. Recently, the NPUAP has updated its pressure ulcer staging system to include DTI:

Deep tissue injury: Injury to the deep layers of tissue due to pressure and/or shear forces under intact skin. Indications of deep damage may appear as a purple discoloration of the skin, resembling a bruise. Tissue may also exhibit a different consistency compared to adjacent areas.

The leading factor for the formation of DTI is the entrapment and compression of tissue between a bony prominence and an external hard surface for extended periods of time (Guthrie and Goulian, 1973; Fennegan, 1983; Swarts et al., 1988; Woolsey and McGarry, 1991; Salcido et al., 1995).

Deep tissue injury is more perilous than surface ulcers as it is difficult to detect and can cause severe damage in bone, ligament, muscle, and fat prior to exhibiting obvious skin signs.

7.4   DETECTION OF DEEP PRESSURE ULCERS

7.4.1   Visual Inspection of the Skin

Pressure ulcer detection relies almost exclusively on the judgment of the nursing staff and attending physicians for individuals being cared for at a clinical institution. The most commonly used technique for detection of a pressure ulcer is frequent inspections of the skin to assess the presence of visible redness or ulcerations. The assessment is typically based on the visual appearance of the skin; however, it is recommended that the visual inspection be accompanied by palpation. Palpation is of particular importance in individuals with darkly pigmented skin, in whom the early changes in skin discoloration and nonblanchable erythema associated with the onset of a superficial pressure ulcer are harder to detect visually (Lyder, 1996; Lyder et al., 1998, 1999; Rosen et al., 2006; Black et al., 2007). A universal system for classifying detected pressure ulcers quantitatively does not exist. However, the most frequently used technique is composed of the four-stage scale set forth by the NPUAP in the United States. A similar four-grade scale developed by the European Pressure Ulcer Advisory Panel (EPUAP) is utilized in Europe (Black et al., 2007).

There are three main limitations associated with skin inspections and the NPUAP scale for pressure ulcer detection and classification: (1) The results are highly subjective and examiner dependent (Bergstrom, 1992; Garber et al., 1996). (2) Although the scale now recognizes the etiology of DTI as a type of pressure ulcer, by the time these deep ulcers exhibit skin signs, large volumes of bone, muscle, and fat would have already been destroyed. (3) Visual inspections are time-consuming and labor-intensive. In addition, measurement of the depth of ulcers for proper assessment of their stage, and description of wound characteristics such as amount of fluid discharge are not commonly performed (Lyder, 2003). These limitations can increase the chance of misclassification and inappropriate treatment of ulcers if no other system is utilized.

7.4.2   Risk Assessment Scales

In addition to frequent skin inspections, a widely used tool that helps not only in the detection of pressure ulcers but also in their prevention, is the use of risk assessment scales such as the Braden, Norton, and Waterlow scales. These scales try to classify individuals based on their risk of developing a pressure ulcer. Based on the assessed risk, resources can be better allocated to attend more carefully and frequently to those individuals at higher risk; this is of particular importance in centers with limited staff and resources dedicated to pressure ulcer detection and prevention. Of these three scales, the Braden scale offers the best validity and reliability and has been used in a larger number of studies compared to the Norton and Waterlow scales (Pancorbo-Hidalgo et al., 2006). The Braden scale evaluates a person's risk of developing a pressure ulcer using six different subscales. These subscales are (1) sensory perception, (2) activity level, (3) mobility, (4) nutrition status, (5) skin's exposure to moisture, and (6) skin's exposure to shear and friction forces. For subscales 1–5 a score ranging from 1 to 4 is given, and for the sixth subscale the score ranges from 1 to 3. Once a score has been given in each subscale, the scores are summed to give a final score that ranges from 6 to 23, with lower scores being associated with a higher risk of developing a pressure ulcer (Braden and Maklebust, 2005). Despite the fact that the score given to the individual in each subscale is still based on the judgment of the caregiver, the use of this scale has improved the prediction of those at risk of developing pressure ulcers (Pancorbo-Hidalgo et al., 2006). The frequency of each assessment varies depending on the individual's overall health and skin condition, as well as the institution's settings; however, it is recommended that it be performed on admission, at least every 48 h for patients in acute care units; on admission and then every 48 h during the first week, weekly for the first month, and then monthly or quarterly for patients in long-term care; and on admission and during every visit for patients in home care (Braden and Maklebust, 2005).

7.4.3 SUPERFICIAL PRESSURE MEASUREMENTS

Prolonged exposure to high loads has been considered the main cause behind the formation of pressure ulcers for a long time. Although there is debate regarding the main source of tissue injury in pressure ulcer formation (excessive mechanical deformation or ischemia), it is agreed that high pressure is the main cause for both processes. For this reason, superficial pressure measurements, which are measurements made at the surface–skin interface, have been a valuable tool in the study of pressure ulcers. By measuring superficial pressures, it is possible to predict which regions of the body are most at risk for developing a pressure ulcer. In 1961, Lindan performed a study that provided pressure measurements of a healthy adult male lying supine, prone, on his side, and seated (Lindan, 1961). Pressure measurements were made by having the person lie down or sit on a "bed" of inverted nails. Each nail was attached to a spring with a specific stiffness, so as the man's weight pressed down on the nails' heads, pressure was calculated by measuring the compression of the springs. In this manner, whole body pressure maps were obtained. Later studies utilized air-filled bladders connected to a pressure transducer to obtain superficial pressure measurements with the objective of comparing the effectiveness of different support surfaces and different sitting postures based on the reduction of pressure each surface and posture provide (Palmieri et al., 1980; Berjian et al., 1983; Rosenthal et al., 1996). As technological advances in electronic sensors took place, resistive and capacitive pressure sensors became common, making pressure-sensing systems more easily available. Commercially available pressure-sensing pads include XSENSOR (Calgary, AB, Canada, www.xsensor.com), TEKSCAN (Boston, MA, www.tekscan.com), FSA (the Netherlands, www.vistamedical.nl), and Novel (Munich, Germany, www.novel.de). Clinically, in addition to comparing support surfaces, the use of superficial pressure measurements has two more applications vital in the detection and prevention of pressure ulcers: (1) It allows the prescription of the best pressure relieving cushion or mattress and/or the best repositioning regime for each individual; (2) It provides an assessment of the risk of developing a pressure ulcer for each person, allowing physicians and nursing staff to focus their attention on the individuals most at risk of developing a pressure ulcer. Although very helpful, superficial pressure measurements have some limitations: (1) Superficial pressure measurements are dependent on the placement of the sensor, therefore, variation in the measurements will arise if the positioning of the person over the sensors is not exactly the same each time. (2) The use of different clothes and different support surfaces will generate pressure variations between sessions, especially if the resolution of the sensors is high. (3) Subject body shape and mass variability can make it difficult to generalize results and obtain statistically valid measurements between subjects, this can even become an issue within subjects if the body characteristics of the person change between measurements. (4) Numerical models studying the propagation of mechanical forces from the surface–skin interface to deeper layers of tissue, indicate that the superficial pressure measurements may not accurately predict the stresses and strains experienced by the deeper layers of tissue (Oomens et al., 2003; Linder-Ganz and Gefen, 2004). This could lead to an improper assessment of people at risk of developing a pressure ulcer based on superficial measurements.

7.4.4 OBJECTIVE METHODS OF PRESSURE ULCER DETECTION

While frequent skin inspections and the use of risk assessment scales are the norm for pressure ulcer detection, over the years, a series of techniques have been proposed to indicate the viability and status of soft tissues subjected to periods of loading, and have assisted in the early detection of pressure ulcers. Laser Doppler flowmetry has been utilized in several studies to measure changes in skin blood perfusion under loading conditions and its relationship to pressure ulcer formation (Ek et al., 1987; Frantz and Xakellis, 1989; Schubert and Fagrell, 1991; Schubert and Heraud, 1994; Colin and Saumet, 1996; Sachse et al., 1998); however, results have been mixed and with great degree of variability. Measurements of transcutaneous gas tensions (T_cPO_2 and T_cPCO_2) (Newson and Rolfe, 1982; Bader, 1990a,b; Colin and Saumet, 1996; Colin et al., 1996; Knight et al., 2001) have provided solid practical education for both patients and care givers (Bogie et al., 1992, 1995; Coggrave and Rose, 2003); however, use of transcutaneous gas tensions has yielded no clear relationship between gas levels of compromised tissue and the onset of progressive tissue breakdown that will ultimately result in a pressure ulcer (Bogie and Bader, 2005). Sweat analyses have also been proposed as indicators of increased risk of developing pressure ulcers (Ferguson-Pell and Hagisawa, 1988; Polliack et al., 1993, 1997; Taylor et al., 1994; Knight et al., 2001). When pressure is applied over a region of the body, sweat secretion in that region is reduced and the concentration of metabolites like lactate and urea is increased. After the removal of pressure, these levels return to normal. Although these results indicate that sweat analyses could present a viable technique for predicting the formation of pressure ulcers, to date they have not received widespread use. During the last decade, magnetic resonance imaging (MRI) has been utilized to assess the damage in deep tissue generated by the external loading of the muscles. MRI provides excellent soft tissue contrast as well as high spatial and temporal resolution of deep tissue (Hencey et al., 1996; Bosboom et al., 2001, 2003; Stekelenburg et al., 2006a,b; Solis et al., 2007; Stekelenburg et al., 2007). It allows for the assessment and quantification of changes in different muscle properties as a result of extended compression of the muscle (Linder-Ganz et al., 2007;

Stekelenburg et al., 2007). While the results indicate that MRI is capable of detecting early morphological and physiological changes that result from extended loading of the muscles, its current moderate availability and high cost have limited its use to experimental testing only.

Given the startling prevalence of pressure ulcers and the great difficulty and expense associated with their treatment, early detection methods of deep tissue damage and objective predictors of individuals at risk are notably lacking. In particular, quantitative methods for the early detection and assessment of DTI prior to their development into open wounds are needed.

7.5   TREATMENT OF PRESSURE ULCERS

Treating pressure ulcers is difficult, often requiring prolonged hospitalization (Grip and Merbitz, 1986). Once a pressure ulcer is detected, it is assessed by documenting its location, size, depth, and amount of exudates, and classified according to the NPUAP staging scale or an equivalent tool (Baranoski, 2006; Thomas, 2006). Once the assessment is complete, the first step for treating a pressure ulcer is the removal of the mechanical forces, namely pressure, shear, and friction, which contributed to its development. Complete relief of pressure from the affected tissue is necessary to allow proper healing of the ulcer and stop its progression. Although necessary, the removal of pressure can be an extremely taxing procedure on the affected individual, since the person is unable to lie down on the affected area. This can become even more difficult when ulcers are present in more than one part of the body. For individuals in wheelchairs in particular, whose mobility is already limited, this can compromise their ability to use the wheelchair as they risk applying pressure to the affected region.

The next step in the treatment process varies depending on the severity of the ulcer. After the removal of pressure, ulcers that do not require debridement can be managed by the application of a variety of local wound dressings. Maintaining an appropriate level of moisture in the wound has been associated with improved healing; toward this end, different types of moist dressings can be used. Moist wound healing dressings can be classified into (1) dressings that absorb exudate, such as alginates, hydrofibers, and foams; (2) dressings that maintain moisture, such as hydrocolloids and transparent films; and (3) dressings that donate moisture, such as hydrogels (Ovington, 2007). Dressings that provide an antimicrobial effect in addition to moisture control, such as silver containing dressings are also available (Ovington, 2007). While there are hundreds of different available dressings, there is no single treatment or dressing that can be universally applied to guarantee healing (Whitney et al., 2001), because the best dressing for each case is dictated by the wound conditions.

If the pressure ulcer already shows signs of necrosis, debridement of the necrotic tissue is recommended to allow proper healing. The debridement of the ulcer can be performed in several ways, such as (Baranoski, 2006) the following:

Surgical debridement: This type of debridement consists of cutting away unviable tissue to clean the wound. Depending on the severity of the ulcer, this can be performed at the bedside if only small amounts of tissue are involved, or in a surgical suite which is usually required in the case of stage IV pressure ulcers.

Mechanical debridement: Examples of this type of debridement include the use of wet-to-dry gauze dressings, whirlpool treatments, or wound irrigation treatments (pulsed lavage) to remove necrotic tissue by force. Of the three, pulsed lavage is the most commonly used method, consisting in the use of a handheld device (syringe) to apply saline solutions at safe pressure levels.

Autolytical debridement: While autolytical debridement takes longer than surgical debridement methods, it is relatively painless and easy to apply. The principle behind this method is to use the enzymes naturally present in the body to soften and breakdown the eschar and degrade the necrotic tissue. These enzymes are selective to necrotic tissue and spare viable tissue. To promote such autolysis, moisture-retaining dressings such as semiocclusive and occlusive (transparent films, hydrocolloids, and hydrogels) dressings are used, as they provide an enclosed space over the wound in which a proper moisture environment facilitates cell movement. This method however, is not appropriate for infected wounds.

Enzymatical debridement: This method utilizes proteolytical enzymes and is best suited for situations when surgical debridement is not possible. Even though this debridement process is slow, it can be utilized on infected wounds. Care must be taken because certain wound cleaners can deactivate the enzymes. While several enzymatical agents are commercially available, they require a prescription and are expensive, which limits their use.

Biological debridement: Maggot larvae are placed in the wound, where they break the necrotic tissue and ingest microorganisms. They help remove bacteria from the wound and promote healing.

Ultrasound-assisted debridement: Necrotic tissue is removed by applying ultrasonic energy through a saline fluid pressure wave.

After debridement is performed, the appropriate dressing is applied and periodical assessments of the wound are made to track its progression. The Pressure Sore Status Tool (PSST) and Pressure Ulcer Scale for Healing (PUSH) are the two most widely used instruments to assess and track the healing of a pressure ulcer. These tools provide a numeric indicator of different characteristics of the pressure ulcer, such as wound size and depth, tissue appearance and coloration, and amount of exudate present (Baranoski, 2006; Thomas, 2006).

Severe ulcers, in which bone, muscle, and skin become necrotic, are often dealt with surgically. Necrotic tissue is excised and a musculocutaneous flap is sometimes used to fill the void created by the excision (Lyder, 2003). The flaps provide wound closure and in some cases supply a sensory patch in an otherwise insensate region that is susceptible to sustained external pressures incurred while seated in a wheelchair. These surgical procedures are technically demanding, and complications involving irregularities in blood supply to the muscle or skin and potential damage to nerves providing sensory input to the flap are relatively high. High recurrence of ulcers following musculocutaneous flap surgeries has also been reported (Lyder, 2003).

Even though debridement and dressings are utilized to treat and heal a localized pressure ulcer, care is taken to ensure the overall health of the patient. Given that a pressure ulcer is a potential entry point for bacteria into the body, the risk of infection is always latent. Infection of the wound can hinder the healing of skin grafts and muscle flaps (Thomas, 2006). More dangerously, an infected wound can lead to bacteremia, which can be lethal, especially in individuals with already compromised health (Galpin et al., 1976; Bryan et al., 1983; Wall et al., 2003). Culture swabs are often obtained from the wound site to quantify the colonization of bacteria and determine its type. To prevent the spread of infection, prophylactic antibiotic treatment is administered as necessary, in particular when there are signs of systemic infection.

An alternative technique to facilitate wound closure, recommended in particular for stage III and IV ulcers with high amounts of exudate, is the use of vacuum-assisted closure (VAC) (Kaufman and Pahl, 2003; Smith, 2004). This technique consists of applying topical negative pressure to the wound surface to promote healing. To apply this technique, a porous foam dressing is placed directly over the wound surface and an adhesive dressing is placed over the foam, creating a contained environment. Negative pressure is achieved by inserting a tube attached to a vacuum pump into the foam dressing. The negative pressure cleans the wound, removing excessive exudate; it also promotes vasodilation, increasing blood flow and promoting granulation. Negative pressure also reduces bacterial colonization in the wound (Argenta and Morykwas, 1997; Morykwas et al., 1997). The use of VAC in the treatment of pressure ulcers induces faster healing rates and better wound closure when compared to hydrocolloid or alginate dressings (Smith, 2004).

Although not widely utilized in the treatment of pressure ulcers, the use of electrical stimulation has shown improved healing in chronic wounds and pressure ulcers (Griffin et al., 1991; Gardner et al., 1999; Reger et al., 1999; Bogie et al., 2000; Houghton et al., 2003; Allen and Houghton, 2004). There is no consensus about the exact mechanism by which electrical stimulation improves healing. Suggested mechanisms include a reduction in bacterial growth due to electrical stimulation (Rowley et al., 1974); facilitation of white cell movement into the wound (Petrofsky et al., 2005); promotion of angiogenesis (Zhao et al., 2004); and an increase in blood flow in the wound area (Petrofsky et al., 2005). The electrical stimulation modalities typically utilized to treat wounds are low-intensity direct current (LIDC), high-voltage pulsed current (HVPC), alternate current (AC), and microamperage electrical stimulation (MES).

A final step in the treatment of pressure ulcers is the monitoring and maintenance of a proper nutritional status of the person. In particular, higher intakes of vitamin C, zinc, and protein have been associated with improved healing (Breslow et al., 1993; Desneves et al., 2005; Lee et al., 2006). Vitamin C helps in the formation of connective tissue and scar formation. Zinc is a component of several enzymes and is required for several metabolic processes. Proteins (amino acids, peptides, polypeptides) are required for the formation of the wound healing matrix, as well as helping to stabilize the intracellular oncotic pressure (Zagoren, 2001).

Even after a pressure ulcer has fully healed, the possibility of recurring pressure ulcers is extremely high, in particular in wheelchair users, in whom Niazi et al. (1997) reported a pressure ulcer recurrence rate of 91%. This exemplifies the need to focus on preventing the initial onset of pressure ulcer formation in those persons at risk.

7.6 PREVENTION OF PRESSURE ULCERS

7.6.1 REPOSITIONING

Given that excessive pressure, shear forces, and friction applied to the tissue around bony prominences are the main cause for pressure ulcer development, prevention methods are aimed at eliminating or reducing these forces. The gold standard for pressure ulcer prevention is the frequent repositioning of the individual to allow periodical relief of pressure in areas at risk (i.e., sacrum, ischial tuberosities, trochanters). At locales where individuals at risk of developing pressure ulcers are under the care of health professionals, for example at hospitals and nursing homes, the staff of the institution plays a vital role in preventing the formation of pressure ulcers. Patients or residents in these institutions who are unable to leave their bed or move independently rely entirely on the institution staff to be repositioned. While there is no conclusive evidence of an ideal repositioning frequency (Thomas, 2001, 2006; Defloor et al., 2005; Vanderwee et al., 2007), traditionally the recommended repositioning time is every 2 h (Baranoski, 2006). This time, however, can vary for each individual, with some people requiring more frequent repositioning (Thomas, 2001, 2006; Baranoski, 2006). In practice, each institution establishes its own pressure ulcer prevention program (Catania et al., 2007; de Laat et al., 2007), with repositioning frequency being determined by the patient's condition, staff's availability, and costs associated with the repositioning (Xakellis et al., 2001; Baranoski, 2006; Thomas, 2006). During repositioning, utmost care is taken to avoid dragging the person against the support surface, thus reducing friction at the skin and shear at the bone–muscle interfaces. For inpatient populations, frequent skin inspections and pressure ulcer risk assessments are also performed by the staff in conjunction with the repositioning program to further reduce the incidence of pressure ulcers. For people confined to bed but living at home, the repositioning and inspections are dependent on the individuals themselves, a relative or a private caregiver.

Repositioning is not only required for individuals in bed, but also for wheelchair users, in particular for individuals with SCI. Frequent postural adjustments to relieve internal pressure when seated, emulating the constant subconscious adjustments performed by able-bodied individuals in reaction to discomfort, are a critical factor in the prevention of pressure ulcers. To this end, wheelchair users are encouraged to adjust their posture regularly. People with paraplegia are trained to perform wheelchair push-ups and those with quadriplegia are trained to perform side leans and front-to-back rocking to relieve ischial tuberosity pressure (Merbitz et al., 1985; Grip and Merbitz, 1986; White et al., 1989). However, for wheelchair users effective prevention through a regime of regular pressure relief is largely dependent on (1) individual compliance, (2) the ease with which the exercises can be performed, and (3) the effectiveness of these adjustments in producing adequate relief of internal pressure at the bone–muscle interface.

7.6.2 SPECIALIZED CUSHIONS AND MATTRESSES

A common and widely used method to aid in the prevention of pressure ulcers is the use of specialized wheelchair cushions, bed mattresses, and overlays to reduce the pressure at the interface between the skin and the chair/bed (Garber, 1979, 1985a,b; Marshall and Overstall, 1983; Ferguson-Pell et al., 1986). Although the use of these special surfaces does not eliminate the need for periodical repositioning, by reducing the interface pressures these devices may allow a person to remain in the same position for a longer period of time without compromising the integrity of the tissue. This is of particular importance for wheelchair users, who perform most of their daily activities sitting in the wheelchair, as well as for institutions where the staff available to aid in the repositioning is limited, and the time between repositions is longer than that usually recommended. Based on their operating mode, support surfaces can be divided into nonpowered and powered systems. Nonpowered systems provide a static redistribution of pressure while powered systems provide a dynamic redistribution of pressure.

7.6.2.1 Nonpowered Pressure Redistribution Surfaces

These surfaces do not require any source of power to function. They are designed to maximize the surface area in contact with the skin, thus reducing the pressure at the skin–surface interface. Also, their compliant surface allows regions of high pressure under bony prominences to sink into the surface, thus diffusing the pressure to surrounding areas (Woolsey and McGarry, 1991). Nonpowered support surfaces can be made of different components including, viscoelastic foams, elastic foams, closed cell foams, open cell foams, and elastomers. They can also be composed of cells or bladders filled with water, air, gel, and viscous fluids. The support surface can be made of any single type of component (Figure 7.5d) or a combination of different components (Figure 7.5c). Specialized wheelchair cushions are currently the only devices available for providing pressure relief while sitting, and are routinely prescribed by physical and occupational therapists.

Air-filled cushions are composed of multiple cells that are inflated to a desired air pressure (Figure 7.5a). The amount of pressure reduction provided by air-filled cushions can be affected by variables such as the size, shape, material, air capacity, and air pressure of the inflated cushion. In particular, the inflating pressure of the cushion has been studied and associated with the cushion's performance. Varying the inflating pressure can change the amount of pressure relief provided by the cushion. Pitfalls of this type of cushion include difficulties to adjust the inflating air pressure by the user and/or caregiver (Hamanami et al., 2004). In addition, if not enough air pressure is utilized to inflate the cushion, the user can "bottom out" in the cushion, eliminating any pressure relief.

Viscoelastic foam mattresses (Figure 7.5e) are made of heat-sensitive foam that allows them to mold to the contour of the body, providing a reduction in the interface pressures and a reduction of friction and shear forces (Beldon, 2002). In a study performed with patients in an acute care setting, the reported benefits of using this type of mattress were a reduction in the ward's pressure ulcer incidence from a range of 3.5% to 4% to less than 1%; however, no direct comparison was made against other pressure relieving systems (Beldon, 2002). Different studies have compared the use of standard hospital mattresses and cushions against mattresses and cushions made from viscoelastic foam in the same population. The results indicate that the use of the specialized support surfaces offers better pressure reduction (Hampton and Collins, 2005), and significantly reduces the incidence of blanchable erythema

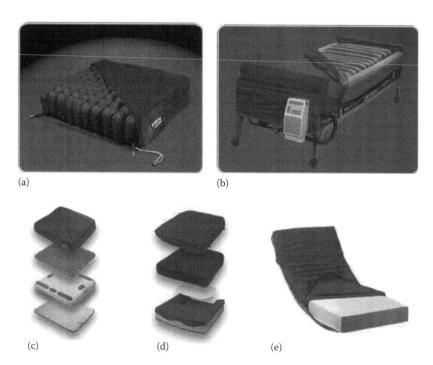

(a)   (b)

(c)   (d)   (e)

FIGURE 7.5 Different types of specialized support surfaces: (a) air-filled cushion, (b) alternating air pressure mattress, (c) gel/foam cushion, (d) foam cushion, and (e) viscoelastic foam mattress.

compared to standard devices; however, in the cases where blanchable erythema developed, the progression of the lesion seemed to be unaffected by the type of support surface utilized (Russell et al., 2003). When comfort was assessed, patients who utilized this type of mattresses found them more comfortable than their standard mattresses (Russell et al., 2003; Hampton and Collins, 2005), or other systems such as the alternating pressure air mattresses (Beldon, 2002; Russell et al., 2003).

7.6.2.2   Powered Pressure Redistribution Surfaces

This type of support surface requires an external source of power to function, whether in the form of batteries or an AC plug. They are capable of providing a dynamic redistribution of pressure, wherein air or water is actively pumped so that the pressure within the supporting surface is continuously changing.

Alternating pressure air systems include cushions, mattresses (Figure 7.5b), and overlays. This type of system is made of air-filled cells through which air is pumped to maintain an alternating interface pressure (Gray, 1999). Some systems are equipped with a liquid crystal display through which adjustments to the alternating cycle can be made. In addition, they can also be equipped with audio alarms in case of electrical or pressure failure (Gray, 1999). Other alternating pressure air systems use variable density foam within the air cells; this makes the flow of air through the cells more subtle, and reduces the unpleasant sensations that some alternating pressure air systems can generate (Gray, 1999).

Some drawbacks of alternating air pressure mattresses include (1) generating a sensation of "seasickness" in some people; (2) they are noisy, which makes sleeping more difficult; and (3) they can be easily damaged (Beldon, 2002). Because the operation of powered wheelchair pressure reduction devices is dependent on compressors and power supplies, these systems can limit the person's mobility and in turn, the users' level of activity (Conine et al., 1989). Reclining and "tilt-in-space" wheelchairs are also available for periodical relief of pressure (Burns and Betz, 1999; Cooper et al., 2000). These types of wheelchairs are designed for individuals who do not have enough upper body strength to perform the recommended periodical wheelchair push-ups and side leans for pressure relief (Burns and Betz, 1999). The wheelchairs are equipped with a motor that tilts the backrest to different angles. The change in inclination shifts the weight bearing of the body from the ischial tuberosities to the sacrum and the back, thus redistributing the pressure with each setting (Burns and Betz, 1999). Drawbacks of this type of chair include the risk of generating shear forces (Cooper et al., 2000), malpositioning for some individuals (Burns and Betz, 1999; Cooper et al., 2000), high cost, and larger size than regular wheelchairs, which limits the accessibility and transportation of the wheelchair (Burns and Betz, 1999).

7.6.3 Alternative Pressure Relieve Systems

Given the importance of preventing the onset of pressure ulcers, continuous investigations into the improvement of standard prevention techniques are conducted, and focus on the development of new support surfaces as well as optimizing existing procedures for pressure ulcer prevention. An alternative prevention technique that has been studied irregularly for the past 15 years is the use of electrical stimulation. While the results of treating developed ulcers with electrical stimulation have been positive, its effectiveness in preventing the development of new ulcers remains unclear. Levine et al. (1989, 1990a,b) first proposed the use of electrical stimulation for preventing the formation of pressure ulcers in people with SCI. Their studies indicated that electrical stimulation generates changes in muscle shape (Levine et al., 1990a), redistribution of pressure at the seating interface (Levine et al., 1989), and increases in blood flow (Levine et al., 1990b). Studies by Bogie et al. (2000), and Rischbieth et al. (1998) indicated that frequent use of electrical stimulation increases muscle mass, which could allow wheelchair users to remain seated for longer periods of time. Increases in transcutaneous oxygen levels have also been reported in a long-term study with a single subject (Bogie et al., 2006). While these studies have focused on the application of electrical stimulation through the use of surface electrodes, placed directly over the skin of the target muscle, electrical stimulation through implanted electrodes has shown similar results (Bogie and Triolo, 2003; Liu et al., 2006a,b). These studies indicated that the benefits obtained through the daily use of an electrical stimulation system (increased blood flow and larger muscle mass) could lead to the prevention of pressure ulcers.

A recent study by Solis et al. (2007) directly investigated the effects of applying intermittent electrical stimulation during periods of increased pressure on the extent of DTI. Their results demonstrated that the volume of DTI is significantly reduced when the muscles are intermittently stimulated during the loading period compared to cases when the muscles were loaded but not stimulated. Intermittent electrical stimulation evoked periodical readjustments of posture that redistributed pressure and increased tissue oxygenation levels, mimicking the effects of voluntary repositioning in able-bodied individuals. Although these results indicate that intermittent electrical stimulation could become a valuable technique for the prevention of pressure ulcers, its testing to date has been limited to animal experimentation and a small number of human volunteers.

7.7   CONCLUSION

Pressure ulcers are a major medical complication associated with prolonged immobilization, affecting individuals who are confined to a bed or dependent on a wheelchair. Once a pressure ulcer develops, its treatment is expensive and can last from several weeks to several months, and requiring surgical interventions in severe cases. Developed ulcers not only greatly affect the quality of life of people affected by them but also can put their overall health at risk, as ulcers tend to develop in individuals who already have a compromised health condition. One of the major difficulties when dealing with pressure ulcers is the inability of current detection techniques to identify DTI promptly. The recent official recognition of DTI as a type of pressure ulcer provides caregivers with a standardized definition for this type of ulcer, which should be considered during the assessments and detection programs at each institution. However, the fact remains that DTI can injure large amounts of tissue before manifesting itself on the skin. It is necessary that more research be dedicated to find new cost-effective methods to detect DTI in its early stages of development, as well as methods to more objectively assess developed ulcers, and predict a person's risk of developing an ulcer.

Of equal importance is the need for more effective methods to prevent the formation of pressure ulcers. Every person at risk of developing a pressure ulcer should be provided with an appropriate pressure redistribution support surface in conjunction with a repositioning program. Many types of support surfaces are currently available and each has its advantages and disadvantages. Nonetheless, an appropriate cushion can be selected for each individual. Undoubtedly, without the use of these specialized surfaces, the incidence rates of pressure ulcers would be significantly higher, especially in institutions where nursing staff is limited, and among wheelchair users.

Better pressure ulcer prevention methods are still needed. Development of new pressure redistribution surfaces that can provide maximal pressure relief around high-risk regions is needed. Emphasis should also be placed on reducing the cost of these surfaces and improving their ease of use to encourage a wider spread of their use. New technologies, such as electrical stimulation systems, which could be utilized alone or in conjunction with existing support surfaces, warrant further research.

REFERENCES

Allen J and Houghton PE. Electrical stimulation: A case study for a stage iii pressure ulcer. *Wound Care Canada* 2: 34–36, 2004.
Appell HJ, Glöser S, Soares JMC, and Duarte JA. Structural alterations of skeletal muscle induced by ischemia and reperfusion. *Basic Applied Myology* 9: 263–268, 1999.

Argenta LC and Morykwas MJ. Vacuum-assisted closure: A new method for wound control and treatment: Clinical experience. *Annals of Plastic Surgery* 38: 563–576, 1997.

Ariëns GA, Bongers PM, Douwes M, Miedema MC, Hoogendoorn WE, van der Wal G, Bouter LM, and van Mechelen W. Are neck flexion, neck rotation, and sitting at work risk factors for neck pain? Results of a prospective cohort study. *Occupational and Environmental Medicine* 58: 200–207, 2001.

Aronovitch SA. Intraoperatively acquired pressure ulcers: Are there common risk factors? *Ostomy Wound Management* 53: 57–69, 2007.

Auvinen J, Tammelin T, Taimela S, Zitting P, and Karppinen J. Neck and shoulder pains in relation to physical activity and sedentary activities in adolescence. *Spine* 32: 1038–1044, 2007.

Bader DL. Effects of compressive load regimens on tissue viability. In: *Pressure Sores— Clinical Practice and Scientific Approach*, ed. Bader DL. Basingstoke: Macmillan Press, 1990a, pp. 191–201.

Bader DL. The recovery characteristics of soft tissues following repeated loading. *Journal of Rehabilitation Research and Development* 27: 141–150, 1990b.

Baranoski S. Raising awareness of pressure ulcer prevention and treatment. *Advances in Skin & Wound Care* 19: 398–405, 2006.

Beldon P. Transfoam Visco: Evaluation of a viscoelastic foam mattress. *British Journal of Nursing* 11: 651–655, 2002.

Bennett G, Dealey C, and Posnett J. The cost of pressure ulcers in the UK. *Age and Ageing* 33: 230–235, 2004.

Benoit RA and Watts C. The effect of a pressure ulcer prevention program and the bowel management system in reducing pressure ulcer prevalence in an ICU setting. *The Journal of Wound, Ostomy, and Continence Nursing* 34: 163–175, 2007.

Bergstrom N. A research agenda for pressure ulcer prevention. *Decubitus* 5: 22–24, 1992.

Berjian RA, Douglass HOJ, Holyoke ED, Goodwin PM, and Priore RL. Skin pressure measurements on various mattress surfaces in cancer patients. *American Journal of Physical Medicine* 62: 217–226, 1983.

Black J, Baharestani MM, Cuddigan J, Dorner B, Edsberg L, Langemo D, Posthauer ME, Ratliff C, Taler G, and (NPUAP). TNPUAP. National Pressure Ulcer Advisory Panel's updated pressure ulcer staging system. *Advances in Skin & Wound Care* 20: 269–274, 2007.

Bogie K and Bader D. Susceptibilitiy of spinal cord-injured individuals to pressure ulcers. In: *Pressure Ulcer Research: Current and Future Perspectives*, eds. Bader D, Bouten C, Colin D, and Oomens C. Heidelberg: Springer-Verlag, 2005, pp. 73–88.

Bogie KM, Nuseibeh I, and Bader DL. Early progressive changes in tissue viability in the seated spinal cord injured subject. *Paraplegia* 33: 141–147, 1995.

Bogie KM, Nuseibeh I, and Bader DL. Transcutaneous gas tensions in the sacrum during the acute phase of spinal cord injury. *Proceedings of the Institution of Mechanical Engineers Part H Journal of Engineering in Medicine* 206: 1–6, 1992.

Bogie KM, Reger SI, Levine SP, and Sahgal V. Electrical stimulation for pressure sore prevention and wound healing. *Assistive Technology* 12: 50–66, 2000.

Bogie KM and Triolo RJ. Effects of regular use of neuromuscular electrical stimulation on tissue health. *Journal of Rehabilitation Research and Development* 40: 469–475, 2003.

Bogie KM, Wang X, and Triolo RJ. Long-term prevention of pressure ulcers in high-risk patients: A single case study of the use of gluteal neuromuscular electric stimulation. *Archives of Physical Medicine and Rehabilitation* 87: 585–591, 2006.

Bosboom EMH, Bouten CV, Oomens CW, Baaijens FP, and Nicolay K. Quantifying pressure sore-related muscle damage using high-resolution MRI. *Journal of Applied Physiology* 95: 2235–2240, 2003.

Bosboom EMH, Bouten CV, Oomens CW, van Straaten HWM, Baaijens FP, and Kuipers H. Quantification and localization of damage in rat muscles after controlled loading; a new approach to study the etiology of pressure sores. *Medical Engineering & Physics* 23: 195–200, 2001.

Bouten CV, Knight MM, Lee DA, and Bader DL. Compressive deformation and damage of muscle cell subpopulations in a model system. *Annals of Biomedical Engineering* 29: 153–163, 2001.

Bouten CV, Oomens CW, Baaijens FP, and Bader DL. The etiology of pressure ulcers: Skin deep or muscle bound? *Archives of Physical Medicine and Rehabilitation* 84: 616–619, 2003.

Braden BJ and Maklebust J. Preventing pressure ulcers with the Braden scale: An update on this easy-to-use tool that assesses a patient's risk. *American Journal of Nursing* 105: 70–72, 2005.

Brandeis GH, Morris JN, Nash DJ, and Lipsitz LA. The epidemiology and natural history of pressure ulcers in elderly nursing home residents. *JAMA* 264: 2905–2909, 1990.

Brandeis GH, Ooi WL, Hossain M, Morris JN, and Lipsitz LA. A longitudinal study of risk factors associated with the formation of pressure ulcers in nursing homes. *Journal of the American Geriatrics Society* 42: 388–393, 1994.

Breslow RA, Hallfrisch J, Guy DG, Crawley B, and Goldberg AP. The importance of dietary protein in healing pressure ulcers. *Journal of the American Geriatrics Society* 41: 357–362, 1993.

Breuls RG, Bouten CV, Oomens CW, Bader DL, and Baaijens FP. Compression induced cell damage in engineered muscle tissue: An in vitro model to study pressure ulcer aetiology. *Annals of Biomedical Engineering* 31: 1357–1364, 2003a.

Breuls RGM, Bouten CV, Oomens CW, Bader DL, and Baaijens FP. A theoretical analysis of damage evolution in skeletal muscle tissue with reference to pressure ulcer development. *Journal of Biomedical Engineering* 125: 902–909, 2003b.

Bryan CS, Dew CE, and Reynolds KL. Bacteremia associated with decubitus ulcers. *Archives of Internal Medicine* 143: 2093–2095, 1983.

Burns SP and Betz KL. Seating pressures with conventional and dynamic wheelchair cushions in tetraplegia. *Archives of Physical Medicine and Rehabilitation* 80: 566–571, 1999.

Cagnie B, Danneels L, Van Tiggelen D, De Loose V, and Cambier D. Individual and work related risk factors for neck pain among office workers: A cross sectional study. *European Spine Journal* 16: 679–686, 2007.

Catania K, Huang C, James P, Madison M, Moran M, and Ohr M. PUPP: The Pressure Ulcer Prevention Protocol interventions. *The American Journal of Nursing* 107: 44–52, 2007.

Coggrave MJ and Rose LS. A specialist seating assessment clinic: Changing pressure relief practice. *Spinal Cord* 41: 692–695, 2003.

Colin D, Loyant R, Abraham P, and Saumet JL. Changes in sacral transcutaneous oxygen tension in the evaluation of different mattresses in the prevention of pressure ulcers. *Advances in Wound Care* 9: 25–28, 1996.

Colin D and Saumet JL. Influence of external pressure on transcutaneous oxygen tension and laser Doppler flowmetry on sacral skin. *Clinical Physiology* 16: 61–72, 1996.

Conine TA, Choi AK, and Lim R. The user-friendliness of protective support surfaces in prevention of pressure sores. *Rehabilitation Nursing* 14: 261–263, 1989.

Cooper RA, Dvorznak MJ, Rentschler AJ, and Boninger ML. Displacement between the seating surface and hybrid test dummy during transitions with a variable configuration wheelchair: A technical note. *Journal of Rehabilitation Research and Development* 37: 297–303, 2000.

Curley MA, Quigley SM, and Lin M. Pressure ulcers in pediatric intensive care: Incidence and associated factors. *Pediatric Critical Care Medicine* 4: 284–290, 2003.

Daniel RK, Priest DL, and Wheatley DC. Etiologic factors in pressure sores: An experimental model. *Archives of Physical Medicine and Rehabilitation* 62: 492–498, 1981.

de Laat EH, Pickkers P, Schoonhoven L, Verbeek AL, Feuth T, and van Achterberg T. Guideline implementation results in a decrease of pressure ulcer incidence in critically ill patients. *Critical Care Medicine* 35: 815–820, 2007.

Defloor T, De Bacquer D, and Grypdonck MH. The effect of various combinations of turning and pressure reducing devices on the incidence of pressure ulcers. *International Journal of Nursing Studies* 42: 37–46, 2005.

Desneves KJ, Todorovic BE, Cassar A, and Crowe TC. Treatment with supplementary arginine, vitamin C and zinc in patients with pressure ulcers: A randomised controlled trial. *Clinical Nutrition* 24: 979–987, 2005.

Dinsdale SM. Decubitus ulcers in swine: Light and electron microscopy study of pathogenesis. *Archives of Physical Medicine and Rehabilitation* 54: 51–56, 1973.

Dinsdale SM. Decubitus ulcers: Role of pressure and friction in causation. *Archives of Physical Medicine and Rehabilitation* 55: 147–152, 1974.

Drummond DS, Narechania RG, Rosenthal AN, Breed AL, Lange TA, and Drummond DK. A study of pressure distributions measured during balanced and unbalanced sitting. *Journal of Bone and Joint Surgery* 64: 1034–1039, 1982.

Edlich RF, Winters KL, Woodard CR, Buschbacher RM, Long WB, Gebhart JH, and Ma EK. Pressure ulcer prevention. *Journal of Long-term Effects of Medical Implants* 14: 285–304, 2004.

Ek AC, Gustavsson G, and Lewis DH. Skin blood flow in relation to external pressure and temperature in the supine position on a standard hospital mattress. *Scandinavian Journal of Rehabilitation Medicine* 19: 121–126, 1987.

Fennegan D. Positive living or negative existence? *Nursing Times* 15: 51–54, 1983.

Ferguson-Pell M, Cochran GVB, Palmieri VR, and Brunski JB. Development of a modular wheelchair cushion for spinal cord injured persons. *Journal of Rehabilitation Research and Development* 23: 63–76, 1986.

Ferguson-Pell M and Hagisawa S. Biochemical changes in sweat following prolonged ischemia. *Journal of Rehabilitation Research and Development* 25: 57–62, 1988.

Ferguson-Pell MW. Design criteria for the measurement of pressure at body support interfaces. *Engineering in Medicine* 9: 209–214, 1980.

Finestone HM, Levine SP, Carlson GA, Chizinsky KA, and Kett RL. Erythema and skin temperature following continuous sitting in spinal cord injured individuals. *Journal of Rehabilitation Research and Development* 28: 27–32, 1991.

Frantz RA and Xakellis GC. Characteristics of skin blood flow over the trochanter under constant, prolonged pressure. *American Journal of Physical Medicine & Rehabilitation* 68: 272–276, 1989.

Galpin JE, Chow AW, Bayer AS, and Guze LB. Sepsis associated with decubitus ulcers. *American Journal of Medicine* 61: 346–350, 1976.

Garber SL. A classification of wheelchair seating. *American Journal of Occupational Therapy* 33: 652–654, 1979.

Garber SL. Wheelchair cushions for spinal cord-injured individuals. *American Journal of Occupational Therapy* 39: 722–725, 1985a.

Garber SL. Wheelchair cushions: A historical review. *American Journal of Occupational Therapy* 39: 453–459, 1985b.

Garber SL and Rintala DH. Pressure ulcers in veterans with spinal cord injury: A retrospective study. *Journal of Rehabilitation Research and Development* 40: 433–441, 2003.

Garber SL, Rintala DH, Rossi CD, Hart KA, and Fuhrer MJ. Reported pressure ulcer prevention and management techniques by persons with spinal cord injury. *Archives of Physical Medicine and Rehabilitation* 77: 744–749, 1996.

Gardner SE, Frantz RA, and Schmidt FL. Effect of electrical stimulation on chronic wound healing: A meta-analysis. *Wound Repair and Regeneration* 7: 495–503, 1999.

Gengenbacher M, Stähelin HB, Scholer A, and Seiler WO. Low biochemical nutritional parameters in acutely ill hospitalized elderly patients with and without stage III to IV pressure ulcers. *Aging Clinical and Experimental Research* 14: 420–423, 2002.

Gilsdorf P, Patterson R, and Fisher S. Thirty-minute continuous sitting force measurements with different support surfaces in the spinal cord injured and able-bodied. *Journal of Rehabilitation Research and Development* 28: 33–38, 1991.

Goldstein B and Sanders J. Skin response to repetitive mechanical stress: A new experimental model in pig. *Archives of Physical Medicine and Rehabilitation* 79: 265–272, 1998.

Grace PA. Ischaemia-reperfusion injury. *British Journal of Surgery* 81: 637–647, 1994.

Gray D. Pressure ulcer prevention and treatment: The transair range. *British Journal of Nursing* 8: 454–458, 1999.

Griffin JW, Tooms RE, Mendius RA, Clifft JK, Vander Zwaag R, and el-Zeky F. Efficacy of high voltage pulsed current for healing of pressure ulcers in patients with spinal cord injury. *Physical Therapy* 71: 433–442, 1991.

Grip JC and Merbitz CT. Wheelchair-based mobile measurement of behavior for pressure sore prevention. *Computer Methods and Programs in Biomedicine* 22: 137–144, 1986.

Gute DC, Ishida T, Yarimizu K, and Korthuis RJ. Inflammatory responses to ischemia and reperfusion in skeletal muscle. *Molecular and Cellular Biochemistry* 179: 169–187, 1998.

Guthrie RH and Goulian D. Decubitus ulcers: Prevention and treatment. *Geriatrics* 28: 67–71, 1973.

Hamanami K, Tokuhiro A, and Inoue H. Finding the optimal setting of inflated air pressure for a multi-cell air cushion for wheelchair patients with spinal cord injury. *Acta Medica Okayama* 58: 37–44, 2004.

Hampton S and Collins F. Reducing pressure ulcer incidence in a long-term setting. *British Journal of Nursing* 14: S6–S12, 2005.

Hencey JY, Vermess M, van Geertruyden HH, Binard JE, and Manchepalli S. Magnetic resonance imaging examinations of gluteal decubitus ulcers in spinal cord injury patients. *Journal of Spinal Cord Medicine* 19: 5–8, 1996.

Houghton PE, Kincaid CB, Lovell M, Campbell KE, Keast DH, Woodbury MG, and Harris KA. Effect of electrical stimulation on chronic leg ulcer size and appearance. *Physical Therapy* 83: 17–28, 2003.

Johanning E. Evaluation and management of occupational low back disorders. *American Journal of Industrial Medicine* 37: 94–111, 2000.

Kabaroudis A, Gerassimidis T, Karamanos D, Papaziogas B, Antonopoulos V, and Sakantamis A. Metabolic alterations of skeletal muscle tissue after prolonged acute ischemia and reperfusion. *Journal of Investigative Surgery* 16: 219–228, 2003.

Kaufman MW and Pahl DW. Vacuum-assisted closure therapy: Wound care and nursing implications. *Dermatology Nursing* 15: 317–320, 323–325, 2003.

Knight SL, Taylor RP, Polliack AA, and Bader DL. Establishing predictive indicators for the status of loaded soft tissues. *Journal of Applied Physiology* 90: 2231–2237, 2001.

Kosiak M. Etiology and pathology of ischemic ulcers. *Archives of Physical Medicine and Rehabilitation* 40: 62–69, 1959.

Kosiak M. Etiology of decubitus ulcers. *Archives of Physical Medicine and Rehabilitation* 42: 19–29, 1961.

Kosiak M, Kubicek WG, Olson M, Danz JN, and Kottke FJ. Evaluation of pressure as factor in production of ischial ulcers. *Archives of Physical Medicine and Rehabilitation* 39: 623–629, 1958.

Krismer M, van Tulder M, and Project. TLBPGotBaJHSfE. Strategies for prevention and management of musculoskeletal conditions. Low back pain (non-specific). *Best Practices and Research Clinical Rheumatology* 21: 77–91, 2007.

Krouskop TA, Noble PC, Garber SL, and Spencer WA. The effectiveness of preventive management in reducing the occurrence of pressure sores. *Journal of Rehabilitation Research and Development* 20: 74–83, 1983.

Kvarnstrom S. Occurrence of musculoskeletal, disorders in a manufacturing industry with special attention to occupational shoulder disorders. *Scandinavian Journal of Rehabilitation Medicine Supplement* 8: 1–114, 1983.

Labbe R, Lindsay T, and Walker PM. The extent and distribution of skeletal muscle necrosis after graded periods of complete ischemia. *Journal of Vascular Surgery* 6: 152–157, 1987.

Lee SK, Posthauer ME, Dorner B, Redovian V, and Maloney MJ. Pressure ulcer healing with a concentrated, fortified, collagen protein hydrolysate supplement: A randomized controlled trial. *Advances in Skin & Wound Care* 19: 92–96, 2006.

Levine SP, Kett RL, Cederna PS, Bowers LD, and Brooks SV. Electrical muscle stimulation for pressure variation at the seating interface. *Journal of Rehabilitation Research and Development* 26: 1–8, 1989.

Levine SP, Kett RL, Cederna PS, and Brooks SV. Electric muscle stimulation for pressure sore prevention: Tissue shape variation. *Archives of Physical Medicine and Rehabilitation* 71: 210–215, 1990a.

Levine SP, Kett RL, Gross MD, Wilson BA, Cederna PS, and Juni JE. Blood flow in the gluteus maximus of seated individuals during electrical muscle stimulation. *Archives of Physical Medicine and Rehabilitation* 71: 682–686, 1990b.

Lindan O. Etiology of decubitus ulcers: An experimental study. *Archives of Physical Medicine and Rehabilitation* 42: 774–783, 1961.

Linder-Ganz E, Engelberg S, Scheinowitz M, and Gefen A. Pressure-time cell death threshold for albino rat skeletal muscles as related to pressure sore biomechanics. *Journal of Biomechanics* 39: 2725–2732, 2006.

Linder-Ganz E and Gefen A. Mechanical compression-induced pressure sores in rat hindlimb: Muscle stiffness, histology, and computational models. *Journal of Applied Physiology* 96: 2034–2049, 2004.

Linder-Ganz E, Shabshin N, Itzchak Y, and Gefen A. Assessment of mechanical conditions in sub-dermal tissues during sitting: A combined experimental-MRI and finite element approach. *Journal of Biomechanics*, 40(7):1443–1454, 2007.

Liu LQ, Nicholson GP, Knight SL, Chelvarajah R, Gall A, Middleton FR, Ferguson-Pell MW, and Craggs MD. Interface pressure and cutaneous hemoglobin and oxygenation changes under ischial tuberosities during sacral nerve root stimulation in spinal cord injury. *Journal of Rehabilitation Research and Development* 43: 553–564, 2006a.

Liu LQ, Nicholson GP, Knight SL, Chelvarajah R, Gall A, Middleton FR, Ferguson-Pell MW, and Craggs MD. Pressure changes under the ischial tuberosities of seated individuals during sacral nerve root stimulation. *Journal of Rehabilitation Research and Development* 43: 209–218, 2006b.

Liu MH, Grimm DR, Teodorescu V, Kronowitz SJ, and Bauman WA. Transcutaneous oxygen tension in subjects with tetraplegia with and without pressure ulcers: A preliminary report. *Journal of Rehabilitation Research and Development* 36: 202–206, 1999.

Lyder CH. Examining the inclusion of ethnic minorities in pressure ulcer prediction studies. *Journal of Wound, Ostomy, and Continence Nursing* 23: 257–260, 1996.

Lyder CH. Pressure ulcer prevention and management. *Journal of the American Medical Association* 289: 223–226, 2003.

Lyder CH, Yu C, Emerling J, Mangat R, Stevenson D, Empleo-Frazier O, and McKay J. The Braden Scale for pressure ulcer risk: Evaluating the predictive validity in Black and Latino/Hispanic elders. *Applied Nursing Research* 12: 60–68, 1999.

Lyder CH, Yu C, Stevenson D, Mangat R, Empleo-Frazier O, Emerling J, and McKay J. Validating the Braden Scale for the prediction of pressure ulcer risk in blacks and Latino/Hispanic elders: A pilot study. *Ostomy Wound Management* 44: 42S–49S; discussion 50S, 1998.

Marshall M and Overstall P. Pressure sores, 2. Mattresses to prevent pressure sores. *Nursing Times* 79: 54, 56, 57, 1983.

Mathus-Vliegen EM. Old age, malnutrition, and pressure sores: An ill-fated alliance. *The Journals of Gerontology Series A Biological Sciences and Medical Sciences* 59: 355–360, 2004.

Merbitz CT, King RB, Bleiberg J, and Grip JC. Wheelchair push-ups: Measuring pressure relief frequency. *Archives of Physical Medicine and Rehabilitation* 66: 433–438, 1985.

Morken T, Riise T, Moen B, Hauge SH, Holien S, Langedrag A, Pedersen S, Saue IL, Seljebo GM, and Thoppil V. Low back pain and widespread pain predict sickness absence among industrial workers. *BMC Musculoskeletal Disorders* 4: 1–8, 2003.

Morykwas MJ, Argenta LC, Shelton-Brown EI, and McGuirt W. Vacuum-assisted closure: A new method for wound control and treatment: Animal studies and basic foundation. *Annals of Plastic Surgery* 38: 553–562, 1997.

Newson TP and Rolfe P. Skin surface PO_2 and blood flow measurements over the ischial tuberosity. *Archives of Physical Medicine and Rehabilitation* 63: 553–556, 1982.

Niazi ZB, Salzberg CA, Byrne DW, and Viehbeck M. Recurrence of initial pressure ulcer in persons with spinal cord injuries. *Advances in Wound Care* 10: 38–42, 1997.

Oomens CW, Bressers OF, Bosboom EM, Bouten CV, and Blader DL. Can loaded interface characteristics influence strain distributions in muscle adjacent to bony prominences? *Computer Methods in Biomechanics and Biomedical Engineering* 6: 171–180, 2003.

Ovington LG. Advances in wound dressings. *Clinics in Dermatology* 25: 33–38, 2007.

Palmieri VR, Haelen GT, and Cochran GV. A comparison of sitting pressures on wheelchair cushions as measured by air cell transducers and miniature electronic transducers. *Bulletin of Prosthetics Research* (Spring): 5–8, 1980.

Pancorbo-Hidalgo PL, Garcia-Fernandez FP, Lopez-Medina IM, and Alvarez-Nieto C. Risk assessment scales for pressure ulcer prevention: A systematic review. *Journal of Advanced Nursing* 54: 94–110, 2006.

Panel NPUA. Pressure ulcers in America: Prevalence, incidence, and implications for the future. An executive summary of the National Pressure Ulcer Advisory Panel monograph. *Advances in Skin & Wound Care* 14: 208–215, 2001.

Peeters EA, Bouten CV, Oomens CW, and Baaijens FP. Monitoring the biomechanical response of individual cells under compression: A new compression device. *Medical & Biological Engineering & Computing* 41: 498–503, 2003.

Peirce SM, Skalak TC, and Rodeheaver GT. Ischemia-reperfusion injury in chronic pressure ulcer formation: A skin model in the rat. *Wound Repair and Regeneration* 8: 68–76, 2000.

Petrofsky J, Schwab E, Lo T, Cúneo M, George J, Kim J, and Al-Malty A. Effects of electrical stimulation on skin blood flow in controls and in and around stage III and IV wounds in hairy and non hairy skin. *Medical Science Monitor* 11: CR309–CR316, 2005.

Polliack A, Taylor R, and Bader D. Analysis of sweat during soft tissue breakdown following pressure ischaemia. *Journal of Rehabilitation Research and Development* 30: 250–259, 1993.

Polliack A, Taylor R, and Bader D. Sweat analysis following pressure ischaemia in a group of debilitated subjects. *Journal of Rehabilitation Research and Development* 34: 303–308, 1997.

Porter JM and Gyi DE. The prevalence of musculoskeletal troubles among car drivers. *Occupational Medicine* 52: 4–12, 2002.

Redelings MD, Lee NE, and Sorvillo F. Pressure ulcers: More lethal than we thought? *Advances in Skin & Wound Care* 18: 367–372, 2005.

Reed RL, Hepburn K, Adelson R, Center B, and McKnight P. Low serum albumin levels, confusion, and fecal incontinence: Are these risk factors for pressure ulcers in mobility-impaired hospitalized adults? *Gerontology* 49: 255–259, 2003.

Reger SI, Hyodo A, Negami S, Kambic HE, and Sahgal V. Experimental wound healing with electrical stimulation. *Artificial Organs* 23: 460–462, 1999.

Richardson RR and Meyer PR Jr. Prevalence and incidence of pressure sores in acute spinal cord injuries. *Paraplegia* 19: 235–247, 1981.

Rischbieth H, Jelbart M, and Marshall R. Neuromuscular electrical stimulation keeps a tetraplegic subject in his chair: A case study. *Spinal Cord* 36: 443–445, 1998.

Robb MJ and Mansfield NJ. Self-reported musculoskeletal problems amongst professional truck drivers. *Ergonomics* 50: 814–827, 2007.

Rosen J, Mittal V, Degenholtz H, Castle N, Mulsant BH, Nace D, and Rubin FH. Pressure ulcer prevention in black and white nursing home residents: A QI initiative of enhanced ability, incentives, and management feedback. *Advances in Skin & Wound Care* 19: 262–268, 2006.

Rosenthal MJ, Felton RM, Hileman DL, Lee M, Friedman M, and Navach JH. A wheelchair cushion designed to redistribute sites of sitting pressure. *Archives of Physical Medicine and Rehabilitation* 77: 278–282, 1996.

Rowley BA, McKenna JM, Chase GR, and Wolcott LE. The influence of electrical current on an infecting microorganism in wounds. *Annals of the New York Academy of Sciences* 238: 543–551, 1974.

Russell LJ, Reynolds TM, Park C, Rithalia S, Gonsalkorale M, Birch J, Torgerson D, and Iglesias C. Randomized clinical trial comparing 2 support surfaces: Results of the prevention of pressure ulcers study. *Advances in Skin & Wound Care* 16: 317–327, 2003.

Sachse RE, Fink SA, and B K. Comparison of supine and lateral positioning on various clinically used support surfaces. *Annals of Plastic Surgery* 41: 513–518, 1998.

Sagach VF, Kindybalyuk AM, and Kovalenko TN. Functional hyperemia of skeletal muscle: Role of endothelium. *Journal of Cardiovascular Pharmacology* 20: S170–S175, 1992.

Salcido R, Fisher SB, Donofrio JC, Bieschke M, Knapp C, Liang R, LeGrand EK, and Carney JM. An animal model and computer-controlled surface pressure delivery system for the production of pressure ulcers. *Journal of Rehabilitation Research and Development* 32: 149–161, 1995.

Salzberg CA, Byrne DW, Cayten CG, van Niewerburgh P, Murphy JG, and Viehbeck M. A new pressure ulcer risk assessment scale for individuals with spinal cord injury. *American Journal of Physical Medicine & Rehabilitation* 75: 96–104, 1996.

Schnelle JF, Adamson GM, Cruise PA, al-Samarrai N, Sarbaugh FC, Uman G, and Ouslander JG. Skin disorders and moisture in incontinent nursing home residents: Intervention implications. *Journal of the American Geriatrics Society* 45: 1182–1188, 1997.

Schubert V and Fagrell B. Postocclusive reactive hyperemia and thermal response in the skin microcirculation of subjects with spinal cord injury. *Scandinavian Journal of Rehabilitation Medicine* 23: 33–40, 1991.

Schubert V and Heraud J. The effects of pressure and shear on skin microcirculation in elderly stroke patients lying in supine or semi-recumbent positions. *Age and Ageing* 23: 405–410, 1994.

Smith N. The benefits of VAC therapy in the management of pressure ulcers. *British Journal of Nursing* 13: 1359–1365, 2004.

Solis LR, Hallihan DP, Uwiera RR, Thompson RB, Pehowich ED, and Mushahwar VK. Prevention of pressure-induced deep tissue injury using intermittent electrical stimulation. *Journal of Applied Physiology* 102: 1992–2001, 2007.

Stekelenburg A, Oomens CW, Strijkers GJ, de Graaf L, Bader DL, and Nicolay K. A new MR-compatible loading device to study in vivo muscle damage development in rats due to compressive loading. *Medical Engineering & Physics* 28: 331–338, 2006a.

Stekelenburg A, Oomens CW, Strijkers GJ, Nicolay K, and Bader DL. Compression-induced deep tissue injury examined with magnetic resonance imaging and histology. *Journal of Applied Physiology* 100: 1946–1954, 2006b.

Stekelenburg A, Strijkers GJ, Parusel H, Bader DL, Nicolay K, and Oomens CW. Role of ischemia and deformation in the onset of compression-induced deep tissue injury: MRI-based studies in a rat model. *Journal of Applied Physiology* 102: 2002–2011, 2007.

Swarts AE, Krouskop TA, and Smith DR. Tissue pressure management in the vocational setting. *Archives of Physical Medicine and Rehabilitation* 69: 97–100, 1988.

Taylor RP, Polliack AA, and Bader DL. The analysis of metabolites in human sweat: Analytical methods and potential application to investigation of pressure ischaemia of soft tissues. *Annals of Clinical Biochemistry* 31: 18–24, 1994.

Thiyagarajan C and Silver JR. Aetiology of pressure sores in patients with spinal cord injury. *British Medical Journal* 289: 1487–1490, 1984.

Thomas DR. Prevention and treatment of pressure ulcers. *Journal of the American Medical Directors Association* 7: 46–59, 2006.

Thomas DR. Prevention and treatment of pressure ulcers: What works? What doesn't? *Cleveland Clinic Journal of Medicine* 68: 704–707, 710–714, 717–722, 2001.

Thomas DR. The role of nutrition in prevention and healing of pressure ulcers. *Clinics in Geriatric Medicine* 13: 497–511, 1997.

Tsuji S, Ichioka S, Sekiya N, and Nakatsuka T. Analysis of ischemia-reperfusion injury in a microcirculatory model of pressure ulcers. *Wound Repair and Regeneration* 13: 209–215, 2005.

Tupling R, Green H, Senisterra G, Lepock J, and McKee N. Effects of ischemia on sarcoplasmic reticulum Ca(2+) uptake and Ca(2+) release in rat skeletal muscle. *American Journal of Physiology—Endocrinology and Metabolism* 281: E224–E232, 2001a.

Tupling R, Green H, Senisterra G, Lepock J, and McKee N. Ischemia-induced structural change in SR Ca^{2+}-ATPase is associated with reduced enzyme activity in rat muscle. *American Journal of Physiology — Regulatory Integrative and Comparative Physiology* 281: R1681–R1688, 2001b.

Vanderwee K, Grypdonck MH, De Bacquer D, and Defloor T. Effectiveness of turning with unequal time intervals on the incidence of pressure ulcer lesions. *Journal of Advanced Nursing* 57: 59–68, 2007.

Wall BM, Mangold T, Huch KM, Corbett C, and Cooke CR. Bacteremia in the chronic spinal cord injury population: Risk factors for mortality. *Journal of Spinal Cord Medicine* 26: 248–253, 2003.

White GW, Mathews RM, and Fawcett SB. Reducing risk of pressure sores: Effects of watch prompts and alarm avoidance on wheelchair push-ups. *Journal of Applied Behavior Analysis* 22: 287–295, 1989.

Whitney JD, Salvadalena G, Higa L, and Mich M. Treatment of pressure ulcers with noncontact normothermic wound therapy: Healing and warming effects. *Journal of Wound, Ostomy, and Continence Nursing* 28: 244–252, 2001.

Woolsey RM and McGarry JD. The cause, prevention, and treatment of pressure sores. *Neurologic Clinics* 9: 797–808, 1991.

Xakellis GC, Frantz RA, Lewis A, and Harvey P. Translating pressure ulcer guidelines into practice: It's harder than it sounds. *Advances in Skin & Wound Care* 14: 249–256, 258, 2001.

Young JS. aBPE. Pressure sores and the spinal cord injured: Part II, Model Systems. *SCI Digest* 3: 11–26, 1981.

Zagoren AJ. Nutritional assessment and intervention in the person with a chronic wound. In: *Chronic Wound Care: A Clinical Source Book for Healthcare Professionals*, eds. DL Kresner and GR Sibbald: HMP Communications, 3rd Edition, 117–126, 2001.

Zanca JM, Brienza DM, Berlowitz D, Bennett RG, Lyder CH, and Panel NPUA. Pressure ulcer research funding in America: Creation and analysis of an on-line database. *Advances in Skin & Wound Care* 16: 190–197, 2003.

Zhao M, Bai H, Wang E, Forrester JV, and McCaig CD. Electrical stimulation directly induces pre-angiogenic responses in vascular endothelial cells by signaling through VEGF receptors. *Journal of Cell Science* 117: 397–405, 2004.

8 Exercise Rehabilitation and Return to Work Following a Cardiac Event

R. G. Haennel and C. R. Tomczak

CONTENTS

8.1 INTRODUCTION

In industrialized countries, coronary artery disease (CAD) accounts for more deaths, disability, and economic loss than any other disease entity.[1] In the United States

243

alone, CAD is responsible for more than 20% of all deaths[2] and accounts for over $350 billion in direct and indirect costs (e.g., wage replacement and lost productivity).[2,3] While CAD remains the leading cause of morbidity and disability, the death rate from myocardial infarction (MI) has declined significantly in the past 30 years. Whether the increased numbers of survivors return to gainful employment has an enormous social and economic implication for both the individual and society. The return to gainful employment is a major goal for many patients and aiding these patients in returning to work is an often-considered important outcome measure of the cost-effectiveness of cardiac rehabilitation programs.

The decision to return to work after a cardiac event is complex, with demographic, socioeconomic, physical, emotional, and medical factors contributing to the decision. This chapter will review the issue of return to work in patients recovering from a cardiac event such as a MI, or coronary artery bypass graft surgery (CABGS). We will examine the typical progression of the patient from the acute event, through rehabilitation, and will examine the various factors that play a crucial role in determining return to work success in patients who have had a cardiac event.

8.2 RISK STRATIFICATION

Following an acute coronary event, risk stratification focuses on assigning the patient into one of three categories: high risk, intermediate risk, and low risk. These strata provide guidelines for both the patient's medical management as well as their vocational rehabilitation. The key elements in risk assessment/stratification include (a) left ventricular dysfunction; (b) functional capacity; (c) the hemodynamic responses to exercise; (d) signs or symptoms of angina; (e) the existence of complex arrhythmias; and (f) depression.[4]

8.2.1 LEFT VENTRICULAR DYSFUNCTION

Ejection fraction (EF) is a key measure of ventricular function. It represents the fraction of blood pumped out by the ventricle with each heartbeat. The term EF applies to both the right and left ventricles; however, without a qualifier, the term refers specifically to the left ventricle. By definition, the volume of blood within a ventricle immediately before a contraction is known as the end-diastolic volume. Similarly, the volume of blood remaining in a ventricle at the end of a contraction is the end-systolic volume. The difference between end-diastolic volume and end-systolic volume (the stroke volume) represents the volume of blood ejected per beat. EF is defined as stroke volume divided by end-diastolic volume and is commonly measured by echocardiography, where the volumes of the heart's chambers are measured during the cardiac cycle. Other methods of measuring EF include cardiac magnetic resonance imaging (MRI), fast scan cardiac-computed axial tomography (CT) imaging, gated single photon emission-computed tomography (SPECT) imaging technique using gamma rays, and the multiple-gated acquisition (MUGA) scan, which involves the injection of a radioisotope into the blood while detecting its flow through the left ventricle. Historically, the gold standard for the measurement of EF is accomplished using ventriculography.

Healthy individuals typically have an EF greater than 55%.[5] If a young healthy person (70 kg) has a resting stroke volume of approximately 70 mL and the left ventricular end-diastolic volume is 110 mL, the EF would approximate 64% (70/110 mL). Damage to the myocardium, such as that sustained during a MI, or as a result of cardiomyopathy, impairs the heart's ability to eject blood and therefore reduces the EF. A significant reduction in the EF (e.g., <30%) will manifest itself clinically as heart failure and will limit a patient's functional ability.[5] The EF is one of the most important predictors of prognosis, as those with significantly reduced EF typically have a poorer medical prognosis and are unlikely to return to work.

8.2.2 FUNCTIONAL CAPACITY

Functional capacity, exercise capacity, and exercise tolerance are generally considered to be synonymous and imply that a maximal effort exercise test has been performed. Functional capacity refers to the ability of an individual to perform aerobic work and is typically defined by maximal oxygen uptake (VO_{2max}). Maximal oxygen uptake is a product of maximal cardiac output and the maximal arteriovenous oxygen content difference. Maximal oxygen uptake is determined from a graded exercise test with open-circuit spirometry. In this procedure, pulmonary ventilation and expired fractions of oxygen (O_2) and carbon dioxide (CO_2) are measured as a patient completes a graded exercise test involving incremental work to fatigue, or signs/symptoms of exertional intolerance.[6] When direct measurement of VO_{2max} is not feasible or desirable, a variety of submaximal and maximal exercise tests can be used to estimate VO_{2max}. These tests estimate VO_{2max} from the linear correlation that exists for VO_2, heart rate, and work rate. A distinction should be made between estimated and measured functional capacity (VO_{2max}). This issue becomes important in patients with CAD; slower VO_2 on-kinetics can create a large discrepancy between estimated and measured VO_{2max} in which the predicted values dramatically overestimate the patient's actual VO_{2max}, especially when aggressive exercise testing protocols are used.[7] In addition, when functional capacity is estimated from work rate achieved rather than directly measured, VO_2 is frequently expressed in metabolic equivalents (METs), where 1 MET represents the resting energy expenditure (approximately $3.5 \, mL \cdot kg^{-1} \cdot min^{-1}$). In these instances, a patient's functional capacity is commonly expressed as a multiple of this resting metabolic rate (METs).

Depending on the severity of the cardiac event, the patient's VO_{2max} may range between 10 and $20 \, mL \cdot kg^{-1} \cdot min^{-1}$ vs. the $30-40 \, mL \cdot kg^{-1} \cdot min^{-1}$ seen in healthy, middle-aged individuals.[8] The reduced VO_{2max} in the CAD patient is primarily attributed to a decrease in maximal cardiac output, secondary to reduced stroke volume, rather than impairment in the peripheral O_2 extraction.[9] As the arteriovenous oxygen content difference does not appear to be affected by CAD, VO_{2max} is considered a good indication of cardiac pump function.[6] With cardiopulmonary exercise testing, it is possible to objectively evaluate and classify the degree of heart failure based on VO_2 at the anaerobic (ventilatory) threshold and at VO_{2max}. Weber and Janicki[10] demonstrated that VO_{2max} correlates with cardiac reserve (Table 8.1).

TABLE 8.1

Weber's Classification of Functional Impairment

Class	Severity	VO$_{2max}$ (mL$\cdot$kg$^{-1}\cdot$min^{-1})	Anaerobic Threshold (VO$_{2max}$) (mL$\cdot$kg$^{-1}\cdot$min^{-1})
A	Mild to none	>20	>14
B	Mild to moderate	16–20	11–14
C	Moderate to severe	10–16	8–11
D	Severe	6–10	5–8
E	Very severe	<6	<4

Source: Weber, K.T. and Janicki, J.S. *Am J Cardiol*, 55, 22A, 1985.

8.2.3 HEMODYNAMIC RESPONSES TO EXERCISE

During incremental aerobic exercise, heart rate increases linearly with metabolic demand. The normal heart rate response to progressive exercise corresponding to 10 ± 2 beats/MET for inactive individuals.[6] The inability to increase heart rate appropriately during exercise is referred to as chronotropic incompetence and is signified by a peak exercise heart rate that is 2 standard deviations (>20 beats$\cdot$min^{-1}) below the age-predicted maximal heart rate for individuals who are limited by volitional fatigue and not taking beta-blockers.[6] Chronotropic incompetence is associated with presence of CAD and poorer prognosis.[11,12] Further, a delayed decrease in the heart rate during the first minute of exercise recovery is also a powerful predictor of overall mortality.[13]

The normal blood pressure response to dynamic exercise consists of a progressive increase in systolic blood pressure, no change or slight decrease in diastolic blood pressure, and a widening of the pulse pressure. Exercise-induced decreases in systolic blood pressure may occur in patients with CAD. This exertional hypotension has been correlated with ischemia, left ventricular dysfunction, and increased risk of subsequent cardiac events.[14,15] The normal postexercise response is a progressive decline in systolic blood pressure, and the diastolic blood pressure may also drop during the postexercise period. The product of heart rate and systolic blood pressure (i.e., the rate pressure product) is another important hemodynamic indicator and is commonly used as an indirect index of myocardial oxygen demand and may be useful for interpreting mechanisms of angina.[16,17]

8.2.4 ANGINA

Coronary atherosclerosis involves a localized accumulation of fibrous tissue within the coronary artery, progressively narrowing the vessel lumen. Ischemia occurs when clinically significant lesions (i.e., >70% of the vessel's cross-sectional area) result in blood flow inadequate to meet myocardial oxygen demand, causing significant ST-segment depression ($\geq$−2 mm) on the electrocardiogram, angina pectoris, or both. Patients with CAD are typically evaluated for evidence of myocardial ischemia before (i.e., from the patient history), during, and after a graded exercise test.

Especially important are symptoms that may represent classic angina pectoris, such as substernal pressure radiating across the chest and/or down the left arm, back, jaw, or stomach, or lower neck pain or discomfort. In one study, post-MI patients who had an ST-segment depression of ≥-2 mm during an incremental exercise test, had a return to work rate 50% lower than for those with less severe ischemic electrocardiographic (ECG) changes.[18]

For a given patient, stable angina predictably occurs with progressive exercise at approximately the same myocardial oxygen demand which can be estimated from the rate pressure product. In contrast, unstable angina may be characterized by an abrupt increase in the frequency of angina, angina at rest, or both. This acceleration of symptoms may herald an impending cardiovascular event and serves as a contraindication to return to work. Accordingly, such patients generally require immediate medical attention. Patients with stable angina pectoris (for whom revascularization is not appropriate) and/or those with an anginal threshold that occurs at a functional capacity greater than 5 METs are candidates for return to work.[19]

8.2.5   COMPLEX ARRHYTHMIAS

Major mechanisms of arrhythmias include increased sympathetic drive and changes in extracellular and intracellular electrolytes, pH, and oxygen tension contribute to disturbances in myocardial and conducting tissue automaticity and reentry. Ventricular arrhythmias such as paired or multiform premature ventricular contractions (PVC) salvos, and ventricular tachycardia, are associated with significant CAD and/or a poor prognosis if they occur in conjunction with signs and/or symptoms of myocardial ischemia such as angina.[20,21]

8.2.6   DEPRESSION

Depression is common among patients recovering from a MI. Approximately one in six post-MI patients experiences major depression and at least twice as many have significant symptoms of depression soon after their cardiac event.[22] Postevent depression is an independent risk factor for increased mortality. Depression is also associated with poor compliance with risk-reducing recommendations, with abnormalities in autonomic tone (that may make patients more susceptible to ventricular arrhythmias), and with increased platelet activation.[22] Depression is also a well-documented predictor of absenteeism, disability, and poor health-related quality of life.[23,24]

In summary, risk stratification is important to distinguish patients who have a poor prognosis from those who have excellent functional capacity. These risk strata also help identify the opposite ends of the spectrum with regard to return to work ability. Some patients may be identified as being likely to return to work without limitations; others could return to work with limitations, while a third group should not or will not be able to return to work because of their medical condition. Table 8.2 illustrates the risk stratification criteria from the American Association of Cardiovascular and Pulmonary Rehabilitation, which integrates the various physiological and psychological factors used in risk assessment.

TABLE 8.2

American Association of Cardiovascular and Pulmonary Rehabilitation (AACVPR) Risk Stratification Criteria for Cardiac Patients

Low Risk	Moderate Risk	High Risk
• No significant left ventricular dysfunction (EF of >50%)	• Moderately impaired left ventricular function (EF = 40%–49%)	• Decreased left ventricular function (EF of <40%)
• Asymptomatic including absence of angina with exertion or recovery. Functional capacity of >7 METs[a]	• Signs/symptoms including angina at moderate levels of exercise (5–6.9 METs) or in recovery.	• Signs/symptoms including angina pectoris at low levels of exercise (<5.0 METs) or in recovery. Functional capacity of <5.0 METs[a]
• No resting or exercise-induced complex arrhythmias		• Survivor of cardiac arrest or sudden death complex ventricular arrhythmias at rest or with exercise
• Uncomplicated MI; CABGS; angioplasty, atherectomy, or stent: Absence of CHF, or signs/symptoms of postevent ischemia		• MI or cardiac surgery complicated by cardiogenic shock, CHF, and/or signs/symptoms of postevent/procedure ischemia
• Normal hemodynamics with exercise or recovery		• Abnormal hemodynamics with exercise (especially flat or decreasing SBP or chronotropic incompetence with increasing workload)
• Absence of clinical depression		• Clinically significant depression
• Low-risk classification is assumed when each of the descriptors in the category is present	• Moderate risk is assumed for patients who do not meet the classification of either high or low risk.	• High-risk classification is assumed with the presence of any one of the descriptors included in this category.

Source: AACVPR. *Guidelines for Cardiac Rehabilitation and Secondary Prevention Programs.* 3rd edn. Champaign, IL: Human Kinetics, 1999.

MI, myocardial infarction; CABGS, coronary artery bypass surgery; CHF, chronic heart failure; SBP, systolic blood pressure.

[a] METs, metabolic equivalent (1 MET = $3.5\,mL \cdot kg^{-1} \cdot min^{-1}$).

8.3 EVALUATION OF THE CARDIAC PATIENT

8.3.1 GRADED EXERCISE TESTING

While angiography and echocardiography are standard techniques used to determine the severity of CAD, the symptom-limited graded exercise test remains the primary tool used to evaluate the patient's functional capacity, anginal threshold, as well as the hemodynamic and ECG responses to exercise.[25] The World Health Organization has indicated that the primary purpose of exercise testing is to determine individual responses to incremental exertion and from this, estimate probable performance during activities of daily living and occupational situations.[26] The graded exercise test has the advantage of reproducibility and quantification of a patient's physiologic responses to known external workloads, which can help assess the patient's return to work potential. Graded exercise testing also has diagnostic and prognostic value in determining objective evidence of myocardial ischemia and provoking life-threatening ventricular arrhythmias. For example, the occurrence of a complex ventricular arrhythmia and of ST-segment displacement during a graded exercise test is predictive of a similar change during activities of daily living of similar intensities.[27]

The measured functional capacity determined from the graded exercise test can be compared to the estimated aerobic requirements of the patient's job to assess expected relevant energy demands. The inability to perform 5 METs of exercise without developing ST-segment changes on the electrocardiogram or arrhythmias has been used as a criterion by the social security administration for disability evaluation.[28] Such patients would be classified as being in a high-risk category.[4]

The value of the symptom-limited graded exercise test in evaluating and counseling patient's for return to work is well established.[29] In a randomized control trial, Dennis et al.[30] reported that the completion of a graded exercise test followed by physician counseling resulted in a significantly earlier return to work for both manual and nonmanual workers. In their study,[30] the efficacy of a graded exercise test in facilitating an early return to work was evaluated approximately 3 weeks after an uncomplicated MI. Patients were previously employed and younger than 60 years. Screening yielded 201 subjects (mean age, 50 years); of these, 99 and 102 subjects were randomized to the intervention or usual-care groups, respectively. Patients in the intervention group, who did not exhibit marked ischemic ST-segment depression (>-2 mm) during the graded exercise test ($n = 91$), were advised to return to work approximately 35–42 days following their MI. Patients in the usual-care group returned to work when they believed it was appropriate. On average, patients in the intervention group went back to work 3 weeks earlier than those who received usual care (51 vs. 75 days) without reported adverse events. These findings suggest that a negative graded exercise test can facilitate an earlier and safe return to work for CAD patients.

Most graded exercise tests are performed on a cycle ergometer or a treadmill. Cycle ergometer protocols have the advantage of yielding better quality ECGs and blood pressure measurements and may be preferred for subjects with poor gait, who are obese, or with orthopedic limitations.[6] Cycle ergometer testing soon after CABGS has been shown to assist in determining a patient's return to work status. Patients who attained a peak power output of ≤60 W on a graded exercise test had a return to work rate less than 50% of those who achieved a power output of ≥120 W.[31] In another study, post-MI patients with a functional capacity of <100 W on a cycle ergometer graded exercise test were less likely to return to work.[32]

The VO_{2max} measured during cycle ergometry has been shown to be 10%–20% below the peak value demonstrated on a treadmill.[33–35] This disparity could unduly influence the return to work decision by implying a low functional capacity. To rectify the discrepancy in VO_{2max} between the two most commonly used testing modalities (cycle ergometers and treadmills), Foster et al.[36] developed the following formula: treadmill METs = 0.98 (cycle ergometer METs) + 1.85. Multiplication of the value obtained from this equation by 3.5 produces a treadmill VO_2 score (in $mL \cdot kg^{-1} \cdot min^{-1}$).

Treadmill protocols involve progressive increases in speed and/or grade. The selection of an appropriate protocol for assessing functional capacity is of critical importance, especially when functional capacity is to be estimated from exercise time or peak work rate. Test protocols with large stage-to-stage increments in energy requirements generally have a weaker relationship between measured VO_2 and work rate.[6] The Balke protocol, which involves modest increases in treadmill elevation at a constant speed, is recommended for this reason.[6] It is important to note that protocols that involve large increments in work with each stage (e.g., Bruce protocol) are more likely to unmask ischemic ECG changes (e.g., ST-segment depression),[37] but are less accurate in estimating a patient's functional capacity.[38]

A patient's functional capacity can also be accurately determined with the use of "ramp-type" protocols, where small increments in work rate occur at intervals of ≤60 s. Regardless of the protocol or modality, the graded exercise test should be tailored to yield a maximum duration of 8–12 min.[39] Even with exercise test protocols using modest increases in workload, results may still indicate a nonlinear relationship between VO_2 and work rate when the test duration is <6 min. Conversely, when the exercise duration is >12 min, subjects may terminate exercise because of specific muscle fatigue or orthopedic factors rather than cardiopulmonary end points. In instances where there is an expectation of >12 min of exercise, a test protocol using a more aggressive approach to increasing workload, (e.g., Bruce protocol) should be considered. The timing of the graded exercise test can also affect outcomes. If a patient completes a graded exercise test shortly after hospital discharge (e.g., 3 weeks), their functional capacity (i.e., VO_{2max}) may be spuriously low because of deconditioning, fatigue, or fear of exertion.[40,41] Finally, grasping the handrail support should not be permitted during a treadmill graded exercise test as this may create a discrepancy between estimated (i.e., from treadmill speed and grade) and actual VO_2.[6]

8.3.2 ARM ERGOMETRY

While most graded exercise tests are completed on a treadmill or cycle ergometer, there are instances where arm ergometry may be preferred. An example of these situations exists when vocational activities predominantly involve dynamic upper extremity effort. Arm ergometer testing is associated with a VO_{2max} that approximates 70%–80% of that observed in the same patient during leg work.[42,43] Similarly, arm exercise produces lower maximal values for heart rate and pulmonary ventilation. These differences relate to the relatively small muscle mass associated with arm exercise. Further, for a given absolute energy expenditure (VO_2), the cardiorespiratory and hemodynamic responses associated with arm ergometry exercise are elevated (vs. leg exercise).[44] These elevated responses may be attributed to a number of factors including reduced mechanical efficiency, the involvement of smaller muscle mass, the static effort required with arm work, increased sympathetic tone, concomitant isometric contraction, and vasoconstriction in the nonexercising leg muscles.[45]

8.3.3 Work Simulation

For many CAD patients, the graded exercise test may be the only test needed to provide realistic advice on return to work potential. However, for patients with borderline functional capacity (e.g., <5 METs) in relationship to the anticipated job demands, those with concomitant left ventricular dysfunction, or those concerned about resuming a physically demanding job, additional work simulation testing may be required.

Although upper extremity static or combined static–dynamic efforts have, in the past, been contraindicated for CAD patients, it appears that such exercise may be less hazardous than previously assumed.[46–48] This may especially be the case in patients with a functional capacity of more than 7 METs and good left ventricular function.[46] Static and combined static–dynamic exercise, generally fail to elicit angina, ischemic ST-segment depression, or significant ventricular arrhythmias among cardiac patients.[47,49,50] The magnitude of the blood pressure response during static and combined static–dynamic exercise depends on the total muscle mass involved,[51] the duration of the muscle contraction, and the tension exerted (relative to the maximal voluntary contraction).[52] Increased subendocardial perfusion, secondary to an elevated diastolic blood pressure, may also contribute to the lower incidence of ischemic responses during static or combined static–dynamic effort. The myocardial oxygen demand (e.g., rate pressure product) may be lower than that observed during maximal dynamic exercise, primarily because of a lower peak heart rate response.[47] Furthermore, the myocardial oxygen supply–demand relationship appears to be favorably altered by superimposing static on dynamic effort such that the rate pressure product at the ischemic threshold is increased.[50] Although left ventricular function deteriorates during progressively increasing workloads (i.e., exercise intensity) in patients with myocardial ischemia, mild ischemia may be tolerated during steady-state exercise without a deterioration of left ventricular function.[49] These reported findings are changing the attitude toward the use of static and combined static–dynamic exercise for CAD patients for both exercise testing and exercise training.

While specialized work simulators (e.g., Baltimore Therapeutic Work Simulator) are available, simple inexpensive tests can be established with ease to evaluate the physiological responses to static and combined static/dynamic exercise.[29] For example, weight carrying or lifting test protocols can be easily modified to meet specific workplace demands.[53] In particular, the American College of Sports Medicine[6] has detailed an interval weight carrying protocol that incorporates work and rest intervals of 1–3 min. During the work intervals, patients walk at a moderate speed (e.g., 2 miles·h^{-1}) while carrying weights in one or both hands. With each stage increment, the patient carries an additional 10 lb (to a maximum load of 50 lb). The metabolic load associated with this protocol ranges from 2.4 to 5 METs. To evaluate the hemodynamic responses to intermittent static effort that employs a light to moderate dynamic load, patients can be asked to repeatedly lift weighted objects (e.g., boxes) from the floor to a higher surface level typically encountered in an individual's workplace environment. Using an interval protocol that includes 6 min work intervals with a 1–3 min rest interval between stages, a self-paced lifting rate with incremental loads ranging from 30 to a maximum of 50 lb (at a rate of 8 lifts·min^{-1}) would yield a metabolic load of the predicted MET level ranging from 3.8 to 4.2.[6]

To make such testing more "real world," additional stresses may be added to the situation. This can be accomplished by fluctuating the work rate of the test, having the patient perform the tasks while wearing work-specific apparel, or completing the test at the work site (with ambulatory monitoring). It is also important that during the actual work simulations that the ECG, heart rate, and blood pressure responses be monitored.

8.3.4 FUNCTIONAL CAPACITY

As previously stated, one of the outcomes of a graded exercise test is an indication of the patient's functional capacity, which is a key indicator for a safe return to work transition. Patients with CAD should work below the metabolic load that evokes signs or symptoms of exertional intolerance, such as ischemic ST-segment depression, angina pectoris, or serious arrhythmias. For most CAD patients, occupational demands are considered appropriate if the 8 h energy expenditure requirement averages 30%–40% of the patient's VO_{2max} (or heart rate reserve)[54,55], and the peak job demands (e.g., 5–45 min) are within guidelines prescribed for a home exercise program (e.g., 80% peak METs or lower).[6] If a return to work is deemed unfeasible due to low functional capacity, patients should be encouraged to enter a formalized cardiac rehabilitation exercise training program. After the completion of this program, the patient should undergo a follow-up graded exercise test to reevaluate their functional capacity.

A patient's functional capacity determined from the graded exercise test can be compared to the estimated aerobic requirements of a particular job or task to assess expected relevant energy demands.[56] With automation, the metabolic requirement of many occupational activities has decreased.[56] The demonstration that the energy requirements for most occupational activities are low (<5 METs)[29,56] and are rarely sustained for more than 2–3 min[57] has facilitated the safe and successful return to work of CAD patients classified as low or intermediate risk. Further, it is estimated that only 5% of patients now perform "heavy" occupational work.[58]

There are however several limitations to the use of energy expenditure as a guide to return to work for CAD patients.[26] One limitation lies in the fact that these energy expenditure tables represent averaged values.[56] Depending on the pace of the activity, previous job training, and work efficiency, the energy expenditure for a given task may vary considerably from person to person. Energy expenditure values also represent the caloric cost during "steady-state" work; most occupational activities are intermittent with rest or relative rest characterizing 30%–45% of work shift.[59,60] Thus, a patient's capacity for certain activities may easily be underestimated. A patient with a functional capacity of 5 METs might be discouraged from returning to an occupation that has an energy requirement of 5 METs, because it may be presumed that the task represents maximal effort; however, if the activity is performed intermittently, with multiple rest intervals, the task could be accomplished at an energy expenditure level well below what is estimated for the task. Finally, factors such as psychological stress, climate, and the activation of muscles not used during the graded exercise test may alter the linear relationship between myocardial and VO_2 demands, creating disproportionate cardiac demands at relatively low levels of energy expenditure. For example, an elevated rate pressure product associated with combined static–dynamic movements such as weight carrying and repeated weight lifting may be camouflaged by the relatively low metabolic requirements associated with these activities.

8.4 CARDIAC REHABILITATION

The American Heart Association considers cardiac rehabilitation to be standard care in the follow-up treatment of patients with CAD.[61] The American Heart Association identifies exercise training and activity prescription, lifestyle modification, and psychosocial/vocational evaluation and counseling as essential rehabilitation program components. Moreover, the American Heart Association has indicated that participation in a comprehensive cardiac rehabilitation program yielded decreased rehospitalization rates and need for cardiac-related medications. Participation in a comprehensive cardiac rehabilitation program also facilitates the transition from patient to worker through the assessment of functional capacity, while improving cardiovascular and muscular fitness, and lifestyle modification.

8.4.1 EXERCISE TRAINING

Following an acute cardiac event, most patients are encouraged to enter a formalized cardiac rehabilitation exercise program. A cardiac rehabilitation program typically involves supervised training three to five times per week and lasts between 8 and 12 weeks. A major objective of the cardiac rehabilitation exercise training program is to improve functional capacity and help patients return to work. Traditional cardiac rehabilitation exercise programs are aerobically based and involve a brief warm-up followed by 30–40 min of aerobic activity and 5–10 min of cool down activity. The warm-up involves some flexibility exercises and low intensity aerobic activity. For the aerobic component, most programs assign an exercise intensity ranging between 40% and 80% of the patient's peak functional capacity (e.g., 40%–80% of VO_{2max} or heart rate reserve), depending on the individual patient's clinical situation. The aerobic activity typically involves continuous activities such as walking, jogging, or stationary cycling. If the program includes resistance training, it is normally initiated after 6 weeks of aerobic training and is usually completed after the aerobic conditioning component of the training session.[62]

The successful completion of a cardiac rehabilitation exercise training program has been shown to improve functional capacity (VO_{2max}) in the range of 11%–56% (mean 20%).[8,63] A substantial portion of this improved functional capacity is attributable to peripheral adaptations within the trained muscles.[8,64,65] Of course, the magnitude of the improvement depends on several factors, including the patient's initial fitness, clinical status, left ventricular function, total volume of exercise accomplished or calories expended, and exercise adherence.[8] From a return to work perspective, a decreased rate pressure product response to submaximal exercise intensity, associated with the completion of such a training program may signify a reduction in myocardial oxygen consumption for a given level of physical work. The improvement in VO_{2max} and decreased heart rate and blood pressure responses to submaximal exercise are especially beneficial for patients with low to marginal functional capacity and those with exercise-induced myocardial ischemia.

Although cardiac rehabilitation exercise programs have been shown to bring about dramatic improvements in functional capacity[40,66] and psychological well-being,[67,68] their success in terms of enhancing the potential for return to work for CAD patients remains controversial.[69] Several nonrandomized-controlled studies have reported higher return to work rates following cardiac rehabilitation exercise training.[70,71] For example, Hedback et al.[72] completed a longitudinal study of cardiac rehabilitation where employment status was evaluated at 5 and 10 years postevent. Patients who received comprehensive cardiac rehabilitation had a significantly higher employment rate at both 5 (51.8% vs. 27.4%, respectively) and 10 years (58.6% vs. 22%, respectively) after the completion of cardiac rehabilitation compared with those receiving standard care. Others have also documented improved return to work rates as a direct result of cardiac rehabilitation. Simchen et al.[73] reported a 2.8-fold increase in return to work rates and a lower drop out rate in post-CABGS patients who participated in cardiac rehabilitation compared with those who did not. In a 5 year follow-up of 228 patients recovering from CABGS, Engblom et al.[74] reported increased return to work rates following participating in a cardiac rehabilitation program. Higher rates of return to work have also been reported in several European randomized-controlled trials.[75,76] However, those findings contrast several randomized control trials that reported no difference in return to work rates following formalized cardiac rehabilitation.[40,77–80] Mital et al.[81] suggested that the return to work potential is not accelerated by improved aerobic capacity, and that return to work rates have not increased in the past 30 years in patients who have undergone cardiac rehabilitation exercise training. The authors[81] suggest that treadmill exercise performance is inadequate as a measure of readiness for return to industrial-type employment. This conclusion is consistent with the findings of others.[82] In their study, Wiklund et al.[82] reported that conventional aerobic training enabled 83% of workers previously engaged in relatively lighter sedentary work to resume employment. However, only 67% of those engaged in physically demanding occupations returned to work. These findings and those of others,[81] suggest that if one of the primary goals of a cardiac rehabilitation program is to return the CAD patient to work, then the formalized exercise program should be tailored to the actual occupation-related tasks with the incorporation of specified occupation-related elements.

8.4.2 Resistance Training

To enhance the return to work potential of CAD patients whose occupation involves upper extremity effort, resistance training should be included in the cardiac rehabilitation conditioning program. In designing a resistance-training program in preparation for returning to work, the program should be individualized according to the occupational demands, as peripheral adaptations are specific to the muscles and action used during training.[83] Accordingly, a theme of training for occupational specificity should be adopted in order to maximize a successful transition. Guidelines for resistance training for CAD patients have been published by the American Heart Association.[62] The major program modifications for CAD patients (vs. healthy adults) are reductions in exercise intensity, a slower progression of the training volume variables, and increased patient monitoring and supervision.[84] Determining the initial load for resistance training may be facilitated with the determination of the patient's one-repetition maximum for a given movement. For CAD populations, the one-repetition maximum refers to the maximum weight the patient can lift comfortably once only, through a complete range of motion and in good form. For CAD patients, the American Heart Association recommends a training intensity of 40%–60% of one-repetition maximum with one set (12–15 repetitions) and 8–10 exercises for both upper and lower extremities 2–3 days per week.[62] Patients engaging in resistance training should have blood pressure monitored during the actual lifting and lowering of the weight (in the nonexercising limb), as postlifting measures may not be valid due to the large decrease in pressure that occurs immediately after the final lift.[85]

The evidence regarding the efficacy of resistance training in cardiac rehabilitation suggests that, after completion of the program, patients demonstrate significant improvements in measures of weight carrying tolerance time and increases in skeletal muscle strength.[86–90] Further, resistance training has been shown to significantly lower peak exercise heart rate and rate pressure product, and improve functional capacity.[91] Moreover, angina, ventricular arrhythmias, and ischemic ST-segment depression occur less frequently during resistance training than during aerobic exercise testing to fatigue.[92–94] Resistance training may also help the patient gain a better appreciation of their ability to perform physical work within reasonable levels of safety. Enhanced self-efficacy, in turn, may lead to a greater willingness on the patient's part to return to work and remain employed for a longer-term following their cardiac event.

In an effort to improve return to work rates in CAD patients, Mital et al.[81] developed a job-simulated program and compared that intervention with a traditional cardiac rehabilitation training program. The study population consisted of 30 subjects who completed a conventional cardiac rehabilitation program and 17 who completed an occupation-simulated cardiac rehabilitation program. Patients were stratified according to gender and the nature of their occupation at the time of their event. The overall stratification of the sample allowed the authors to study the effect that an occupation-simulated cardiac rehabilitation training program had on both men and women performing two very different categories of work (medium to very heavy occupational tasks vs. sedentary light tasks). The training activities included flexibility exercises, dexterity exercises, and strength-oriented upper- and whole-body exercises. The upper- and whole-body exercises involved industrial tasks encompassing lifting, lowering, carrying, pushing, pulling, holding, and stair climbing. The results showed that 100% of patients in the occupation-simulated program returned to work compared with 60% of the conventional cardiac rehabilitation program patients. The second component of the study explored return to work outcomes of the occupation-simulated group and identified key factors that influenced return to work.[95] The researchers reported that of the 17 participants who returned to work, 80% were "mostly to very satisfied" with their occupations and 76% believed that their supervisor was willing to listen to their work-related concerns. Among those who did not return to work, most were unaware of alternative occupations with their employers in the case that they were unable to return to their previous position. The investigators suggested that the skills of a vocational rehabilitation specialist may be significant in facilitating the return to work potential for employees requiring occupational-site accommodation.[95]

8.4.3   VOCATIONAL COUNSELING

Patients who fail to return to work within 6 months following an MI or CABGS are unlikely to do so beyond this time point.[96] Shrey and Mital's[95] finding that the longer the convalescence, the less likely the patient will resume employment, lends support for the need to recognize workers at risk for not returning to work as early as possible. Facilitating an earlier return to work, particularly among low-risk patients, could result in a significant savings in disability compensation. Further, some patients classified as high-risk on the basis of impaired left ventricular function demonstrate a relatively well-preserved physical work capacity and, thus, are capable of gainful employment.[97] However, those who have strenuous occupations may require occupation modifications or reassignment. The goals of vocational rehabilitation therefore are to evaluate whether returning to work is safe and realistic and to expedite the resumption of gainful employment. Early discussion of work-related issues with patients, preferably prior to hospital discharge, may help establish reasonable return to work expectations. Discussion with the patient may include an occupation analysis to ascertain workplace demands, individualize rehabilitation to address to workplace demands and concerns, establishment of tentative time lines for work evaluation and resumption, and identifying occupation-related needs or contacts.[98]

A systematic vocational assessment in rehabilitation may provide important information to the decision-making process for the physician and the patient's employer. Indeed, many patients fail to return to work because they lack the medical assurance that they can resume vocational activities safely. Early intervention by health care professionals may help anticipate, identify, and modify barriers to returning to work and alleviate, at least in part, the anxiety often found in such patients.[99] As Prior and Cupper[100] suggested, "early intervention may help to prevent patients from assuming inappropriate disability perspectives and behaviors that can become difficult to change once adopted" (p. 44). This feedback and the interaction between the patient, their health care providers, employer, and disability case manager, provides the greatest probability and builds confidence in the decision to return to work.

8.4.4   DETERMINANTS OF WORK RESUMPTION

Over the last 30 years, research has dispelled the myth that cardiac patients are unemployable. Rates of returning to work are reported to vary between 47% and 93%, depending upon the CAD population study, interventions, follow-up, and endpoint (i.e., outcome) criteria.[101–106,130] The optimal time to return to work varies with type of cardiac event or interventional procedure, associated complications, and prognosis, but most uncomplicated patients can return to work within 8 weeks following their cardiac event. Importantly, the time for returning to work and resuming full activities following a cardiac event has progressively decreased since the 1970s.[4,30] Froelicher et al.[101] reported that 21% of post-MI patients return to work by week 3, 62% returned to work between weeks 4 and 12, and only 6% did not return to work following their cardiac event.

Whether a patient returns to work following a cardiac event is a complex question which has been studied extensively.[30,72,104,106–110] A number of factors have been shown to predict return to work. Smith and O'Rourke[104] studied 151 post-MI patients and found that education level, employment related to physical activity, severity of the MI, and perception of health status were the only significant predictors of returning to work. Further analysis indicated that >70% of those who returned to work completed high school and maintained occupations that did not require heavy physical activity. Interviews of post-CABGS patients suggest that the reasons for not resuming work are rarely based solely on cardiac findings. Only 30%–40% of the post-CABGS patients studied indicated that their cardiac-related problems kept them from resuming work.[111] Indeed, it has been estimated that demographic and socioeconomic factors account for almost half of the variance in return to work rates, while physical and emotional functioning account for 29%, and medical-related factors predict 20% of the variance in returning to work.[112]

8.4.4.1   Demographic Factors

Older patients, particularly those over 60 years, are less likely to return to work.[96,113] In a 2-year follow-up study with 100 post-MI patients who participated in a cardiac rehabilitation program, the best biological predictor of returning to work was age.[113] Boudrez et al.[114] investigated return to work rates in 295 patients (under age of 60 years) following their initial MI. Of those who worked before their MI, 85% returned to work. The key return to work determinants in that study were age, perceived importance of occupation, support from friends, and participation in a comprehensive cardiac rehabilitation program.

Gender differences also exist in the return to work rate following a cardiac event. Women are generally older than men at the time of their first cardiac event, are diagnosed with more severe CAD, and have a longer convalescence period. All three factors negatively contribute to their time until returning to work.[96,98] Mital et al.[115] suggest that women experience more depressive symptoms following an acute MI and that this likely contributes to the lower return to work rate. The authors suggested that women, particularly married women, may be discouraged from returning to work and that women may have a different attachment to their occupation compared to men.[96] It is important to note however, that women also experience a lower referral rate and poorer adherence to cardiac rehabilitation programs.[116] This latter issue is an active area of investigation.

A higher level of education favors success in returning to work. Of patients returning to work following CABGS, three times as many had completed high school compared to postoperatively retired patients.[117] Occupation also plays an important role in determining success in returning to work. There is a higher rate of returning to work for nonmanual labor occupations, many of whom have graduate or postgraduate training.[98,102,118] This may reflect the fact that many nonmanual labor occupations are motivated by intrinsic and extrinsic factors. In most instances, a major factor determining returning to work is directly related to education level, as 65% of patients not working postcardiac event and treatment maintained manual labor occupations.[119]

8.4.4.2   Socioeconomic Factors

Societal factors are major determinants in the return to work decision. For example, employer attitudes about adjusting work loads and employer return to work policies may impact on the return to work rates following a cardiac event. The availability of disability benefits may also significantly act as a deterrent in returning to work.[120] In situations where a patient is able to maintain their lifestyle from retirement funds or disability payments, the desire to return to work may be marginalized. In addition, labor market factors, such as the level of unemployment and related employment opportunities, also influence return to work rates.[105] Concern for the patient's well-being or lack of encouragement by their family may influence the decision to return to work.[121] The optimal situation is for the family to have appropriate information, lend support, and participate in both the patient's rehabilitation and the decision-making process for returning to work.[122]

8.4.4.3 Physical Functioning

Functional classification based on physical functioning affects return to work rates. In one study that followed CABGS patients 1-year postsurgery, Petrie et al.[123] reported that a major determinant of returning to work was the patient's functional class at 6 months following surgery. Functional classifications, such as the commonly employed New York Heart Association[124] (NYHA) (Table 8.3), are often used to characterize patients with cardiac disease. For example, patients determined to be NYHA functional class I (Table 8.3) are considered to be low risk and have a favorable prognosis for returning to work.[19] This classification of patients are typically

TABLE 8.3
NYHA Functional Classifications

NYHA Classification	Description	METs[19]	Work Classification[28]
I	Cardiac patients with no limitations of physical activity. They can perform ordinary physical activity without undue fatigue or symptoms	>5	Medium to heavy
II	Cardiac patients with slight to moderate limitations of physical activity. They may experience fatigue or symptoms (e.g., dyspnea, angina) during *ordinary* physical activity.	3–4	Light to medium
III	Cardiac patients with moderate to great limitations of physical activity. They may experience fatigue or symptoms (e.g., dyspnea, angina) during *lighter* than ordinary physical activity.	2–3	Sedentary to light
IV	Cardiac patients unable to carry out any physical activity. They experience symptoms (e.g., dyspnea, angina) at rest and cannot perform any physical activity without discomfort.	≤2	Sedentary

Source: Criteria Committee of the New York Heart Association. *Diseases of the Heart and Blood Vessels: Nomenclature and Criteria for Diagnosis.* 6th ed. Boston, MA Little Brown and Co., 1953, pp. 112–113.

capable of performing ordinary physical activities without undue fatigue or cardiac symptoms, and normally have a functional capacity of 5 METs or greater.[4] These individuals typically have no limitations with regard to occupational activities or occupational conditions (e.g., driving, shift work, temperature, humidity, etc.). According to Hellerstein,[19] functional capacity corresponds to the classification of medium work,[28] which permits occasional lifting of 25–50 lb and frequent lifting and carrying of objects weighing up to 25 lb.[28] Patients in NYHA functional class II (who fatigue or experience cardiac symptoms such as angina or dyspnea during ordinary activity) typically have a functional capacity of 3–4 METs and are capable of returning to light work with some modest activity limitations. This may include restricting lifting to 20 lb at a time with frequent lifting/carrying of objects up to 10 lb or less. Hellerstein[19] suggests that patients in NYHA functional class I or II are physically capable of returning to full time employment (e.g., 8 h · day^{-1}). Patients in NYHA functional class III (those who experience fatigue or cardiac symptoms with lighter than ordinary activity) have a markedly greater reduction in occupational limitation. For these individuals, a low aerobic capacity (2–3 METs) may restrict their return to work potential to more sedentary-type occupational tasks with a maximum lift/carry weight of 10 lb that is limited to several times/hour.[19] These patients may also find it best to restrict their work to part-time. Finally, CAD patients who are NYHA functional class IV (those who exhibit symptoms of angina or dyspnea at rest) are unlikely to return to work unless their medical status can be improved.

8.4.4.4 Emotional Functioning

From a vocational perspective, self-efficacy refers to the patient's perception of the ability to return to work successfully.[125] Most cardiac rehabilitation patients with a positive outlook manage to return to their previous occupations within 10 weeks.[126] The patient's expectations of future vocational status have also been shown to be an important predictor for returning to work.[123] Patients who anticipated few future work problems have been shown to have a higher return to work rate compared to those who have negative expectations.[98,127,128] Petrie et al.[123] studied the relationship between the post-MI patients' perception of their illness, and their subsequent time to returning to work. Those who perceived their illness as transient and less serious returned to work earlier and were generally able to resume work within 6 weeks.

The patient's desire to work following a cardiac event is an important psychological predictor.[129] Patients who are working productively at the time of their cardiac event are more likely to return to work sooner and remain at work longer.[98] A study by Boll et al.[130] reported that the preoperatively expressed desire to return to work following their CABGS procedure, in addition to an optimistic attitude with concrete plans for the future, positively correlated with returning to work. If a person feels like a significant contributor to the success of a business or profession, then that person is motivated by their occupation, and thus the fears and anxieties about returning to work may be attenuated.[131,132] In a study examining return to work for low back pain patients, high physical and psychological occupational demands and low supervisory support were each associated with a 20% lower return to work rate.[133] In contrast, high occupational control, particularly regarding work and rest periods, was associated with a 30% higher return to work rate.[133]

Sykes et al.[106] suggested that the preillness occupational environment is another important determinant in returning to work for the CAD patient. The findings of Sykes et al.[106] showed improved quality of life at 1 year following discharge for MI patients who had returned to work compared with those who had not. These authors cautioned however, that returning to work may not be the unequivocally positive outcome that it is generally accepted to be. Patients in their study were more likely to return to work if they had greater independence in making decisions concerning how they carry out their occupational responsibilities, were less depressed, and had more social interaction opportunity at work. Thus, preevent job satisfaction, and relationships with employers and coworkers influence the return to work decision.[131]

Stress has been described as an excessive environmental demand combined with inadequate coping resources that yields the presence of emotional distress or characteristic patterns of maladaptive behaviors, or both.[134] Many patients cite stressors as important contributors to their cardiac disease.[102] Theorell et al.[135] reviewed several studies that showed an association between stressful environments and the risk of MI. The investigations included 127 men who returned to work following an MI and reported an increased death rate in those who returned to high stress jobs. It has been suggested that high stress can precipitate a hypercoagulable state that favors focal thrombosis and, as a consequence, the development and progression of CAD.[136,137] Elevated work stress has also been correlated with a lower return to work rate postcardiac event.[105]

While individuals who return to work early following a cardiac event are more likely to attribute their MI to occupational stressors, Abbot and Berry[138] note that these same patients are more likely to find their work challenging and interesting despite the heavy workload. Rost and Smith[139] studied the relationship between early return to work following an initial MI and the patient's subsequent emotional well-being and reported that 63% of the patients who had been employed at the time of their initial event returned to work by 4 months and remained employed 12 months later. Those patients who returned to work displayed significantly lower levels of emotional distress than patients who did not return to work, and this was independent of multiple indicators of initial physical and psychological adjustment. These findings suggest that the trajectory of emotional adaptation following an acute cardiac event differs for individuals who do vs. those who do not return to work (Table 8.4).

8.4.4.5 Medical Factors

Numerous medical factors are predictive of returning to work. While most CABGS patients can return to their premorbid functional capacity (VO_{2max}), the results of surgery, with respect to return to work, have been disappointing. In a study of 1252 patients, 20% did not return to work post revascularization and long-term maintenance of work was more closely related to demographics and job characteristics than with the type of revascularization and severity of illness.[102,140]

The severity and type of MI are important predictors of returning to work.[141] Patients who have clinically evident severe pump failure or left ventricular dysfunction, with or without angina pectoris, have a poorer prognosis and are less likely to return to work.[141] The number of previous cardiac events also influences subsequent

---

TABLE 8.4

Factors that Positively Influence the Decision to Return to Work

Demographic factors

Younger than 60 years of age

Male gender

Socioeconomic factors

Postgraduate education

"White collar" work

Working prior to the event

Needs the income

Physical–emotional factors

Functional capacity greater than 7 METs

Perceives illness as less serious/transient

High self efficacy for work

High job satisfaction

Manageable work stress

Supportive family

Medical factors

Low-risk patient

First cardiac event

Good left ventricular function

No comorbid conditions

Low NYHA classification

---

work status.[98,102,118] Patients who fail to return to work are more likely to have had an MI or CABGS before the current event and less relief of angina postoperatively than those who resume occupational activities.[118] Thus, while surgical and medical interventions are effective in relieving symptoms of angina pectoris and increasing exercise tolerance, the efficacy of these interventions alone in returning cardiac patients to their premorbid position in society has been less than optimal.[142]

8.5   CONCLUSIONS

The decision to return to work following a cardiac event is complex and should involve the patient, their family, physician, and employer. Risk assessment will help distinguish patients who have a poor prognosis for returning to work from those who are physically capable of returning to full or part-time employment. For patients returning to more physically demanding occupations, additional procedures such as exercise testing, evaluation of the occupational energy requirements, and simulated work testing may aid in formulating a return to work prescription. This work prescription should be integrated into a comprehensive cardiac rehabilitation program. Given that the energy requirements for most occupational activities are considered to be relatively low,[29] and that functional capacity is not likely the limiting factor for most patient's ability to return to work, a modified approach to exercise rehabilitation that includes simulated occupational tasks may be warranted. Finally, the vocational counseling component of cardiac rehabilitation needs to address the psychosocial factors that appear to play a prominent role in determining whether a CAD patient will indeed return to work.

REFERENCES

1. Murray CJ and Lopez AD. Mortality by cause for eight regions of the world: Global Burden of Disease Study. *Lancet* 1997;349(9061):1269–1276.
2. American Heart Association. *Heart Disease and Stroke Statistics—2002 Update.* Dallas, TX: American Heart Association, 2002.
3. Phillips L, Harrison T, and Houck P. Return to work and the person with heart failure. *Heart Lung.* 2005;34(2):79–88.
4. DeBusk R. The Stanford University cardiac rehabilitation program. *J Myocardial Isch.* 1990;2:28.
5. Braunwald E. *Heart Disease. A Textbook of Cardiovascular Medicine.* 5th edn. Philadelphia, PA: W.B. Saunders Co., 1997.
6. ACSM. *ACSM's Guidelines for Exercise Testing and Prescription.* 7th edn. New York: Lippincott Williams and Wilkins, 2006.
7. Myers J, Buchanan N, Walsh D, et al. Comparison of the ramp versus standard exercise protocols. *J Am Coll Cardiol.* 1991;17(6):1334–1342.
8. Pina IL, Apstein CS, Balady GJ, et al. Exercise and heart failure: A statement from the American Heart Association Committee on exercise, rehabilitation, and prevention. *Circulation* 2003;107(8):1210–1225.
9. Franklin BA and Rubenfire M. Exercise testing in coronary artery disease: Mechanisms of improvement. *Pract Cardiol.* 1980;6:84–99.
10. Weber KT and Janicki JS. Cardiopulmonary exercise testing for evaluation of chronic cardiac failure. *Am J Cardiol.* 1985;55(2):22A–31A.
11. Lauer MS, Francis GS, Okin PM, Pashkow FJ, Snader CE, and Marwick TH. Impaired chronotropic response to exercise stress testing as a predictor of mortality. *JAMA* 1999;281(6):524–529.
12. Brener SJ, Pashkow FJ, Harvey SA, Marwick TH, Thomas JD, and Lauer MS. Chronotropic response to exercise predicts angiographic severity in patients with suspected or stable coronary artery disease. *Am J Cardiol.* 1995;76(17):1228–1232.
13. Cole CR, Blackstone EH, Pashkow FJ, Snader CE, and Lauer MS. Heart-rate recovery immediately after exercise as a predictor of mortality. *N Engl J Med.* 1999;341(18):1351–1357.
14. Comess KA and Fenster PE. Clinical implications of the blood pressure response to exercise. *Cardiology* 1981;68(4):233–244.
15. Irving JB, Bruce RA, and DeRouen TA. Variations in and significance of systolic pressure during maximal exercise (treadmill) testing. *Am J Cardiol.* 1977;39(6):841–848.
16. Gobel FL, Norstrom LA, Nelson RR, Jorgensen CR, and Wang Y. The rate-pressure product as an index of myocardial oxygen consumption during exercise in patients with angina pectoris. *Circulation* 1978;57(3):549–556.
17. Kitamura K, Jorgensen CR, Gobel FL, Taylor HL, and Wang Y. Hemodynamic correlates of myocardial oxygen consumption during upright exercise. *J Appl Physiol.* 1972;32(4):516–522.
18. Weintraub M, Jacoby J, and Wigler J. The prognostic value of ECG stress test in postmyocardial infarction patients [abstract]. Paper presented at World Congress on Cardiac Rehabilitation, February 1981, Jerusalem.

19. Hellerstein H. Work evaluation. In: Wenger NK and Hellerstein HK, eds. *Rehabilitation of the Coronary Patient*. New York: Churchill Livingstone, 1992:523–542.

20. Ellestad MH, Cooke BM Jr., and Greenberg PS. Stress testing: Clinical application and predictive capacity. *Prog Cardiovasc Dis*. 1979;21(6):431–460.

21. Fuller T and Movahed A. Current review of exercise testing: Application and interpretation. *Clin Cardiol*. 1987;10(3):189–200.

22. Ziegelstein RC. Depression in patients recovering from a myocardial infarction. *JAMA* 2001;286(13):1621–1627.

23. Ladwig KH, Roll G, Breithardt G, Budde T, and Borggrefe M. Post-infarction depression and incomplete recovery 6 months after acute myocardial infarction. *Lancet* 1994;343(8888):20–23.

24. Sykes DH, Hanley M, Boyle DM, Higginson JD, and Wilson C. Socioeconomic status, social environment, depression and postdischarge adjustment of the cardiac patient. *J Psychosom Res*. 1999;46(1):83–98.

25. Franklin BA. Pitfalls in estimating aerobic capacity from exercise time or workload. *Appl Cardiol*. 1986;14:25–26.

26. Hellerstein HK and Franklin B. Exercise testing and prescription. In: Wenger NK and Hellerstein HK, eds. *Rehabilitation of the Coronary Patient*. 2nd edn. New York: Churchill Livingstone, 1984.

27. Walling A, Trembly GJ, John J, et al. Evaluating the rehabilitation potential of a large population of post-myocardial infarction patients: Adverse prognosis for women. *J Cardiopulmonary Rehabil*. 1988;8:99.

28. U.S. Department of Health and Human Services. *Disability Evaluation under Social Security*. SSA Publication No. 05-100089. February 1986. Sect. 404.1567, Physical Requirements. CFR, Ch.111 U.S. Dept. of Health and Human Services, Washington, DC, 1989.

29. Sheldahl LM, Wilke NA, and Tristani FE. Evaluation and training for resumption of occupational and leisure-time activities in patients after a major cardiac event. *Med Exerc Nutr Health*. 1995;4:273–289.

30. Dennis C, Houston-Miller N, Schwartz RG, et al. Early return to work after uncomplicated myocardial infarction. Results of a randomized trial. *JAMA* 1988;260(2):214–220.

31. Roskamm H, Gohlke H, and Samek I. Long-term effects of aortocoronary bypass surgery on exercise tolerance and vocation rehabilitation. Paper presented at World Congress on Cardiac Rehabilitation, July, 1981, Jerusalem.

32. Velasco J, Tormo V, and Ridocci F. Return to work after a comprehensive cardiac rehabilitation program. *J Cardiac Rehabil*. 1983;3:735–738.

33. Miyamura M and Honda Y. Oxygen intake and cardiac output during maximal treadmill and bicycle exercise. *J Appl Physiol*. 1972;32(2):185–188.

34. Williford HN, Sport K, Wang N, Olson MS, and Blessing D. The prediction of fitness levels of United States Air Force officers: Validation of cycle ergometry. *Mil Med*. 1994;159(3):175–178.

35. Lockwood PA, Yoder JE, and Deuster PA. Comparison and cross-validation of cycle ergometry estimates of VO_{2max}. *Med Sci Sports Exerc*. 1997;29(11):1513–1520.

36. Foster C, Pollock ML, Rod JL, Dymond DS, Wible G, and Schmidt DH. Evaluation of functional capacity during exercise radionuclide angiography. *Cardiology* 1983;70(2):85–93.

37. Starling MR, Crawford MH, and O'Rourke RA. Superiority of selected treadmill exercise protocols predischarge and six weeks postinfarction for detecting ischemic abnormalities. *Am Heart J*. 1982;104(5 Pt 1):1054–1060.

38. Haskell WL, Savin W, Oldridge N, and DeBusk R. Factors influencing estimated oxygen uptake during exercise testing soon after myocardial infarction. *Am J Cardiol*. 1982;50(2):299–304.

39. Myers J, Buchanan N, Smith D, et al. Individualized ramp treadmill. Observations on a new protocol. *Chest* 1992;101(5 Suppl.):236S–241S.
40. DeBusk RF, Houston N, Haskell W, Fry G, and Parker M. Exercise training soon after myocardial infarction. *Am J Cardiol.* 1979;44(7):1223–1229.
41. Savin W, Haskell RJ, and Houston-Miller N. Improvement in aerobic capacity soon after myocardial infarction. *Am Heart J.* 1981;44:1223–1229.
42. Balady GJ, Weiner DA, McCabe CH, and Ryan TJ. Value of arm exercise testing in detecting coronary artery disease. *Am J Cardiol.* 1985;55(1):37–39.
43. Franklin BA. Exercise testing, training and arm ergometry. *Sports Med.* 1985;2(2):100–119.
44. Toner MM, Glickman EL, and McArdle WD. Cardiovascular adjustments to exercise distributed between the upper and lower body. *Med Sci Sports Exerc.* 1990;22(6):773–778.
45. McArdle WD, Katch FI, and Katch VL. *Exercise Physiology: Energy, Nutrition and Human Performance.* 6th edn. Philadelphia, PA: Lippincott Williams & Wilkins, 2007.
46. Fardy P. Isometric exercise and the cardiovascular system. *Phys Sports Med.* 1981;309:45–54.
47. Ferguson R, Cote P, and Bourassa M. Coronary blood flow during isometric and dynamic exercise in angina pectoris patients. *J Can Rehabil.* 1981;1:21–27.
48. DeBusk R, Pitts W, Haskell W, and Houston N. Comparison of cardiovascular responses to static–dynamic effort and dynamic effort alone in patients with chronic ischemic heart disease. *Circulation* 1979;59(5):977–984.
49. Foster C, Gal RA, Murphy P, Port SC, and Schmidt DH. Left ventricular function during exercise testing and training. *Med Sci Sports Exerc.* 1997;29(3):297–305.
50. DeBusk RF, Taylor CB, and Agras WS. Comparison of treadmill exercise testing and psychologic stress testing soon after myocardial infarction. *Am J Cardiol.* 1979;43(5):907–912.
51. Mitchell JH, Payne FC, Saltin B, and Schibye B. The role of muscle mass in the cardiovascular response to static contractions. *J Physiol.* 1980;309:45–54.
52. Lind A and McNichol G. Muscular factors which determine cardiac responses to sustained and rhythmic exercise. *Can Med Assoc J.* 1967;96:706–715.
53. Sheldahl L, Wilke N, and Tristani F. Response to repetitive static–dynamic exercise in patients with coronary artery disease. *J Cardiopulm Rehabil.* 1985;5:139.
54. Lewis SF, Taylor WF, Graham RM, Pettinger WA, Schutte JE, and Blomqvist CG. Cardiovascular responses to exercise as functions of absolute and relative work load. *J Appl Physiol.* 1983;54(5):1314–1323.
55. Rodahl K. Methods for the assessment of physical work capacity and physical workload. In: Rodahl K, ed. *The Physiology of Work.* London: Taylor & Francis, 1989:51–72.
56. Ainsworth BE, Haskell WL, Whitt MC, et al. Compendium of physical activities: An update of activity codes and MET intensities. *Med Sci Sports Exerc.* 2000;32 (9 Suppl.):S498–504.
57. Franklin B and Hellerstein HK. Realistic stress testing for activity prescription. *J Cardiovasc Med.* 1982;7:570.
58. DeBusk RF, Blomqvist CG, Kouchoukos NT, et al. Identification and treatment of low-risk patients after acute myocardial infarction and coronary-artery bypass graft surgery. *N Engl J Med.* 1986;314(3):161–166.
59. Ford AB and Hellerstein HK. Work and heart disease. I. A physiologic study in the factory. *Circulation* 1958;18(5):823–832.
60. Ford AB, Hellerstein HK, and Turell DJ. Work and heart disease. II. A physiologic study in a steel mill. *Circulation* 1959;20:537–548.

61. Balady G, Fletcher B, Froelicher ES, Hartley LH, Krauss RM, and Oberman A. Cardiac Rehabilitation programs: A statement for health care professionals from the American Heart Association. *Circulation* 1994;90:1602–1610.
62. Pollock ML, Franklin BA, Balady GJ, et al. AHA Science Advisory. Resistance exercise in individuals with and without cardiovascular disease: Benefits, rationale, safety, and prescription: An advisory from the Committee on Exercise, Rehabilitation, and Prevention, Council on Clinical Cardiology, American Heart Association; Position paper endorsed by the American College of Sports Medicine. *Circulation* 2000;101(7):828–833.
63. Thompson PD. The benefits and risks of exercise training in patients with chronic coronary artery disease. *JAMA* 1988;259(10):1537–1540.
64. Lampert E, Mettauer B, Hoppeler H, Charloux A, Charpentier A, and Lonsdorfer J. Skeletal muscle response to short endurance training in heart transplant recipients. *J Am Coll Cardiol.* 1998;32(2):420–426.
65. Zoll J, N'Guessan B, Ribera F, et al. Preserved response of mitochondrial function to short-term endurance training in skeletal muscle of heart transplant recipients. *J Am Coll Cardiol.* 2003;42(1):126–132.
66. Coats AJ. Exercise training in heart failure. *Curr Control Trials Cardiovasc Med.* 2000;1(3):155–160.
67. Taylor CB, Houston-Miller N, Ahn DK, Haskell W, and DeBusk RF. The effects of exercise training programs on psychosocial improvement in uncomplicated postmyocardial infarction patients. *J Psychosom Res.* 1986;30(5):581–587.
68. Oldridge NB. Cardiac rehabilitation services: What are they and are they worth it? *Compr Ther.* 1991;17(5):59–66.
69. Gheorghiade M, Cody RJ, Francis GS, McKenna WJ, Young JB, and Bonow RO. Current medical therapy for advanced heart failure. *Heart Lung.* 2000;29(1):16–32.
70. Hertzeanu HL, Shemesh J, Aron LA, et al. Ventricular arrhythmias in rehabilitated and nonrehabilitated post-myocardial infarction patients with left ventricular dysfunction. *Am J Cardiol.* 1993;71(1):24–27.
71. Gutmann MC, Knapp DN, Pollock ML, Schmidt DH, Simon K, and Walcott G. Coronary artery bypass patients and work status. *Circulation* 1982;66(5 Pt 2):III33–III42.
72. Hedback B, Perk J, and Wodlin P. Long-term reduction of cardiac mortality after myocardial infarction: 10-year results of a comprehensive rehabilitation programme. *Eur Heart J.* 1993;14(6):831–835.
73. Simchen E, Naveh I, Zitser-Gurevich Y, Brown D, and Galai N. Is participation in cardiac rehabilitation programs associated with better quality of life and return to work after coronary artery bypass operations? The Israeli CABG Study. *Isr Med Assoc J.* 2001;3(6):399–403.
74. Engblom E, Korpilahti K, Hamalainen H, Ronnemaa T, and Puukka P. Quality of life and return to work 5 years after coronary artery bypass surgery. Long-term results of cardiac rehabilitation. *J Cardiopulm Rehabil.* 1997;17(1):29–36.
75. Lamm G, Denolin H, Dorossiev D, and Pisa Z. Rehabilitation and secondary prevention of patients after acute myocardial infarction. WHO collaborative study. *Adv Cardiol.* 1982;31:107–111.
76. Schiller E and Baker J. Return to work after a myocardial infarction: Evaluation of planned rehabilitation and of a predictive rating scale. *Med J Aust.* 1976;1(23):859–862.
77. Bengtsson K. Rehabilitation after myocardial infarction. A controlled study. *Scand J Rehabil Med.* 1983;15(1):1–9.
78. Carson P, Phillips R, Lloyd M, et al. Exercise after myocardial infarction: A controlled trial. *J R Coll Physicians Lond.* 1982;16(3):147–151.

79. Mayou R, MacMahon D, Sleight P, and Florencio MJ. Early rehabilitation after myocardial infarction. *Lancet* 1981;2(8260–8261):1399–1402.
80. Marra S, Paolillo V, Spadaccini F, and Angelino PF. Long-term follow-up after a controlled randomized post-myocardial infarction rehabilitation programme: Effects on morbidity and mortality. *Eur Heart J.* 1985;6(8):656–663.
81. Mital A, Shrey DE, Govindaraju M, Broderick TM, Colon-Brown K, and Gustin BW. Accelerating the return to work (RTW) chances of coronary heart disease (CHD) patients: Part 1. Development and validation of a training programme. *Disabil Rehabil.* 2000;22(13–14):604–620.
82. Wiklund I, Sanne H, Vedin A, and Wihelmsson C. Determinants of RTW one year after a first myocardial infarction. *J Cardiopulm Rehabil.* 1985;5:62–72.
83. Stolz I. Practical aspects of identifying and correcting worksite stress in post-infarction patients returning to work. *Eur Heart J.* 1988;9:82–83.
84. Feigenbaum MS and Pollock M. Strength training: Rationale for current guidelines for adult fitness programs. *Phys Sportsmed.* 1997;24:44–64.
85. Wiecek EM, McCartney N, and McKelvie RS. Comparison of direct and indirect measures of systemic arterial pressure during weightlifting in coronary artery disease. *Am J Cardiol.* 1990;66(15):1065–1069.
86. Kelemen MH. Resistive training safety and assessment guidelines for cardiac and coronary prone patients. *Med Sci Sports Exerc.* 1989;21(6):675–677.
87. Sparling PB, Cantwell JD, Dolan CM, and Niederman RK. Strength training in a cardiac rehabilitation program: A six-month follow-up. *Arch Phys Med Rehabil.* 1990;71(2):148–152.
88. Ghilarducci LE, Holly RG, and Amsterdam EA. Effects of high resistance training in coronary artery disease. *Am J Cardiol.* 1989;64(14):866–870.
89. Butler RM, Palmer G, and Rogers FJ. Circuit weight training in early cardiac rehabilitation. *J Am Osteopath Assoc.* 1992;92(1):77–89.
90. McCartney N, McKelvie RS, Haslam DR, and Jones NL. Usefulness of weightlifting training in improving strength and maximal power output in coronary artery disease. *Am J Cardiol.* 1991;67(11):939–945.
91. Haennel RG, Quinney HA, and Kappagoda CT. Effects of hydraulic circuit training following coronary artery bypass surgery. *Med Sci Sports Exerc.* 1991;23(2):158–165.
92. Faigenbaum AD, Skrinar GS, Cesare WF, Kraemer WJ, and Thomas HE. Physiologic and symptomatic responses of cardiac patients to resistance exercise. *Arch Phys Med Rehabil.* 1990;71(6):395–398.
93. Featherstone JF, Holly RG, and Amsterdam EA. Physiologic responses to weight lifting in coronary artery disease. *Am J Cardiol.* 1993;71(4):287–292.
94. Sheldahl LM, Wilke NA, Tristani FE, and Kalbfleisch JH. Response of patients after myocardial infarction to carrying a graded series of weight loads. *Am J Cardiol.* 1983;52(7):698–703.
95. Shrey DE and Mital A. Accelerating the return to work (RTW) chances of coronary heart disease (CHD) patients: Part 2—development and validation of a vocational rehabilitation programme. *Disabil Rehabil.* 2000;22(13–14):621–626.
96. Shanfield SB. Return to work after an acute myocardial infarction: A review. *Heart Lung.* 1990;19(2):109–117.
97. Litchfield RL, Kerber RE, Benge JW, et al. Normal exercise capacity in patients with severe left ventricular dysfunction: Compensatory mechanisms. *Circulation* 1982;66(1):129–134.
98. Gutmann M, Sheldahl L, Tristani F, et al. Returning the patient to work. In: Pollock M, Schmidt D, eds. *Heart Disease and Rehabilitation.* 3rd edn. Champaign, IL: Human Kinetics, 1995:405–421.

99. Mitchell D. Principles of vocational rehabilitation: A contemporary view. In: Long C, ed. *Prevention and Rehabilitation in Ischemic Heart Disease.* Baltimore: Williams & Wilkins, 1981:314–344.

100. Prior P and Cupper L. Behavioural, psychosocial and vocational issues in cardiovascular disease. In: Stone J, Arthur H, eds. *Canadian Guidelines for Cardiac Rehabilitation and Cardiovascular Disease Prevention.* Winnipeg: Canadian Association of Cardiac Rehabilitation, 2004:28–52.

101. Froelicher ES, Kee LL, Newton KM, Lindskog B, and Livingston M. Return to work, sexual activity, and other activities after acute myocardial infarction. *Heart Lung.* 1994;23(5):423–435.

102. Mark DB, Lam LC, Lee KL, et al. Identification of patients with coronary disease at high risk for loss of employment. A prospective validation study. *Circulation* 1992;86(5):1485–1494.

103. Dennis C. Vocational capacity with vocational impairment. In: Scheer S, ed. *Medical Perspectives in Vocational Assessment of Impaired Workers.* Rockville, MD: Aspen Publishers, 1990:301–334.

104. Smith GR Jr. and O'Rourke DF. Return to work after a first myocardial infarction: A test of multiple hypotheses. *JAMA* 1988;259(11):1673–1677.

105. Maeland JG and Havik OE. Return to work after a myocardial infarction: The influence of background factors, work characteristics and illness severity. *Scand J Soc Med.* 1986;14(4):183–195.

106. Sykes D, Hanley M, Boyle D, and Higginson J. Work strain and the post-discharge adjustment of patients following a heart attack. *Psychol Health.* 2000;15:609–623.

107. Kempen GI, Sanderman R, Miedema I, Meyboom-de Jong B, and Ormel J. Functional decline after congestive heart failure and acute myocardial infarction and the impact of psychological attributes. A prospective study. *Qual Life Res.* 2000;9(4): 439–450.

108. Manocchia M, Keller S, and Ware JE. Sleep problems, health-related quality of life, work functioning and health care utilization among the chronically ill. *Qual Life Res.* 2001;10(4):331–345.

109. Lewin R. Return to work after MI, the roles of depression, health beliefs and rehabilitation. *Int J Cardiol.* 1999;72(1):49–51.

110. Brody DS, Hahn SR, Spitzer RL, et al. Identifying patients with depression in the primary care setting: a more efficient method. *Arch Intern Med.* 1998;158(22):2469–2475.

111. Anderson A, Barboriak J, Hoffman R, Mullen D, and Walker J. Return to work following coronary artery bypass surgery: Age and sex, specific incidence, and main factors. In: Walter P, ed. *Return to Work after Coronary Artery Bypass Surgery: Pyschological and Economic Aspects.* New York: Springer-Verlag, 1985:3–12.

112. Iacovino V and Cupper L. Factors affecting return to work as identified by cardiac patients. *J Cardiopulm Rehabil.* 1996;16(5):330.

113. Siegrist K and Broer M. Employment after the first myocardial infarct and rehabilitation. *Sozial-und Praventivmedizin.* 1997;42(6):358–366.

114. Boudrez H, De Backer G, and Comhaire B. Return to work after myocardial infarction: results of a longitudinal population based study. *Eur Heart J.* 1994;15(1):32–36.

115. Mital A, Desai A, and Mital A. Return to work after a coronary event. *J Cardiopulm Rehabil.* 2004;24(6):365–373.

116. Ades PA, Waldmann ML, Polk DM, and Coflesky JT. Referral patterns and exercise response in the rehabilitation of female coronary patients aged greater than or equal to 62 years. *Am J Cardiol.* 1992;69(17):1422–1425.

117. Walter O, Thies B, and Gerhardt U. Patienten nehmen nach einer Koronaroperation ihre Arbeit wieder auf? *Med Klin.* 1983;78:276–280.

118. Lundborn J, Myhre H, Ystgaard B, et al. Factors influencing return to work after aortocoronary bypass surgery. *Scand J Thoracic Cardiovasc Surg.* 1992;26:187–192.

119. Rothlin M, Seiber R, and Senning A. Can aortocoronary bypass surgery improve return to work? In: Walter P, ed. *Return to Work after Coronary Artery Bypass Surgery: Pyschological and Social Aspects.* New York: Springer-Verlag, 1985: 323–331.

120. Sagall E. Legal aspects of rehabilitation after myocardial infarction and coronary artery bypass surgery. In: Wengler N, ed. *Rehabilitation and the Coronary Patient.* New York: John Wiley & Sons, 1984:493–511.

121. Mulcahy R, Kennedy C, and Conroy R. The long-term work record of post-infarction patients subjected to an informal rehabilitation and secondary prevention programme. *Eur Heart J.* 1988;9(Suppl. L):84–88.

122. Riegel BJ. Contributors to cardiac invalidism after acute myocardial infarction. *Coron Artery Dis.* 1993;4(2):215–220.

123. Petrie KJ, Weinman J, Sharpe N, and Buckley J. Role of patients' view of their illness in predicting return to work and functioning after myocardial infarction: Longitudinal study. *BMJ* 1996;312(7040):1191–1194.

124. Criteria Committee of the New York Heart Association. *Diseases of the Heart and Blood Vessels: Nomenclature and Criteria for Diagnosis.* 6th ed. Boston, MA Little Brown and Co., 1953, pp. 112–113.

125. Bandura A and Cervone D. Differential engagement of self-reactive influences in cognitive motivation. *Organ Behav Hum Des Process.* 1986;38:92–113.

126. Sarrafzadegan N, Habibi HR, Mirdamadi A, Maghsodlo S, and Sadegi K. Cardiac Rehabilitation exercise programme: Return to work as an outcome assessment. *Atherosclerosis* 1998;136(S1):84.

127. Mittag O, Kolenda KD, Nordman KJ, Bernien J, and Maurischat C. Return to work after myocardial infarction/coronary artery bypass grafting: Patients' and physicians' initial viewpoints and outcome 12 months later. *Soc Sci Med.* 2001;52(9):1441–1450.

128. Boudrez H and De Backer G. Recent findings on return to work after an acute myocardial infarction or coronary artery bypass grafting. *Acta Cardiol.* 2000;55(6):341–349.

129. Samkange Zeeb F, Altenhoner T, Berg G, and Schott T. Predicting non-return to work in patients attending cardiac rehabilitation. *Int J Rehab Res.* 2006;29(1):43–49.

130. Boll A, Klatt L, Koch J, and Langbehn AF. Psychosocial factors influencing return to work after coronary artery bypass surgery (CABS). *Int J Rehabil Res.* 1987;10(4 Suppl. 5):145–154.

131. Brines J, Salazar MK, Graham KY, and Pergola T. Return to work experience of injured workers in a case management program. *Aaohn J.* 1999;47(8):365–372.

132. Cay EL and Walker DD. Psychological factors and return to work. *Eur Heart J.* 1988;9 (Suppl. L):74–81.

133. Krause N, Dasinger LK, Deegan LJ, Rudolph L, and Brand RJ. Psychosocial job factors and return-to-work after compensated low back injury: A disability phase-specific analysis. *Am J Ind Med.* 2001;40(4):374–392.

134. Blumenthal JA, Bradley W, Dimsdale JE, Kasl SV, Powell LH, and Taylor CB. Task Force III: Assessment of psychological status in patients with ischemic heart disease. *J Am Coll Cardiol.* 1989;14(4):1034–1042.

135. Theorell T, Perski A, Orth-Gomer K, Hamsten A, and de Faire U. The effects of the strain of returning to work on the risk of cardiac death after a first myocardial infarction before the age of 45. *Int J Cardiol.* 1991;30(1):61–67.

136. Hillbrand M and Spitz R. *Lipids, Health and Behaviour,* Vol. 30. Washington, DC: American Psychological Association, 1997:61–67.

137. Frimerman A, Miller HI, Laniado S, and Keren G. Changes in hemostatic function at times of cyclic variation in occupational stress. *Am J Cardiol.* 1997;79(1):72–75.

138. Abbott J and Berry N. Return to work during the year following first myocardial infarction. *Br J Clin Psychol.* 1991;30(Pt 3):268–270.
139. Rost K and Smith GR. Return to work after an initial myocardial infarction and subsequent emotional distress. *Arch Intern Med.* 1992;152(2):381–385.
140. Mark DB, Lam LC, Lee KL, et al. Effects of coronary angioplasty, coronary bypass surgery, and medical therapy on employment in patients with coronary artery disease. A prospective comparison study. *Ann Intern Med.* 1994;120(2):111–117.
141. Burgess AW, Lerner DJ, D'Agostino RB, Vokonas PS, Hartman CR, and Gaccione P. A randomized control trial of cardiac rehabilitation. *Soc Sci Med.* 1987;24(4):359–370.
142. Hlatky MA, Haney T, Barefoot JC, et al. Medical, psychological and social correlates of work disability among men with coronary artery disease. *Am J Cardiol.* 1986;58(10):911–915.
143. AACVPR. *Guidelines for Cardiac Rehabilitation and Secondary Prevention Programs.* 3rd edn. Champaign, IL: Human Kinetics, 1999.
144. Dafoe WA, Franklin BA, and Cupper L. Vocational issues: Maximizing the patient's potential for returning to work. In: Pashkow FJ, Dafoe WA, eds. *Clinical Cardiac Rehabilitation: A Cardiologists' Guide.* Baltimore, MD: Williams and Wilkins, 1999:304–323.

Section C

Musculoskeletal Disorders

9 Musculoskeletal Disorders of the Upper Extremity and Ergonomic Interventions

Andris Freivalds

CONTENTS

9.1   EXTENT OF THE PROBLEM

In terms of the estimated magnitude of the musculoskeletal disorders (MSDs), the 1988 National Health Interview Survey found a prevalence of almost 15% for the U.S. population (Lawrence et al., 1998), which stayed relatively constant at 13.9% for the 1995 survey (Praemer et al., 1999). However, the Social Security Supplemental Security Income survey of 1998 did indicate a noticeable increase in prevalence with age, 16.9% for those 50–59 years of age and 23.9% for those 60–65 years of age. In terms of upper limb MSDs, the 1988 National Health Interview Survey found a prevalence of 9.4% in the hand or wrist, with 1.5% being specifically carpal tunnel syndrome and 0.4% being tendinitis (Tanaka et al., 1995). Interestingly when based on reported symptoms, the prevalence for carpal tunnel syndrome can be as high as 14.4%, but when referred for a clinical diagnosis the prevalence drops to 2.7% (Atroshi et al., 1999). A historical trend in MSDs is provided by the Occupational Safety and Health Administration in the Form 300 data. The number of cases labeled "disorders associated with repeated trauma" was relatively steady from 1976 to 1982 at around 22,000, then increased sharply to 332,100 by 1994, at which point there was a gradual reduction to 246,700 by 1999. This recent decline was speculated to have occurred as a result of a better recognition of such MSDs and the implementation of industrial health and safety programs (Conway and Svenson, 1998).

9.2   COMMON MUSCULOSKELETAL DISORDERS AND THEIR ETIOLOGY

There are a large variety of MSDs that have some commonality both in the physiological or anatomical characteristics and in the general location of the problem (see Figure 9.1). For introducing and describing common MSDs it is best to categorize them by the anatomical characteristics, while later, in providing more detailed scientific evidence for risk factors, it is best to categorize them by joints. It would not be unusual for a complaining worker or the medically untrained ergonomist lump medically different disorders into one collective "shoulder" disorder, since, probably, neither can identify the disorder more specifically. From the anatomical viewpoint, MSDs can be classified into six basic types: tendon, muscle, nerve, vascular, bursa, and bone/cartilage.

9.2.1   TENDON DISORDERS

The tendon is the part of the muscle and the surrounding fascia transmitting force from the muscle that attaches to the bone and produces joint motion. In places where there is a great deal of movement (e.g., fingers, wrist, shoulder) the tendon may pass through a sheath that protects and lubricates the tendon to reduce friction. When this sheath and the tendon within become inflamed, it is termed tenosynovitis. When a tendon without the sheath becomes inflamed, it is termed tendinitis. This inflammation can progress to the point of having microtrauma or even visible fraying of the tendon fibers. Sometimes, the disorders are further identified by the sublevel where found on the tendon. Enthesopathy or insertional tendinitis occurs at the tendon–bone interface with relatively little inflammation. A common one is enthesopathy of the extensor

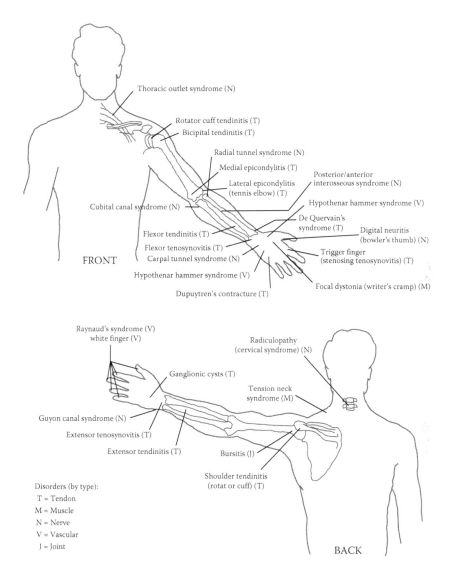

Thoracic outlet syndrome (N)

Rotator cuff tendinitis (T)
Bicipital tendinitis (T)

Radial tunnel syndrome (N)
Medial epicondylitis (T)

Posterior/anterior
interosseous syndrome (N)

Lateral epicondylitis
(tennis elbow) (T)

Hypothenar hammer syndrome (V)

Cubital canal syndrome (N)

De Quervain's
syndrome (T)

Digital neuritis
(bowler's thumb) (N)

Flexor tendinitis (T)

Flexor tenosynovitis (T)

Carpal tunnel syndrome (N)

Trigger finger
(stenosing tenosynovitis) (T)

Hypothenar hammer syndrome (V)

FRONT

Dupuytren's contracture (T)

Focal dystonia (writer's cramp) (M)

Raynaud's syndrome (V)
white finger (V)

Radiculopathy
(cervical syndrome) (N)

Ganglionic cysts (T)

Tension neck
syndrome (M)

Guyon canal syndrome (N)

Extensor tenosynovitis (T)

Extensor tendinitis (T)

Bursitis (J)

Shoulder tendinitis
(rotat or cuff) (T)

Disorders (by type):
T = Tendon
M = Muscle
N = Nerve
V = Vascular
J = Joint

BACK

FIGURE 9.1 Examples of MSDs which may be work related. (Reproduced from Kuorinka, I. and Forcier, L., *Work Related Musculoskeletal Disorders (WMSDs): A Reference Book for Prevention*, Taylor & Francis, London, 1995. With permission.)

carpi radialis brevis from the lateral epicondyle, resulting from forceful, twisting motions, which then is referred to as lateral epicondylitis, or more commonly as tennis elbow. Peritendinitis refers to the inflammation of the tendon proper, where there is no tendon sheath, while the inflammation of the muscle–tendon interface is termed myotendinitis. Although, technically they are all different disorders, they are often found together and exhibit similar symptoms of localized pain and tenderness and are typically collectively referred to as tendinitis. Two common examples of tendinitis are bicipital tendinitis, or inflammation of the long head of the biceps tendon as it passes over the head of the humerus through the bicipital groove caused by hyperabducting the elbow or forceful contractions of the biceps, and rotator cuff tendinitis, inflammation of tendons of various muscles around the shoulder (supraspinatus, infraspinatus, teres minor) caused from abducted arms or arms raised above the shoulders.

Acute cases of tenosynovitis may develop localized swelling, a narrowing or stenosing of the sheath, and even the formation of a nodule on the tendon, causing the tendon to become temporarily entrapped or triggered as it attempts to slide through the sheath. If this occurs in the index finger, typically used in repeatedly and forcefully activating a power tool, it is colloquially termed trigger finger. Many times, upon attempting to straighten the finger and stretching the tendon, the tendon will crackle or crepitate leading to the more complete term of stenosing tenosynovitis crepitans. Other examples of tenosynovitis in the hand include DeQuervain's disease with inflammation of the tendons of the abductor pollicis longus and extensor pollicis brevis of the thumb. Repetitive forceful motions of the thumb in a variety of tasks, even games, lead to such problems and also to names popularized in the media referring back to those tasks, e.g., Atari or Nintendo thumb (Reinstein, 1983). Dupuytren's contracture is formation of nodules in the palmar fascia, an extension of the tendon of the palmaris longus muscle, leading to triggering of the ring and little fingers. Tenosynovitis of the flexor tendons (carpi, digitorum profundus, and superficialias) within the wrist from repeated forceful wrist motion may lead to carpal tunnel syndrome. Similarly repeated opening of scissors or other tools may lead to tenosynovitis in the extensor tendons in the fingers. A by-product of tenosynovitis is the excess release of synovial fluid which may collect and form fluid-filled ganglionic cysts that appear as nodules under the skin on the surface of the hand.

The mechanism of injury for tendon disorders depends on a variety of factors, some of which have been studied in animals. Exercise with controlled conditions can have positive long-term effects by increasing tendon cross-sectional area and strength. Remodeling of the tendon can occur with the laying down of additional fibrocartilaginous tissue (Woo et al., 1980). However, when the exercise becomes excessive (high rates of loading in rabbits), there are degenerative changes in the tendon with increased number of capillaries, inflammatory cells, edema, microtears, and separation of fibers consistent with pathology of tendinosis in humans. Elevated temperatures and hypoxia in the core of the tendon may play a role in these degenerative changes (Backman et al., 1990). When a tendon experiences compressive loading in addition to tension, e.g., curving around a bone or ligament as in the Armstrong and Chaffin (1978) tendon-pulley model, the tendon becomes transformed from linear bands of collagen fascicles into irregular patterned fibrocartilage with changes in the proteoglycans (Malaviya et al., 2000). Coincidentally, tendon strength, at least in rats, decreases with age (Simonsen et al., 1995).

9.2.2 MUSCLE DISORDERS

Muscle disorders start as simple muscle soreness or pain, termed myalgia, in workers, both old and especially new, performing unaccustomed strenuous or repetitive work. The affected area will be sore and tender to touch because of microstrain and inflammation of the tissue, termed myositis. If the work is soon stopped (e.g., a one-time job or a weekend activity), relief will occur in several days. If the work is continued in a gradual manner (i.e., a break-in period), generally, a conditioning process occurs, the muscle heals, becomes accustomed to task, and becomes more resistant to injury. However, if the work is continued in an excessive manner (i.e., few rest periods, frequent overtime), the muscle strain and myalgia become chronic and the disorder becomes myofascial pain syndrome. The muscle may spasm, dysfunction, and temporary disability may result. In chronic stages, the disorder is characterized by chronically painful spastic muscles, tingling sensations, nervousness and sleeplessness and is termed fibromyalgia or fibrositis. It is aggravated by both repeated activities and also, paradoxically, by rest; it may be worse upon rising in the morning. Another characteristic of fibromyalgia is the presence of trigger points, small areas of spastic muscle that is tender to touch surrounded by unaffected muscle. Pressure on these trigger points will often result in pain shooting up or down the extremity. Details on trigger points and treatments of these disorders can be found in Travell and Simons (1983).

One specific and rather common myofascial syndrome is the tension-neck syndrome, characterized by pain and tenderness in the shoulder and neck region for clerical workers and small-parts assemblers, who typically are slightly hunched forward for better visibility and have contracted the upper back (trapezius) and neck muscles (Kuorinka and Forcier, 1995). More active and excessive muscle contraction may lead to writer's cramp or focal dystonia. It was first noticed in Victorian England in scriveners who were responsible for copying contracts by hand using quills gripped firmly. The resulting spasms were first described in detail by Wilks (1878) and later by others (Sheehy and Marsden, 1982) resulting from the repetitive forceful contractions of the hand with complications induced by cocontractions of the forearm flexors and extensors. The problem is that individuals tend to overgrip tools or other objects by as much as a factor of 5. The problem is further exacerbated by carpal tunnel syndrome or other neurological disorders, which reduce sensory feedback and increase overgripping to a factor of 10 (Lowe and Freivalds, 1999).

The mechanism of injury for muscle disorders is quite different from tendon disorders. Typically, muscle injury occurs as the result of excessive external forces on the passive structures, mainly connective tissue, rather than from overuse. Excessive muscle use will result in muscle fatigue limiting contractile capability before cellular damage can occur. This fatigue is due to intramuscular pressure exceeding capillary pressure (about 30 mmHg), causing ischemia and hypoxia to the active muscle fibers (Sjøgaard and Søgaard, 1998), which then may contribute to alterations in the intracellular pH, lactic acid, calcium and potassium concentrations and may upset overall homeostasis (Sjøgaard and Jensen, 1997). Eccentric contractions, in which external loads cause the sarcomeres to length during active cross-bridging, are also likely to cause structural damage, inflammation, hemorrhaging, and loss of force-generating capacity (McCully and Faulkner, 1985). Based on an exponential relationship that exists between stress and the number of cycles, with greater stress requiring fewer cycles, there should be a theoretical stress limit, below which injury could be avoided (Warren et al., 1993). However, no such value has been derived for human muscle. There are also indications that passive stretch (Noonan et al., 1994) and vibration (Necking et al., 1966) contribute to muscle injury. As for tendons, there are age-related changes in skeletal muscle, with a gradual decrease in strength starting at age 40 years and increasing more dramatically after age 65 years (Faulkner et al., 1990).

9.2.3 NERVE DISORDERS

Nerve entrapment occurs between two different tissues, muscles, bones, ligaments, or other structures, and may be due to a variety of diseases, such as hyperthyroidism or arthritis, vascular disorders or edema, in addition to chronic work-related trauma. During entrapment, pressure on the nerve will impair blood flow and oxygenation of the Schwann cells and the myelin sheath with consequent affects on axonal transport system and production of action potentials. If the pressure is high enough, mechanical blocking of the depolarization process will occur (Lundborg, 1988). A complicating factor is that entrapment at one location of the nerve (which may be up to 1 m in length) increases the susceptibility to further injury at points either distal or proximal to the first location, due to impairment of the axonal flows of ions. This multiple entrapment, known as the double crush syndrome, makes it even more important that ergonomists consider the whole extremity when analyzing a job and diagnosing potential problems.

The most common nerve entrapment of the upper limbs is carpal tunnel syndrome. The carpal tunnel is formed by eight carpal bones on the dorsal side and the transverse carpal ligament (flexor retinaculum, which serves to prevent bowstringing) on the palmar side of the wrist (see Figure 9.2). Through this tunnel, in a tight fit, pass various blood vessels, flexor tendons, and the median nerve, which innervates the index and middle fingers and parts of the thumb and ring finger. Any additional increase in the contents of the tunnel will increase the pressure on the median nerve with consequent disruption of nerve conduction. This may occur in pregnant females when additional water retention results in swelling of the contents of carpal tunnel (Punnett et al., 1985) or in clerical, assembly, garment, and food processing workers from forceful repetitive wrist flexions/extensions or ulnar/radial deviations. The resulting friction of the tendons when sliding through their sheaths wrapped around the carpal tunnel bones or ligaments in the Armstrong and Chaffin (1978) tendon-pulley model (presented in Section 14.3.1) is compensated by additional secretions of synovial fluid. This causes swelling, increases resting carpal canal pressures by up to a factor of 3 (Okutsu et al., 1989), and compresses the median nerve resulting in shooting pains, especially at night, tingling and numbness, and loss of fine motor control to the above-mentioned fingers.

Two other nerves, ulnar and radial, pass through the wrist area, although, not through the carpal tunnel. The ulnar nerve enters the hand at Guyon's canal on the medial (little finger) side, innervating the little finger and part of the ring finger. Sometimes the ulnar nerve is entrapped leading to the Guyon canal syndrome with tingling and numbness of the associated fingers. The ulnar nerve may also be trapped further back in either the ulnar groove or the cubital tunnel formed by the two heads of the flexor carpi ulnaris near the elbow in the cubital tunnel syndrome as a result of direct pressure on the area from resting the elbows on sharp table edges or twisting motions at the elbow. Symptoms include pain and soreness at the medial elbow and tingling and numbness in the associated fingers. An acute blow to the ulnar nerve at the ulnar groove results in the "funny bone" sensation.

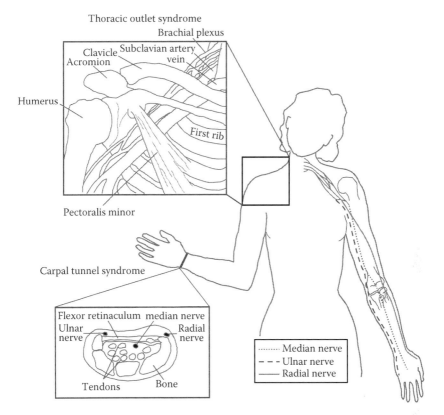

FIGURE 9.2 Carpal tunnel and thoracic outlet syndromes. (Reproduced from Kuorinka, I. and Forcier, L., *Work Related Musculoskeletal Disorders (WMSDs): A Reference Book for Prevention*, Taylor & Francis, London, 1995. With permission.)

The radial nerve also passes into the forearm just below the lateral epicondyle near the head of the radius. Compression of the nerve due to a contracted muscle or bones will result in localized pain and tenderness and tingling and numbness in the thumb, termed the radial tunnel syndrome. A similar effect will result from an entrapment of a deep branch of the radial nerve (interosseous) within the supinator muscles of the forearm in the Arcade of Frohse in the posterior interosseous syndrome. This condition will also show a weakness in extensor muscles for the wrist and little finger.

The median nerve can similarly be trapped both at the elbow, in the pronator teres syndrome, and in the forearm, in the anterior interosseous syndrome. In the first case, the median nerve is trapped beneath the two heads of the pronator teres muscle, due to inflammation and swelling of muscle from constant pronation as in the classic "clothes wringing" motion. Symptoms include spasm and tightness of the pronator teres muscle resulting in pain on the palm side of forearm and symptoms distally that are similar to those of carpal tunnel syndrome and may result in misdiagnosis. The only difference is that the palmar cutaneous branch of median nerve branches off before the carpal tunnel. Therefore it will produce impaired sensations in the palm in the pronator teres syndrome but not the carpal tunnel syndrome (Parker and Imbus, 1992). In the second case, the anterior interosseus branch of the median nerve can be compressed by the deep anterior forearm muscles from overuse. Since the nerve innervates muscles in midforearm and the flexor pollicis longus, symptoms include pain in the front of the forearm and difficulty producing an O-shaped pattern in a thumb-index fingertip pinch (Parker and Imbus, 1992).

Further back on the upper limb, the thoracic outlet syndrome is entrapment of the brachial plexus (and also the subclavian artery and vein) in one or more different sites: the scalenus muscles in the neck, between the clavicle and first rib and between the chest wall and the pectoralis minor muscle. Symptoms include numbness or tingling and pain in the arm and hand, especially on the ulnar side. Even the spinal nerve roots that form the brachial plexus (cervical vertebrae C5, C6, C7, and C8) may be compressed between the intervertebral openings in cervical radiculopathy. These openings may narrow due to degenerative disc disease or arthritis, which may be further exacerbated by repetitive neck motions. Symptoms include tingling and numbness and pain radiating to various locales determined by the innervation of the appropriate nerve root.

In a different type of nerve disorder, digital neuritis, direct pressure while grasping tools (e.g., scissors) or other items with sharp edges may result in inflammation and swelling of the underlying nerve and eventual numbness in the associated digit. Again the aggravating task or item may lead to descriptive colloquial names such as bowler's thumb (Howell and Leach, 1970; Dunham et al., 1972) or cherry pitter's thumb (Viegas and Torres, 1989).

Extraneural compression pressures as low as 30 mmHg decrease intraneural flow and impair axonal transport within peripheral neurons. After several hours of compression, inflammation leads to fibrin deposits, proliferation of fibroblasts, which after several days leads growth of fibrous tissues. After 1 week, demyelination and axonal degeneration are observed, with the degree of injury correlated with the external pressure (Dyck et al., 1990). Chronic nerve compression in rats shows a similar etiologic pattern ending in nerve fiber degeneration (Sommer et al., 1993; Mosconi and Kruger, 1996). Vibration exposure shows similar edema formation, demyelination, and ultimately nerve degeneration both experimentally induced in rats (Chang et al., 1994) as well as from occupational exposure in humans (Strömberg et al., 1997). Although experimental studies on spinal nerve root compression are much less common than for peripheral nerves, the injury mechanisms appear to be similar. Direct acute mechanical compression leads to intraneural edema and subsequent fibrosis (Rydevik et al., 1976). Chronic nerve compression may be less severe with changes evolving gradually allowing for adaptation of the axons and vasculature. On the other hand, the compression leads to an increase in neurotransmitters that stimulate pain transmission (Cornefjord et al., 1997).

9.2.4 VASCULAR DISORDERS

In vascular disorders, one or more of three different factors, vibration, cold temperatures, and direct pressure, cause ischemia of the blood supply to nerves and muscle resulting in hypoxia to the tissue with tingling, numbness and loss of fine control. In the hand–arm vibration syndrome (HAVS) vibration (e.g., from power tools) activates the smooth muscle surrounding arterioles causing a clamping action and loss of blood flow (ischemia) to the hand, resulting in a blanching or the colloquial white finger syndrome. This will also result in numbness and an inability to perform precision work. Cold temperatures have a very similar ischemic effect on the arterioles through a local vasoconstrictor reflex. However, some individuals, especially women in northern climates, have an especially pronounced response leading to painful sensations, termed Raynaud's syndrome. The prevalence for HAVS increases markedly when there is a combination of vibration from power tool usage in cold environments, e.g., railroad work (Yu et al., 1986), stone cutting (Taylor et al., 1984), mining (Hedlund, 1989), and forestry work (Olsen and Nielsen, 1988). Vibration also happens to be a major factor in carpal tunnel syndrome.

Direct pressure on the circulatory vessels can also cause ischemia and loss of fine motor control, effects similar to vibration or cold. This can occur in the thoracic outlet syndrome, where the subclavian vessels are in close proximity to the brachial plexus and are similarly entrapped within the shoulder area, or in the hypothenar hammer syndrome, where the ulnar artery is compressed against the hypothenar eminence (muscle below the little and ring fingers) during hand hammering.

9.2.5 BURSA DISORDERS

Bursitis is inflammation of bursae, closed sacs filled with synovial fluid. Bursae are usually located in areas with potential for friction and help facilitate the motion of tendons and muscles over bone protuberances, especially around joints. Bursitis may be caused by friction, trauma, inflammatory diseases such as rheumatoid arthritis, and by bacteria. In the upper limbs, it is found at the elbow (olecranon bursa) and the shoulder (subacromial bursitis), the latter developing as part of the degeneration of the rotator cuff tendons. The most common occupationally induced bursitis, however, is in the knee (prepatellar bursitis) found in carpet layers due to the kneeling posture and use of the knee kicker (Thun et al., 1987).

9.2.6 BONE AND CARTILAGE DISORDERS

Arthritis can be of two forms: rheumatoid arthritis, which is a generalized inflammatory process associated with diseases such as gout, and osteorthritis, which is a degenerative process of joint cartilage. Despite an increase in cartilage water content and increased synthesis of proteoglycans, the cartilage decreases in thickness, with increased trauma to subchondral bone resulting in sclerosis. How the process begins is quite unclear. Many cases are idiopathic, having no clear predisposing factors, while other cases may occur as a result of specific trauma or injury to the joint. There is some evidence that repetitive work such as lifting may contributed to osteoarthritis severity in the shoulder joint (Stenlund et al., 1992).

9.3 UPPER EXTREMITY MODELS

Considering that the human hand alone has some 27 bones, 20 major joints, 33 major muscles, and 8 tendon pulley sheaths per digit, modeling the upper extremity completely can be quite difficult. Only simple basic models will be presented here, to serve as a starting point for understanding the complexities of the system and the potential sources for development of MSDs.

9.3.1 STATIC TENDON-PULLEY MODELS

Landsmeer (1960, 1962) developed three biomechanical models for finger flexor tendon displacements, in which the tendon–joint displacement relationships are determined by the spatial relationships between the tendons and joints. In Model I (see Figure 9.3a), he assumed that the tendon is held securely against the curved articular surface of the proximal bone of the joint, and the proximal articular surface can be described as a trochlea. Such a model is particularly useful in describing extensor muscles. The tendon displacement relationship is described by

$$x = R\theta \tag{9.1}$$

where
   x is the tendon displacement
   R is the distance from the joint center to the tendon
   θ is the joint rotation angle

However, if the tendon is not held securely, it may be displaced from the joint when the joint is flexed and will settle in a position along the bisection of the joint angle (see Figure 9.3). Model II is useful for describing tendon displacement in intrinsic muscles as

$$x = 2R\sin(\theta/2) \tag{9.2}$$

Landsmeer's (1960) Model III depicts a tendon running through a tendon sheath held securely against the bone, which allows the tendon to curve smoothly around the joint (see Figure 9.3c). The tendon displacement is described by

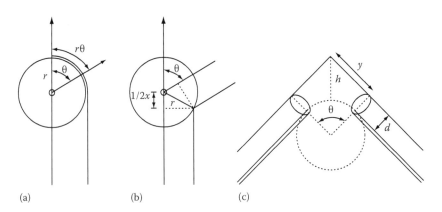

(a)   (b)   (c)

FIGURE 9.3 Landsmeer's tendon models: (a) Model I, (b) Model II, and (c) Model III. (Adapted from Landsmeer, J.M.F., *Ann. Rheumat. Dis.*, 21, 164, 1962.)

$$x = 2\left[y + \tfrac{1}{2}\theta \left(d - y / \tan \tfrac{1}{2}\theta \right) \right] \tag{9.3}$$

where
  y is the tendon length to joint axis measured along long axis of bone
  d is the distance of tendon to the long axis of bone

For small angles of flexion ($\theta < 20°$), $\tan \theta$ is almost equal to θ, and Equation 9.3 simplifies to

$$x = d\theta \tag{9.4}$$

Armstrong and Chaffin (1979) proposed a static model for the wrist based on Landsmeer's (1962) tendon Model I and LeVeau's (1977) pulley-friction concepts (see Figure 9.4). Armstrong and Chaffin (1978) found that, when the wrist is flexed, the flexor tendons are supported by flexor retinaculum on the volar side of the carpal tunnel. When the wrist is extended, the flexor tendons are supported by the carpal bones. Thus, deviation of the wrist from neutral position causes the tendons to be displaced against and past the adjacent walls of the carpal tunnel. They assumed that a tendon sliding over a curved surface is analogous to a belt incurring friction forces while wrapped around a pulley. The radial reaction force on the ligament or the carpal bones, F_R, can be characterized as follows:

$$F_R = 2F_T e^{\mu\Theta} \sin(\theta/2) \tag{9.5}$$

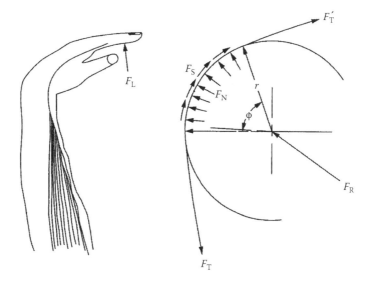

FIGURE 9.4 Armstrong tendon-pulley model for the wrist. (Reproduced from Chaffin, D.B., Andersson, G.B.J., and Martin, B.J., *Occupational Biomechanics*, 4th edn., John Wiley & Sons, New York, 2006. With permission.)

where

F_R is the radial reaction force
F_T is the tendon force or belt tension
μ is the coefficient of friction between tendon and supporting tissues
θ is the wrist deviation angle (in radians)

The resulting normal forces on the tendon exerted by the pulley surface can be expressed per unit arc length as

$$F_N = \frac{2\,F_T e^{\mu\Theta} \sin\left(\theta/2\right)}{R\theta} \tag{9.6}$$

where

F_N is the normal forces exerted on tendon
R is the radius of curvature around supporting tissues

For small coefficient of frictions, comparable to what is found in joints ($\mu < 0.04$) and for small angles of θ, Equation 9.6 reduces to the simple expression:

$$F_N = F_T / R \tag{9.7}$$

Thus F_N is a function of only the tendon force and the radius of curvature. As the tendon force increases or the radius of curvature decreases (e.g., small wrists), the normal supporting force exerted on tendon increases. F_R, on the other hand, is independent of radius of curvature but is dependent on the wrist deviation angle.

This tendon-pulley model provides a relatively simple mechanism for calculating the normal supporting force exerted on tendons that are a major factor in work related musculoskeletal disorders (WRMSDs). However, this model does not include the dynamic components of wrist movements such as angular velocity and acceleration, which might be risk factors in WRMSDs.

9.3.2 DYNAMIC TENDON-PULLEY MODELS

Schoenmarklin and Marras's (1990) dynamic biomechanical model extended Armstrong and Chaffin's (1979) static model to include dynamic component of angular acceleration (see Figure 9.5). The dynamic model is two-dimensional in that only the forces in flexion and extension plane are analyzed. This model investigates the effects of maximum angular acceleration on the resultant reaction force that the wrist ligaments and carpal bones exert on tendons and their sheaths.

Key forces and movements in the model include the reaction force at the center of the wrist (W_x and W_y), the couple or moment (M_w) required to flex and extend the wrist, and the inertial force ($M \times A_n$ and $M \times A_t$) and inertial moment ($I \times \ddot{\Theta}$) acting around the hand's center of mass. For equilibrium, the magnitude of moment around the wrist in the free body diagram must equal the magnitude of moment acting around the hand's center of mass in the moment acceleration diagram:

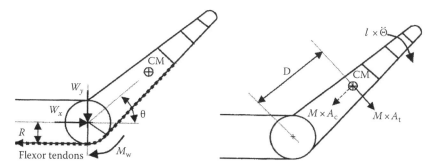

FIGURE 9.5 Dynamic tendon-pulley model for the wrist. (Adapted from Schoenmarklin, R.W. and Marras, W.P., *Proceedings of the Human Factors Society 34th Annual Meeting*, Santa Monica, CA: Human Factors Society, 1990, pp. 805–809.)

$$F_T \times R = (M \times A_t + M \times A_n) \times D + I \times \ddot{\Theta} \qquad (9.8)$$

where
  M is the mass
  A_t is the tangential acceleration
  A_c is the centripetal acceleration
  F_T is the tendon force
  I is the moment of inertia of the hand in flexion and extension
  $\ddot{\Theta}$ is the angular acceleration

Thus, the hand is assumed to accelerate from a stationary posture, so, the angular velocity is theoretically zero, resulted in zero centripetal force ($A_c = V^2/R = 0$). Then,

$$F_t \times R = (M \times A_t) \times D + I \times \ddot{\Theta} \qquad (9.9)$$

$$F_t \times R = (M \times D \times \ddot{\Theta}) \times D + I \times \ddot{\Theta} \qquad (9.10)$$

$$F_t = \frac{(M \times D^2 + I) \times \ddot{\Theta}}{R} \qquad (9.11)$$

$$F_R = 2 \times \left(\frac{(M \times D^2 + I) \times \ddot{\Theta}}{R} \right) \times \sin\left(\frac{\theta}{2}\right) \qquad (9.12)$$

where
    R is the radius of curvature of the tendon
    D is the distance between the center of mass of hand and wrist
    M is the weight of hand
    θ is the wrist deviation angle

The above equations indicate that the resultant reaction force, F_R, is a function of angular acceleration, radius of curvature, and wrist deviation. Thus, exertion of wrist and hand with greater angular acceleration and deviated wrist angle would result in greater total resultant reaction forces on the tendons and supporting tissues than exertions with small angular acceleration and neutral wrist position. According to Armstrong and Chaffin (1979), increases in resultant reaction force would increase the supporting force that the carpal bones and ligaments exert on the flexor tendons, therefore increasing the chance of inflammation and risk of carpel tunnel syndrome (CTS). Therefore, these results might provide theoretical support to why angular acceleration variable can be considered a risk factor of WRMSDs.

The advantage of Schoenmarklin and Marras (1990) model is that it does include the dynamic variable of angular acceleration into assessment of resultant reaction force on the tendons. But the model is two-dimensional, and it does not consider the coactivation of antagonistic muscles in wrist joint motions. This points to the need for further model developments to account for additional physiological factors.

9.4 ERGONOMIC INTERVENTIONS IN HAND TOOLS

Since tools, as we know them, were developed as extension of the upper extremities to reinforce the strength and the effectiveness of these limbs, this section will focus primarily on ergonomic interventions in hand tools. Approximately 6% of all compensable work injuries and 10% of all industrial injuries in the United States are caused by the use of hand tools (Mital and Sanghavi, 1986; Aghazadeh and Mital, 1987). This means over 73,000 injuries involving at least 1 work day lost amounting to over $10 billion annually in costs (Bureau of Labor Statistics, 1995). The most injured body parts by both nonpowered and powered hand tools were the upper extremities (59.3% and 51.0%, respectively) followed by back, trunk, and lower extremities. Fingers accounted for 56% of upper extremity injuries or about 30% of all body parts (Aghazadeh and Mital, 1987).

9.4.1 GENERAL TOOL PRINCIPLES

1. An efficient tool has to fulfill some basic requirements (Drillis, 1963): It must perform effectively the function for which it is intended. Thus an axe should convert a maximum amount of its kinetic energy into useful chopping work, separate cleanly wood fibers and be easily withdrawn.
2. It must be properly proportioned to the body dimensions of the operator to maximize efficiency of human involvement.
3. It must be designed to the strength and work capacity of the operator. Thus allowances have to be made for the gender, training, and physical fitness of the operator.

4. It should not cause undue fatigue, i.e., it should not demand unusual postures or practices that will require more energy expenditure than necessary.
5. It must provide sensory feedback in the form pressure, some shock, texture, temperature, etc. to the user.
6. The capital and maintenance cost should be reasonable.

9.4.2 ANATOMY AND TYPES OF GRIP

The human hand is a complex structure of bones, arteries, nerves, ligaments, and tendons. The fingers are controlled by the extensor carpi and flexor carpi muscles in the forearm. The muscles are connected to the fingers by tendons which pass through a channel in the wrist, formed by the bones of the back of the hand on one side and the transverse carpal ligament on the other. Through this channel, called the carpal tunnel, pass also various arteries and nerves. The bones of the wrist connect to two long bones in the forearm, the ulna, and the radius. The radius connects to the thumb side of the wrist and ulna connects to the little finger side of the wrist. The orientation of the wrist joint allows movement in only two planes, each at 90° to the other. The first gives rise to palmar flexion and dorsiflexion. The second movement plane gives ulnar and radial deviation. The ulna and radius of the forearm connect to the humerus of the upper arm. The biceps brachii, brachialis, and brachoradialis control elbow flexion and to some degree supination (outward rotation) of the wrist. The triceps acts as an elbow extensor.

Probably the most unique feature of the above upper extremity is the manual, dexterity produced by the hand. Napier (1956) defined the prehensile movements of the human hand in terms of a power grip and a precision grip. In a power grip the tool, whose axis is more or less perpendicular to the forearm, is held in a clamp formed by the partly flexed fingers and the palm, with opposing pressure being applied by the thumb (see Figure 9.6). There are three subcategories of the power

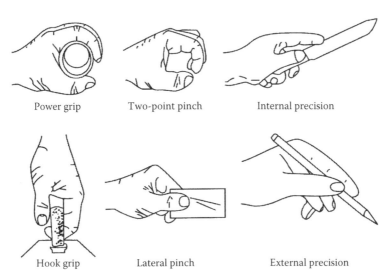

FIGURE 9.6 Types of grip. (Reproduced from Freivalds, A., *Occupational Ergonomic Handbook*, W. Karwowski and W. S. Marras (ed.), New York: CRC Press, 1999, pp. 461–478. With permission.)

grip, differentiated by the line of action of force: (1) force parallel to the forearm, as in sawing; (2) force at an angle to forearm, as in hammering; and (3) torque about the forearm, as when using a screwdriver. As the name implies, the power grip is used for power or for holding heavy objects (Bendz, 1974).

In a precision grip, the tool is pinched between the flexor aspects of the fingers and the opposing thumb. The relative position of the thumb and fingers determines how much force is to be applied and provides sensory surface for receiving feedback necessary to give the precision needed. There are two types of precision grip (see Figure 9.6): (1) internal, in which the shaft of the tool (e.g., knife) passes under the thumb and is thus internal to the hand; and (2) external, in which the shaft (e.g., pencil) passes over the thumb and is thus external to the hand. The precision grip is used for control. There is also the hook grip, which is used to support weight by the fingers only, as in holding a box, a lateral pinch, as in holding a key, a pulp or tip pinches, depending if the pulpy part or nails of the fingers touch. A finer gradation of grips is also possible, as presented by Kroemer (1986). Note that all of these pinches have a significantly decreased strength capability as compared to the power grip (see Table 9.1) and, therefore, large forces should never be applied using pinch grips.

One theory of gripping forces has been described by Pheasant and O'Neill (1975). The hand gripping a cylindrical handle forms a closed system of forces in which portions of the digits and palm are used, in opposition to each other, to exert compressive forces on the handle (Figure 9.7). The strength of the grip (G) may be defined as the sum of all components of forces exerted normal to the surface of the handle:

$$G = \Sigma g \tag{9.13}$$

When exerting a turning action on the handle, the maximum torque, at the moment of hand slippage, is given by

$$T = SD \tag{9.14}$$

where
   T is the torque
   S is the total frictional or shear force
   D is the handle diameter

TABLE 9.1

Relative Forces for Different Types of Grips

Grip	Male (N)	Female (N)	% of Power Grip
Power grip	400	228	100
Tip pinch	65	45	18
Pulp pinch	61	43	17
Lateral pinch	109	76	30

Source: Adapted from An, K.N., Askew, L.J., and Chao, E.Y. Biomechanics and functional assessment of upper extremities, in W. Karwowski (ed.) *Trends in Ergonomics/Human Factors III*, Amsterdam: Elsevier, pp. 573–580, 1986.

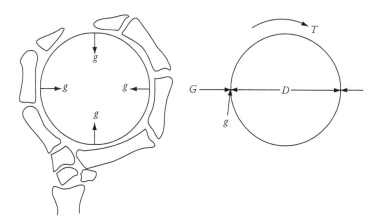

FIGURE 9.7 The mechanics of gripping. (Reproduced from Freivalds, A., *Int. Rev. Ergon.* 1, 43, 1987. With permission.)

and *S* can be defined by

$$S = \mu G \tag{9.15}$$

where μ is the coefficient of friction.

Thus torque is directly dependent upon handle diameter and indirectly upon diameter squared, since the gripping force also depends on the circumference of the handle gripped. This was confirmed experimentally by Pheasant and O'Neill (1975). For thrusting motions in the direction of the long axis of the handle, the diameter is not involved and determination of maximum force is more complicated. For handles larger than the grip span diameter, the gripped area no longer increases in proportion of the diameter. An analysis of such conditions was performed by Replogle (1983) who concluded that for handles up to twice the grip span diameter the relative ungripped area of the handle increases, reducing the effective gripped area. Torque is then dependent on handle diameter as follows:

$$T = \frac{3d^2(4-d)}{(d+2)^2} \tag{9.16}$$

where *d* is the ratio of handle diameter to grip span diameter. For larger handle diameters the expression for torque becomes much more complicated (Replogle, 1983).

The individual fingers do not contribute equally to force production in a power grip. The middle finger is the strongest at 28.7% of the grip force, followed by the index, ring, and little fingers, with percentage contributions of 26.5%, 24.6%, and 20.2%, respectively (Kong and Freivalds, 2003). Similar values have been found by An et al. (1978), Amis (1987), Ejeskar and Örtengren (1981), Chen (1991), and Radhakrishnan and Nagaravindra (1993).

These different finger force contributions may be explained by the mechanical characteristics of bone and muscle. From the bone point of view, the middle finger is at the center of the hand and longer than the others and, thus, may have the mechanical advantage over the other fingers. The index and the ring fingers are located about the same distance from the center of the hand and, consequently, exert a similar amount of force. The little finger is the farthest from the center of the hand, and, therefore, may have a mechanical disadvantage over the other fingers when gripping.

From the muscle point of view, each finger has different muscle characteristics such as mass, volume, and length of muscle fibers. Brand et al. (1981) reported that the mass or volume of muscle is proportional to the total work capacity and showed that the flexor digitorum superficialis (FDS) of the middle finger has the largest mass fraction of total weight, followed by the flexor digitorum profundus (FDP) of the middle finger. The FDS of the little finger has the lowest mass fraction. Ketchum et al. (1978) also reported that the FDS of the middle finger was strongest and the combined force of both the superficialis and the profundus tendons was also the strongest in the middle finger, followed by the index, ring, and little finger.

Phalange force distributions are also nonuniform. The force imposed by the distal phalange (35.9%) was significantly higher than that imposed by the middle (32.4%) and the proximal (31.7%) phalanges in the gripping task (Kong and Freivalds, 2003). These findings are confirmed by An et al. (1978), Amis (1987), Chao et al. (1989), and Lee and Rim (1990). Note that these results only apply to a gripping task. For a pulling task utilizing a power grip, a greater amount of the force is applied by the proximal (37.6%) and middle (33.6%) phalanges and lesser amount by the distal phalange (28.8%) (Kong and Freivalds, 2003). Note also that female power grip force is roughly 70% of male power grip force (see Figure 9.3).

9.4.3   BIOMECHANICS OF PRECISION GRIP AND FRICTION

Precision or pinch grip can be modeled as follows (see Figure 9.8). The application force (F_A) is transmitted to the workpiece (in addition to the tool weight) through the

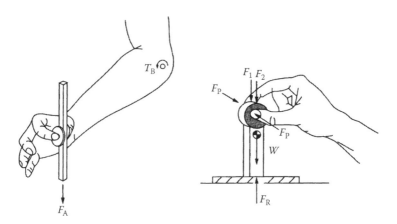

FIGURE 9.8   Forces of a precision grip. (Reproduced from Lowe, B.D. and Freivalds, A., *Ergonomics*, 42, 550, 1999. With permission.)

axis of the tool. In static equilibrium, a reactive force (F_R) is directionally opposite and equal in magnitude to the application force plus the weight of the tool (W):

$$F_R = F_A + W \tag{9.17}$$

When F_A is applied, the tendency for the reactive force, F_R, to push the tool upward through the grasp, is resisted by the frictional forces (F_{f1} and F_{f2}) between the fingertip surfaces and tool grip surface material. The sum of these frictional forces must be greater than the force applied with the tool (F_A) to resist the slip. In this paradigm, the frictional forces at each digit (F_f) are a result of the pinch forces normal to the tool surface (F_P) multiplied by the static coefficient of friction (μ) between the digital pulpar skin and the tool grip surface material. Further, the forces applied by the thumb and index finger (F_{P1} and F_{P2}) are equal in magnitude and opposite in direction (due to net zero horizontal translation of the tool) so that the total frictional force downward is equal to $2\mu F_P$:

$$F_{f1} + F_{f2} \geq F_R - W \tag{9.18}$$

$$2\mu F_P \geq F_R - W \tag{9.19}$$

Provided that the tool does not slip within the grip, $2F_{p(task)}$ must be greater than the minimum pinch force required to prevent slip, $2F_{p(slip)}$. At the instant of slip, $2F_{p(slip)}$ is directionally opposite and equal in magnitude to ($F_R - W$), so the coefficient of friction can be defined by

$$2F_{P(slip)}\mu = F_R - W \tag{9.20}$$

$$\mu = \frac{F_R - W}{2F_{P(slip)}} \tag{9.21}$$

Conversely, if μ is known, calculation of the minimum required pinch force (pinch force at slip) as a function of reactive force F_R is

$$F_{p(slip)} = \frac{F_R - W}{2\mu} \tag{9.22}$$

The pinch force safety margin (SM) is defined as the excessive pinch force (sum of thumb and index finger force) exceeding the minimum pinch force resisting slip ($2F_{p(slip)}$):

$$SM = 2F_{p(task)} - 2F_{p(slip)} \tag{9.23}$$

$$SM = 2F_{p(task)} - \frac{F_R - W}{\mu} \tag{9.24}$$

The SM can be an unreliable measure of excess grip force because it relies on the skin coefficient of friction, which can be difficult to measure and generally is estimated. One can also define a force ratio as the ratio of grip to application forces. The force ratio is not dependent on unreliable estimates of frictional coefficients, but, since it is a unitless ratio, it cannot provide any information on the absolute magnitude of excess grip force (Lowe and Freivalds, 1999).

The coefficient of friction between the digital pulpar skin and the grip surface has been measured by determining peak shear force as a function of normal (pinch) force (Buchholz et al., 1988). The subjects pinched, between alcohol-cleansed (to remove oils) thumb and index fingertips, an instrumented "tool." Based on visual feedback of force displayed on an oscilloscope, the subjects attempted to maintain a constant normal (pinch) force while slowly pulling upward on the clamped tool, which also measured axial force. As the upward pull force increased, the fingertip shear forces were estimated from axial forces on the tool. Eventually the fingertips slipped, with the ratio of the maximum axial force immediately preceding the slip to the sum of the two normal forces yielding the coefficient of friction. The coefficients ranged approximately from 0.25 to 0.55 for different materials, with large inter- and intrasubject variabilities. Cloth and suede material exhibited higher values as compared to aluminum. Also, the coefficient of friction was inversely related to the pinch force applied by the digits, decreasing approximately 0.1 per each 30 N of pinch force. The calculation of the coefficient of friction is further complicated by the difficulties subjects had in maintaining a constant pinch force and avoiding the reflexive pinch force increase or a slip reflex, which occurs approximately 75 ms after the onset of slip between the fingertips and the object (Cole and Abbs, 1987; Johansson and Westling, 1987).

Later research found very similar results but with significantly lower values of friction for older adults (Cole, 1991; Lowe and Freivalds, 1999). This could be attributed to the reduced eccrine sweat gland output (Cole, 1991), but with regular cleansing of the fingertip surfaces, this should not be a major factor. An alternative explanation may be related to skin deformation characteristics and changes in the viscoelasticity of the pulpar skin that may occur with age. Young skin viscoelastic properties deviate considerably from Amonton's laws (Comaish and Bottoms, 1971), aging would only exacerbate that. The deviations Amonton's laws were demonstrated quite dramatically by Bobjer et al. (1993) in measuring coefficients of friction for textured and nontextured surfaces contaminated with oil and lard. In many conditions, they found coefficients of friction well above the theoretical limit of 1.0.

The results also presented trade-off problems for designers of hand tools. Smooth, nontextured handles produced highest coefficients of friction for clean hands ($\mu = 1.4$), but lowest coefficients of friction ($\mu = 0.2$) when the hands were contaminated, as one would reasonably expect. By adding texture, the friction was increased for contaminated conditions, perhaps, by channeling them away. However, with normal (cleansed with alcohol) hands, any texture decreased the coefficient of friction, perhaps because of the decreased area of contact with the skin. Perhaps the optimum situation with acceptable coefficients of friction for all conditions (approximately uniform at $\mu = 0.75$) were achieved with a coarse texture of alternating 2 mm ridges and 2 mm grooves (Bobjer et al., 1993).

9.4.4 GRIP FORCE COORDINATION

Coordination was defined by Athènes and Wing (1989) as "the way in which different motor acts are coupled with regard to their temporal and spatial characteristics to allow for a more efficient motor performance." Neurophysiological studies of grip force coordination in simple lift and hold maneuvers have revealed that individuals apply a higher grip force than demanded by mechanical conditions (mainly friction) of the external object (Johansson and Westling, 1984; Westling and Johansson, 1984). The higher grip force represents a SM (Johansson, 1991), or buffer, against unanticipated perturbing forces or slip of the tools from the grip. The minimum ratio of grip force to the load force (external force demand) is governed by mechanical conditions of the hand–object interface and the force which is transmitted through the grasped object to its external environment. The actual ratio of these forces is scaled above this minimum slip force to achieve an adequate margin of safety. The scaling of the ratio of these forces determines the efficiency of an individual's grip force coordination and represents a clear trade-off between maintaining a margin of safety and minimizing excess grip force on the object.

Under conditions in which there is impairment of the sensory nerves, such as anesthesia of the digital pulpy areas, subjects have experienced difficulties in modulating grip force in parallel with the load force (Johansson et al., 1992). Microneurographic recordings from the afferent tactile mechanoreceptors have shown that cutaneous feedback from these receptors is critical in transmitting information regarding the conditions preceding slip at the grip interface (Westling and Johansson, 1987). When, the mechanoreceptors are anesthetized, individuals lose this feedback. Similarly, Cole (1991) observed force coordination impairments in elderly individuals that were attributed to an age-related decrement in tactile sensibility.

Compression neuropathies of the median nerve, such as carpal tunnel syndrome, result in decreased tactile sensitivity of the thumb and first digits (Jackson and Clifford, 1989) and could be hypothesized to consequently also degrade the ability to coordinate pinch grip, resulting in higher grip force levels. Reviews of epidemiological studies have suggested that force exertions exceeding 15%–20% of an individual's maximum voluntary contraction (MVC) maybe linked with MSDs (Kroemer, 1989, 1992). This suggestion appears to be based on previous findings that force exertions below 15% MVC are associated with an essentially infinite endurance time while recovery periods are needed for larger exertions (Monod and Scherrer, 1965; Rohmert, 1973).

The effects of a deficit in grip force coordination efficiency relative to a 15% MVC threshold is illustrated conceptually in Figure 9.9 (Lowe and Freivalds, 1999). Two individuals (A and B) of equivalent maximum strength may actually exert very different grip forces when performing identical tasks. The model illustrates that the employee who exerts a higher grip force as a result of reduced grip force coordination efficiency (higher SM) has an amplified risk. When the force requirement is below the risk threshold, an individual with reduced grip force coordination efficiency may apply a grip force above the threshold purely as a result of the SM. For those individuals who

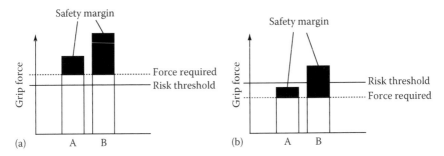

FIGURE 9.9 Conceptual model of the relationship between the required force, SM, and risk threshold. (a) Employee B exerts only 29% higher grip force on the tool, but the grip force exceeding the risk threshold is 83% higher than that of employee A. (b) Employee B's grip force, which exceeds the risk threshold, is attributable exclusively to a higher SM while employee A's grip force is below the risk threshold. (Reproduced from Lowe, B.D. and Freivalds, A., *Ergonomics*, 42, 550, 1999. With permission.)

already are slightly impaired with a median nerve entrapment disorder would exhibit even higher grasp forces and would have even greater risk.

Grip coordination was tested further by Lowe and Freivalds (1999) with an instrumented hand tool (shown in Figure 9.4) on seven patients diagnosed with CTS and seven matched controls. The subjects were required to track a sinusoidal target force (varying both in amplitude and frequency between conditions) presented on an oscilloscope display by applying a tool application force (F_A). The application force and pinch force ($2F_P$) were recorded (see Figure 9.10) and used to calculate two measures of grip coordination. The modulation index indicated the percentage of maximum pinch force as it modulated between the minimum and maximum tool application force:

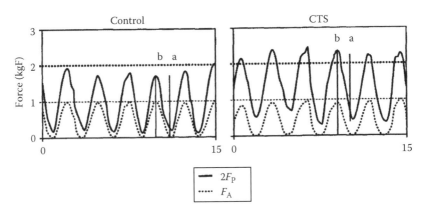

FIGURE 9.10 Grip force ($2F_P$) and application force (F_A) performance for a typical control group subject (left panel) and CTS group subject (right panel). The modulation index is the ratio of the lengths of line segments a (difference between maximum and minimum pinch forces) and b (peak pinch force). (Reproduced from Lowe, B.D. and Freivalds, A., *Ergonomics*, 42, 550, 1999. With permission.)

$$\text{Modulation index} = \frac{F_{\text{Pmax(t)}} - F_{\text{Pmin(t)}}}{F_{\text{Pmax(t)}}} \tag{9.25}$$

The modulation index ranged from 0 (no grip force modulation) to 1 (most efficient grip force modulation). The force ratio represented the ratio of total grip force to the applied force, integrated over one period of the application force cycle:

$$\text{Force ratio} = \int \frac{2F_{\text{P(t)}}}{F_{\text{R(t)}}}\, \mathrm{d}t \tag{9.26}$$

On average, the CTS group exerted significantly higher pinch forces at equivalent levels of application force and modulated their grip force less, indicating a lower efficiency of grip force coordination. More specifically, the mean value for the modulation index was 12.4% lower for the CTS group, while the force ratio was 54% higher for the CTS group. The link between median nerve compression and decreased grip coordination is hypothesized to be an adaptive, compensatory rescaling of the force ratio to a higher SM. The increased force ratio (and SM) serves a larger buffer against localized slips which may be "undetected" by a less sensitive afferent system. The higher grip forces indicate higher flexor tendon forces as they glide within the carpal tunnel, further aggravating the compression of the medium nerve through the tendon-pulley model (see Section 9.3.1). For example, Chao et al. (1976) estimated the flexor digitorum profundus tendon forces to be 4.32 times the external force measured at the fingertip. A 54% average increase in the force ratio for CTS patients as compared to controls would now yield tendon forces as 6.5 times the external force, further accelerating the risk for further injury. However, by increasing the friction characteristics of the tool surface (in this case, suede material) the force ratio for CTS patients was reduced significantly almost to the same level as found in controls (Lowe and Freivalds, 1999).

9.4.5   STATIC LOADING AND WRIST POSTURE

When tools are used in situations in which the arms must be elevated or tools have to be held for extended periods, muscles of the shoulders, arms, and hands may be loaded statically, resulting in fatigue, reduced work capacity and soreness. Abduction of the shoulder with corresponding elevation of the elbow will occur if work has to be done with a straight tool on a horizontal workplace. An angled tool reduces the need to raise the arm (Eastman Kodak, 1983). A good example of such a tool is the redesigned soldering iron described by Tichauer and Gage (1977).

Prolonged work with arms extended can produce soreness in the forearm for assembly tasks done with force. By rearranging the workplace so as to keep the elbows at 90° most of the problem can be eliminated. Similarly, continuous holding of an activation switch can result in fatigue of the fingers and reduced flexibility. Thus tool activation forces should be kept low to reduce this loading, or a power grip bar instead of a single-finger trigger should be used. For a two-handled tool, a spring-loaded return saves the fingers from having to return the tool to its starting position (Eastman Kodak, 1983).

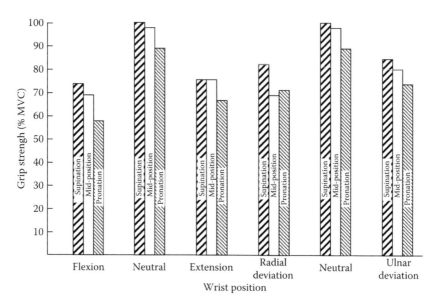

FIGURE 9.11   Grip strength as a function of wrist and forearm position. (Adapted from Terrell, R. and Purswell, J., The influence of forearm and wrist orientation on static grip strength as a design criterion for hand tools, in *Proceedings of the Human Factors Society, 20th Annual Meeting*, Santa Monica, CA: Human Factor Society, pp. 28–32, 1976.)

As the wrist is moved from its neutral position there is loss of grip strength (Terrell and Pursewell, 1976). Starting from a neutral wrist position, full pronation decreases grip strength by 12%, full flexion/extension by 25%, and full radial/ulnar deviation by 15% (See Figure 9.11). This degradation of maximum grip strength available can be quantified by

$$\% \text{Grip strength} = 95.7 + 4.3 \text{ PS} + 3.8 \text{ FE} - 25.2 \text{ FE}^2 - 16.8 \text{ RU}^2 \qquad (9.27)$$

where
    PS = 1 if the wrist is fully pronated or supinated and 0 if in a neutral position
    FE = 1 if the wrist is fully flexed or extended and 0 if in a neutral position
    RU = 1 if the wrist is fully in radial or ulnar deviate and 0 if in a neutral position

Furthermore, awkward hand positions may result in soreness of the wrist, loss of grip and, if sustained for extended periods of time, occurrence of WRMSDs. To reduce this problem, the workplace of the tools should be redesigned to allow for straight wrist, i.e., lowering work surfaces and edges of containers, tilting jigs toward the hand, etc., using a pistol grip on knives (Armstrong et al., 1982), using a pistol handle on powered tools for vertical surfaces and in-line handles for horizontal surfaces (Armstrong, 1983), and putting a bend in the tool handle to reflect the axis of grasp such as the Tichauer and Gage (1977) pliers.

TABLE 9.2
Maximal Static Finger Flexion Forces

Digit	Maximum Force (N)	% Force of Thumb
Thumb	73	100
Index	59	81
Middle	64	88
Ring	50	69
Little	32	44

Source: Adapted from Hertzberg, H., *Human Engineering Guide*, Washington, DC: U.S. Government Printing Office, pp. 467–584, 1973.

If the index finger is used excessively for operating triggers, symptoms of trigger finger develop. Trigger forces should be kept low, preferably below 10 N (Eastman Kodak, 1983) to reduce the load on the index finger. Two or three finger-operated controls are preferable. Finger strip controls are even better, because they require the use of more and stronger fingers. Absolute finger flexion strengths are shown in Table 9.2.

9.4.6 HANDLES FOR SINGLE-HANDLED TOOLS

A cutout handle should be large enough to provide space for all four fingers. Hand breadth across the metacarpals ranges from 71 mm for a 5% female to 97 mm for a 95% male (Garrett, 1971). Thus 100 mm may be a reasonable minimum, but 125 mm may be more comfortable (Konz and Johnson, 2000). Eastman Kodak (1983) recommended 120 mm. If the grip is enclosed or gloves are used, even larger openings are recommended. For an external precision grip, the tool shaft must be long enough to be supported at the base of the first finger or thumb. A minimum value of 100 mm is suggested (Konz and Johnson, 2000). For an internal precision grip, the tool should extend past the palm, but not so far as to hit the wrist (Konz and Johnson, 2000). It is interesting to note that screwdriver torque was experimentally found to be proportional to the handle grip length (Magill and Konz, 1986).

For a power grip on screwdrivers Rubarth (1928) recommended a diameter of 40 mm. Basing their recommendation on empirical judgments of stair rails, Hall and Bernett (1956) suggested 32 mm. Based on minimum electromyograms (EMG) activity Ayoub and LoPresti (1971) found a 51 mm handle diameter to be best. However, based on the maximum number of work cycles completed before fatigue and on the ratio of grip force to EMG activity, they suggested a 38 mm diameter. Pheasant and O'Neill (1975) found that muscle strength deteriorates when using handles greater than 50 mm in diameter. Rigby (1973) recommended 38 mm for full encirclement of the hand and heavy loads. For handles on boxes, Drury (1980) found diameters of 31–38 mm to be best in terms of least reduction in grip strength. Using various handles of noncircular cross-section, Cochran and Riley (1982, 1986) found largest thrust forces in handles of 130 mm circumference (or 41.4 mm equivalent circular diameter) for both males and females. For manipulation, however, the smallest handles of 22 mm were found to be best (Cochran and Riley, 1983). Replogle (1983), in validating his gripping model, found maximum torques at twice the grip span diameter. With average spans of about 25 mm, this yields a handle diameter of 50 mm. Based on company experience, Eastman Kodak (1983) recommended 30–40 mm with an optimum of 40 mm for power grips and 8–16 mm with an optimum of 12 mm for precision grips.

Based on the above data, one could summarize that handle diameters should be in the range of 31–50 mm with the upper end best for maximum torque and the lower end for dexterity and speed. However, it would also be best to size the handle to each individual's hand size. This was first succinctly observed by Fox (1957) in that a handle which allows some overlap between the thumb and index finger may be better than a larger handle that matches the individual's grip diameter. Grant et al. (1992) later confirmed that handles 1 cm smaller than the inside grip diameter maximized grip strength as compared to handles 1 cm larger or those matching the inside grip diameter.

Kong et al. (2004) went further by defining normalized handle size (NHS) as the ratio of the handle circumference to hand length, as measured from the wrist crease to the tip of the middle finger. Thirty subjects, ranging from 5th percentile females to 95th percentile males, with hand lengths ranging from 160 to 205 mm, gripped a variety of handle sizes in several different tasks. This resulted in NHS ranging from 45% to 90%. Maximum grip forces and minimum subjective ratings of perceived exertion were obtained roughly in the range of 50%–55% NHS or absolute handle sizes in the range of 30.6–39.2 mm, depending on the individuals hand length. A more detailed analysis indicated that a better match yet is for the handle size to conform to individual finger lengths, with the ratio of the handle circumference to the length of finger ranging from 90% to 110%. This would result in a handle shape that is of an asymmetrical double frustum shape described further in the next section.

As early as 1928, Rubarth investigated handle shape and concluded that, for a power grip, one should design for maximum surface contact so as to minimize unit pressure of the hand. Thus a tool with a circular cross-section was found to give largest torque. Pheasant and O'Neill (1975) concluded that the precise shape of handles was irrelevant and recommended simple knurled cylinders. Evaluation of handle shape on grip fatigue in manual lifting (which is a different action than for tool use) did not indicate any significant differences in shapes (Scheller, 1983). Maximum pull force, though, was obtained with a triangular cross-section, apex down. For thrusting forces, the circular cross-section was found to be worst and a triangular best (Cochran and Riley, 1982). However for a rolling type of manipulation, the triangular shape was slowest (Cochran and Riley, 1983). A more comprehensive study indicated that no one shape may be perfect, and that shape may be more dependent on the type of task and motions involved than initially thought (Cochran and Riley, 1986). A rectangular shape of width: height ratios, from 1:1.25 to 1:1.50 appeared to be a good compromise. A further advantage of a rectangular cross-section is that the tool does not roll when placed on a table (Konz and Johnson, 2000). It should also be noted that handles should not have the shape of a true cylinder except for a hook grip. For screwdriver type tools, the handle end is rounded to prevent undue pressure at the palm and for hammer type tools the handle may have some flattening curving to indicate the end of the handle.

In a departure from the circular, cylindrically shaped handles, Bullinger and Solf (1979) proposed a more radical design using a hexagonal cross-section, shaped as two truncated cones joined at the largest ends. Such a shape fits the contours of the palm and thumb best in both precision and power grips and yielded highest torques (9 N m) in comparison with more conventional handles. A more detailed study by Kong et al. (2004) identified four asymmetric double frustum cone handle sizes that would fit most of the adult population:

Small—corresponding to a 5th percentile female hand (160 mm)

Medium—corresponding to a 50th percentile female/5th percentile male hand (175 mm)

Large—corresponding to a 50th percentile male/95th percentile female hand (190 mm)

Extra large—corresponding to a 95th percentile male hand (205 mm)

The double frustum shape, with thick ends joined, allows one handle to fit all four fingers naturally. The index and middle fingers are larger, thus the slant of the top cone is less (6.9°) than for the bottom cone (15.4°). The total length of the handle is 130 mm, i.e., 65 mm for each cone.

A final note on shape is that T-handles yield much better performance than straight screwdriver handles. Pheasant and O'Neill (1975) reported as much as 50% increase in torque. Optimum handle diameter was found to be 25 mm and optimum angle was 60°, i.e., a slanted T (Saran, 1973). The slant allows the wrist to remain straight and thus generate larger forces.

For centuries, wood was the material of choice for tool handles. Wood was readily available, and easily worked. It has good resistance to shock and to thermal and electrical conductivity and has good frictional qualities even when wet. Since wooden handles can break and stain with grease and oil, there has been a shift to plastic and even metal. Plastic handles are typically knurled or cross-hatched with grooves to improve the hand/tool frictional interface (Pheasant and O'Neill, 1975).

Such grooved fiberglass handles were evaluated with respect to traditional wooden handles by Chang et al. (1999). Although the focus was primarily on weight and efficiency of shoveling, with hollow handles requiring 12% less energy expenditure than solid handles, the subjects rated the grooved fiberglass handles more acceptable than wooden handles in terms of tactile feeling and slipperiness.

Metal should be covered with rubber or leather to reduce shock and electrical conductance and increase friction (Fraser, 1980). Such a resilient covering may also aid in the reduction of hand discomfort. Fellows and Freivalds (1991) found that a 4 mm foam covering on wooden handled garden tools provided a significantly more uniform grip force distribution and lower ratings of perceived discomfort as compared to plain wooden handles. Unfortunately, in most cases, the total grip forces were higher for the foam-covered handles due to an excessive deformation of the foam and a "loss of control" feeling in the subjects. The authors hypothesized that a thinner layer of foam would have provided more control, but still maintained a better grip force distribution.

As discussed in Section 9.4.5, deviations of the wrist from the neutral position under repetitive load can lead to a variety of cumulative trauma disorders as well as decreased grip strength (see Figure 9.11). Therefore angulation of tool handles, e.g., power tools, may be necessary so as to maintain a straight wrist. The handle should reflect the axis of grasp, i.e., about 78° from the horizontal, and should be oriented so that the eventual tool axis is in line with the index finger (Fraser, 1980). This principle was first applied to pliers by Tichauer and Gage (1977) and then later to soldering irons, knives, and other tools.

9.4.7 HANDLES FOR TWO-HANDLED TOOLS

Grip strength and the resulting stress on finger flexor tendons vary with the size of the object being grasped. A maximum grip strength is achieved at about 45–80 mm (Pheasant and Scriven, 1983). The smaller values of 45 mm were obtained on a dynamometer with parallel sides (Pheasant and Scriven, 1983), whereas the larger values of 75–80 mm were obtained on a dynamometer with handles angled inwards (see Figure 9.9). This relationship can be modeled as

$$\% \text{ Grip strength} = 100 - 0.11S - 10.2S^2 \tag{9.28}$$

where S is the given grip span minus optimum grip span in cm.

Also, as is seen in Figure 9.12, there is quite a large variation in strength capacity over the population. To accommodate this population variability, maximal grip requirements should be limited to less than 90 N.

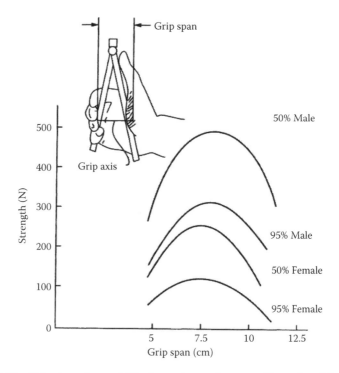

FIGURE 9.12 Grip strength capability for various grip spans. (Reproduced from Greenberg, L. and Chaffin, D.B., *Workers and Their Tools*, Pendell, Midland, MI, 1976. With permission.)

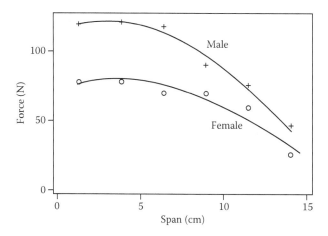

FIGURE 9.13 Pulp pinch strength capability for various grip spans. (Adapted from Heffernan, C. and Freivalds, A., *Appl. Ergon.*, 31, 409, 2000.)

A similar effect is found for pinch strength (see Figure 9.13). However, the overall four-point pulp pinch force is at a much more reduced force level (approximately 17% of power grip, see Figure 9.10 for other types of pinches) and drops sharply beyond a 4–5 cm pinch span (Heffernan and Freivalds, 2000).

9.4.8 OTHER TOOL CONSIDERATIONS

Alternating hands permits reduction of local muscle fatigue. However, in many situations this is not possible as the tool use is one-handed. Furthermore, if the tool is designated for the user's preferred hand, which for 90% of the population is the right hand, then 10% are left out (Konz, 1974). Laveson and Meyer (1976) gave several good examples of right-handed tools that cannot be used by a left-handed person, i.e., a power drill with side handle on the left side only, a circular saw, and a serrated knife leveled on one side only.

A few studies have compared task performance using dominant and nondominant hands. Shock (1962) indicated the nonpreferred hand grip strength to be 80% of the preferred hand grip strength. Miller and Freivalds (1987) found right-handed males to show a 12% strength decrement in the left hand while right-handed females showed a 7% strength decrement. Surprisingly both left-handed males and females had nearly equal strengths in both hands. He concluded that left-handed subjects were forced to adapt to a right-handed world. Using time study ratings, Konz and Warraich (1985) found decrements, ranging from 9% for an electric drill to 48% for manual scissors, for ratings using the nonpreferred hand as opposed to the preferred hand.

A series of studies were performed by Mital and colleagues to examine various tool and operator factors on torque capability (Mital, 1985, 1986; Mital et al., 1985; Mital and Sanghavi, 1986). In general, unless the posture is extreme, i.e., standing versus lying, torque exertion capability was not affected substantially. The height at which torque was applied had no influence on peak torque exertion capability.

On the other hand, torque exertion capability decreased linearly with increasing reach distance. Another interesting requirement for proper tool usage is the volume or space envelope generated during operation of the tool. Comprehensive data on a variety of tools have been collected by Baker et al. (1960).

The weight of a hand tool will determine how long it can be held or used and how precisely it can be manipulated. For tools held in one hand with the elbow at 90° for extended periods of time, Greenberg and Chaffin (1976) recommend a load of no more that 2.3 kg. A similar value is suggested by Eastman Kodak (1983). For precision operations, tool weights greater than 0.4 kg are not recommended unless a counterbalanced system is used. Heavy tools, used to absorb impact or vibration, should be mounted on a truck to reduce effort for the operator (Eastman Kodak, 1983).

9.4.9   Efficiency of Striking Tools

Axes and hammers are striking tools designed to transmit a force to an object by direct contact and thereby change its shape or drive it forward. The tool's efficiency in doing this may be defined as the ratio of the energy utilized in striking to the energy available in the stroke. Using geometric methods, Drillis et al. (1963) showed that the tool's efficiency could be defined by

$$\eta = 1 - \frac{S^2}{\rho_1^2} \tag{9.29}$$

where
  η is the efficiency
  S is the distance from the mass center to the line of action (OB in Figure 9.3)
  ρ_1 is the radius of gyration with respect to the center of action

For the efficiency to be 100%, the center of mass should coincide with the line of action, which is impossible with a shafted tool. In the hand axe of stone-age man, the total energy of the stroke movement was converted into useful energy giving maximum efficiency, although the force was fairly weak. The opposite extreme is a uniform rod held at one end, which has an efficiency of only 25% but provides quite a bit more relative force.

Two comparable formulae for tool efficiency were developed by Gorjatschkin (1924, cited in Drillis et al., 1963). The first related tool efficiency to the ratio of S to the tool length, L:

$$\eta = 1 - 1.5 \frac{S}{L} \tag{9.30}$$

Again this indicates that the efficiency increases as the ratio of S to L increases. Physically this is achieved by placing the mass center as close as possible to the center of action, i.e., increasing the mass of the tool head relative to the handle. A second way of expressing the above observation is to relate the mass of the handle to the total mass:

$$\eta = 1 - 0.75 \frac{m_1}{m_1 + m_2} \qquad (9.31)$$

where
   m_1 is the mass of handle
   m_2 is the mass of tool head

Drillis et al. (1963) indicated that efficiencies for typical striking tools ranged from 0.8 to 0.95 for axes, from 0.7 to 0.9 for hammers, from 0.55 to 0.85 for scutches, and from 0.3 to 0.65 for hoes.

Regarding impacting tools such as hammers, the efficiency of impact and recoil are very important. When two bodies collide, the ratio between their relative velocity after impact to that before impact is defined as the coefficient of restitution. This can be used to derive the energy of recoil and eventually the efficiency of impact (Drillis et al., 1963).

In the case of forging this can be defined as

$$\eta = \frac{1}{1 + m_0/m} \qquad (9.32)$$

where
   m_0 is the mass of hammer
   m is the mass of other object (e.g., forging and anvil)

The aim is to transform as much of the kinetic energy of the hammer into deforming the object's shape as possible. Thus the mass of the hammer should be small relative to the mass of the forging and anvil. On the other hand, in driving a nail the intent is to transform the kinetic energy of the hammer into the kinetic energy of the nail. Then the mass of the hammer should be great in relation to the mass of the nail and the efficiency becomes

$$\eta = \frac{1}{1 + m/m_0} \qquad (9.33)$$

The overall efficiency of the system including the operator becomes the product of the efficiency of the tool, the efficiency of the stroke movement, the efficiency of impact, and the physiological efficiency of the human operator. This latter factor can range from a low of 3%–4% for relatively static tasks such as shoveling (Freivalds, 1986) to a high of 25%–30% for dynamic tasks such as cycling (Lehmann, 1953). Drillis et al. (1963) computed the overall efficiency of hammering a 6 in. (15 cm) nail into a wooden block as 57%, not counting the physiological efficiency. Using an average value of 15% for physiological efficiency, overall system efficiency reduces to 8.6%.

The effect of the weight of the head on swing characteristics dynamics of striking tools, especially axes, was further investigated by Widule et al. (1978) and Corrigan et al. (1981). Using cinematography they analyzed the dropping motion of the subjects using four axes with head weights of 0.85, 1.6, 2.2, and 3.6 kg.

Accelerations as well as kinetic energy for various points of interest were calculated frame by frame from the film.

The results supported the hypothesis that an increase in head weight led to an increase in kinetic energy. However, a noticeable drop-off in angular velocity and kinetic energy was found for the heaviest axe. Thus there appeared to be a limit to the ability of an individual to achieve rotational inertia and adding additional mass may have been counterproductive in terms of physiological energy costs. The authors concluded that the heavy axes (heads ranging from 2.2 kg and above) used to clear the American forests in the late 1800s, although more taxing in terms of energy expenditure, were more efficient in clearing forests. Rapid bursts of energy were used to chop down a tree, and necessary rest periods could be obtained during preparation of the cut, sharpening the axe and chopping off branches. The authors also concluded that the American axe, distinguished from the European axe by its possession of a poll (a lump of metal at the rear of the head—see Figure 9.14A) was more efficient. The poll counterbalanced the protruding blade and gave the axe better handling characteristics.

Such observations were confirmed by Drillis et al. (1963) based on his survey of 521 axes used in Latvia. Average head weight was found to be 1.4 kg or about 2% of the user's weight. Average handle length was found to be 0.6 m or about 35% of the user's height. He concluded that these values compared very favorably to folk norms. Optimum swing height to achieve maximum kinetic energy for wood splitting was found to be approximately 1.1 m.

Some variations on these optimum values were noted by German work physiologists. In a study of sledgehammers, Meyer (1930) examined hammers ranging in weight from 4.4 to 10.6 kg. He concluded though that to get a more lively action (i.e., increased acceleration) one should use lighter hammers. Gläser (1933, cited in Lehmann, 1953) investigated axes with head weights under 2 kg for forestry use. He found the opposite and concluded that the "most lively action" was to be achieved using axes weighing 3–4 kg. A mitigating factor is that the Germans most likely measured the weight of the whole implement. Subtracting approximately 0.6–0.8 kg for the handle yields values more closely in line with the other studies.

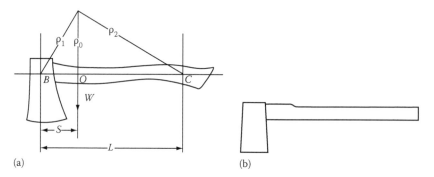

(a)   (b)

FIGURE 9.14 (a) Determination of striking tool efficiency (American axe); O=mass center, B=center of action, C=center of percussion (ideal point for holding), L=length of the tool, W=weight of the tool (b) European axe. (Reproduced from Freivalds, A., *Int. Rev. Ergon.*, 1, 43, 1987. With permission.)

9.5 CONCLUSIONS

Over the centuries tools have been used to accomplish a variety of objectives, typically in agriculture and industry. Many have incorporated folk norms and have evolved into fairly efficient instruments, while others have remained virtually unchanged for centuries. These latter tools, coupled with the increased robot-like motions required of operators on assembly lines, have led to an increase in a variety of MSDs. Hopefully, some of this information will be useful in redesigning tools or selecting the proper tools for more efficient and injury free work.

Problems

1. Complete the development of Landsmeer's Model III, i.e., derive Equation 9.3.
2. Compare the differences in tendon forces predicted by the three Landsmeer models.
3. Plot the relative torque produced as handle diameter increases from practically zero to double the grip span diameter.
4. What is the loss in grip strength for an average male using channel-lock pliers with a grip span of 10 cm held in full ulnar deviation (as would be the case for most work on a horizontal work surface)?
5. What is the loss of efficiency for a cheap hammer that is made completely of cast iron as compared to a hammer with a very light weight handle? (*Hint*: Assume the center of gravity for the first hammer is at the midposition of the handle.)

REFERENCES

Aghazadeh, F. and Mital, A. 1987 Injuries due to hand tools, *Applied Ergonomics*, 18, 273–278.

Amis, A.A. 1987 Variation of finger forces in maximal isometric grasp tests on a range of cylindrical diameters, *Journal of Biomedical Engineering*, 9, 313–320.

An, K.N., Cooney, W.P., Chao, E.Y., and Linscheid, R.L. 1978 Functional strength measurement of normal fingers, *ASME Advances in Bioengineering*, pp. 89–90.

An, K.N., Askew, L.J., and Chao, E.Y. 1986 Biomechanics and functional assessment of upper extremities, in W. Karwowski (ed.), *Trends in Ergonomics/Human Factors III*, Amsterdam: Elsevier, pp. 573–580.

Armstrong, T.J. 1983 *An Ergonomic Guide to Carpal Tunnel Syndrome*, Akron, OH: American Industrial Hygiene Association.

Armstrong, T.J. and Chaffin, D.B. 1978 An investigation of the relationship between displacements of the finger and wrist joints and the extrinsic finger flexor tendons, *Journal of Biomechanics*, 11, 119–128.

Armstrong, T.J. and Chaffin, D.B. 1979 Some biomechanical aspects of the carpal tunnel, *Journal of Biomechanics*, 12, 567–570.

Armstrong, T.J., Foulke, J.A., Joseph, B.S., and Goldstein S.A. 1982 Investigation of cumulative trauma disorders in a poultry processing plant. *American Industrial Hygiene Association Journal*, 43, 103–116.

Athènes, S. and Wing, A., 1989, Knowledge-directed coordination in reaching for objects in the environment, in Wallace, S.A. (ed.)., *Perspectives on the Coordination in Movement*, Amsterdam: North Holland, pp. 284–301.

Atroshi, I., Gummesson, C., Johnsson, R., Ornstein, E., Ranstam, J., and Rosen, I. 1999 Prevalence of carpal tunnel syndrome in a general population, *Journal of the American Medical Association*, 282, 153–158.

Ayoub, M. and LoPresti, P. 1971 The determination of an optimum size cylindrical handle by use of electromyography, *Ergonomics*, 14, 509–518.

Backman, C., Boquist, L., Friden, J., Lorentzon, R., and Toolanen, G. 1990 Chronic achilles paratenonitis with tendinosis: An experimental model in the rabbit, *Journal of Orthopaedic Research*, 8, 541–547.

Baker, P.T., McKendry, J.M., and Grant, G. 1960 Volumetric requirements for hand tool usage, *Human Factors*, 2, 156–162.

Bendz, P. 1974 Systematization of the grip of the hand in relation to finger motor, systems, *Scandinavian Journal of Rehabilitation Medicine*, 6, 158–165.

Bobjer, O., Johansson, S.E., and Piguet, S. 1993 Friction between hand and handle. Effects of oil and lard on textured and non-textured surfaces; perception of discomfort, *Applied Ergonomics*, 24, 190–202.

Brand, P.W., Beach, R.B., and Thompson, D.E. 1981 Relative tension and potential excursion of muscles in the forearm and hand, *Journal of Hand Surgery*, 6, 209–218.

Buchholz, B., Frederick, L.J., and Armstrong, T.J. 1988 An investigation of human palmar skin friction and the effects of materials, pinch force and moisture, *Ergonomics*, 31, 317–325.

Bullinger, H.J. and Solf, J.J. 1979 *Ergonomische Arbeitsmittel-gestaltung II—Handgeführte Werkzeuge - Fallstudien* (Ergonomic improvements to dangerous hand tools), Dortmund: Bundesanstalt fur Arbeitsschutz und Unfallforschung.

Bureau of Labor Statistics. 1995 *Reports on Survey of Occupational Injuries and Illnesses in 1977–1994*, Washington DC: U.S. Department of Labor.

Chaffin, D. B., Andersson, G. B. J., and Martin, B.J. 2006 *Occupational Biomechanics*, 4th edn., New York: John Wiley & Sons.

Chang, K.Y., Ho, S.T. and Yu, H.S. 1994 Vibration induced neurophysiological and electron microscopical changes in rat peripheral nerves, *Occupational and Environmental Medicine*, 51, 130–135.

Chang, S.R., Park, S., and Freivalds, A. 1999 Ergonomic evaluation of the effects of handle types on garden tools, *International Journal of Industrial Ergonomics*, 24, 99–105.

Chao, E.Y.S., An, K.N., Cooney, W.P., and Linsheid, R.L. 1989 *Biomechanics of the Hand: A Basic Research Study*, Singapore: World Scientific.

Chao, E.Y., Opgrande, J.D., and Axmear, F.E. 1976 Three-dimensional force analysis of finger joints in selected isometric hand functions, *Journal of Biomechanics*, 9, 387–396.

Chen, Y. 1991 An evaluation of hand pressure distribution for a power grasp and forearm flexor muscle contribution for a power grasp on cylindrical handles, Unpublished Ph.D. Dissertation, Lincoln, NE: University of Nebraska.

Cochran, D.J. and Riley, M.W. 1982 An evaluation of handle shapes and sizes, in *Proceedings of the Human Factors Society*, 26th Annual Meeting, Santa Monica, CA, Human Factor Society, pp. 408–412.

Cochran, D.J. and Riley, M.W. 1983 An examination of the speed of manipulation of various sizes and shapes of handles, in *Proceedings of the Human Factors Society*, 27th Annual Meeting, Santa Monica, CA, Human Factor Society, pp. 432–436.

Cochran, D.J. and Riley, R.W. 1986 The effects of handle shape and size on exerted forces, *Human Factors*, 27, 295–301.

Cole, K.J. 1991 Grasp force control in older adults, *Journal of Motor Behavior,* 23, 251–258.

Cole, K.J. and Abbs, J.H. 1987 Kinematic and electromyographic responses to perturbation of a rapid grasp, *Journal of Neurophysiology*, 57, 1498–1510.

Comaish, S. and Bottoms, E. 1971 The skin and friction: deviations from Amonton's laws and the effects of hydration and lubrication, *British Journal of Dermatology*, 84, 37–43.

Conway, H. and Svenson, J. 1998 Occupational injury and illness rates, 1992–1996: Why they fell, *Monthly Labor Review*, 121, November, 36–58.

Corrigan, D.L., Foley, V., and Widule, C.J. 1981 Axe use efficiency—A work theory explanation of an historical trend, *Ergonomics*, 24, 103–109.

Cornefjord, M., Sato, K., Olmarker, K., Rydevik, B., and Nordborg, C. 1997 A model for chronic nerve root compression studies. Presentation of a porcine model for controlled, slow-onset compression with analyses of anatomic aspects, compression onset rate, and morphologic and neurophysiologic effect, *Spine*, 22, 946–57.

Drillis, R.J. 1963 Folk norms and biomechanics, *Human Factors*, 5, 427–441.

Drillis, R., Schneck, D. and Gage, H. 1963 The theory of striking tools, *Human Factors*, 5, 467–478.

Drury, C.G. 1980 Handles for manual materials handling, *Applied Ergonomics*, 11, 35–42.

Dunham, W., Haines, G., and Spring, J.M. 1972 Bowler's thumb ulnovolar neuroma of the thumb, *Clinical Orthopaedics*, 83, 99–101.

Dyck, P.J., Lais, A.C., Giannini, C., and Engelstad, J.K. 1990 Structural alterations of nerve during cuff compression, *Proceedings of the National Academy of Sciences*, 87, 9828–9832.

Eastman Kodak Company. 1983 *Ergonomic Design for People at Work*, Belmont, CA: Lifetime Learning Publications, pp. 140–159.

Ejeskar, A., and Örtengren, R. 1981 Isolated finger flexion force—A methodological study, *British Society for Surgery of the Hand*, 13, 223–230.

Faulkner, J.A., Brooks, S.V., and Zerba, E. 1990 Skeletal muscle weakness and fatigue in old age: Underlying Mechanisms, *Annual Review of Gerontology and Geriatrics*, 10, 147–166.

Fellows, G.L. and Freivalds, A. 1991 Ergonomics evaluation of a foam rubber grip for tool handles, *Applied Ergonomics*, 22, 225–230.

Fox, K. 1957 The Effect of Clothing on Certain Measures of Strength of Upper Extremities. (Report EP-47). Natick, MA: Environmental Protection Branch, U.S. Army Quartermaster Research and Development Center.

Fraser, T.M. 1980 *Ergonomic Principles in the Design of Hand Tools*, Occupational Safety and Health Series, No. 44, Geneva: International Labour Office.

Freivalds, A. 1986 The ergonomics of shovelling and shovel design—An experimental study, *Ergonomics*, 29, 19–30.

Freivalds, A. 1987 The ergonomics of tools, *International Reviews of Ergonomics*, 1:43–75.

Freivalds, A. 1999 Ergonomics of hand tools, *Occupational Ergonomics Handbook*, W. Karwowski and W.S. Marras (ed.), New York: CRC Press, pp. 461–478.

Garrett, J. 1971 The adult human hand: some anthropometric and biomechanical considerations, *Human Factors*, 13, 117–131.

Gläser, H. 1933 *Beiträge zur Form der Waldsäge und zur Technik des Sägens* (Contributions to the design of forestry saws and sawing techniques), Dissertation Eberswalde.

Gorjatschkin, W. 1924 Theory of striking hand tools, *Herald of Metal Industry*, Moscow, No. 4 (in Russian).

Grant, K.A., Habes, D.J., and Steward, L.L. 1992 An analysis of handle designs for reducing manual effort: The influence of grip diameter, *International Journal of Industrial Ergonomics*, 10, 199–206.

Greenberg, L. and Chaffin, D.B. 1976 *Workers and Their Tools*, Midland, MI: Pendell.

Hall, N.B. and Bernett, E.M. 1956 Empirical assessment of handrail diameters, *Journal of Applied Psychology*, 40, 381–382.

Hedlund, U. 1989 Raynaud's phenomenon of fingers and toes of miners exposed to local and whole-body vibration and cold, *International Archives of Occupational & Environmental Health*, 61, 457–461.

Heffernan, C. and Freivalds, A. 2000 Optimum pinch grips in the handling of dies, *Applied Ergonomics*, 31, 409–414.

Hertzberg, H. 1973 Engineering anthropometry, in H. van Cott and R. Kincaid (eds.) *Human Engineering Guide*, Washington, DC: U.S. Government Printing Office, pp. 467–584.

Howell, E. and Leach, R.E. 1970 Bowler's thumb, *Journal of Bone and Joint Surgery*, 52A, 379–381.

Jackson, D.A. and Clifford, J.C. 1989 Electrodiagnosis of mild carpal tunnel syndrome, *Archives of Physical Medicine Rehabilitation*, 70, 199–204.

Johansson, R.S. 1991 How is grasping modified by somatosensory input?, in Humphrey, D.R. and Freund, H.J. (eds.)., *Motor Control: Concepts and Issues*, Chichester: John Wiley, pp. 331–355.

Johansson, R.S. and Westling, G. 1984 Roles of glabrous skin receptors and sensorimotor memory in automatic control of precision grip when lifting rougher or more slippery objects, *Experimental Brain Research*, 56, 550–564.

Johansson, R.S. and Westling, G. 1987 Signals in tactile afferents from the fingers eliciting adaptive motor responses during precision grip, *Experimental Brain Research*, 66, 141–154.

Johansson, R.S., Huger, C., and Bäckström, L. 1992 Somatosensory control of precision grip during unpredictable pulling loads, III. Impairments during digital anesthesia, *Experimental Brain Research*, 89, 204–213.

Ketchum L.D., Thompson D., Pocock G., Wallingford D. 1978. A clinical study of forces generated by the intrinsic muscles of the index finger and the extrinsic flexor and extensor muscles of the hand, *Journal of Hand Surgery*, 3, 571–578.

Kong, Y.K. and Freivalds, A. 2003 Evaluation of meat-hook handle shapes, *International Journal of Industrial Ergonomics*, 32, 12–23.

Kong, Y.K., Freivalds, A., and Kim, S.E. 2004 Evaluation of handles in a maximum gripping task, *Ergonomics*, 47, 1350–1364.

Konz, S. 1974 Design of handtools, in *Proceedings of the Human Factors Society*, 18th Annual Meeting, Santa Monica, CA, Human Factor Society pp. 292–300.

Konz, S. and Johnson, S. 2000 *Work Design*, 5th edn., Scottsdale, AZ: Holcomb Hathaway, Inc.

Konz, S. 1986 Bent hammer handles, *Human Factors*, 27, 317–323.

Konz, S. and Warraich, M. 1985 Performance differences between the preferred and non-preferred hand when using various tools, in Brown, I.D., Goldsmith, R. Coombes, K. and Sinclair, M.A., (eds.)., Ergonomics International '85, London: Taylor & Francis, pp. 451–453.

Kroemer, K.H.E. 1986 Coupling the hand with the handle: An improved notation of touch grip and grasp, *Human Factors*, 27, 337–339.

Kroemer, K.H.E. 1989 Cumulative trauma disorders: their recognition and ergonomics measures to avoid them, *Applied Ergonomics*, 20, 274–280.

Kroemer, K.H.E. 1992 Avoiding cumulative trauma disorders in shops and offices, *American Industrial Hygiene Association Journal*, 53, 596–604.

Kuorinka, I. and Forcier, L. 1995 *Work Related Musculoskeletal Disorders (WMSDs): A Reference Book for Prevention*, London: Taylor & Francis.

Landsmeer, J.M.F. 1960 Studies in the anatomy of articulation, *Acta Morphologica Nederlands*, 3–4, 287–303.

Landsmeer, J.M.F. 1962 Power grip and precision handling, *Annals of Rheumatoid Diseases*, 21, 164–170.

Laveson, J.K. and Meyer, R.P. 1976 Left out "lefties" in design, in *Proceedings of the Human Factors Society*, 20th Annual Meeting, Santa Monica, CA, Human Factor Society, pp. 122–125.

Lawrence, R.C., Helmick, C.G., Arnett, F.C., Deyo, R.A., Felson, D.T., Giannini, E.H., Heyse, S.P., Hirsch, R., Hochberg, M.C., Hunder, G.G., Lian, M.H., Pillemer, S.R., Steen, V.D., and Wolfe, F. 1998 Estimates of the prevalence of arthritis and selected musculoskeletal disorders in the United States, *Arthritis and Rheumatism*, 41, 778–799.

Lee, J.W. and Rim, K. 1990 Maximum finger force prediction using a planar simulation of the middle finger, *Proceedings of the Institute of Mechanical Engineers*, 204, 167–178.

Lehmann, G. 1953 *Praktische Arbeitsphysiologie* (Practical Work Physiology), Stuttgart: Thieme, pp. 182–197.

LeVeau, B. 1977 *William and Lissner Biomechanics of Human Motion*, Philadelphia: W.B. Saunders.

Lowe, B.D. and Freivalds, A. 1999 Effect of carpal tunnel syndrome on grip force coordination on hand tools, *Ergonomics*, 42, 550–564.

Lundborg, G. 1988 *Nerve Injury and Repair*, Edinburgh: Churchill Livingstone.

Magill, R. and Konz, S. 1986 An evaluation of seven industrial screwdrivers, in *Trends in Ergonomics/Human Factors*, vol. III, W. Karwowski (ed.), Amsterdam: Elsevier, pp. 597–604.

Malaviya, P., Butler, D.L., Boivin, G.P., Smith, F.N., Barry, F.P., Murphy, J.M., and Vogel, K.G. 2000 An in vivo model for load-modulated remodeling in the rabbit flexor tendon, *Journal of Orthopaedic Research*, 18, 116–125.

McCully, K.K. and Faulkner, J.S. 1985 Injury to skeletal muscle fibres of mice following lengthening contractions, *Journal of Applied Physiology*, 59, 119–126.

Meyer, F. 1930 Arbeitsgrösse, Arbeitsaufwand und Arbeitsökonomie beim hantieren schwerer Hammer, *Arbeitsphysiologie*, 3, 529.

Miller, G. and Freivalds, A. 1987 Gender and handedness in grip strength, in *Proceedings of the Human Factors Society*, 31st Annual Meeting, Santa Monica, CA, Human Factor Society, 1987, pp. 906–909.

Mital, A. 1985 Effects of tool and operator factors on volitional torque exertion capabilities of individuals, in *Ergonomics International '85*, I.D. Brown, R. Goldsmith, K. Coombes and M. A. Sinclair (eds.), London: Taylor & Francis, pp. 262–264.

Mital, A., Sanghavi, N., and Huston, T. 1985 A study of factors defining the operator-hand tool system at the work place, *International Journal of Production Research*, 23, 297–314.

Mital, A. 1986 Effect of body posture and common hand tools on peak torque exertion capabilities, *Applied Ergonomics*, 17, 87–96.

Mital, A. and Sanghavi, N. 1986 Comparison of maximum volitional torque exertion capabilities of males and females using common hand tools, *Human Factors*, 27, 283–294.

Mosconi, T. and Kruger, L. 1996 Fixed-diameter polyethylene cuffs applied to the rat sciatic nerve induce a painful neuropathy: Ultrasound morphometric analysis of axonal alterations, *Pain*, 64, 37–57.

Monod, H. and Scherrer, J. 1965 The work capacity of a synergic muscular group, *Ergonomics*, 8, 329–338.

Napier, J. 1956 The prehensile movements of the human hand, *Journal of Bone and Joint Surgery*, 38B, 902–913.

Necking, L.E., Lundstrom, R., Dahlin, L.B., Lundborg, G., Thornell, L.E., and Friden, J. 1966 Tissue displacement is a causative factor in vibration-induced muscle injury, *Journal of Hand Surgery (Br)*, 21, 753–757.

Noonan, T.J., Best, T.M., Seaber, A.V., Garrett, W.E. 1994 Identification of a threshold for skeletal muscle injury, *American Journal of Sports Medicine*, 22, 257–261.

Okutsu, I., Ninomiya, S., Hamanaka, I., Kuroshima, N., and Inanami, H. 1989 Measurement of pressure in the carpal canal before and after endoscopic management of carpal tunnel syndrome, *Journal of Bone and Joint Surgery*, 71A, 679–683.

Olsen, N. and Nielsen, S.L. 1988 Vasoconstrictor response to cold in forestry workers: A prospective study, *British Journal of Industrial Medicine*, 45, 39–42.

Parker, K.G. and Imbus, H.R. 1992 *Cumulative Trauma Disorders*, Chelsea, MI: Lewis Publishers.

Pheasant, S.T. and O'Neill, D. 1975 Performance in gripping and turning—A study in hand/handle effectiveness, *Applied Ergonomics*, 6, 205–208.

Pheasant, S.T. and Scriven, J. G. 1983 Sex differences in strength—Some implications for the design of handtools, in Coombes, K. (ed.)., *Proceedings of the Ergonomics Society's Conference 1983*, London: Taylor & Francis, pp. 9–13.

Praemer, A., Furner, S., Rice, D.P. 1999 *Musculoskeletal Conditions in the United States*, Rosemont, IL: American Academy of Orthopaedic Surgeons.

Punnett, L., Robins, J.M., Wegman, D.H., and Keyserling, W.M. 1985 Soft-tissue disorders in the upper limbs of female garment workers, *Scandinavian Journal of Work, Environment & Health*, 11, 417–425.

Radhakrishnan, S., and Nagaravindra, M.C. 1993 Analysis of hand forces in health and disease during maximum isometric grasping of cylinders, *Medicine and Biological Engineering and Computing*, 31, 372–376.

Reinstein, L. 1983 DeQuervain's stenosing tenosynovitis in a video game player, *Archives of Physical Medicine and Rehabilitation*, 64, 434–435.

Replogle, J.0. 1983 Hand torque strength with cylindrical handles, in *Proceedings of the Human Factors Society*, 27th Annual Meeting, Santa Monica, CA, Human Factor Society, pp. 412–416.

Rigby, L.V. 1973 Why do people drop things? *Quality Progress*, 6, 16–19.

Rohmert, W. 1973 Problems in determining rest allowances, *Applied Ergonomics*, 4, 91–95.

Rubarth, B. 1928 Untersuchung zur Festgestaltung von Handheften für Schraubenzieher und ähnliche Werkzeuge (Research on handles for screwdrivers and similar tools), *Industrielle Psychotechnik*, 5, 129–142.

Rydevik, B., Lundborg, G., and Nordborg, C. 1976 Intraneural tissue reactions induced by internal neurolysis, *Scandinavian Journal of Plastic and Reconstructive Surgery*, 10, 3–8.

Saran, C. 1973 Biomechanical evaluation of T-handles for a pronation supination task, *Journal of Occupational Medicine*, 15, 712–716.

Scheller, W.L. 1983 The effect of handle shape on grip fatigue in manual lifting, in *Proceedings of the Human Factors Society*, 27th Annual Meeting, Santa Monica, CA, Human Factor Society, pp. 417–421.

Sheehy, M.P. and Marsden, C.D. 1982 Writer's cramp—A focal dystonia, *Brain*, 105, 461–480.

Schoenmarklin, R.W. and Marras, W.P. 1990 A dynamic biomechanical model of the wrist joint, in *Proceedings of the Human Factors Society*, 34th Annual Meeting, Santa Monica, CA: Human Factors Society, pp. 805–809.

Shock, N. 1962 The physiology of aging, *Scientific American*, 206, 100–110.

Simonsen, E.B., Klitgaard, H., and Bojsen-Moller, F. 1995 The influence of strength training, swim training and ageing on the Achilles tendon and m. soleus of the rat, *Journal of Sports Sciences*, 13, 291–295.

Sjøgaard, G. and Jensen, B.R. 1997 Muscle pathology with overuse, in Ranney, D. (ed.)., *Chronic Musculoskeletal Injuries in the Workplace*, Philadelphia: W.B. Saunders, pp. 17–40.

Sjøgaard, G. and Søgaard, K. 1998 Muscle injury in repetitive motion disorders, *Clinical Orthopaedics and Related Research*, 351, 21–31.

Sommer, C., Gailbraith, J.A., Heckman, H.M., and Myers, R.R. 1993 Pathology of experimental compression neuropathy producing hyperesthesia, *Journal of Neuropathology and Experimental Neurology*, 52, 223–233.

Stenlund, B., Goldie, I., Hagberg, M., Hogstedt, C., and Marions, O. 1992 Radiographic osteoarthrosis in the acromioclavicular joint resulting from manual work or exposure to vibration, *British Journal of Industrial Medicine*, 49, 588–593.

Strömberg, T., Dahlin, L.B., Brun, A., and Lundborg, G. 1997 Structural nerve damage at wrist level in workers exposed to vibration, *Occupational and Environmental Medicine*, 54, 307–311.

Tanaka, S., Wild, D.K., Seligman, P.J., Haperin, W.E., Behrens, V.J., and Putz-Anderson, V. 1995 Prevalence and work-relatedness of self-reported carpal tunnel syndrome among U.S. workers' analysis of the Occupational Health Supplement data of the 1988 National Health Interview Survey, *American Journal of Industrial Medicine*, 27, 451–470.

Taylor, W., Wasserman, D., Behrens, V., Reynolds, D., and Samueloff, S. 1984 Effect of the air hammer on the hands of stonecutters. The limestone quarries of Bedford, Indiana, revisited, *British Journal of Industrial Medicine*, 41, 289–295.

Terrell, R. and Purswell, J. 1976 The influence of forearm and wrist orientation on static grip strength as a design criterion for hand tools, in *Proceedings of the Human Factors Society*, 20th Annual Meeting, Santa Monica, CA, Human Factor Society, pp. 28–32.

Thun, M., Tanaka, S., Smith, A.B., Halperin, W.E., Lee, S.T., Luggen, M.E., and Hess, E.V. 1987 Morbidity from repetitive knee trauma in carpet and floor layers, *British Journal of Industrial Medicine*, 44, 611–620.

Tichauer, E.R. and Gage, H. 1977 Ergonomic principles basic to hand tool design, *Journal of the American Industrial Hygiene Association*, 38, 622–634.

Travell, J.G. and Simons, D.G. 1983 *Myofascial Pain and Dysfunction—The Trigger Point Manual*, Baltimore: Williams & Wilkins.

Viegas, S.F. and Torres, F.G. 1989 Cherry pitter's thumb. Case report and review of the literature, *Orthopaedic Review*, 18, 336–338.

Warren, G.L., Hayes, D.A., Lowe, D.A., Prior, B.M., and Armstrong, R.B. 1993 Material fatigue initiates eccentric contraction-induced injury in rat soleous muscle, *Journal of Applied Physiology*, 464, 477–489.

Westling, G. and Johansson, R.S. 1984 Factors influencing the force control during precision grip, *Experimental Brain Research*, 53, 277–284.

Westling, G. and Johansson, R.S. 1987 Responses in glabrous skin mechanoreceptors, *Experimental Brain Research*, 66, 128–140.

Widule, C.J., Foley, V. and Demo, F. 1978 Dynamics of the axe swing, *Ergonomics*, 21, 925–930.

Wilks, S. 1878 *Lectures on Diseases of the Nervous System*, London: Churchill, pp. 452–460.

Woo, S.L., Ritter, M.A., Amiel, D., Sanders, T.M., Gomez, M.A., Kuei, S.C., Garfin, S.R., and Akeson, W.H. 1980 The biomechanical and biochemical properties of swine tendons—Long term effects of exercise on digital extensors, *Connective Tissue Research*, 7, 177–183.

Yu, Z.S., Chao, H., Qiao, L., Qian, D.S., and Ye, Y.H. 1986 Epidemiologic survey of vibration syndrome among riveters, chippers and grinder in the railroad system of the People's Republic of China, *Scandinavian Journal of Work, Environment & Health*, 12, 289–292.

10 Ergonomic Risk Assessment for Musculoskeletal Disorders of the Upper Extremity: State of the Art

Troy Jones and Shrawan Kumar

CONTENTS

10.1 INTRODUCTION

A large body of evidence supporting the role of workplace physical exposures in the causation of musculoskeletal injuries (MSIs) is now available (U.S. Department of

Health and Human Services, 1997). A number of mechanisms of injury causation based on established physiologic principles have been proposed (Kumar, 2001). A systematic review of epidemiologic literature examining the relationship of physical exposures to MSIs has found that in most specific MSI conditions, the risk associated with combined physical exposures is greater than the risk associated with the physical exposures alone (U.S. Department of Health and Human Services, 1997). Given it is the combination of physical exposures which are most strongly related to precipitation of MSI, a model of MSI causation is needed, which is able to account for the relative role of the individual exposure variables. A validated model of MSI causation is needed to enable ergonomic practitioners to identify jobs at increased risk of MSI. Should a model of MSI causation be able to correctly identify jobs associated with high rates of MSI it follows that the model will have correctly accounted for the relative role of the physical exposures and may be used to evaluate the relative risk associated with those exposures.

Observational ergonomic risk assessments (ERAs) are based on models of MSI causation, which consider the combined effect of physical exposures. ERAs are used by practicing ergonomists to gain insight into how the physical exposures of the job interact to precipitate MSIs. ERAs have been identified as the best method, considering the constraints of practice, by which ergonomic practitioners may establish a basis for identifying priorities for intervention (David, 2005). Up to 83.1% of practicing professional ergonomists make use of ERAs to assess the risk associated with manual material handling tasks (Dempsey et al., 2005).

At present, multiple risk assessment methods of unique structures have been proposed and the research field has been divided in the pursuit of validating competing models. As a result of the current state of disagreement there is a need to focus the research area by identifying the model of MSI causation best able to predict risk of injury and identify problem exposures. Identification of the model of injury causation "best" able to predict MSI will allow the field to move forward toward refining a model of risk prediction which accurately accounts for the role of physical exposures in the precipitation of MSIs. Refinement of the models of injury causation and their validation is needed to improve our understanding of how physical exposures may interact to precipitate MSIs. An improved understanding of the relationship between physical exposures and MSIs is needed to improve our ability to design effective prevention initiatives and reduce both the human and financial impact of MSIs. It is the intent of this chapter to review the current state of literature examining upper extremity ERAs. An appreciation of the current state of research is necessary for practitioners to select the most appropriate method for a given industrial setting.

Five risk assessment methods have been selected for discussion in this chapter. The risk assessment methods considered here are the Rapid Upper Limb Assessment (RULA, McAtamney and Corlett, 1993), Rapid Entire Body Assessment (REBA, Hignett and McAtamney, 2000), the quantitative version of the American Conference of Governmental Industrial Hygienists Threshold Limit Value for monotask hand work (ACGIH TLV, University of Michigan, 2005), the Strain Index (SI, Moore and Garg, 1995), and the Concise Exposure Index (OCRA, Colombini, 1998; Grieco, 1998; Occhipinti, 1998).

10.2 REVIEW OF CURRENT STATE OF RESEARCH

In order to outline the process of identifying the "best" method of risk assessment it is first necessary to understand how the lack of consensus between risk assessment models is possible. It is hypothesized here that the current limited agreement between methods is primarily due to differences in the "expert opinion" of authors, the limited ability of authors to set risk level scores, and the lack of consensus in studies of predictive validity regarding the definition of morbidity.

10.2.1 MODEL STRUCTURE

Selection of exposure variables to be considered in the risk assessment and the roles of those variables is made based upon the author's interpretation of biomechanical, physiological, and epidemiologic literature. Because each author's interpretation of the literature is free to vary there is no agreement between authors as to how exposure variables such as repetition, force, or posture should be weighted and how the magnitude of the interactions should be quantified in assessments of risk (Winkel and Westgaard, 1992). Only in the case of the SI have the authors set the weights of variables considering the findings of an experimental study in the same worker population upon which the predictive validity of the assessment was established (Moore and Garg, 1994). The general lack of objective processes used by authors in setting the relative weights of variables suggests that the authors have relied on an underlying theoretical orientation to define model structure. A model structure capable of describing risk associated with MSIs in general is sought as it is not the intent of observational ERAs to examine risk associated with specific conditions. It is assumed that both current global theories of MSI causation (Kumar, 2001) and current theories of the pathomechanisms of injury to muscle, ligament/tendon, and nervous tissue (Forde et al., 2002) have been considered in selecting relevant variables and setting relative variable roles. Given the structure of the methods has been set primarily based on the opinion of the authors, it is reasonable that a level of disagreement between methods exists.

10.2.2 DETERMINING MODEL STRUCTURE

10.2.2.1 Practical Considerations

Before setting the structure of a method the authors must consider the validity of the measure and the practical implication of misclassifying the risk and the consequent output variability between evaluators.

10.2.2.1.1 False Positives

The implication of misclassifying an at-risk job as safe is greater than misclassifying a safe job as at-risk. The definitions of morbidity used in studies of the association between risk output and morbidity generally err on the side of identifying safe jobs as at-risk (false-positive predictions).

10.2.2.1.2 Reliability

The implication of risk output varying significantly between evaluators is of primary importance. Variability in risk assessment scores both within and between evaluators is primarily the result of measurement error due to a lack of clear definition and stringent methods of measurement of relevant variables. Authors have sought to control for measurement error resulting from exposure assessment via observation through two methods of approximation. In one method, the authors adopt broad classification categories specific to each exposure variable to maximize the chance the recorded exposure will correspond to actual exposure and correlate to subsequent evaluations (e.g., RULA shoulder postures are assessed in up to 45° increments). The risk of using broad classifications, however, is that the groupings of exposure may not accurately capture the role of the exposure variable in the precipitation of MSI. In the second method, authors recommend multiple evaluators assess each job and use consensus scores in the determination of risk. The consensus method lacks precision however, as there is no guarantee that a consensus score will be more accurate than the score of an individual evaluator. The proponents of this method have gone on to study the psychometric properties of the assessments resulting from studies using multiple evaluators and controlled exposure records. The results of this study design, while an important first step, do not reflect the limitations imposed on worksite evaluators performing assessments based on observation. Most often the ideal angle of observation, ideal focal length, ideal resolution, and multiple evaluators are not available. Because of these "real world" limitations the psychometric properties resulting from such study designs cannot be assumed to reflect those attainable in worksite application. Thus both methods of approximation inherently lack accuracy and create considerable output variability between evaluators. Output variability affects both the validity and reliability of the assessment methods.

10.2.3   MODEL OUTPUT

The output of ERAs may be roughly broken down into four levels.

1. *Component scores*: Scores specific to body regions or physical exposure variables. Component scores are weighted by the method to reflect the relative importance of the exposure variable in the prediction model. Component scores are interpreted by the evaluator to identify and prioritize problem exposures.
2. *Combined component scores*: An intermediate level of interpretation where the combined role of two or more variables (e.g., posture and force) is assessed. Combined component scores may be weighted by the method to reflect the relative importance of the exposure variable in the prediction model. Component scores are interpreted by the user to identify combinations of problem exposures.
3. *Risk index score*: Raw "risk" output.
4. *Risk level or criterion score*: Final score representing the degree of risk associated with performance of the job.

10.2.3.1   Risk Output

Worksite evaluators interpret the assessment's risk output to determine the degree of risk present in a job. Risk outputs include raw "risk index" scores and either multiple "risk levels" or a single "criterion score." Criterion or risk level scores are determined by selecting risk index cut-points, which differentiate between groups of risk (e.g., no risk, moderate risk, and high risk). Risk index cut-points may be set subjectively, reflecting the expert opinion of the authors and possibly a focus group, or objectively by studying the relationship between risk index scores and morbidity. The RULA, REBA, and quantitative ACGIH TLV methods have used expert opinion to set risk levels. Risk index cut-points of the SI and OCRA procedures have also been set primarily based on expert "opinion," however both methods have also considered the results of objective studies.

The criterion score of the SI has been set based on the subjective inspection of relationship between risk index scores and incidence as reported by Moore and Garg (1994) however, logistic modeling of SI scores and MSI incidence information has been used to support the criterion score selected (Knox and Moore, 2001). The procedures used to select the risk level cut-points in the OCRA assessment are less clear. Risk level cut points originally described by Occhipinti (1998) for the OCRA procedure were selected based on a subjective review of relationship between OCRA scores and incidence of MSI. Occhipinti and Colombini (2004) report the use of an "original approach" to revise the OCRA risk level cut-points. While the use of an "original method" suggests an objective process has been used the precise method of selection used remains unclear, as a complete description of the methodology used has been published in the Italian language only.

At present, expert opinion has primarily been used to set criterion and risk level scores. Objective examination of the ability of the risk level cut-points selected to differentiate between levels of risk present are needed to refine the current risk index cut-points that result in broad risk level scores. Refining risk index cut points is hypothesized to result in an increased ability to differentiate between levels of risk present in jobs. Comparison of the relative ability of multiple ERA methods to differentiate between the level of risk present in jobs will lead to conclusions regarding the strength of the models of MSI causation upon which the assessments are based.

10.2.3.2　Challenges to Using Objective Means to Set Risk Level Scores

Risk index cut-points identified by objective means are set based upon an examination of the relationship between risk index scores and incidence of MSI in multiple jobs representing different levels of risk. The relationship is studied by examining the location of each job with respect to risk index score and morbidity. The plot of risk assessment scores and morbidity information is then analyzed to differentiate between groups of jobs, where the groups reflect different levels of risk. Risk index cut-points, which define the levels of risk, are then set. The ability of the authors to differentiate between groups, and thus set cut-points, is limited by (1) practical considerations (described above), (2) inaccuracy of exposure data collected via observation, and (3) resolution of morbidity data.

10.2.3.2.1　Inaccuracy of Exposure Data Collected via Observation

ERA techniques are traditionally calculated based on exposure assessments performed by observation. A body of literature is currently available, which describes the significant measurement error resulting from exposure assessment via observation

(Bao et al., 2006a; Lowe, 2004). Inaccuracy resulting from the discrepancy between exposure measurements obtained via observation and actual exposures affects the accuracy of risk assessments in a compound manner (multiple variables considered). The "real world" limitations imposed on workplace exposure measurement by observation, combined with the literature base documenting measurement error due to observation, suggests accurate and reliable risk assessment performance, such as is required to evaluate risk index cut-points, requires exposure assessment by quantified means. Quantified tools such as electromyography and electrogoniometry are the current gold standard objective measures in exposure assessment. Application of electromyography and electrogoniometry within the worksite results in significantly lower levels of measurement error than are obtained in exposure assessment based on observation.

A series of studies performed by Jones and Kumar (2007c,d, 2008b,c) based the calculation of the five ERAs compared on the quantified physical exposure information previously described by Jones and Kumar (2006, 2007a,b, 2008a). Collection of exposure information via quantitative means allowed Jones and Kumar (2007c,d, 2008b,c) to examine the effect of multiple definition of the posture and exertion variable on ERA scores. Across all ERA methods examined varying posture variable definition resulted in significantly different component or combined component scores. Defining range of motion required to perform a job by the postures required to perform the primary task only vs. the peak postures observed reduced risk index output by as much as 83% (Jones and Kumar, 2008c). Definition of the exertion variable was also observed to have a significant effect on component, combined component, and risk index scores on all methods examined across all jobs. In some cases definition of the exertion variable was observed to result in significantly different risk level output.

Quantification of the physical exposures required to perform at-risk jobs in multiple workers also allowed Jones and Kumar (2007c,d, 2008b,c) to examine the effect of variability in exposures between workers on ERA output. Coefficient of variation values describing the variation in risk assessment multiplier scores observed between workers performing the same job reported by Jones and Kumar (2007c,d, 2008b,c) suggest that assessment of one worker performing a repetitive job will perhaps be insufficient to arrive at risk assessment scores representative of that job.

Assessment of the population of workers available at the four facilities assessed by Jones and Kumar (2006, 2007a,b, 2008a) allowed the sample size required to arrive at risk assessment scores (component, combined component, risk index, and risk level), which reflect the group mean to be calculated (Figure 10.1). In this chapter, an alpha level of 0.05 was used to calculate the number of worker assessments required to derive an average value falling within one category level of the population mean. Table 10.1 describes the mean and range of worker assessments necessary to arrive at the population mean considering all jobs and all subjects across facilities assessed. Review of Table 10.1 illustrates that while only one worker assessment

$$n = \left[\frac{(Z\,\alpha/2)\sigma}{E} \right]$$

FIGURE 10.1 Sample size calculation.

TABLE 10.1

Number of Worker Assessments Required to Arrive at a Mean Score Representative of the Population Mean

Method	Component	Combined Component	Risk Index	Risk Level
RULA	1 (1–2)	1 (1–4)	1 (1)	1
REBA	1 (1–2)	2 (1–6)	5 (1–6)	1
ACGIH TLV	1 (1–4)			1
SI	1 (1–2)			1
OCRA	3 (1–11)			1

Range of values observed across jobs in brackets.

may be needed to arrive at a risk level representative of the job, and more than one assessment may be required to arrive at representative component or combined component scores. Importantly, values reported in Table 10.1 reflect those derived using the scoring categories of the assessments. For example, the SI posture component score has five ordinal scoring categories, each of which is assigned a multiplier value by the authors. The ordinal scoring levels were used to derive the values reported in Table 10.1 to provide insight on the ability of the evaluator to arrive at the scoring category representing the population mean. Arriving at the population mean scoring category is important as exposures are frequently prioritized for intervention based on component or combined component scores which may vary by worker assessed.

Using Figure 10.2 to illustrate the implications of the inaccuracy of observational exposure assessments on an author's ability to set risk index cut points, we see that while the true representative job score lies in the middle of the concentric circles (corresponding to sources of measurement error) a score obtained from a single worker based on an observational exposure assessment is free to fall anywhere within the circles. The implication of measurement error is a decreased ability to

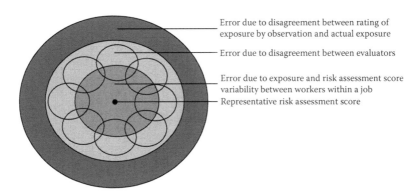

FIGURE 10.2 Sources of measurement error in exposure measurement via observation.

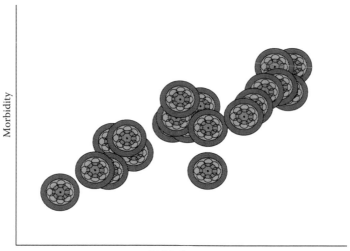

FIGURE 10.3 Effect of measurement error due to observation on setting risk index cut-points.

identify groups of workers and derive cut-points corresponding to different levels of risk by objective means (Figure 10.3). The inability to set risk index cut-points by objective means has resulted in broad risk levels or single criterion scores set by sub-jective means. Broad risk level scores set to minimize the chance of misclassifying at-risk jobs as safe have been easily correlated to "safe" measures of morbidity. The limited ability to identify groups by objective means combined with the adoption of safe morbidity classifications has resulted in the validation of several models of MSI causation of unique structure.

There is currently a lack of consensus between authors regarding the physical exposures to be considered in predicting risk and the relative role of those variables in the model of MSI precipitation upon which they are based. This lack of consensus makes examination of the comparability of risk output from multiple assessments in the same worker population(s) necessary. This necessity is heightened by the fact that up to 83.1% of practicing ergonomists make use of observational ERAs and the implication of disagreement between methods is the inappropriate assignment of risk and/or identification of problem exposures (Dempsey et al., 2005).

10.2.3.2.2 Morbidity

Morbidity may be defined as the rate of incidence of MSI conditions. In order to establish the predictive validity of an assessment method risk output is compared to a measure of morbidity. Should the assessment demonstrate an association between increasing risk output scores and increasing morbidity, the assessment has estab-lished a measure of predictive validity. Both the morbidity event and the definition of morbidity itself influence the relationship between risk output and morbidity.

Three event types have been used by past studies to define morbidity: report of discomfort consistent with MSI, recorded incidence of MSI (may include inci-dence of discomfort), or diagnosis of MSI based on medical examination. Inclusion of reported discomfort as an event indicating incidence of MSI must be done with caution as discomfort is a subjective experience known to vary by individual. The risk of including reported discomfort events in morbidity classifications is that false-positive cases result when discomfort not indicative of MSI and/or unrelated to the job are considered in morbidity classifications. The effect of false-positives in examinations of the relationship between risk assessment scores and morbidity is a reduced ability to differentiate between groups of subjects (safe and at-risk jobs). Defining events to be considered in morbidity classifications based on diagnosed conditions by health professionals minimizes the chance of false-positives and is therefore the gold standard.

Morbidity has been defined in a number of ways in the literature. In some cases morbidity is defined simply as the report of discomfort and predictive validity that is established by studying the association between discomfort and risk assessment scores. In these cases the association is evaluated with measures of association such as the chi-square test of independence or the Fischer's exact test. In some cases, the prevalence of conditions is considered and the definition of morbidity is based on the percentage of subjects reporting symptoms or diagnosed with conditions. In these cases examinations of the relationship between risk assessment scores and morbidity information are based measuring the relationship between prevalence of morbidity events in the population and risk assessment scores with prediction models such as linear and logistic regression. In these cases predictive validity is demonstrated by positive associations and high levels of explained variance. In other cases, authors define "at-risk jobs" based on a definition of morbidity related to a "trigger value." For example, authors may define an "at-risk job" as one in which a single morbidity event was recorded in the period reviewed (a one incident trigger corresponds to an incident rate >0). In these cases the relationship between risk assessment scores and morbidity are examined by selecting a cut-point value (criterion score), which best differentiates between two groups defined by the morbidity classification (safe and at-risk jobs). In these cases, a dichotomous risk outcome (safe or at-risk) is selected and justified by maximizing the diagnostic property of interest (e.g., sensitivity). Given the authors have dichotomized both risk output (at-risk vs. not at-risk) and morbidity outcome (positive or negative based on trigger value) predictive validity of the assessment is studied by examining the diagnostic properties of the assessment and establishing the association between risk classification and morbidity. Definition and derivation of the diagnostic properties used to evaluate predictive validity in cases where both a dichotomous risk outcome and morbidity classification is present are illustrated in Figure 10.4. When predictive validity of the assessment is examined in this way, the value of the criterion cut-point is influenced by the definition of morbidity. If a one incident trigger (incidence rate >0) is selected to define morbidity, the criterion cut-point will tend to be lower and the sensitivity of the test will tend to be higher at the expense of specificity. Sensitivity of the test will tend to be higher at the expense of specificity in these cases because one can expect cases where the morbidity event has occurred not as a result of the job to be included as positive cases (false-positives). Practically then, a one incident trigger morbidity definition maximizes the risk assessment's ability to determine a job is "at-risk" at the expense of the risk assessments ability to find jobs which are not "at-risk." While this is a valid approach, it follows that jobs which are not at increased risk of MSIs are more

Risk	Morbidity	
assessment	Positive	Negative
Risk	a (True positive)	b (False positive)
No risk	c (False negative)	d (True negative)

$$\text{Sensitivity} = \frac{a}{a+c}$$

$$\text{Specificity} = \frac{d}{b+d}$$

$$\text{Positive predictive value} = \frac{a}{a+b}$$

$$\text{Negative predictive value} = \frac{d}{c+d}$$

Sensitivity: The risk assessment's ability to identify the job as at-risk when morbidity is assessed present.

Specificity: The risk assessment's ability to identify the job as not at-risk when no morbidity is present.

Positive predictive value: The likelihood that the job assessed at-risk actually was associated with morbidity.

Negative predictive value: The likelihood that the job assessed as not at-risk was not associated with morbidity.

FIGURE 10.4   Diagnostic properties.

often identified as at-risk and exposures levels which may not be related to incidence of MSI are examined for intervention. Using a multi-incident trigger (or specified incidence rate) to define morbidity potentially decreases the sensitivity of the test and increases its specificity by correctly identifying a higher proportion of true negative cases. Accurate definition of a multi-incident trigger is best done based upon an understanding of the prevalence of the conditions of interest in the occupation. If the prevalence of the conditions of interest in the nonexposed population is known, the examiner is able to set the trigger value to reflect increases in prevalence hypothesized to result from work-related physical exposures. Should the specified multi-incident trigger (incidence rate) underestimate the number of conditions due to workplace exposures, an increased number of false-positives will result decreasing the specificity of the test (ability to indicate no risk when morbidity is not present). Should the specified multi-incident trigger (incidence rate) overestimate the number of conditions due to workplace exposures, an increased number of false-negative values will result influencing sensitivity (ability to indicate risk when morbidity is present). The key challenge to setting the multi-incident trigger is defining the prevalence of MSI conditions in the normal population. Prevalence of MSI conditions in the normal population is often poorly understood and therefore our ability to determine the rate at which MSIs may be due to workplace physical exposures is limited. The limited ability to precisely define the prevalence of MSIs in the nonexposed population justifies the use of "safe" morbidity definitions (one incident trigger).

10.3   SELECTION OF AN APPROPRIATE ERGONOMIC RISK ASSESSMENT TECHNIQUE

The previous general discussion of the practical and methodological issues faced by the authors of risk assessment methods has emphasized the need for objective studies of predictive validity seeking to refine risk assessment methods. The information constraints faced by authors has resulted in the current state where the validity of multiple risk assessment methods of unique structure has been established and selection of the most appropriate assessment in a given application is difficult. No studies are currently available, which have examined the comparative predictive validity of multiple assessment methods based on the same definition of morbidity in the same worker population. Such studies are needed to objectively identify the most appropriate assessment for a given application.

10.3.1 SELECTION OF AN ERGONOMIC RISK ASSESSMENT BASED ON CONTENT VALIDITY

Knox and Moore (2001) have defined content validity, as the concept applies to ERAs, as follows: to be consistent with or derived from relevant physiological, biomechanical, and epidemiological principles. The content validity of ERAs which consider physical exposures related to MSI causation is established by the evidence base linking physical exposures to MSIs. The content validity of the methods is also established by defining model structure based on a theoretical orientation which reflects current theories of MSI injury causation. All of the assessment techniques examined in this chapter consider physical exposures related to MSIs of the upper extremity. The number of exposures considered by the methods and the relative role of those exposures in the model of MSI causation upon which the methods are based vary however. An evaluation of the content validity of the different methods is dependent on a comparison of the level of evidence supporting the role of the exposure variables in the causation of MSI vs. the exposures considered and the relative roles of those variables in the ERA method. Figure 10.5 illustrates the findings of

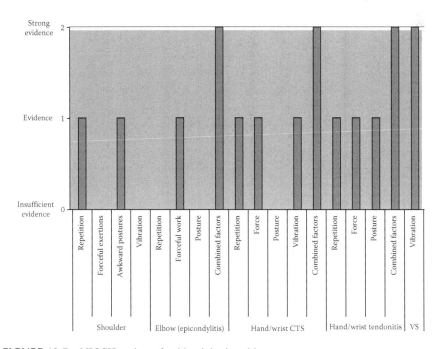

FIGURE 10.5   NIOSH review of epidemiologic evidence.

TABLE 10.2
Physical Exposures Considered by Method

Methodology	Force	Repetition	Posture	Vibration	Combined Factors
RULA	√	√	√		√
REBA	√	√	√		√
OCRA	√	√	√	√	√
SI	√	√	√		√
ACGIH TLV	√	√			√

Physical Exposures Considered spans Force, Repetition, Posture, Vibration, Combined Factors.

the 1997 review of epidemiologic evidence linking physical exposures to MSIs of the upper extremity and Table 10.2 describes the variables considered by the risk assessment examined.

10.3.2   SELECTION OF AN ERGONOMIC RISK ASSESSMENT BASED ON PREDICTIVE VALIDITY

Knox and Moore (2001) have defined predictive validity, as the concept applies to ERAs, as follows: to exhibit a reasonable ability to discriminate between adverse and nonadverse exposures. External validity is an extension of predictive validity and describes the assessments ability to be applicable to a variety of circumstances of exposure (Knox and Moore, 2001). The predictive validity of multiple ERA methods has been established. Generally the predictive validity of the ERA methods has been established by three methods: (1) examining the association between risk output and reported discomfort, (2) examining the association between dichotomized risk output and morbidity (defined by a single incident trigger), and (3) examining the association between risk output and prevalence of MSI conditions. Selection of the most appropriate ERA by the worksite evaluator for the application in question requires the evaluator examine the evidence of predictive validity specific to each method. Consideration must be given to the following factors in an examination of the strength of studies of predictive validity:

1. Population studied and the relationship to population of interest
2. Variables examined
3. Exposure assessment technique used
4. Morbidity definition
5. Statistical techniques
6. Results

Table 10.3 describes the current studies of predictive validity by method according to the criteria above.

TABLE 10.3

Studies of Predictive Validity

Method	Study	Population	Variables Examined	Exposure Assessment	Morbidity Classification	Statistics Used	Results	Interpretation
RULA	Massaccesi et al. (2003)	77 garbage truck drivers	Ergonomic: RULA variables	Performed via observation. 1 evaluator	Discomfort as assessed by body part discomfort survey.	Association between reported pain, aches, or discomfort and corresponding RULA body part scores assessed with the χ^2-test of independence.	Neck and trunk score associated with pain. Upper arm, lower arm, wrist scores associated with pain.	RULA neck and trunk scores associated with pain in garbage truck drivers. Association between upper arm, lower arm, or wrist pain and RULA scores not established in this population.
	Shuval and Donchin (2005)	84 visual display terminal workers. Computer programmers, managers, administrators, and marketing specialists	Ergonomic: RULA variables Individual: Nordic questionnaire Work organizational: Nordic questionnaire (Kourinka et al., 1987) Stress:	Performed via observation. 1 evaluator. Two direct observations of each job. Mean score resulting from two observations used.	Upper extremity musculoskeletal symptoms assessed via the Nordic questionnaire.	Predictive ability of RULA scores on hand/wrist/finger symptoms studied with logistic regression while calculating the odds ratio (OR) of the different categories compared to the reference category.	An increase of 1 point in the RULA risk index score increased risk of reporting hand/wrist/ finger symptoms by 3.2 times.	Association between the RULA score and reported symptoms established in VDT users. We do not know how predictive RULA score is of symptoms overall

(continued)

TABLE 10.3 (continued)
Studies of Predictive Validity

Method	Study	Population	Variables Examined	Exposure Assessment	Morbidity Classification	Statistics Used	Results	Interpretation
				Questionnaire (Toviana, 1999).			Strength of prediction model not described (r^2).	(what % of the variance is explained) because the factors have been considered individually.
ACGIH TLV	Latko et al. (1999) *nonquanti-fied technique	352 workers from three manufacturing companies	109 exposure variables analyzed: 10 anthropometry parameters, 25 medical history parameters, 5 demographic parameters, 13 psychosocial parameters, 4 tobacco use parameters, and 53 ergonomic parameters.	The HAL repetition assessment technique (Latko, 1997) was performed via observation. 4 evaluators. Repetition modeled as three categories (low/medium/high) and as a continuous variable (0–10). The relationship between repetition (assessed by HAL) and the conditions	Assessed via four techniques: 1. Worker questionnaire. (Cohen et al., 1983; Karasek, 1985; Franzblau et al., 1997). 2. Physical medical examination (Fine and Silverstein, 1995). 3. Electrodiagnostic testing. 4. Anthropometric measurements.	The relationship between the five health outcomes (nonspecific discomfort, tendonitis, carpal tunnel syndrome (CTS) symptoms only, CTS symptoms, and electro-physiology) and the independent variables was assessed using a three step process. 1. Univariate analysis to establish relationship 2. Multiple variable logistic analyses were	Repetitiveness of work was found to be significantly associated with prevalence of reported discomfort in the wrist, hand, or fingers, tendonitis in the distal upper extremity, and symptoms consistent with carpal tunnel syndrome. An association was also found between	Repetition as assessed by HAL was a significant term in the prediction models of reported discomfort, tendonitis, and carpal tunnel syndrome. Importantly however, only repetition was evaluated and it was evaluated using the HAL assessment and not the quantitative assessment

Reference	Sample	Exposure variables	Method	Outcome measures	Analysis	Results	Comments
	was of interest. Multiple workers for each job?				used to eliminate those variables within each group (anthropometry, medical history, demographic, psychosocial, tobacco, and ergonomic) which did not contribute significantly to the explained variance. 3. Multivariate logistic analyses formation of a predictive model which accounts for multiple groups of variables.	repetitiveness of work and carpal tunnel syndrome, indicated by the combination of positive electrodiagnostic results and symptoms consistent with carpal tunnel syndrome. Strength of prediction models are not described.	presented by the University of Michigan (2005)
Franzblau et al. (2005)	908 workers from seven different job sites. Four manufacturing operations (office furniture manufacturing, industrial container manufacturing,	Ergonomic: TLV variables Individual factors: age, gender, body mass index	Observational method of Latko used to rate repetition and force required in jobs. 4 evaluators.	Presence of condi tions of interest (wrist/hand/finger symptoms, elbow/forearm symptoms, wrist/hand/finger tendonitis, elbow/forearm tendonitis, carpal tunnel syndrome diagnosed	Chi-square test was used to examine the associations. Evidence of a linear trend was assessed with the Mantel-Haenszel chi-square test of linear trend.	The prevalence of symptoms in the wrist/hand/fingers or elbow/forearm was not related to increases in TLV levels. Presence of tendonitis in the wrist/hand/fingers was not	Associations between TLV levels and elbow/forearm tendonitis and carpal tunnel syndrome were established. TLV risk level dichotomization scheme used to

(continued)

TABLE 10.3 (continued)
Studies of Predictive Validity

Method	Study	Population	Variables Examined	Exposure Assessment	Morbidity Classification	Statistics Used	Results	Interpretation
		automobile parts manufacturing, and spark plug manufacturing) and three employers involving office or computer-related jobs (an insurance claims processing center and two government computer data entry facilities)			by hand diagrams, CTS diagnosed by median mononeuropathy, CTS diagnosed by hand diagrams and electro diagnostic studies) assessed via three techniques: 1. Electrodiagnostic studies 2. Self-administered questionnaire 3. Physical examination		related to TLV level. Presence of elbow/forearm tendonitis was related to TLV risk level. Presence of carpal tunnel syndrome was related to TLV risk level. The sensitivity and specificity for the TLV with respect to all outcomes ranged from 0.29 to 0.59 and 0.67 to 0.73, respectively.	calculate diagnostic properties reported not described. Exposure assessment performed with observational scales not the quantitative assessment presented by the University of Michigan (2005)
Werner et al. (2005)		501 active workers from seven different job sites. Four manufacturing operations	Ergonomic: TLV variables (repetition and force), posture Individual: age, gender, medical	TLV used process not described but taken to be identical to Fanzblau et al. (2005)	Upper extremity body part discomfort survey score.	The relationship of multiple variables to body part discomfort was examined. Univariate analysis was followed by	Workers with ACGIH TLV risk levels of 2 or 3 were 2.14 times more likely to develop	Very low explained variance indicating the factors considered do not predict the outcome well. Association

Author (year)	Subjects	Variables	Assessment / TLV	Analysis	Results	Comments
	(office furniture manufacturing, industrial container manufacturing, automobile parts manufacturing, and spark plug manufacturing) and three employers involving office or computer-related jobs (an insurance claims processing center and two government computer data entry facilities)	history, obesity, smoking history, exercise levels. Psychosocial: skill discretion decision authority, coworker support, job insecurity, job satisfaction, perceived stress. Electrophysiologic variables were also included as independent variables.	(same population of workers).	logistic regression modeling to determine the most predictive model for incident cases from baseline data	discomfort over time compared to the control group (OR 2.14). Strength of the prediction model $r^2 = 0.14$	between discomfort and TLV level established. Exposure assessment performed with observational scales not the quantitative assessment presented by the University of Michigan (2005)
Gell et al. (2005)	432 workers from seven different job sites. Four manufacturing operations (office furniture manufacturing, industrial container manufacturing,	Ergonomic: TLV variables (repetition and force), posture Individual: age, gender, medical history, obesity, smoking history, exercise levels. Psychosocial:	TLV used process not described but taken to be identical to Fanzblau et al. 2005 (same population of workers).	Presence of carpal tunnel syndrome assessed via 3 techniques: 1. Electrodiagnostic studies 2. Self-administered questionnaire 3. Physical examination. Multivariate logistic regression was performed using new onset of CTS as the dependent variable to create a predictive model based on data from the initial screening.	No significant difference in proportion of subjects rating above TLV level 2 between incident and control groups. Multiple logistic regression yielded	TLV level not observed to be a significant predictor of carpal tunnel syndrome not established with statistically significant findings in this study

(continued)

TABLE 10.3 (continued)
Studies of Predictive Validity

Method	Study	Population	Variables Examined	Exposure Assessment	Morbidity Classification	Statistics Used	Results	Interpretation
		automobile parts manufacturing, and spark plug manufacturing) and three employers involving office or computer-related jobs (an insurance claims processing center and two government computer data entry facilities)	skill discretion decision authority, coworker support, job insecurity, job satisfaction, perceived stress. Electrophysiologic variables were also included as independent variables.				a model for prediction ($r^2 = 0.25$) but TLV level 3 was not a significant predictor.	Exposure assessment performed with observational scales not the quantitative assessment presented by the University of Michigan 2005.
SI	Moore and Garg (1995)	25 jobs within a pork processing plant possible to examine more then one worker in the majority of cases.	Ergonomic: SI variables	Performed via observation. 1 evaluator	Review of OSHA logs and employee medical records. Specific conditions were identified by review but events included symptoms of non specific disorders. One incident trigger was used.	Diagnostic properties calculated as per Figure 10.4	Criterion value of 5 results in sensitivity of 0.92 and specificity of 1.0	Association between SI hazard classification and morbidity definition established in pork processing jobs.

| Moore et al. (2001). | 56 jobs. 28 from manufacturing (16 from chair assembly, 12 from hose and hose connector fabrication and assembly). 28 from poultry processing | Ergonomic: SI variables in addition to vibration, localized compression, cold, and use of gloves | Performed via observation. 2 raters for each job. | OSHA 200 logs, one incident trigger used. | Association between hazard classification and morbidity was assessed using Peason's chi-square or Fishers exact test. Strength of association was reported with estimated ORs. Diagnostic properties calculated as per Figure 10.4 | SI estimated OR (108.5). Sensitivity and specificity of the SI 0.9 and 0.93, respectively | Association between SI hazard classification and morbidity definition established in chair and hose manufacturing as well as poultry processing. |
| Knox and Moore (2001) | 28 turkey processing jobs. | Ergonomic: SI variables | Performed via observation. 2 raters for each job. | OSHA 200 logs, one incident trigger used. | Evidence of association was assessed using the likelihood ratio (LR) test for independence strength of association and was reported as the OR. If at least one cell had a count less than 5 Fishers exact test | Analysis 1 (left and right upper extremity considered separately). Relationship between morbidity and hazard assessed sig. with OR of 22. The sensitivity specificity, positive predictive value and negative predictive value were 0.86, 0.79, 0.92, and 0.65, respectively. | Association between SI hazard classification and morbidity definition established in turkey processing. |

(continued)

TABLE 10.3 (continued)
Studies of Predictive Validity

Method	Study	Population	Variables Examined	Exposure Assessment	Morbidity Classification	Statistics Used	Results	Interpretation
						was used to determine statistical significance. Diagnostic properties calculated as per Figure 10.4.	Analysis 2 (job score represented by highest upper extremity score): OR 50 sensitivity, specificity, positive predictive value, and negative predictive value were 0.91, 0.83, 0.95, and 0.71 respectively.	
	Rucker and Moore (2002)	28 jobs assessed: 10 jobs at a hose connector plant and 18 jobs at a chair manufacturing plant.	Ergonomic: SI variables	Performed via observation. 2 raters for each job.	OSHA 200 logs, one incident trigger used.	Evidence of association was assessed using the LR test for independence strength of association and was reported as the OR. If at least one cell had a count less than 5 Fishers exact test was	Analysis 1 (left and right upper extremity considered separately). Relationship between morbidity and hazard assessed sig. with OR of 73.3 and an LR of 21.5). The sensitivity specificity, positive predictive value, and	Association between SI hazard classification and morbidity definition reestablished in hose and chair manufacturing.

Study	Population	Variables	Exposure assessment	Health outcome	Statistical analysis	Results
					used to determine statistical significance.	negative predictive value were 1.0, 0.84, 0.47, and 1.0, respectively. Analysis 2 (job score represented by highest upper extremity score): OR 106.6, LR 19.1 sensitivity, specificity, positive predictive value and negative predictive value were 1.0, 0.91, 0.75, and 0.75, respectively.
Bovenzi et al. (2005)	Female workers performing sanding manually or using orbital sanders (17 furniture plants: 3 groups orbital sanders A, both orbital and hand group B, hand only C) or office work	Ergonomic: SI variables in addition to vibration Individual: age, smoking drinking, height, weight, body mass index	Ergonomic variables assessed via observation. 2 raters for each job. Vibration: accelerometers	Medical interview and physical examination used to assess presence of to Raynaud's phenomenon and CTS	Univariate analysis performed to compare groups and variables significantly different were included in a multivariate regression analysis. The chi-square statistic or the Fishers exact test was applied to data in the 2×2 contingency tables.	Log-binomial regression analysis showed that the occurrence of sensorineural symptoms and CTS increased significantly with the increase of SI score. It was estimated that the risk for CTS increased by a factor of 1.09 SI scores related to CTS, and symptoms in the wrist, elbow, and shoulder.

(continued)

TABLE 10.3 (continued)
Studies of Predictive Validity

Method	Study	Population	Variables Examined	Exposure Assessment	Morbidity Classification	Statistics Used	Results	Interpretation
		462 workers exposed to repetitive activities of the upper limbs and 749 workers not exposed in eight manufacturing industries				Log binomial regression analysis used to assess the relationship between health complaints and individual and exposure variables.	for each unit of increase in the SI score. Similar results were obtained for shoulder, elbow, and wrist musculoskeletal complaints.	
OCRA	Grieco (1998)		Ergonomic: OCRA variables	Analyzed using the methods proposed by Occhipinti (1998) and Colombini (1998). No further description	An index was derived equal to the total number of work-related musculoskeletal disorders of the upper limb over the total number of limbs at increased risk. Disorders of the shoulder elbow wrist and hands were identified based on questionnaire (Menoni 98).	The degree of association between the morbidity scheme and the OCRA scores were examined using the simple and multiple regression functions.	A significant prediction equation was derived using simple regression equation: $y_1 = 0.614 + 0.858x_1$ y = Sum of all WRMSD/total number of limbs at risk and x = exposure index (OCRA). $r^2 = 0.88$	The linear association between the % of disorders present and OCRA index is established.

10.3.3 SELECTION OF AN ERGONOMIC RISK ASSESSMENT BASED ON CONCURRENT VALIDITY

Concurrent validity of ERA techniques is established by correlating the findings of one valid test to another. Should two methods have independently established predictive validity the agreement between those should be high. Possible confounders in these examinations however are differences in the populations in which the methods have demonstrated predictive validity, differences in morbidity definition used, etc. Three studies are currently available, which have examined the agreement between methods. Drinkaus et al. (2003) compared the SI and the RULA assessment and found poor agreement (kappa score of 0.11). Bao et al. (2006b) compared the ACGIH TLV (nonquantitative method) and the SI and found poor to moderate agreement (weighted kappa score 0.45). Jones and Kumar (2007e) compared the RULA, REBA, quantitative ACGIH TLV, SI, and OCRA based on quantified exposure measurement. The findings of Jones and Kumar (2007e) indicate that agreement between methods varies from moderate to low and is in some cases affected by the definition of exposure variables used.

10.4 CONCLUSION

ERAs are used by practicing ergonomists to identify jobs at-risk of MSI and to identify and prioritize exposures for intervention in prevention efforts. Given the current human and financial impact of MSIs and the established role of physical exposures in their precipitation, research seeking to improve the ability of ERAs to predict injury is of paramount importance. Direct comparison of the validity of ERAs is not presently possible given the lack of studies examining the methods based on standardized criteria. At present therefore, selection of the most appropriate methodology requires the evaluator consider the evidence of content, predictive, and concurrent validity supporting each method. Among the models and methodologies considered here, significant deficiencies are present in each one of them. The situation begs for additional original, rigorous, and objective studies to make a meaningful impact.

REFERENCES

Bao S., Howard N., Spielholz P., and Silverstein B. 2006a. Quantifying repetitive hand activity for epidemiological research on musculoskeletal injuries—part I: Individual exposure assessment. *Ergonomics* 49(4): 381–392.

Bao S., Howard N., Spielholz P., and Silverstein B. 2006b. Quantifying repetitive hand activity for epidemiological research on musculoskeletal injuries—part II: Comparison of different methods of measuring force level and repetitiveness. *Ergonomics* 49(4): 381–392.

Bovenzi M., Della Vedova A., Nataletti P., Alessandrini B., and Poian T. 2005. Work-related injuries of the upper limb in female workers using orbital sanders. *International Archives of Occupational and Environmental Health* 78(4): 303–310.

Chohen S., Kamarck T., and Mermelstein, R. 1983. A global measure of perceived stress. *Journal of Health Social Behavior* 24: 385–396.

Colombini D. 1998. An observational method for classifying exposure to repetitive movements of the upper limbs. *Ergonomics* 41(9): 1261–1289.

David G.C. 2005. Ergonomic methods for assessing exposure to risk factors for work-related musculoskeletal disorders. *Occupational Medicine* 55: 190–199.

Dempsey P.G., McGorry R.W., and Maynard W.S. 2005. A survey of methods used by certified professional ergonomists. *Applied Ergonomics* 36: 489–503.

Drinkaus P., Sesek R., Bloswick D., Bernard T., Walton B., Joseph B., Reeve G., and Counts J.H. 2003. Comparison of ergonomic risk assessment outputs from Rapid Upper Limb Assessment and the Strain Index for tasks in automotive assembly plants. *Work* 21(2): 165–172.

Fine L.J. and Silverstein B.A. 1995. Work-related disorders of the neck and upper extremity. In: Levy BS, Wegman DH (Eds.). *Occupational Health: Recognizing and Preventing Work Related Disease*. Boston, MA: Little Brown. P. 470–490.

Forde M.A., Punnett L., and Wegman D.H. 2002. Pathomechanisms of work-related musculoskeletal disorders: Conceptual issues. *Ergonomics* 45(9): 619–630.

Franzblau A., Salerno D.F., Armstrong T.J., and Werner R.A. 1997. Test-retest reliability of an upper extremity discomfort questionnaire in an industrial population. *Scandinavian Journal of Work and Environment Health* 23: 299–307.

Franzblau A., Armstrong T.J., Werner R.A., and Ulin S.S. 2005. A cross-sectional assessment of the ACGIH TLV for hand activity level. *Journal of Occupational Rehabilitation* 15(1): 57–67.

Gell N., Werner R.A., Franzblau A., Ulin S.S., and Armstrong T.J. 2005. A longitudinal study of industrial and clerical workers: Incidence of carpal tunnel syndrome and assessment of risk factors. *Journal of Occupational Rehabilitation* 15(1): 47–55.

Grieco A. 1998. Application of the concise exposure index (OCRA) to tasks involving repetitive movements of the upper limbs in a variety of manufacturing industries: Preliminary validations. *Ergonomics* 41(9): 1347–1356.

Hignett S. and McAtamney L. 2000. Rapid entire body assessment (REBA). *Applied Ergonomics* 31(2): 201–205.

Jones T. and Kumar S. 2006. Assessment of physical demands and comparison of multiple exposure definitions in a repetitive high risk sawmill occupation: Saw-filer. *International Journal of Industrial Ergonomics* 36: 819–827.

Jones T. and Kumar S. 2007a. Assessment of physical demands and comparison of multiple exposure definitions in a repetitive sawmill job: Board edger operator. *Ergonomics* 50(5): 676–693.

Jones T. and Kumar S. 2007b. Assessment of physical demands and comparison of exposure definitions in a repetitive sawmill occupation: Trim-saw operator. *Work* 28(2): 183–196.

Jones T. and Kumar S. 2007c. Comparison of ergonomic risk assessments in a repetitive high risk sawmill occupation: Saw-filer. *International Journal of Industrial Ergonomics*. 37: 744–753.

Jones T. and Kumar S. 2007d. Comparison of ergonomic risk assessments in a repetitive mono-task sawmill occupation: Board edger operator. In press.

Jones T. and Kumar S. 2007e. Comparison of ergonomic risk assessment output in four sawmill jobs. Submitted to *Human Factors*, May 2007.

Jones T. and Kumar S. 2008a. Assessment of physical demands and comparison of exposure definitions in a high risk mono-task sawmill occupation: Lumber grader. *International Journal of Industrial Ergonomics*. In revision.

Jones T. and Kumar S. 2008b. Comparison of ergonomic risk assessments in a high risk repetitive mono-task sawmill occupation: Trim saw operator. *Work*. In press.

Jones T. and Kumar S. 2008c. Comparison of ergonomic risk assessments in a high risk mono-task sawmill occupation: Lumber grader. Submitted to *International Journal of Industrial Ergonomics*, June 2008.

Karasek R. 1985. Job content questionnaire and user's guide. Rev. 1.1. Lowell, MA: University of Massachusetts.

Knox K. and Moore J.S. 2001. Predictive validity of the Strain Index in turkey processing. *Journal of Occupational and Environmental Medicine/American College of Occupational And Environmental Medicine* 43(5): 451–462.

Kourinka B., Jonsson B., Kilbom A., Vinterberg H., Biering-Sorensen F., Andersson G., and Jorgensen K. Standardized Nordic questionnaires for the analysis of musculoskeletal symptoms. *Applied Ergonomics* 18, 233–237.

Kumar S. 2001. Theories of musculoskeletal injury causation. *Ergonomics* 44: 17–47.

Latko W.A., Armstrong T.J., Franzblau A., Ulin S.S., Werner R.A., and Albers J.W. 1999. Cross-sectional study of the relationship between repetitive work and the prevalence of upper limb musculoskeletal injuries. *American Journal of Industrial Medicine* 36(2): 248–259.

Latko W.A., Armstrong T.J., Foulke J.A., Herrin G.D., Rabourn R.A., and Ulin S.S. 1997. Development and evaluation of an observational method for assessing repetition in hand tasks. *American Industrial Hygiene Association Journal* 58: 278–285.

Lowe B.D. 2004. Accuracy and validity of observational estimates of wrist and forearm posture. *Ergonomics* 47: 527–554.

Massaccesi M., Pagnotta A., Soccetti A., Masali M., Masiero C., and Greco F. 2003. Investigation of work-related injuries in truck drivers using RULA method. *Applied Ergonomics* 34(4): 303–307.

McAtamney L. and Corlett N.E. 1993. RULA: A survey method for the investigation of work-related upper limb injuries. *Applied Ergonomics* 24: 91–99.

Moore J.S. and Garg A. 1994. Upper extremity injuries in a pork processing plant: Relationships between job risk factors and morbidity. *American Industrial Hygiene Association Journal* 55(8): 703–715.

Moore J.S. and Garg A. 1995. The Strain Index: A proposed method to analyze jobs for risk of distal upper extremity injuries. *American Industrial Hygiene Association Journal* 56: 443–458.

Moore J.S., Rucker N.P., and Knox K. 2001. Validity of generic risk factors and the Strain Index for predicting nontraumatic distal upper extremity morbidity. *American Industrial Hygiene Association Journal* 62(2): 229–235.

Occhipinti E. 1998. OCRA: A concise index for the assessment of exposure to repetitive movements of the upper limbs. *Ergonomics* 41: 1290–1311.

Occhipinti E. and Colombini D. 2004. The OCRA method: updating of reference values and prediction models of occurence of work-related musculoskeletal diseases of the upper limbs (UL-WMSDs) in working populations exposed to repetitive movements and exertions of the upper limbs. *La Medicina Del Lavoro* 95(4): 305–319.

Rucker N. and Moore J.S. 2002. Predictive validity of the Strain Index in manufacturing facilities. *Applied Occupational And Environmental Hygiene* 17(1): 63–73.

Shuval K. and Donchin M. 2005. Prevalence of upper extremity musculoskeletal symptoms and ergonomic risk factors at a Hi-Tech company in Israel. *International Journal of Industrial Ergonomics* 35(6): 569–581.

Toviana Y.Y., 1999. HiTech stress questionnaire. *HiTech Life*, September–October, 21–24, Hebrew.

University of Michigan Rehabilitation Engineering Research Center. 2005. ACGIH TLV for mono-task hand work, evaluating the TLV. Available online at: http://umrerc.engin.umich.edu/jobdatabase/RERC2/HAL/EvaluatingTLV.htm (Accessed January 21, 2005).

US Department of Health and Human Services. 1997. B.P. Bernard (Ed.). Musculoskeletal injuries and workplace factors: A critical review of epidemiologic evidence for work-related musculoskeletal injuries of the neck, upper extremity and low back. Cincinnati, OH: Public Health Service Centers for Disease Control and Prevention, National Institute for Occupational Safety and Health.

Werner R.A., Franzblau A., Gell N., Ulin S.S., and Armstrong T.J. 2005. Predictors of upper extremity discomfort: A longitudinal study of industrial and clerical workers. *Journal of Occupational Rehabilitation* 15(1): 27–35.

Winkel J. and Westgaard R. 1992. Occupational and individual risk factors for shoulder-neck complaints: Part II. The scientific basis (literature review) for the guide. *International Journal of Industrial Ergonomics* 10: 85–104.

11 Musculoskeletal Disorders of the Neck and Shoulder and Ergonomic Interventions

Murray E. Maitland

CONTENTS

11.1 INTRODUCTION

This chapter deals specifically with the cervical spine, shoulder girdle, and glenohumeral joint as potential sources of a worker's symptoms caused by posture-related or repetitive movement injury. Neck and shoulder pain caused by prolonged posture or repetitive stress can occur in diverse occupations such as supermarket cashiers [32], newspaper office employees [9], sewing machine operators [28], automobile

339

assembly line workers [44], or people working at telephone call center [47]. It seems that people in any workplace cannot be considered to be protected from neck or shoulder problems. In fact, very disparate working postures and levels of physical stress appear to be associated with a high incidence and prevalence of shoulder and neck pain.

The prevalence of occupational neck and shoulder problems, measured in cross-sectional studies by questionnaire, seems vast. In a recently published study of newspaper employees, data for the year 2001 indicates that 75% of 813 employees reported some level of neck pain and 61% reported shoulder pain [9]. Leclerc et al. [32] found the prevalence of shoulder pain in 598 workers in a variety of occupations to be 59%. Similar findings seem consistent across cultures. For example, 1041 computer users at Nigerian university campuses were surveyed. Seventy-three percent of the respondents reported neck pain and 63% reported shoulder pain [1]. Whether employees are engaged in physically demanding work [26], sedentary occupations, or an activity of moderate physical stress, neck and shoulder pain appears to be common.

Isolating a simple anatomical source of worker symptoms is not possible as there is a chain of structures undergoing prolonged stresses in the workplace. A pattern of dysfunction develops because people have a consistent anatomical makeup. Yet, a similar clinical presentation of two individuals can be the result of different underlying pathologies. For example, in a descriptive study of 58 individuals on a waiting list for physical therapy treatment of shoulder impingement syndrome (SIS), magnetic resonance imaging (MRI) identified a wide range of shoulder pathologies including supraspinatus muscle tears and glenoid labral tears [4].

Unfortunately, current research in neck and shoulder ergonomics does not provide detailed differential diagnoses to draw cause–effect relationships [45]. Even with detailed physical examination, it is difficult to determine the time course and interplay of various factors from cross-sectional studies. A group of 485 patients whose chief complaints were work-related upper extremity pain and other upper extremity symptoms underwent a thorough physical examination [41]. The patients had a broad range of clinically identifiable physical problems. Many of the patients demonstrated protracted shoulders (78%), head-forward position (71%), thoracic outlet syndrome (70%), shoulder impingement (13%), and peripheral muscle weakness (70%) [41]. Since this is a cross-sectional case series, the time courses of these problems are not clear.

This chapter presents a cross-section of current concepts in the examination and intervention of work-related neck and shoulder pain. Despite controversies and lack of consensus concerning different aspects of neck and shoulder ergonomics, there is a rapid increase in the breadth and depth of published literature. In particular, there is a growing body of literature pertaining to the interaction between intrinsic (musculoskeletal), environmental, and psychosocial factors as it relates to neck and shoulder symptoms [32,62,63]. In this chapter, the postural and functional anatomical chain from thoracic spine to the glenohumeral joint will be considered as potential intrinsic predisposing factors. Extrinsic environmental factors combined with work demands and the environment will be considered. Interventions should be directed at minimizing the predisposing factors, mechanisms of injury, and the perpetuating factors that are identified through examination.

11.2 SPINE, SHOULDER GIRDLE, AND SHOULDER POSTURE

Posture is generally thought of as relatively long-term, static positioning of the body segments. Habitual patterns of thoracic, scapular, and humeral posture will alter intra-articular and extra-articular stresses. For an individual, the effects of posture are cumulative from occupation, recreation, and sleeping. While external aids, like chairs, are important to a person's posture, there are common patterns of posture that are believed to be associated with symptoms.

In a clinical environment, evaluating the effects of standing posture on the cervical spine and shoulder starts at the feet. For sitting posture, normally the pelvis would be the starting point. This is a process of identifying the relative position and motions along anatomical segments and then considering the consequences. A kinematic chain, in anatomical terms, can be understood as the physiological, performance, or functional effects as a consequence of the position of one anatomical segment relative to another segment. When interpreting positions and motions, we often are attempting to understand the kinetic chain, defined as the effects of forces and torques across anatomical segments. As other chapters in this book cover the lower extremities and lumbar spine, we will begin with the implications of thoracic spine posture on shoulder function.

While the fundamental ergonomic principles used to identify risk factors for repetitive strain injury, including frequency, intensity, and duration, are equally valid for the neck and shoulder regions, long-term postures are perhaps more relevant to determine neck and shoulder pain compared to other regions. Walker-Bone and Cooper [62] concluded from their recent review that abnormal posture combined with repetition contribute markedly to work-related conditions of the neck and upper extremity.

Figure 11.1 illustrates two markedly different sitting postures. Traditionally we think of an ideal posture in the sagittal plane as maintaining the ear lobe over the acromion process. The cervical spine is traditionally thought to form a gentle curve concave posteriorly. The thoracic spine is idealized as a gentle curve concave anteriorly. If one were to draw a vertical line from the ear downward, it should fall near the greater trochanter of the femur. Theoretically, the center of gravity of the

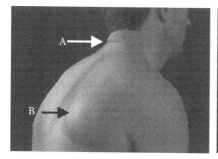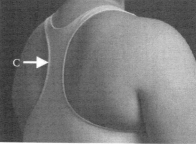

FIGURE 11.1 Slouch and erect sitting postures. These images highlight three postural differences between the two subjects: A marked crease at the C6–C7 region of the cervical spine (A), a forwardly rotated, winged right scapula (B), and a flat thoracic spine (C).

head should be close to the skeletal base of support (e.g., the cervical bodies) in order to minimize the torque acting on each articulation. The articulations should be in a midrange, not at the end point of flexion or extension in the sagittal plane. The male subject in Figure 11.1 demonstrates a high degree of thoracic kyphosis and consequently the cervical spine must have excessive extension to position the eyes. The ears are far ahead of the acromion process. The female in Figure 11.1 demonstrates that a flat midthoracic and increased upper thoracic and lower cervical spine flexion spine is her normal posture. Neither posture matches the traditionally ideal posture. Both spinal postures have consequences on the scapular position described below.

A relatively passive activity led to a cumulative strain injury of my shoulder in my days as a graduate student in anatomy. Certainly, the problem rated as injury because the symptoms were significant and it interfered with other aspects of my life including writing. Processing tissue samples for electron microscopic analysis kept my right upper extremity elevated. It seems odd that the stress of making glass knives or sectioning tissue would be more injurious to my shoulder compared to competitive cross-country skiing. The answer to this paradox is associated with the long-term static positioning.

11.3 PRINCIPLES OF POSTURE IN THE THORACIC SPINE

Slouching is a common habitual posture during sitting or standing. Slouching is a postural habit of increasing the thoracic curvature and can be corrected because it is reversible. When the increased thoracic spinal curve is structural, it is described as kyphosis. Normal thoracic curvature, measured as the angle between the superior–inferior axis of the first thoracic vertebrae and the twelfth thoracic vertebrae, has been reported to be between 20° and 40° depending on the age and gender of the individual [21]. Once the thoracic curvature reaches 50° and is uncorrectable by conscious effort, it is considered abnormal. Abnormal thoracic curvature can be associated with several disease processes such as Scheuerrnann disease, osteoporosis as well as inflammatory disease or trauma. Aging appears to cause an increase in thoracic kyphosis [50].

A cross-sectional MRI study of 169 subjects found that the anterior height/posterior height ratio of the thoracic vertebral bodies gradually declined in older individuals [23]. The authors concluded the nature of vertebral shape changes and the prevalence of disk-degenerative findings across the life span. The study found more abnormal findings in the annuli, nuclei, and disk margins increasing with increasing age.

Extrapolating from research on lumbar spine biomechanics, increased spinal anteroposterior (sagittal plane) curvature is correlated to an increase in torques acting on each spinal segment [11]. The torque required to stabilize the lumbar spine can double between a slightly extended position and a flexed position in part because the distance from the fulcrum of the segments' masses increase. The force produced by the erector spinae must also increase because in a flexed spinal posture, the lever arm lengths of the lumbar erector spinae may decrease by up to 13.3% [11]. Excessive muscle activation causes increased spinal joint loads and may prevent optimal motion.

Respiration also affects the stability of the spine. Shirley et al. [53] measured the stiffness of the lumbar spine with breathing. Increased lumbar spinal stiffness was related to the respiratory effort and was greatest during maximum expiration. Intra-abdominal pressure unloads the lumbar spine about 10% and is most effective in a flexed position [53]. The lungs perform in a similar stiffening function in the thoracic spine compared to the abdominal contents on the lumbar spine.

Breast size seems to be a factor affecting posture, especially thoracic kyphosis and lumbar lordosis angles. Large breasts can be associated with physical symptoms such as chronic neck, shoulder, and back pain, as well as stiff neck [19].

Lateral curvatures of the thoracic spine are common and become more common in aging populations. In a study of 75 elderly volunteers without spinal health problems and never having a diagnosis of scoliosis, 68% of the subjects could be classified as having a scoliosis [51]. In the study population, averaging 70 years of age, the average Cobb angle was 17°. Previous reports note a prevalence of adult scoliosis from 2% to 32% depending on the population that was studied [51]. Theoretically, scolosis can be associated with mechanical changes at the articulations, causing tension on the convex side and compression on the concave side of the curve.

The thoracic spine, along with the ribs, forms the base of support for the scapula and cervical spine. Figure 11.1 illustrates increased thoracic kyphosis with increased anterior tilt of the scapula. This position of increased curvature of the thoracic spine has direct effects on these other regions. Finley and Lee [20] studied 16 adult volunteers who were symptom-free. In a within-subject repeated measures research design, they used electromagnetic tracking sensors to study motion of the scapula in slouched vs. erect posture. Increased thoracic kyphosis significantly altered the kinematics of the scapula during humeral elevation. Primarily, slouching reduced lateral rotation of the scapula, which prevents upward mobility of the acromion process [20].

11.4 CERVICAL SPINE POSTURE

Head forward posture is considered to be mechanically stressful because of increased torque on the spine, increased muscle tension to balance the torque, and increased compression of the spinal structures. Head forward posture can be measured by the angle between the horizontal line passing through C7 and a line extending from the tragus of the ear to C7. This is the craniovertebral angle. A smaller craniovertebral angle indicates a greater forward head posture. In a case–control study of 20 subjects with headaches and 20 age-matched controls without headaches, forward head posture was associated with chronic tension-type headaches. The duration of the headaches was also related to the forward head posture [18].

Head-forward posture can have an effect on neck motion. A case–control study of 272 subjects with radiographically normal spines subdivided this population into five groups based on each subject's normal posture. Lateral radiographs of maximal extension and flexion were used to study the segmental kinematics of the spine. Initial static alignment of the cervical curvature was associated with differences in dynamic kinematics of the cervical spine during cervical flexion–extension [59].

Generally clinicians assume that structural changes of the spine produce postural positions that are unchanging, and that people in general have a static preferred neck posture. However, head-forward positions for people may vary. Dunk et al. [15] studied the reliability of two-dimensional spinal postural measurements in three planes. Photographic methods were use to gather data from 14 individuals for three trials per session over three sessions. Large variability within subjects was observed in the head-forward and other positions. Intraclass correlation coefficients for the cervical neck angles in three planes were poor ranging from 0.13 to 0.44. On the one hand, this study is discouraging because identifying postural correlates with symptoms will be difficult. On the other hand, the study demonstrates that posture may be easily modified given the right circumstances.

11.5 SCAPULAR FUNCTION

To the external observer, as a person elevates his/her upper extremity, the changing position of the arm, forearm, and hand can be seen relative to the trunk. It is difficult for the external observer to appreciate the link between the clavicle and the humeral head. This is the scapular segment between the acromion process to the glenoid fossa. The flat portion of the scapula, with attachments of the trapezius, levator scapulae, rhomboids, serratus anterior, and pectoralis minor acts like a sesamoid bone enveloped with strong muscles [33]. As large torques are supported by the upper extremity, large moment arms of muscles acting on the body of the scapula help to position the scapular segment. While the analogy of the scapula being like a sesamoid bone may not be perfectly correct, the analogy emphasizes the interplay by opposing muscle forces acting on the flat body of the scapula that increases the muscle torques about the acromioclavicular joint.

The integrated motion of the clavicle, scapula, and humerus at the acromioclavicular joint and the glenohumeral joint is called glenohumeral rhythm. Clinically, there has been increasing emphasis on glenohumeral rhythm and shoulder problems since the ratio between scapulothoracic motion and glenohumeral motion is often altered in patients with shoulder symptoms [29]. The glenohumeral rhythm has a normal pattern depending on the degree of upper extremity elevation and the activity performed (especially changes in forces acting on the upper extremity). Kibler [29] in his recent review proposes that abnormal glenohumeral rhythm is causative of SIS. However, most of Kiber's [29] supporting evidence comes from case–control studies. For example, Hébert et al. [25] performed a case–control study of 41 subjects with SIS and 10 subjects without shoulder pain, examining scapular and humeral motions using motion analysis. The symptomatic and asymptomatic shoulders of subjects with unilateral SIS were similar, but both shoulders of subjects with SIS differed from the shoulders of healthy subjects [25]. The authors contend that the magnitude and direction of asymmetry of the scapula during abduction or elevation of the upper extremity is indicative of either a cause of shoulder pain or an undesirable compensation. Other case–control studies support the relationship between SIS and abnormal scapular motion [35].

The dynamic position of the scapula may have a relationship with the ultimate range of motion of the glenohumeral joint in all planes. A case–control study of 23 individuals who participated in overhead throwing activities examined motion in the scapula and internal rotation at the glenohumeral joint [5]. Posterior glenohumeral joint capsule tightness is one of the factors that has been theorized to play a role in motions of both segments. The study found that a glenohumeral internal rotation deficit of 20% and abnormal anterior tilt during movement at the glenohumeral joint were significantly related.

Figure 11.1 illustrates anterior tilting and winging of the scapula in the male subject. The anterior tilting is sometimes thought to be caused by tightness in the pectoralis minor muscle [6]. The subject also has chronic serratus anterior weakness caused by an idiopathic long thoracic nerve palsy.

11.6 HUMERUS

The glenohumeral joint is typically described as a shallow ball and socket joint with the socket deepened by a fibrocartilage labrum. To complicate the ball and socket arrangement of the humerus on the scapula, there is a bony shelf over the superior portion on the "socket" side of the joint, the acromion process. On the "ball" side, the greater tubercle is another obstacle that limits symmetrical rotation in all three dimensions. Consequently some positions of the glenohumeral joint are limited [30] and potentially injurious to the shoulder. In addition, intrinsic changes to the glenohumeral joint, such as posterior or anterior stiffness, cause changes in glenohumeral rhythm as well as changes in the way the humeral head moves relative to the glenoid fossa [34].

Klopčar et al. [30] used shoulder girdle and shoulder anatomical information to model the arm-reachable workspace in three dimensions. The resulting volume is not symmetrical. Klopčar et al. [30] illustrate that various shoulder pathologies change the arm-reachable volume in a complex three-dimensional manner.

When the person's elbow is extended, the hand is rotated in the horizontal plane primarily by shoulder rotation rather than forearm pronation and supination. In positions of the arm-reachable workspace around 90° of flexion and above, commonly called impingement positions, positioning the palm down can cause shoulder pain for susceptible people. Clinical and physical tests of the shoulder joint take advantage of positions that can provoke symptoms in impingement tests such as the Kennedy-Hawkins tests. When people reach to shoulder height or above, they may rotate their palms downward, and may be aggravating their shoulders by reproducing the impingement tests in their working or home environments.

Clinically, the preferred workspace for the upper extremity is a short diagonal arc. The highest medial position would be similar to touching the index finger to the nose. The most inferolateral position is similar to the anatomical position with the arms abducted to about 30° in the coronal plane. Arm positions to avoid include horizontal abduction and adducted positions.

11.7 DISEASE AND INJURY IN THE SHOULDER AS IT APPLIES TO ERGONOMICS

Intrinsic factors, as part of the individual, interact with the working environment to culminate in neck and shoulder pain in some cases. So far, the discussion has been about the relative joint positions in posture in relatively healthy individuals.

However, many workers have injuries and diseases that accumulate over their working life, whether caused by their working activities or not. The following section will cover some of the common problems either caused by the working environment or that are prevalent in the general population.

11.8   ROTATOR CUFF DISEASE AND INJURY

While many are familiar with the rotator cuff muscles (supraspinatus, infraspinatus, teres minor, and subscapularis) with regard to their role in producing rotation at the glenohumeral joint movement, these muscles have several other functions in the shoulder. Since the tendons of the rotator cuff are bound to the shoulder joint capsule, tears in the rotator cuff tendons can cause shoulder instability. Also, coordination of upward motion of the glenohumeral joint requires muscular coordination, especially the rotator cuff. The rotator cuff applies an upward rotation of the humerus relative to the scapula, and certain muscles of the group stabilize the humerus against an upward translation caused by the deltoid [52]. Degenerative changes associated with aging, or injuries associated with sports, and the loss of rotator cuff functions are difficult to disassociate from injuries in the workplace.

Rotator cuff disorders are the most commonly diagnosed cause of shoulder pain and dysfunction in working adults aged over 30 years. Rotator cuff problems have been shown to be a major source of morbidity in working populations. In Washington State, the incidence of workers' compensation rotator cuff syndrome claims (15.3 per 10,000 full-time equivalent workers) is the most common disorder [54]. In France's Pays de la Loire region, 80 occupational physicians evaluated 2685 men and women [48]. The most frequent disorder or the upper extremity was diagnosed as rotator cuff syndrome followed by carpal tunnel syndrome and lateral epicondylitis. Overall, 6.8% of men were diagnosed with rotator cuff syndrome compared with 9% of the women. The diagnosis of rotator cuff syndrome increases dramatically with increasing age. For males in the age of 50–59 years category, this diagnosis was used for 33% of upper extremity disorders in this population [48]. A group of workers at high risk for rotator cuff syndrome was studied to determine whether there was an association between dose of overhead work and the diagnosis of rotator cuff syndrome. The 136 male machinists, car mechanics, and house painters participants were aged 40–50 years and had been employed in their trades for not less than 10 years. There was a significant exposure–response relationship found in rotator cuff degenerative tears [58].

Rotator cuff dysfunction causes specific weakness, creates instability of the shoulder joint, and changes how the shoulder is used. In particular, changes to the rotator cuff affect glenohumeral rhythm [38]. As a result, common patterns at work are altered.

11.9   NERVE ENTRAPMENTS

Many places along the length of upper extremity peripheral nerves, from the cervical spine to the fingers, pressure can cause sensory symptoms and weakness. Any of the upper extremity nerves can be affected and there are several common patterns of neuropathy. Many people are familiar with pain, sensory symptoms, and weakness that can be caused by pressure at the cervical spine. There are many

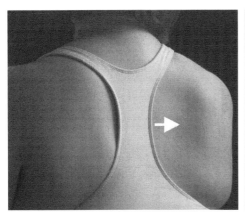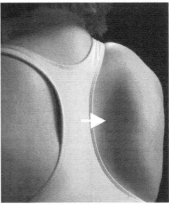

FIGURE 11.2 A subject with idiopathic long thoracic nerve palsy. In the left image there is no forces applied to the upper extremity. In the right image, a force is applied to the hand. The arrows identify the region between the medial border of the scapula and the spinous processes of the thoracic spine.

more problematic locations through the shoulder girdle and past the shoulder joint. Pratt [43] identified at least seven possible nerve entrapment sites in the proximal upper extremity. Also, viruses, metabolic diseases, and many other problems can cause specific peripheral nerve problems. For example, winging of the scapula (Figure 11.2) is commonly caused by long thoracic nerve injury or disease. For many patients, the source of this pathology is unclear. The relationship between repetitive motion and nerve dysfunction is controversial. However, there is a long list of diagnoses that are circumstantially linked to nerve stretch, nerve compression, or other nerve trauma caused by repetitive motion. Working positions may be related to these problems.

A depressed shoulder girdle may be one postural factor related to compression as nerve structures pass from the thorax to the upper extremity, resulting in the potential for thoracic outlet syndrome. This is very controversial as a diagnosis. However, the potential for neurovascular structures to undergo pressure-induced pathology associated with posture has been identified in some case studies [2].

Repetitive or prolonged shoulder protraction may place the median nerve at risk of injury. Julius et al. [27] studied eight people in postural positions using high-frequency ultrasound images to study median nerve movement. Nerve movement was reduced through the shoulder region when the shoulder was protracted and other joints were moved. The authors concluded that a protracted scapula may adversely affect median nerve function and increase the risk of developing upper quadrant pain.

Extreme movements into shoulder flexion, extension, or horizontal abduction may be sufficient to cause neural tension. Case histories demonstrate that repetitive movements and trauma at the end of range can be associated with subsequent weakness and sensory changes. For example, Streib [57] documents three cases where repetitive arm activity at work combined with a sudden forceful contraction and stretch of the arm muscles led to delayed radial nerve palsy.

Double nerve crush syndrome is a term used to indicate the potential of multiple entrapments contributing to the overall nerve dysfunction. This is a controversial concept with some studies supporting a proximal entrapment contributing to distal entrapment neuropathies and some studies refuting this concept. The double crush hypothesis proposes that a proximal lesion along an axon predisposes it to injury at a more distal site along its course through impaired axoplasmic flow. A study of 277 patients with C6, C7, or C8 radiculopathies did not support increased frequency of distal entrapment syndromes coincident with proximal nerve entrapment [31]. On the other hand, a case–control study using MRI found a higher incidence of narrowed cervical foramens in people suffering from carpal tunnel syndrome [42].

Overall neuromuscular health is the result of metabolic and other processes. For example, scapular winging is a common finding in the general population and most often it has been attributed to long thoracic nerve palsy. Scapular winging is also a hallmark feature in other neuromuscular disorders: viral infections, facioscapu- lohumeral dystrophy, scapuloperoneal dystrophy, Emery–Dreifuss muscular dystro- phy, congenital myopathies, myotonic dystrophy, and acid maltase deficiency [17]. Attributing a work-related cause and excluding other potential causes requires a detailed examination process.

11.10 SHOULDER INSTABILITY

There are many possible diagnoses that identify specific direction or pathologies associated with instability at the glenohumeral articulation. While some diagno- ses indicate gross disruption of joint stability, some of these diagnoses indicate a subtle change in the mechanism of connective tissues that stabilize the ball and socket geometry of the joint. The term "minor instability" [8] has been used to indicate a dysfunction of glenohumeral articulation, especially in combination with microtrauma that gives rise to shoulder symptoms. The syndrome of minor instabil- ity accents the common clinical concept that the shallow ball and socket geometry of the glenohumeral joint requires effective soft tissue and muscular function.

The general population has a range of flexibility in the connective tissues. The generalized ligamentous laxity of the glenohumeral joint is believed to increase the risk of shoulder pain in certain activities. Figure 11.3 illustrates the consequence of an inferiorly directed force on the upper extremity in a person with hyperflexibility. To date, studies do not appear to use this factor in the analysis of workplace injuries.

11.11 DIABETES MELLITUS

The peripheral neural and musculoskeletal systems are indicative of a person's over- all health. The hormonal and metabolic balance of the body is evidenced by neuro- musculoskeletal changes in the periphery. Diabetes mellitus is one example of this generalization.

In a study of over 3000 Finnish workers, insulin-dependent diabetes mellitus was associated with rotator cuff syndrome [39]. In a study of patients with bilateral-frozen shoulders, 42% had diabetes [40]. It appears that diabetes mellitus has effects on the histology and vascular structure in the periphery. Hypertrophic and hyperemic syno- vitis was observed in the arthroscopic findings of diabetic-frozen shoulders [49].

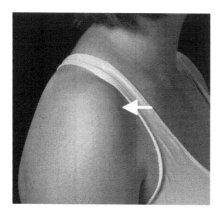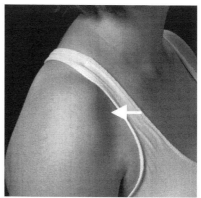

FIGURE 11.3 Generalized laxity of the shoulder is identified by an inferior directed force at the elbow. The arrow highlights the superior edge of the humeral head as it sinks relative to the acromion process.

11.12 ERGONOMIC FACTORS, WORKSTATION SETUP, AND INTERVENTIONS

Currently the status of research is not precise enough to give cause–effect relationships between predisposing factors, the mechanism of injury and anatomical pathology that gives rise to workers' symptoms. Punnett and Wegman [45] conclude in their review that many studies are merely identifying regions of symptoms by self-report. They call this a good first step but limited in the ability to formulate a mechanism-based intervention plan exposure assessment that has too often been limited due to crude indicators and inadequate diagnosis [45]. However, there are indicators that the intrinsic physical capacity, perceived exertion, awkwardness, postural stress, and environmental issues faced by the worker might be identified and modified.

There appears to be ergonomic issues that are different for women compared to men that need to be identified and accommodated. For example, a cross-sectional study [12] compared work technique and self-reported musculoskeletal symptoms between men and women performing the same type of work tasks within a metal industry. The study used videotape of 55 workers. A higher proportion of women than men reported shoulder symptoms. Women spent more time on household activities than men, which indicates a higher total workload in paid and unpaid work. Women also handled materials with hands at and above shoulder height more frequently. The authors concluded that workplace design factors were probably a reason for differences in working technique between men and women [12].

Rocha et al. [47] used a self-report study design to assess 108 call center operators. They found that perception of the workstations varied between women compared to men. About 50% or the female operators thought the height of the table was good or excellent, the height of the chair was good or excellent for 63%, but the visibility of the video terminal was good or excellent for only 20% of the female operators. About 43% of female operators had neck or shoulder symptoms compared to 8% of the male operators who also had a more favorable impression of the workstations.

11.13   REACHING

Based on the preceding discussion, it would appear that to reduce neck and shoulder pain, the ideal reach in the working environment would have some standard characteristics. The thoracic spine would be supported in a way that would avoid slouching. The cervical spine would be held erect. The scapula would be slightly retracted and posteriorly rotated. The head of the humerus would avoid and anteriorly translated and internally rotated position. The arm would function in the ideal reachable space described above that comes to the midline of the body in a short arc. In addition, one must consider the environmental and psychological stress on the working individual.

Many working environments do not match the ideal circumstances for the neck and shoulder. Figure 11.4 illustrates some common ergonomic problems in an experimental laboratory setup. In a crowded laboratory, bench space is at a premium so often areas are crowded and are multifunctional. In the figure, an experimental apparatus is set high on a shelving unit and is blocked by other equipment. A relatively short person is required to reach above and between objects to pipette. In the same laboratory environment, reaching is awkward (Figure 11.5). Traditional organization of glassware, drying racks, and chemicals makes long reaches inevitable. Depending on the person's physical capacity, intrinsic health, number of repetitions, and psychosocial factors, this setup could precipitate neck and shoulder problems. In the laboratory environment, simple ergonomic changes might reduce neck and shoulder risk.

Monitor placement during computer use is another issue that might be easy to remedy if there was consensus on the correct position. Straker and Mekhora [56] noted that current postural recommendations for people at computer workstations are

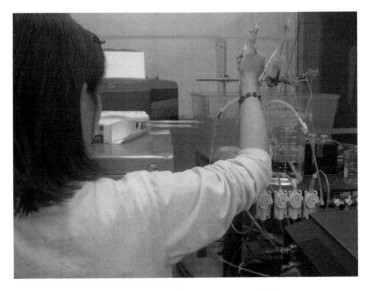

FIGURE 11.4   An actual laboratory working environment illustrating several ergonomic considerations for the neck and shoulder.

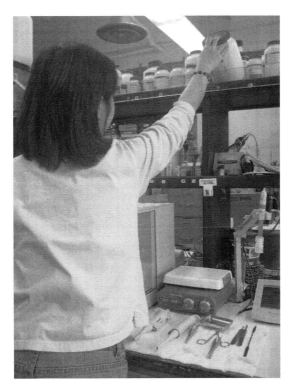

FIGURE 11.5   Reaching in a laboratory environment.

conflicting. They compared musculoskeletal demands, visual demands, and comfort of two different postures. They found significant differences in body postural angles for the two monitor positions. They also found a significant difference in the normalized cervical erector spinae activity measured by electromyography between the two postures. In another study, more neck and shoulder symptoms and disorders were reported when monitor placement causes neck extension [37].

Associated with the monitor position, the presence of armrests on chairs was significantly associated with a lower risk for neck and shoulder symptoms or disorders [37]. Postural support for the shoulder girdle and shoulder means providing workers with a means of resting their arms, either on the work surface or the armrests of their chair [10]. Research supports the practice of placing the keyboard and mouse so that workers can keep their elbows near the torso [55].

11.14   REPETITIVE TASKS

Repetition has often been mentioned as an important contributing factor to neck and shoulder pain. Like many of the details in this field, controversy exists about role of repetitive loading in combination with range of motion and force in causing symptoms. However, there appears to be some evidence for increased risk related to the repetitive nature of a stressful activity. For example, Frost et al. [22] carried out a cross-sectional study of 1961 workers in repetitive work exposure–response analyses relating levels of shoulder loads with the prevalence of dominant shoulder tendonitis showed positive associations for repetition, force requirements, and lack of micro-pauses. Interventions could reduce the number of repetitions or allow for pauses between repetitions. Pauses can be within the task or by switching tasks.

Long hours of keyboarding in the working environment are known to increase the risk of neck and shoulder symptoms. Since many people are using keyboards for recreational and activities of daily living, there is an extension of ergonomic factors beyond the workplace. There may be a place for intervening in the home working environment for certain individuals.

A study evaluated the effects on work-related neck and upper-limb disorders among computer workers prompted (by a software program) to take regular breaks and perform physical exercises [60]. A group of 268 computer workers with complaints in the neck or an upper limb from 22 office locations were randomized into a control group and two intervention groups. One intervention group was prompted to take extra breaks and one intervention group was prompted to perform exercises during the extra breaks. More subjects in the intervention groups than in the control group reported recovery (55% vs. 34%) from their complaints and fewer reported deterioration (4% vs. 20%) [60].

Individuals can also learn to control their posture and muscle activity. Eleven females without neuromuscular disorders were trained with biofeedback during standardized computer work [36]. The biofeedback training led to significant decreases in trapezius muscle activity measured by electromyography and lower ratings of perceived exertion. The authors felt that biofeedback may change muscle synergies during computer work [36].

Certain employment categories are notorious for neck and shoulder problems. Among these, dentistry stands out. Alexopoulos et al. [3] used a questionnaire to study the 12-month prevalence of musculoskeletal disorders of 430 dentists in Greece. They found that 62% of dentists reported at least one musculoskeletal complaint during the 12-month time period and 30% had chronic complaints. Low back pain was most common. In the upper extremity, hand symptoms were reported most often followed by shoulder (20%) and neck (26%) symptoms. Strenuous (awkward) posture was cited by 52.3% of the dentists as contributing to their symptoms.

Bovenzi [7] recently reviewed the health disorders caused by occupational exposure to whole-body vibration and hand-transmitted. Long-term occupational exposure to intense vibration was found to be associated with an increased risk for disorders including shoulder and neck symptoms. However, the epidemiological link between vibration and proximal upper extremity problems was determined to be weak [7]. Alexopoulos et al. [3] also found that the frequent use of vibrating tools was identified as an important risk factor and vibration was correlated to shoulder pain.

11.15 WORKPLACE ENVIRONMENT

Beyond physical demands of the working activity, psychosocial and environmental demands can impact neck and shoulder symptoms. Physical comfort of the worker may contribute to the overall problem. Rocha et al. [47] found that the thermal environment (comfort) was found to be associated with neck shoulder pain for call center workers. Only 28% of call center workers thought the thermal comfort of the environment was good or excellent.

Harkness et al. [24] studied 1081 newly employed subjects in 12 diverse occupational settings. The subjects were employed in jobs that required prolonged working with hands at or above shoulder level. For these workers, the psychosocial exposures, those who reported low job satisfaction, low social support, and monotonous work, had an increased risk of new-onset widespread pain including the neck and shoulder [24]. Identification of perceived environmental or psychosocial stressors may be a step toward appropriate interventions for neck and shoulder pain.

11.16   TOOLS

Engineering a solution may involve the workstation but it may also be necessary to adjust the tools for the job. There has been a long history of ingenious methods to make work easier, and some of these tools make work less injurious. For example, Duke et al. [14] studied the use of angled pliers in computer parts installation. The authors used motion analysis of 16 participants during jumper installation. Change in tool design significantly reduced shoulder elevation in specific task. The benefit of the tool design was task-dependent.

Apples are hand-harvested by workers who carry them from the tree to a bin in buckets weighing as much as 19 kg. Earle-Richardson et al. [16] compared muscle exertion (using electromyography) of back and shoulder muscles for apple pickers using different carrying systems. Their approach was to use a hip belt system to decrease stress from shoulder straps. Laboratory volunteers were studied under intervention and control conditions, in two postures. The belt system significantly reduced electromyographic activity but the effectiveness of the intervention depended on the postural position where it was most effective in a spinal flexion position.

Both of these studies demonstrate the goals of improving posture and reducing force through devices.

11.17   EMPLOYEE WELLNESS PROGRAMS

Improving the psychosocial well-being of the worker may be accomplished in part by a physical wellness program. Increasing the physical capacity of the worker through wellness programs should be a direction for future research. Therapeutic exercise studies have identified specific shoulder girdle and shoulder strengthening programs where the number of exercise can be minimized. In particular, these exercise programs focus on sets of muscles that tend to be weaker due to aging or sedentary lifestyles such as the rotator cuff and deltoid muscles [46] and the serratus anterior [13]. In our society, and even in exercising populations, the rotator cuff rarely is activated at a level adequate for causing hypertrophy or even maintaining the strength.

11.18   CONCLUSIONS

At this time, there is increasing epidemiological research and other literature to identify some potential causes of neck and shoulder symptoms associated with the workplace, and their treatments. Unfortunately neither the mechanisms of worker injury nor the mechanisms to eliminate these injuries have been studied with sufficient detail. The Cochrane Collaboration report on ergonomic interventions [61] found that there is limited evidence for adding breaks during computer work but interventions are not supported by strong evidence. Verhagen et al. [61] recently stated that despite good intentions of approaches to work-related neck and shoulder pain, the cost–benefit analyses of these interventions are not adequate.

The recent literature covers intrinsic, ergonomic, and environmental variables. For example, Werner et al. [63] summarized interaction of personal and ergonomic variables of 501 active industrial and clerical workers over a 5 year time period. The factors found to have the highest predictive value for identifying a person who is likely to develop an upper extremity tendonitis included age over 40 years, a body mass index over 30, a complaint at baseline of a shoulder or neck discomfort, a history of carpal tunnel syndrome, and a job with a higher shoulder posture rating. The risk profile identifies both ergonomic and personal health factors as risks and both categories of factors may be amenable to prevention strategies.

The chapter has covered interactions between posture, physical health, and the workplace environment. The premise of this discussion has been that there needs to be an assessment and treatment of these interacting variables.

REFERENCES

1. Adedoyin RA, Idowu BO, Adagunodo RE, and Idowu PA. Musculoskeletal pain associated with the use of computer systems in Nigeria. *The Internet Journal of Pain, Symptom Control and Palliative Care* 2004;3, available at *http://www.ispub.com/ostia/index.php?xmlFilePath=journals/ijpsp/vol3n2/computer.xml.*
2. Al-Shekhlee A and Katirji B. Spinal accessory neuropathy, droopy shoulder, and thoracic outlet syndrome. *Muscle & Nerve* 2003;28:383–385.
3. Alexopoulos EC, Stathi I-C, and Charizani F. Prevalence of musculoskeletal disorders in dentists. *BioMedical Central Musculoskeletal Disorders* 2004;5:16.
4. Ardic F, Kahraman Y, Kacar M, Kahraman MC, Findikoglu G, and Yorgancioglu ZR. Shoulder impingement syndrome: Relationships between clinical, functional, and radiologic findings. *American Journal of Physical Medicine and Rehabilitation* 2006;85:53–60.
5. Borich MR, Bright JM, Lorello DJ, Cieminski CJ, Buisman T, and Ludewig PM. Scapular angular positioning at end range internal rotation in cases of glenohumeral internal rotation deficit. *Journal of Orthopaedic and Sports Physical Therapy* 2006;36:926–934.
6. Borstad JD. Resting position variables at the shoulder: Evidence to support a posture-impairment association. *Physical Therapy* 2006;86:549–557.
7. Bovenzi M. Health risks from occupational exposure to mechanical vibration. *La Medicina del Lavoro* 2006;97:535–541.
8. Castagna A, Nordenson U, Garofalo R, and Karlsson J. Minor shoulder instability. *The Journal of Arthroscopic and Related Surgery* 2007;23:211–215.
9. Cole DC, Hogg-Johnson S, Manno M, Ibrahim S, Wells RP, and Ferrier SE. Reducing musculoskeletal burden through ergonomic program implementation in a large newspaper. *International Archives of Occupational and Environmental Health* 2006;80:98–108.
10. Cook C and Kothiyal K. Influence of mouse position on muscular activity in the neck, shoulder and arm in computer users. *Applied Ergonomics* 1998;29:439–443.
11. Daggfeldt K and Thorstenssona A. The mechanics of back-extensor torque production about the lumbar spine. *Journal of Biomechanics* 2003;36:815–825.

12. Dahlberg R, Karlqvist L, Bildt C, and Nykvist K. Do work technique and musculoskeletal symptoms differ between men and women performing the same type of work tasks? *Applied Ergonomics* 2004;35:521–529.

13. Decker MJ, Hintermeister RA, Faber KJ, and Hawkins RJ. Serratus anterior muscle activity during selected rehabilitation exercises. *American Journal of Sports Medicine* 1999;27:784–791.

14. Duke K, Mirka GA, and Sommerich CM. Productivity and ergonomic investigation of bent-handle pliers. *Human Factors* 2004;46:234–243.

15. Dunk NM, Chung YY, Sullivan Compton D, and Callaghan JP. The reliability of quantifying upright standing postures as a baseline diagnostic clinical tool. *Journal of Manipulative and Physiological Therapeutics* 2004;27:91–96.

16. Earle-Richardson G, Jenkins PL, Freivalds A, et al. Laboratory evaluation of belt usage with apple buckets. *American Journal of Industrial Medicine* 2006;49:23–29.

17. Felice KJ, North WA, Moore SA, and Mathews KD. FSH dystrophy 4q35 deletion in patients presenting with facial-sparing scapular myopathy. *Neurology* 2000;54:1927–1931.

18. Fernandez-de-las-Penas C, Alonso-Blanco C, Cuadrado ML, Gerwin RD, and Pareja JA. Trigger points in the suboccipital muscles and forward head posture in tension-type headache. *Headache* 2006;46:454–460.

19. Findikcioglu K, Findikcioglu F, Ozmen S, and Guclu T. The impact of breast size on the vertebral column: A radiologic study. *Aesthetic Plastic Surgery* 2007;31:23–27.

20. Finley MA and Lee RY. Effect of sitting posture on 3-dimensional scapular kinematics measured by skin-mounted electromagnetic tracking sensors. *Archives of Physical Medicine and Rehabilitation* 2003;84:563–568.

21. Fon GT, Pitt MJ, and Thies AC Jr. Thoracic kyphosis: Range in normal subjects. *American Journal of Roentgenology* 1980;134:979–983.

22. Frost P, Bonde JPE, Mikkelsen S, et al. Risk of shoulder tendinitis in relation to shoulder loads in monotonous repetitive work. *American Journal of Industrial Medicine* 2002;41:11–18.

23. Goh S, Tan C, Price RI, et al. Influence of age and gender on thoracic vertebral body shape and disc degeneration: An MR investigation of 169 cases. *Journal of Anatomy* 2000;197:647–657.

24. Harkness EF, Macfarlane GJ, Nahit E, Silman AJ, and McBeth J. Mechanical injury and psychosocial factors in the work place predict the onset of widespread body pain: A two-year prospective study among cohorts of newly employed workers. *Arthritis & Rheumatism* 2004;50:1655–1664.

25. Hébert LJ, Moffet H, McFadyen BJ, and Dionne CE. Scapular behavior in shoulder impingement syndrome. *Archives of Physical Medicine and Rehabilitation* 2002;83:60–69.

26. IJzelenberg W and Burdorf A. Risk factors for musculoskeletal symptoms and ensuing health care use and sick leave. *Spine* 2005;30:1550–1556.

27. Julius A, Lees R, Dilley A, and Lynn B. Shoulder posture and median nerve sliding. *BioMedical Central Musculoskeletal Disorders* 2004;5:23.

28. Kaergaard A and Andersen JH. Musculoskeletal disorders of the neck and shoulders in female sewing machine operators: Prevalence, incidence, and prognosis. *Occupational and Environmental Medicine* 2000;57:528–534.

29. Kibler WB. Scapular involvement in impingement: Signs and symptoms. *Instructional Course Lectures* 2006;55:35–43.

30. Klopčar N, Tomšič M, and Lenarčič J. Kinematic model of the shoulder complex to evaluate the arm-reachable workspace. *Journal of Biomechanics* 2007;40:86–91.

31. Kwon HK, Hwang M, and Yoon DW. Frequency and severity of carpal tunnel syndrome according to level of cervical radiculopathy: Double crush syndrome? *Clinical Neurophysiology* 2006;117:1256–1259.

32. Leclerc A, Chastang J-F, Niedhammer I, Landre M-F, and Roquelaure Y. Incidence of shoulder pain in repetitive work. *Occupational and Environmental Medicine* 2004;61:39–44.

33. Levin SM. The scapula is a sesamoid bone. *Journal of Biomechanics* 2005;38:1733–1734.

34. Lin J, Lim HK, and Yang J-L. Effect of shoulder tightness on glenohumeral translation, scapular kinematics, and scapulohumeral rhythm in subjects with stiff shoulders. *Journal of Orthopaedic Research* 2006;24:1044–1051.

35. Ludewig PM and Cook TM. Alterations in shoulder kinematics and associated muscle activity in people with symptoms of shoulder impingement. *Physical Therapy* 2000;80:276–291.

36. Madeleine P, Vedsted P, Blangsted AK, Sjřgaard G, and Sjřgaard K. Effects of electromyographic and mechanomyographic biofeedback on upper trapezius muscle activity during standardized computer work. *Ergonomics* 2006;49:921–933.

37. Marcus M, Gerr F, Monteilh C, et al. A prospective study of computer users: II. Postural risk factors for musculoskeletal symptoms and disorders. *American Journal of Industrial Medicine* 2002;41:236–249.

38. Mell AG, LaScalza S, Guffey P, Ray J, Maciejewski M, and Carpenter JE. Effect of rotator cuff pathology on shoulder rhythm. *Journal of Shoulder and Elbow Surgery* 2005;14:58S–64S.

39. Miranda H, Viikari-Juntura E, Heistaro S, Heliövaara M, and Riihimäki H. A population study on differences in the determinants of a specific shoulder disorder versus nonspecific shoulder pain without clinical findings. *American Journal of Epidemiology* 2005;161:847–855.

40. Pal B, Anderson J, Dick WC, and Griffiths ID. Limitation of joint mobility and shoulder capsulitis in insulin- and non-insulin-dependent diabetes mellitus. *British Journal of Rheumatology* 1986;25:147–151.

41. Pascarelli EF and Hsu YP. Understanding work-related upper extremity disorders: Clinical findings in 485 computer users, musicians, and others. *Journal of Occupational Rehabilitation* 2001;11:1–21.

42. Pierre-Jerome C and Bekkelund SI. Magnetic resonance assessment of the double-crush phenomenon in patients with carpal tunnel syndrome: A bilateral quantitative study. *Scandinavian Journal of Plastic and Reconstructive Surgery and Hand Surgery* 2003;37:46–53.

43. Pratt N. Anatomy of nerve entrapment sites in the upper quarter. *Journal of Hand Therapy.* 2005;18:216–230.

44. Punnett L, Gold J, Katz JN, Gore R, and Wegman DH. Ergonomic stressors and upper extremity musculoskeletal disorders in automobile manufacturing: A one year follow up study. *Occupational and Environmental Medicine* 2004;61:668–674.

45. Punnett L and Wegman DH. Work-related musculoskeletal disorders: The epidemiologic evidence and the debate. *Journal of Electromyography & Kinesiology* 2004;14:13–23.

46. Reinold MM, Wilk KE, Fleisig GS, et al. Electromyographic analysis of the rotator cuff and deltoid musculature during common shoulder external rotation exercises. *Journal of Orthopaedic and Sports Physical Therapy* 2004;34:385–394.

47. Rocha LE, Glina DMR, Marinho MdF, and Nakasato D. Risk factors for musculoskeletal symptoms among call center operators of a back in São Paulo, Brazil. *Industrial Health* 2005;43:637–646.

48. Roquelaure Y, Ha C, Leclerc A, et al. Epidemiologic surveillance of upper-extremity musculoskeletal disorders in the working population. *Arthritis & Rheumatism* 2006;55(5):765–778.

49. Ryu J-D, Kirpalani PA, Kim J-M, Nam K-H, Han C-W, and Han S-H. Expression of vascular endothelial growth factor and angiogenesis in the diabetic frozen shoulder. *Journal of Shoulder and Elbow Surgery* 2006;15:679–685.

50. Schwab F, Lafage V, Boyce R, Skalli W, and Farcy JP. Gravity line analysis in adult volunteers: Age-related correlation with spinal parameters, pelvic parameters, and foot position. *Spine* 2006;31:E959–E967.

51. Schwab F, Dubey A, Gamez L, et al. Adult scoliosis: Prevalence, SF-36, and nutritional parameters in an elderly volunteer population. *Spine* 2005;30:1082–1085.

52. Sharkey NA, Marder RA, and Hanson PB. The entire rotator cuff contributes to elevation of the arm. *Journal of Orthopaedic Research* 1994;12:699–708.

53. Shirley D, Hodges PW, Eriksson AEM, and Gandevia SC. Spinal stiffness changes throughout the respiratory cycle. *Journal of Applied Physiology* 2003;95:1467–1475.

54. Silverstein B, Viikari-juntura E, and Kalat J. Use of a prevention index to identify industries at high risk for work-related musculoskeletal disorders of the neck, back, and upper extremity in Washington State, 1990–1998. *American Journal of Industrial Medicine* 2002;241:149–169.

55. Straker L, Pollock C, and Mangharam J. The effect of shoulder posture on performance, discomfort and muscle fatigue whilst working on a visual display unit. *International Journal of Industrial Ergonomics* 1997;20:1–10.

56. Straker L and Mekhora K. An evaluation of visual display unit placement by electromyography, posture, discomfort and preference. *International Journal of Industrial Ergonomics* 2000;26:389–398.

57. Streib E. Upper arm radial nerve palsy after muscular effort: Report of three cases. *Neurology* 1992;42:1632–1634.

58. Svendsen SW, Gelineck J, Mathiassen SE, et al. Work above shoulder level and degenerative alterations of the rotator cuff tendons: A magnetic resonance imaging study. *Arthritis & Rheumatism* 2004;50:3314–3322.

59. Takeshima T, Omokawa S, Takaoka T, Araki M, Ueda Y, and Takakura Y. Sagittal alignment of cervical flexion and extension: Lateral radiographic analysis. *Spine* 2002;27:E348–E355.

60. van den Heuvel SG, de Looze MP, Hildebrandt VH, and The KH. Effects of software programs stimulating regular breaks and exercises on work-related neck and upper-limb disorders. *Scandinavian Journal of Work and Environmental Health* 2003;29:106–116.

61. Verhagen AP, Karels C, Bierma-Zeinstra SMA, et al. Ergonomic and physiotherapeutic interventions for treating work-related complaints of the arm, neck or shoulder in adults. *Cochrane Database of Systematic Reviews* 2006;3:CD003471. DOI: 10.1002/14651858. CD003471.pub3.

62. Walker-Bone K and Cooper C. Hard work never hurt anyone: or did it? A review of occupational associations with soft tissue musculoskeletal disorders of the neck and upper limb. *Annals of Rheumatic Disease* 2005;64:1391–1396.

63. Werner RA, Franzblau A, Gell N, Ulin SS, and Armstrong TJ. A longitudinal study of industrial and clerical workers: Predictors of upper extremity tendonitis. *Journal of Occupational Rehabilitation* 2005;15:37–46.

12 Work-Related Low Back Pain: Biomechanical Factors and Primary Prevention

Jaap H. van Dieën and Allard J. van der Beek

CONTENTS

12.1   INTRODUCTION

In this chapter, we will discuss the possibilities for the prevention of low back pain (LBP) and disability due to LBP from a biomechanical perspective. We will focus on LBP with unknown causes, as in the large majority of cases of LBP, standard diagnostic techniques do not reveal specific causes. Aspecific LBP is not exclusively a biomechanical problem and from that perspective, we can only give a partial account of the state of knowledge with respect to LBP and its prevention. However, mechanical loading of the low back has been shown to be a risk factor for LBP and mechanical loading often provokes pain in patients with LBP. Therefore, insight into the mechanics of the low back can help to design and optimize preventive measures. Finally, we will give an overview of the epidemiologic evidence regarding the effectiveness of interventions aiming at primary prevention of LBP.

12.2   LOW BACK PAIN

LBP is one of the most common causes of lost or restricted working hours in the industrialized world. In the general population, the annual incidence is about 5% [1] and the lifetime prevalence has been estimated at around 70% [2]. In subpopulations exposed to high mechanical loads on the low back (during occupational activities), the prevalence appears to be even higher [3,4].

    LBP is probably a phenomenon of all times and all cultures. However, the way in which LBP is approached varies widely over time and cultures. In the mid-nineteenth century, the idea that LBP was a consequence of tissue damage due to physical injury gained popularity in Europe, in particular due to the high prevalence among railway workers [5]. The problem, however, was and still is that the presence of tissue damage is difficult to verify objectively. This led to a change in perception of the problem in which, at the end of the nineteenth century, LBP was considered mainly a form of "hysteria" [5].

    In the early twentieth century, with the advance of orthopedics as a medical profession, LBP was again viewed as a predominantly physical problem. Protrusion of the intervertebral disk and stages of disk injury preceding a detectable protrusion became to be seen as primary causes of LBP and at the end of the 1960s compression forces on the spine were regarded as the cause of these injuries [6]. In line with this rationale, bed rest and surgery, the latter in case of the presence of a detectable protrusion, became widely used treatments [7]. When disk protrusion or other disorders could not be found, a psychosomatic disorder was implied in the view of many researchers [5]. Then, as it became clear that x-ray diagnostics did not lead to verification of disk (or other) injury in most cases, the idea of LBP as a psychosomatic problem again gained momentum.

One of the first large-scale prospective studies on LBP, the so-called "Boeing study" [8] revealed a stronger relationship of LBP with job dissatisfaction and other psychological factors than with physical workload. Although this study was criticized for the way in which physical workload was quantified [9] and in spite of the fact that psychosocial variables account for a only a small percentage of the incidence of LBP [10,11], the conclusion that psychosocial factors were the main determinants of LBP became influential.

Up to date, the cause of LBP remains elusive in most cases; only in about 10% of the cases of LBP, a specific diagnosis is made [12–14]. The main symptoms of aspecific LBP are pain and limitations in the execution of activities of daily living. In addition, loss of strength, stiffness, and a reduced range of motion are in some cases reported, but appear in general only weakly associated with LBP [7]. The complaints can be episodic or continuously present. Often a distinction is made between acute (<6 weeks), subacute (6–12 weeks), and chronic complaints (>12 weeks). The majority of patients attending to the general practitioner in connection with LBP recovers fairly quickly without specific treatment and falls in the first or second category. The median period to recovery is 7 weeks, and after 12 weeks, only 35% of the population still has symptoms [15]. However, relapses are common, with 60%–75% relapsing within 1 year [2,15,16]. In a minority of subjects (10%), LBP becomes a chronic problem and persists even 1 year after the first visit to the general practitioner [15].

Statistics from the UK indicate that most people continue to work with LBP, with sick leave occurring in only 5%–10% of the cases [17]. Nevertheless, the economic costs associated with LBP are high. In the Netherlands, direct costs (sick leave and disability compensation and medical costs) in 1991 were estimated at 1.7% of the gross national product or €4.1 billion [18]. Of those LBP patients on sick leave, 67% resumed work after 1 week, 84% after 1 month, and 97% after 1 year [19]. The probability of work resumption after 2 years appears to be almost nonexistent [19,20].

12.3 PREVENTION

Interventions can generally be categorized into the three main prevention types: (1) primary prevention, (2) secondary prevention, and (3) tertiary prevention. The first category (primary prevention) concerns those interventions that intend to diminish the incidence of symptoms/disorders in a healthy (working) population. Interventions of the second category (secondary prevention) aim at recovery from early symptoms, for instance found after screening, and at a reduced risk of recurrence of symptoms and disorders. Interventions of the third category (tertiary prevention) intend to reduce symptoms/disorders and/or to prevent (further) worsening of disorders including the improvement of the patient's ability to cope with disabilities resulting from the disorders. In the secondary prevention category, the purpose from the company perspective is reduction of production loss while at work due to early low back symptoms (i.e., reduction of so-called presenteeism). In the last-mentioned category (tertiary prevention) the purpose from the company perspective is reduction of sick leave due to low back disorders (i.e., reduction of absenteeism). Thus, prompt and effective interventions to promote early return to work after an episode of sick leave or vocational rehabilitation to promote a patient's occupational adjustment to their irremediable conditions are tertiary prevention.

The target population of biomechanical interventions aiming at primary prevention is most of the time a group of workers. For instance, an educational back school program for all employees of a distribution center, or ergonomic changes of an assembly line resulting in decreased workload of all assembly workers involved. However, measures can also be aimed at individual workers. For instance, the ergonomic redesign of a specific workstation of a tall worker. Interventions for secondary or tertiary prevention are more often focusing on individuals, i.e., workers with early low back symptoms. For instance, back schools for those workers who are at risk of being absent from work due to their early symptoms can be mentioned as an example of secondary prevention. Therapeutic interventions, such as physiotherapy, chiropractic treatment or pain management, for chronic pain patients can be mentioned as examples of tertiary prevention focusing on individuals. In this chapter, the focus will be mainly on primary prevention.

Interventions can aim at the worksite or at the workforce, but can also have a much wider scope. From the community perspective, many interventions can be considered. For instance, legislation with respect to topics such as manual lifting can have an enormous impact on the actual biomechanical exposures of the individual workers. Moreover, technological developments and subsequent implementation of these developments can be regarded as ergonomic interventions with a wide scope, for which the health effects can hardly be underestimated.

Table 12.1 presents an overview of interventions categorized into organizational ergonomics, physical ergonomics, and individual worker interventions. In the broad sense, these types of intervention are oriented at organizational strategies, workplace design and layout, and worker capacity, respectively. For each of the categories examples are shown, without the purpose of being completely comprehensive.

12.4   RISK FACTORS FOR LBP

In this section, we will give an overview of the evidence that can be found in the scientific literature with regard to the association between LBP and work-related physical factors, work-related psychosocial factors, and individual risk factors. The issue of risk factors for LBP is neither well understood nor consistently documented. However, there are systematic reviews of the literature, in which epidemiologic studies were retrieved according to well-described inclusion and exclusion criteria. This overview will only be based on this type of systematic reviews, while narrative reviews will not be taken into account. Also, in some of the systematic reviews, the strength of the evidence was assessed, based on the methodological quality of the included studies and the consistency of the findings of these studies. Consequently, levels of evidence were reported for each of the reviewed risk factors (see Table 12.2). For instance, for the association of a risk factor with LBP the conclusion could be: "strong evidence," "moderate evidence," "insufficient evidence," or "no evidence." However, it should be noted that this "level" is just a grading of the strength of the evidence; it is an indicator of confidence in the conclusion,

TABLE 12.1

An Overview of Three Different Types of Intervention Aimed at Prevention of LBP

Organizational ergonomics interventions

- Organizational measures, such as job enlargement, work groups, job rotation, reorganization of an assembly line, or modification of the production system
- Administrative controls, such as preemployment selection, or employee restriction
- Light duty or other modified work programs for absent workers returning to work
- Guidelines and protocols, for example, occupational health surveillance or return to work after reporting sick

Physical ergonomics interventions

- Ergonomic redesign and/or technical engineering modifications of workstations
- Machinery, equipment, tools, parts, etc.
- Availability of manual handling aids such as lifting devices

Individual worker interventions

- Training in work methods, such as lifting technique
- Physical activity, physical exercise, and employee fitness programs
- Improving awareness regarding safety and ergonomics
- Availability of personal protective equipment (e.g., back belts/lumbar supports, or safety shoes)

For each of the categories organizational ergonomics interventions, physical ergonomics interventions, and individual worker interventions examples are given.

rather than its effect size. In fact, most well-documented risk factors for LBP have rather small effect sizes, which logically will compromise the potential effect of preventive interventions.

12.4.1 WORK-RELATED PHYSICAL FACTORS

Five systematic reviews summarized epidemiologic research on the association between manual materials handling, mainly consisting of manual lifting, and LBP [21–25]. Table 12.2 generally shows that there is "strong evidence" that lifting/ manual materials handling are associated with LBP. Two of these systematic reviews also paid attention to exposure to patient handling in particular, and both concluded "moderate evidence" for the association between patient handling and LBP [23,24]. For occupational exposure to carrying, pushing and pulling the picture seems to be less clear.

Three systematic reviews concluded "strong evidence" for the association between awkward postures of the trunk, which includes bending and twisting, and LBP [22,23,25], while the level was just "evidence" in another review [21].

The levels of evidence for exposure to heavy physical work are ranging between "evidence" [21] and "moderate evidence" [23] up to "strong evidence" [22,25]. However, the question of what is exactly meant by heavy physical work remains

TABLE 12.2

An Overview of Systematic Reviews Regarding the Association between Work-Related Risk Factors and (Low) Back Pain

	Bernard [21]	Burdorf and Sorock [22][a]	Kuiper et al. [24][a]	Hoogendoorn et al. [23,29]	Linton [30]	NRC/IoM [25][b]	Hartvigsen et al. [11]
Work-related physical factors							
Lifting/forceful movement	Strong evidence	Strong evidence	Moderate evidence	Strong evidence			
Manual materials handling			Moderate evidence			Strong evidence	
Patient handling			Moderate evidence	Moderate evidence			
Awkward posture/bending and twisting	Evidence	Strong evidence		Strong evidence		Strong evidence	
Heavy physical work	Evidence	Strong evidence		Moderate evidence		Strong evidence	
Whole body vibration	Strong evidence	Strong evidence		Strong evidence		Strong evidence	
Static work posture	Insufficient evidence	Mixed evidence				Mixed evidence	
Standing/walking				No evidence			
Prolonged sitting				No evidence			
Work-related psychosocial factors							
Job demands/workload	Evidence			Insufficient evidence	Strong evidence	Strong evidence	Moderate evidence[c]
Work pace		No evidence		Insufficient evidence	Moderate evidence	Strong evidence	
Low job control	Limited evidence	Mixed evidence		Insufficient evidence	Moderate evidence	Moderate evidence	
Monotonous work/job content	Mixed evidence			Insufficient evidence	Strong evidence	Strong evidence	

Poor social support at work	Insufficient evidence	No evidence	Strong evidence	Strong evidence	Strong evidence	Moderate evidence[c]
(Mental) stress		Insufficient evidence		Strong evidence	Strong evidence	Insufficient evidence
Perceived ability to work				Strong evidence	Strong evidence	
Job dissatisfaction	Evidence	Mixed evidence	Strong evidence	Strong evidence	Strong evidence	Moderate evidence[c]
Belief that work is dangerous				Moderate evidence	Moderate evidence	
Emotional effort at work				Moderate evidence	Moderate evidence	

[a] These authors did not report "levels of evidence." This interpretation is based on the text of the authors(s).

[b] NRC/IoM, National Research Council/Institute of Medicine. This report did not report "levels of evidence" for work-related physical factors. This interpretation is based on the findings for work-related physical factors and the "levels of evidence" that were given for comparable findings on work-related psychosocial factors, for which "levels of evidence" were reported.

[c] In these cases moderate evidence was found for no association between the (categories of) work-related psychosocial factors and LBP.

unanswered in all of these systematic reviews. In fact, it has been elegantly proven that the "true" risk estimate for heavy physical work is close to the value 1, when corrected for exposure to manual materials handling and frequent bending or twisting of the trunk [26]. Hence, we conclude that heavy physical work cannot be separated from other exposures such as manual materials handling and awkward postural load, and that heavy physical work by itself is probably not associated with LBP.

The conclusion regarding exposure to whole-body vibration is unambiguous: there is "strong evidence" for its association with LBP [21–23,25].

There are three systematic reviews on the association between sitting-while-at-work and LBP [23,27,28]. The conclusions of these reviews are clear: the epidemiologic literature does not show evidence for the popular opinion that prolonged sitting by itself is associated with LBP. However, sitting in combination with exposure to whole-body vibration and/or awkward postures seems to be associated with LBP [27,28]. It is unclear whether prolonged sitting adds to the risk of LBP for those being exposed to whole-body vibration and/or awkward postures [28]. This is important to find out since whole-body vibration as well as awkward trunk postures are associated with LBP, even without sitting.

Finally, there is insufficient evidence that occupational exposure to static working postures is associated with LBP [21,22,25] and no evidence that exposure to standing/walking is associated with LBP [23].

In conclusion, there is solid epidemiologic evidence for three work-related physical factors to be associated with LBP: manual lifting/manual materials handling, awkward trunk postures, and whole-body vibration. Other work-related physical factors, including the "risk factors" heavy physical work, static working posture, standing/walking, and prolonged sitting, seem by themselves not to be associated with LBP.

12.4.2 Work-Related Psychosocial Factors

The evidence for the associations between work-related psychosocial factors and LBP is less straightforward than for work-related physical factors. Table 12.2 indicates that the levels of evidence reported for the association of the work-related psychosocial factors with LBP are highly inconsistent among the six different systematic reviews [11,21,22,25,29,30]. Particularly, the conclusion for the association between poor social support at work and LBP varied very much: three reviews concluded "strong evidence" [25,29,30], one review concluded "insufficient evidence"[21], another review concluded "no evidence" [22], and the most recent review even concluded "moderate evidence for no association" [11]. In general, the largest disagreement can be found between the most recent review and those published in 2001: Hartvigsen and colleagues [11] concluded "moderate evidence for no association" for psychosocial factors that were found to be associated with LBP in the other two reviews (either "moderate evidence" or "strong evidence") [25,30].

On the one hand, two points of critique can be mentioned as to the systematic review of Hartvigsen and colleagues [11]. First, it is incorrect to conclude that there is evidence for no association. In science, the empirical finding that the null hypothesis (no association) cannot be rejected in favor of the alternative hypothesis (association) does not necessarily mean that the null hypothesis is true. Second, in this review many conceptually different factors were lumped together into one single category. This meant, for instance, that variables such as job security, conflicting demands, pace, work content, work control, qualitative demands, quantitative demands, decision latitude, skill discretion, and work monotony were grouped into the category "organizational aspects of work." Then, the evidence was reported for that category, including all studies reporting on one or more of these variables. It is plausible that negative findings for variables that indeed have no association with LBP outnumber positive findings for those that are associated with LBP.

On the other hand, Hartvigsen et al. based, far more than Linton and NRC/IoM did, the conclusions of their review on the methodological quality of the included studies. This can only partly explain the different conclusions, since the methodological quality of the included studies was also taken into account by Hoogendoorn et al., who concluded either "insufficient evidence" or "strong evidence" for the associations between work-related psychosocial factors and LBP. Another obvious explanation for the inconsistent conclusions is that different studies were included in the different reviews. Hartvigsen et al. only included prospective cohort studies that were published from 1990 up to 2002; studies with other study designs and those published before 1990 were excluded. In the early 2000s several prospective cohort studies were published on the topic. In fact, 10–13 of the 18 studies included by Hartvigsen et al. could not have been included in the three reviews published in 2000 or 2001, simply because these studies were published later than the literature search for these reviews was performed.

In summary, the epidemiologic evidence for the associations between work-related psychosocial factors and LBP is far from conclusive. Although it is plausible that high job demands and poor social support at work play a role in the occurrence of LBP, more research is needed to verify or falsify this conclusion.

12.4.3 INDIVIDUAL FACTORS

There are no systematic reviews evaluating epidemiologic research on the association between individual factors and LBP. Hence, we have based this overview on available narrative reviews [31–34]. By far the most powerful risk factor for a new episode of LBP is a previous history of LBP [31,32], indicating that primary prevention of LBP is essential. Another important individual factor that has been reported to be associated with LBP is age, whereas the effect size is smaller for gender and smoking [31–34].

Of the many anthropometric variables, body height and body weight have most frequently been studied. For body height, conflicting evidence was reported as to its association with LBP [32]. For body weight, mixed evidence was found. It was concluded that the majority of epidemiologic studies revealed no or weak adverse effects for body weight or any other measure of body mass [32–34]. However, the effects were substantial for the most obese individuals [32,34].

There is evidence for a negative association between strength of back and abdominal muscles and the occurrence of LBP [32,33]. However, it has been stressed that there is only evidence for measures referring to relative strength (i.e., ratio of physical job demands to worker's physical capacity), whereas measures referring to absolute strength (e.g., isometric or isokinetic trunk strength) are not associated with LBP [32]. Besides, it is unlikely that measures of aerobic fitness (i.e., maximum oxygen uptake or other indicators of cardiorespiratory capacity) are associated with LBP [32].

In conclusion, there is epidemiologic evidence that previous history of LBP, age, gender, smoking, obesity, and relative strength of back and abdominal muscles are associated with the occurrence of LBP.

12.5   MECHANICAL LOADING AND LBP

In this section, we will review the mechanisms underpinning the associations between established risk factors and LBP as reviewed in the previous section. The fundamental assumption made is that some form of injury is relevant to the pathophysiology of LBP. Specifically these injuries are presumed to be of mechanical origin. While this assumption cannot be proven for aspecific LBP—in fact, LBP would not be aspecific, if this were proven—the overview of risk factors makes the assumption plausible. We will further address the validity of this assumption by briefly reviewing the literature on the relationship between injury and LBP. Subsequently, we will discuss possible injury mechanisms and next we will describe how these mechanisms are related to the most important risk factors identified in Section 12.4.

12.5.1   INJURY AND LBP

As discussed above, no diagnosis is made in the majority of LBP cases. Nevertheless, in some studies, it was attempted to identify injured structures or tissues with techniques that are not routinely applied in the diagnostic process. In most of these studies, patient selection was not random. The participating patients usually had LBP that was considered aspecific and chronic, and most had undergone several diagnostic and treatment procedures with limited or no success.

12.5.1.1   Intervertebral Disk and Endplates

The vertebrae of the human spinal column are connected by intervertebral disks. The disks consist of an outer ring of fibers connecting the two vertebrae, organized in lamellae, the annulus fibrosus, which surrounds a gel-like nucleus, containing a high percentage of water. The boundary layer of the disk and the vertebra is called the endplate and consists of cartilage and bone. The disks confer flexibility to the spine and transmit forces from vertebra to vertebra.

Although the specificity and sensitivity of positive findings on x-ray diagnostics are low, a relationship between LBP and x-ray signs of intervertebral disks degeneration does exist [35]. In addition, studies employing more advanced diagnostic techniques, such as diskography, do indicate that structural damage in the disk is present in a considerable fraction (80%–94%) of LBP cases [36,37]. Moreover, this structural damage is a quite specific finding by itself, and highly specific when appearing combined with provocation of pain on mechanical stimulation of the disk [38]. Using very strict criteria for a positive diskogram (structural abnormalities, plus pain reproduction, plus negative results at other disk levels), positive results were found in

26%–39% of the chronic LBP cases studied [39,40]. In addition, evidence of ruptures in the annulus fibrosus determined postmortem was related to a history of LBP [41].

Postmortem studies have shown that (repaired) damage to the endplate is a very common phenomenon [42–46]. This type of damage is usually not visible with x-ray or other imaging modalities [47–51], although very large injuries sometimes show up on magnetic resonance imaging (MRI) and are in these cases clearly related to pain [50,52–55]. The morphological findings described are related to pain provocation upon increasing the pressure in the intervertebral disk [36,37,54,56,57].

Kuslich and coworkers [58,59] asked patients, after mechanical stimulation during surgery for LBP with radiating pain to the leg, if pain was experienced and if so whether this pain resembled their usual LBP. Among those structures most frequently provoking LBP were the outer annulus fibrosus (33%–71%) and the end-plates (33%–61%). In conclusion, in a substantial part of the population with LBP, the origin of the pain appears to be the annulus fibrosus or the endplate. The pressure increase caused by diskography would provoke both structures [56].

12.5.1.2 Facet Joints

The facet joints have also been implicated in LBP. Blocking nociceptive afference from these joints by injection of local anesthetics, a method that has been shown to be quite specific provided that strict control measures are taken, reduced back pain by more than 50% in 15%–40% of the cases studied [40,60–62]. Also mechanical provocation during surgery caused pain resembling normally experienced LBP in 15%–30% of the patients studied [58,59].

It is known that osteoarthrotic changes of these joints are common [63], but whether mechanical injury plays a part in the causation of these is obscure. Some indication that injury of these joints can occur has been obtained in postmortem investigations of spines of young adults who had died after severe trauma, e.g., in car accidents. Injuries not visible on standard radiography were found in a high percentage of joints. Facet joint injuries were almost entirely absent in a comparable group of young subjects with no recent history of major trauma, but resembled some of the "age-related changes" seen in older subjects [64].

12.5.1.3 Ligaments

It has been suggested that subfailure injury of spinal ligaments can be an important cause of LBP [65,66]. Partial or complete tears of the interspinous ligament are frequently observed during low back surgery [67]. Moreover, electrical stimulation of this structure has been shown to cause LBP and pain radiating to the legs [68]. Also mechanical stimulation of the interspinous and supraspinous ligaments during surgery caused concordant pain in 6%–25% of the cases studied [58]. Diagnostic blocks of these ligaments, performed without control measures for false-positive findings, were positive in 10%–14% of the cases [69,70].

12.5.1.4 Instability

Instability of the spine is considered a cause of LBP by many clinicians as well as in the biomechanical literature [71,72]. Unfortunately, it is often unclear what exactly is meant with the term instability [73]. Mechanically, instability can be unambiguously and quantitatively defined, but a qualitative description of this mechanical definition suffices for the present discussion. A mechanically stable system will return to the vicinity of its intended configuration after a perturbation. Hence, when unstable any perturbation will cause the system to move to a configuration far away from the intended configuration. It is important to realize that perturbations are always present, and therefore an unstable system cannot function. For example, when a child is building a tower of blocks, the tower will usually be stable when only a few blocks have been stacked. However, at a certain number of blocks, let us say five, the tower will be unstable and collapse even without any notable perturbation. Slight movement of the building or of the surrounding air can be sufficient. Connecting the blocks by elastic straps may allow building a tower of five blocks high. The added stiffness of the connections between the blocks can stabilize the system. The higher the stiffness of the connections, the higher the tower that can be built. Suppose that a tower of blocks connected with elastic straps is unstable, when it consists of seven blocks. After the collapse of this tower, another advantage of the straps may become apparent. Failure of the tower is less catastrophic than before, because the straps limit the motion of the blocks and some structural integrity remains. The system (a tower of seven blocks) is still considered unstable though, because the final displacement from the intended state is bigger than the perturbation.

Obviously, the spine can be compared to a tower of blocks and the ligaments, intervertebral disks and facet joint capsules joining the vertebrae can be compared to elastic straps. Injury of the connecting structures, which reduces their stiffness [74–77], will increase the probability of a loss of stability. When the spine is unstable, excessive rotations of segments will occur and pain and (further) injury may be provoked [71,72]. White and Panjabi [78] proposed a clinical definition of spinal instability: "a loss of the spine's ability to maintain its patterns of displacement under physiologic loads so there is no neurologic deficit, major deformity, or incapacitating pain." Note that the measurable criterion of a final displacement being smaller than the perturbation in the mechanical definition is replaced by the clinically relevant, but not directly measurable criterion, so that neurological deficits, deformity, and pain are avoided.

Muscles also connect the vertebrae and hence stiffness of muscle tissue contributes to the stability of the spine. In itself the spine with ligaments and disks is unstable already under loads that are lower than upper body mass [79]. Hence, muscular contributions are required to stabilize the spine. Muscle stiffness can be increased by increasing coactivation of agonistic and antagonistic muscles, such that the net moment around a joint remains unchanged. Thus, the stability of the spine can be controlled by the central nervous system. Moreover, we so far only considered the elastic forces that provide an instantaneous force that tends to return the system to its previous configuration. Biological systems also encompass feedback control mechanisms, like reflexes, that tend to return the system to the intended (not necessarily the previous) configuration, based on sensory information and with some delay. This implies that the quality of sensory feedback will affect stability of the spine. Importantly, pain and fatigue have been implicated to degrade proprioceptive afferent information [80]. Moreover, the importance of active muscular control implies that muscle strength and the rate at which muscles can develop force determine spine stability. Consequently, trunk muscle fatigue and deconditioning of trunk muscle may be indirect causes of (recurrence of) LBP.

12.5.2 INJURY MECHANISMS

The morphological changes associated with LBP that have been described in the previous sections are not necessarily caused by mechanical injury. It is difficult in most cases to distinguish between age-related degenerative changes and injury. Clearly nonmechanical factors, for example genetic factors, play an important role in disk degeneration [81]. Interactions between genetic, age-related, and mechanical factors are likely to occur. Nevertheless, the literature on risk factors clearly suggests that mechanical loading is one of the causes of LBP and this is further supported by directly determined relationships between mechanical loading and LBP [82].

In the following discussion, we will describe which types of mechanical loading might contribute to the morphological changes described above. The evidence for injury mechanisms stems mainly from mechanical tests on cadaver material and to a limited extent from in vivo animal experiments. Obviously there may be some limitations in applying these data to the living human tissue. A puzzling paradox regarding spinal injury comes to the fore when considering the source of the mechanical loads that the spine is exposed to. Obviously, the spine is directly loaded by gravity on the upper body and inertial forces when the upper body accelerates. However, these forces are much lower than the forces produced by the trunk muscles. One might expect some balance to exist between the forces that the muscles spanning the lumbar spine can generate and the strength of the spinal tissues. Associations between physical activity and strength of spinal tissues [83,84] support such an assumption. A relationship between muscle strength and spinal strength makes it difficult to conceive how muscle force could injure the spine. However, it should be kept in mind that, in general, repeated submaximal loading of tissues could lead to injury. Furthermore, it is conceivable that in some cases uncontrolled extreme forces are produced, for example, when one loses balance during performance of a task that already requires high muscle forces [85]. Finally, adaptation to increased loading is much faster in muscle tissue than in the intervertebral disk and in the vertebrae, which might cause an increased injury risk in a period during which physical demands are rapidly increased as when starting in a physically demanding job [86].

12.5.2.1 Intervertebral Disk and Endplates

In the 1950s and 1960s, when protrusion of the intervertebral disk was seen as a major cause of LBP, many researchers started to investigate the mechanisms that could lead to a disk protrusion. Various authors performed mechanical tests on so-called motion segments, two vertebrae with all the connecting soft tissues. Testing was initially done in compression. It was found that compression forces in between 2,000 and 10,000 N cause fractures of the endplates and underlying bone, but do not cause disk protrusion [87–91]. Repeated submaximal compression caused similar damage as supramaximal loading [92,93]. There is no consensus in the literature on the effect of posture on the probability of endplate fractures. Whereas one study showed no effect of flexion on compressive strength in single loading cycles [94], a study on porcine spine segments did find an effect on the number of cycles to failure in repetitive loading [95]. In spite of the absence of protrusion, the type of damage induced by compression has been hypothesized to be an important cause of LBP [96]. Furthermore, it has been shown in animal studies that endplate injuries cause subsequent degeneration of the intervertebral disk [97].

Bending of the spine causes tensile force in the ligaments and lamellae of the intervertebral disks on the concave side. Extreme forward bending (hyperflexion) combined with high compression can cause a rupture of the posterior annulus fibrosus [98,99]. Repetitive submaximal bending combined with high compression forces can cause a similar type of injury [100,101] and the probability of injury appears to increase when the movement is asymmetric [100,102,103]. It should be noted that most motion segments tested in the studies cited here failed with an endplate fracture and only a minority showed annulus failure.

It has been assumed that torsion of the spine plays a role in the causation of tears in the intervertebral disk. Torsion causes shearing between lamellae of the annulus fibrosus as well as tensile forces in half of the lamellae. The shearing between lamellae could lead to concentric tears or clefts between the lamellae that are often seen with diskography [36,37]. Such concentric tears have been shown to cause disk degeneration in an animal model [104], but it is not sure whether these tears lead to pain directly. The tensile forces could lead to radial tears in the annulus that can also be visualized with diskography [36,37]. Farfan et al. [105] concluded that torsion could induce such tears when the torsion angle between two lumbar vertebrae exceeds 2°–3°. However, Adams and Hutton [106] have argued against this conclusion. In their experiments, damage to the facet joints occurred long before disk injury occurred. It is conceivable that the disparity between these studies arises in part from the axis of rotation that was imposed in the tests. A later study has shown damage to the annulus fibrosus after repeated torsion at only 1.5° [107]. Moreover, torsion was found to increase the probability of annulus fibrosus failure in repetitive flexion/extension cycles under compression [103]. In conclusion, the possibility that torsion contributes to injury of the intervertebral disk can certainly not be ruled out.

12.5.2.2 Facet Joints

The facet joints are compressed by anterior shear forces on the spine and one-sided compression occurs under torsion. It is conceivable that such joint compression could lead to damage to the articular cartilage, but this has not been sufficiently studied. In vitro tests on the strength of spinal motion segments mostly caused a bony failure [108–112] that is comparable to spondylolysis, which can be a specific, but not frequently occurring, cause of LBP [113,114]. It is however, possible that cartilage damage occurred prior to this bony failure, but this requires further research. Adams et al. [94] reported that motion segments compressed while in extension showed mechanical signs of damage at relatively low compression forces (approximately 500 N). It was not studied which structures were injured, but damage to facet joints appears plausible. Some authors have argued that osteoarthritis of the facet joints is secondary to disk degeneration [46,63] probably due to the fact that facet joints will carry more compression when the disk is degenerated [115,116].

12.5.2.3 Ligaments

The supraspinous and intraspinous ligaments can be ruptured due to extreme flexion of the spine [98]. In addition, animal experiments indicate that sustained submaximal flexion causes subfailure injuries to these ligaments that trigger inflammatory responses and muscular hyperexcitability and spasms [65].

12.5.3 MECHANISMS BEHIND RISK FACTORS

12.5.3.1 Mechanical Loading in Manual Lifting

As discussed above, manual lifting is one of the risk factors for LBP. During lifting the spine is exposed to high compression forces, high anterior shear forces, especially on the lower lumbar segments, and often undergoes considerable deformation in bending, sideward bending, and twisting. As mentioned above, compression as well as bending and torsion can be a cause of injury that may lead to LBP. The peak compression forces during a lifting movement have been estimated by means of biomechanical models to reach levels within the range in which endplate fractures can occur [117–119]. In contrast, spine bending angles in vivo appear to be well within the range of maximal flexion observed in vitro, suggesting that other (possibly muscular) tissue provides a margin of safety against excessive bending [120,121]. However, the bending angles found during lifting have been implicated to reduce the fatigue strength in compression as described above [95] and repetitive lifting has also been suggested to potentially cause failure of the annulus fibrosus [100,122,123]. In addition, bending as often occurs in lifting, may cause substantial stresses in the supraspinous and intraspinous ligaments [124], which may lead to subfailure injury as described above. Epidemiologic studies have associated heavy lifting in general with disk degeneration [125], and bending and twisting during lifting to disk protrusion [126].

12.5.3.2 Mechanical Loading in Awkward Trunk Postures

Unfortunately, it is in most cases impossible to directly relate the risk factor awkward trunk posture as defined in epidemiologic studies to mechanical loading, due to uncertainty about definitions or incomplete operationalization. In general, posture can be defined as the orientation of body segments in space and in relation to each other. This definition assumes body segments to be rigid links, whose orientation with respect to a neighboring segment is determined by rotations about three axes in one joint. With respect to the trunk, this assumption is clearly not correct. Reflecting the fact that the motions causing this orientation are in reality not pure rotations, they are called forward/backward bending, lateral bending, and twisting in accordance with ISO 11226 [127]. This terminology is also used in most epidemiologic studies. However, the effects of a trunk posture are not only determined by the angles between segments, but also by the orientation of the trunk with respect to the gravitational field. The angles with respect to the gravitational axis system will be referred to as forward inclination and sideward inclination. The third degree of freedom in the gravitational system is irrelevant in terms of the effects of posture on an individual. However, when rotating the trunk around a vertical axis while standing and keeping the feet fixed, individuals do also rotate the pelvis in the hip joints. Therefore, the overall rotation of the trunk is not equal to twisting. Most epidemiologic papers on trunk posture lack a clear description of the definition of posture used. For example, it can be unclear whether trunk bending refers to pure bending, to inclination, or to both, or whether twisting angles include pelvis rotation or not. Moreover, the above definitions can be unambiguously used only for postures or movements in a primary plane or about a primary axis.

For an extensive review on the effects of trunk posture on trunk loading we refer to Ref. [128]. Here we will focus on trunk bending and twisting, which have been associated with LBP, as described above. Assuming that trunk bending in most cases coincides with trunk inclination, this association can partially be understood by the fact that to maintain a forward inclined posture substantial trunk extensor muscle force is required. This will cause substantial compression forces on the spine. A recent study estimated that bending over to ground level even without any lifting could entail compression forces as high as 3.5 kN [129]. Hence in particular frequent bending may be a cause of endplate fractures.

In contrast, the magnitude of the mechanical loads on the spine due to the maintenance of sustained postures is generally limited such that these tissue loads will not directly cause injury. However, it is conceivable that the time-dependent deformation (creep) of tissues in repetitive or sustained exposure causes subfailure injury. Cyclic and static flexion cause creep of facet joint capsules and ligaments [130,131]. Such creep has also been found to occur after prolonged sitting in a flexed posture [132] and has been shown to cause alterations in muscle activity that appeared comparable to those coinciding with subfailure injuries in animal experiments as described above [133,134]. Ligament creep in addition will decrease spine stiffness and may affect sensory feedback [65]. These two factors combined can cause a decreased stability of the spine and might predispose the spine to injury.

Fatigue development in trunk muscles is substantially faster with any forward inclination [135,136]. In addition, trunk exertions in a twisted posture result in more rapid development of muscle fatigue than exertions in neutral postures [137]. Thus, muscle forces required to maintain nonneutral trunk postures can cause or accelerate fatigue development, which may reduce control over spine posture and movement and thus cause instability.

12.5.3.3 Mechanical Loading and Whole-Body Vibration

Exposure to whole-body vibration causes cyclic bending and compression of the lumbar spine [138]. Sandover [139] hypothesized that these cyclic loading modes could cause damage to the annulus fibrosus and endplate, respectively. Later model studies to estimate the magnitude of the compression forces induced by whole-body vibration partially support this assumption and showed that the magnitude of the forces on the spine is proportional to the acceleration levels and strongly depends on the frequency of the exposure, with the highest forces occurring for whole-body vibration at frequencies around 4–5 Hz [140,141]. Both types of failure could underpin the relationship between disk degeneration shown on x-ray and exposure to whole-body vibration [125].

In addition, to these direct effects whole-body vibration may negatively affect spinal stability through an increase in trunk muscle activity [142,143], which might accelerate fatigue development and through adverse effects on proprioceptive feedback [144] and spinal reflexes [145] and as such indirectly contribute to spinal injury. However, effects of whole-body vibration on muscle activity have been debated [146] and the frequency of vibrations that most affect proprioceptive feedback is higher than the frequency of vibrations typically associated with LBP.

12.5.3.4   Mechanical Loading and Psychosocial Factors

Psychosocial factors can interact with the physical risk factors. Obviously, time pressure can cause an increase in the volume of work performed and hence increase intensity, frequency, and duration of mechanical loads on the back. In addition, several studies of Marras and coworkers [147–149] have shown that psychosocial stressors can slightly increase mechanical back load in tasks such as lifting due to an overall increase in muscle activity. Alternative pathways are that work-related psychosocial factors may trigger (sustained) stress reactions, which on its turn may cause physiological responses that contribute to LBP. Furthermore, these stress reactions may cause a different appraisal of the mechanical load, which may contribute to an increased risk of LBP as well [150].

12.6   BIOMECHANICAL EFFICACY OF PREVENTIVE MEASURES

In the preceding sections, it was argued that tissue damage is a possible cause of cases of aspecific LBP and potential injury mechanisms were described. Compression forces and tissues stresses in bending and twisting were identified as potential mechanisms underpinning the risk factors for LBP. The efficacy of interventions aimed at reducing the risk of LBP can thus be assessed by measuring or estimating these mechanical parameters and quantitative predictions of the efficacy of interventions can be made. The value of this approach is supported by a review of intervention studies that showed that health effects were partially predictable from changes in mechanical exposure [151]. Net moments around the lumbar spine provide a good indicator of compression forces as well as of the required muscle force, which determines fatigue development [119]. The net moment is therefore used below as an additional indicator of back load. In addition to these mechanical parameters, we will more qualitatively discuss effects with respect to factors such as muscle fatigue that may influence spine stability. Finally, the probability of injury is always determined by the difference between the mechanical load and the capacity to bear this load. Therefore, the final section will deal with determinants of capacity that could be targeted in interventions.

12.6.1   Determinants of Low Back Load in Manual Lifting

As described above, manual lifting could lead to clinically relevant injuries due to the high compression forces it causes and due to the high bending stresses, occurring when lifting coincides with substantial trunk flexion. Twisting of the trunk during lifting can further increase the probability of injury. The efficacy of different interventions aimed at reducing the risk of LBP can thus be assessed by measuring effects on these parameters.

An extensive literature on back load during lifting in terms of peak net moments and compression forces and trunk bending and twisting angles exists, in which the following potential determinants have been studied:

1. The vertical position of the hands at the initiation of the lift
2. The horizontal distance between the low back and the hands at the initiation of the lift
3. The mass of the object
4. The velocity of lifting
5. Asymmetry of lifting
6. Lifting style or technique
7. Wearing a lumbar support
8. Tilting the object before lifting
9. One-handed versus two-handed lifting
10. Team lifting
11. Number of lifts (fatigue effects)

In the following, each of these determinants will be discussed separately. Wherever possible, a quantitative estimate of the effect of each of the determinants will be provided such that the efficacy of different intervention measures can be gauged. These quantitative estimates are mostly based on a recent comprehensive literature review [152]. To be able to compare all results between determinants, effect size will be expressed relative to a reference task, for which we will assume a peak net moment of 200 Nm. Other effects on other parameters such as spine bending and twisting as well as fatigue development will be discussed more qualitatively.

The vertical position of the hands at the initiation of the lift determines the peak net moment because the peak moment occurs shortly after the initiation of the lift. It does determine back load because it determines the amount of trunk inclination, which, given the high mass of the trunk, has a major effect on the net moment that has to be produced by the trunk muscles. The effect across different studies can be summarized based on regression as −261 Nm or −143% per meter difference in vertical position [152]. To illustrate the meaning of this figure, consider the following example. Suppose that the vertical hand position at lift initiation can be increased from 0 to 0.5 m, for example, by making handles in a (approximately 0.5 m high) box that has to be lifted from the floor. The regression coefficient of −260 then implies that a 130 Nm decrease in net moment can be achieved, which roughly corresponds to a decrease in compression force of 17 × 130 = 2210 N [119]. Considering that the maximum compression strength of lumbar spine segments is more or less normally distributed with a range of 2,000–10,000 N [90], this effect is very substantial. Obviously reducing the vertical position will also reduce trunk bending and hence reduce the loads on the annulus fibrosus and spinal ligaments, but these effects have not been quantified as yet. In conclusion, vertical position has a major influence on back load in lifting.

The horizontal distance between the low back and the hands at the initiation of the lift determines the moment arm that the load has with respect to the low back and often also has an effect on trunk inclination, as the trunk is inclined to reach forward. The effect across different studies can be summarized based on regression as 160 Nm or 80% per meter difference in horizontal distance [152]. Since large horizontal distances can require trunk bending to reach the load to be lifted, reductions of this distance will reduce trunk bending as was described for the vertical position. The effect on bending of the spine has not been studied extensively, but a study by Dolan et al. [121] suggests an effect of 84% per meter distance. However, Gill et al. [153] who measured bending of the lower lumbar spine instead of the whole lumbar spine found no effect of horizontal distance in lifting low-lying loads [153]. In conclusion, horizontal distance has a substantial effect on back load especially when considering net moments and compression forces.

The mass of the object to be lifted has a limited effect on net moments produced by the trunk muscles of 5 Nm or 2.5% per kg [152]. The effect on bending of the spine has not been studied extensively, but a study by Dolan et al. [121] suggests an effect of 1.5% per kg object mass. This implies that substantial decreases in load mass are required to obtain relevant reductions in back load. In addition, when load masses are reduced often proportionally more lifts need to be performed to maintain productivity [154] and as stated above repetitive loading on the spine increases the risk of injury.

The effects of movement velocity on back loads across various trunk extension exertions were reviewed by Davis and Marras [118]. They concluded that a monotonic and substantial increase with velocity occurs. However, the limited control over velocities in the studies reviewed and the wide range of tasks included precluded precise quantitative estimation of the effects on net moments and compression forces. Faber et al. [152] concluded that slower and faster lifting than normal (self-selected) decreases back load by about 5% and increases it by about 10%, respectively.

The effects of asymmetry have been less well studied up to date. Most studies on asymmetry have focused on lifting loads that are placed outside the sagittal plane. To lift the object, subjects in this kind of lifting tasks use a combination of pelvis rotation and trunk bending, lateral bending, and twisting to bring the hands to the object [155]. It was found that asymmetric lifting up to 60° of asymmetry causes net moments to be more asymmetric, but total net moments were not affected [155]. However, another study estimated 9%, 13%, and 24% increases in spinal compression relative to symmetric lifting for asymmetries of 30°, 60°, and 90° [156]. Although higher compression forces can occur at equal net moments due to cocontraction, these results are apparently contradictive and further study is needed. Trunk muscles appeared to fatigue at a higher rate when lifting asymmetrically (at 90°) than when lifting symmetrically [157]. Finally, twisting of the spine itself has been implicated as a source of spinal injuries as discussed above and although quantitative estimates of the effect are still uncertain, it seems that twisting during lifting is best avoided.

Lifting style or lifting technique has been the topic of a large number of studies, which usually compared stoop (knees extended, trunk bent) and squat (knees bent, trunk extended) lifting. In practice, squat lifting is often advised, while self-selected techniques are usually in between stoop and squat lifting [158]. A comprehensive review of the literature comparing back load in stoop and squat lifting appeared in 1999 [117]. It was concluded that only limited differences (less than 10%) between back load in stoop and squat lifting exist and when differences were found these were often opposite to the expected effects, i.e., low back load was lower in stoop lifting. In terms of low back load, self-selected lifting techniques appear intermediate between stoop and squat, therefore effects relative to self-selected lifting are even smaller. Moreover, Gill et al. [153] recently showed that bending in the lower lumbar spine was not different between the stoop and squat styles when lifting low-lying objects. Other recent studies showed that lifting style interacts with, for example, the vertical position of the load, such that no single advice can be given [159,160]. These findings combined suggest that the effect of lifting style defined as squat or stoop lifting on back load can be considered negligible. For a novel and promising approach toward interventions aimed at lifting style, see Ref. [161].

Wearing lumbar supports or back belts has been advocated as a means to reduce low back load during lifting. The assumed mechanisms are that the support would lower required trunk muscle forces by creating an extension moment or by increasing abdominal pressure and that the belt would restrict the amount of bending and twisting occurring. A systematic review, published in 2000, revealed significant effects on range of motion in forward bending and twisting of rigid supports, whereas elastic supports did not have a significant effect on twisting range of motion. No effects were found on intra-abdominal pressure and trunk muscle activity [162]. The variability of the effects between and within studies was large, with some subjects showing effects opposite of the expected effects. The increased trunk stiffness provided by a lumbar support not only restricts the range of trunk motion, but may also help to prevent spinal instability [163,164]. Some recent studies confirmed the effect on range of motion in lifting [165,166]. Furthermore, a recent study, in which a very stiff support (as used by competitive weight lifters) was used, reported a 10% decrease in compression forces on the spine [167]. The fact that this type of belt is quite uncomfortable to wear and that effect was found only when combining the use of the support with a special breathing technique suggests that this cannot be transferred to working situations. In conclusion, the effect of lumbar supports appears to be limited to restricting the range of motion (whether due to perturbations or not) and the intervention does not have the desired effect in all subjects.

Two studies from the same group indicated that tilting an object before actually lifting it can reduce back load by 9%–17% [168,169]. The effects on back load of one-handed versus two-handed lifting have been reported in two studies. Marras and Davis [156] reported that spinal compression was 5% lower in one-handed lifting, when the object was placed in the midsagittal plane, and this effect increased to 21%, when lifting was 60° asymmetric. Kingma and Dieën [170] compared one-handed and two-handed lifting in lifting over an obstacle and found a decrease in net moments by 10% and of compression forces by 18% for one-handed lifting. The reduction in both parameters was as high as 37% when the upper body was supported with the free hand.

Team lifting, i.e., lifting an object with two people instead of single-handedly, has been studied only in a limited number of studies. Therefore only preliminary conclusions with respect to efficacy can be drawn. Dennis and Barret [171] reported a 20% reduction in peak net moment when lifting an object together instead of single-handedly. In a follow-up study, they reported that differences in standing height between team members did not negatively affect peak loads [172]. Marras et al. [173] reported approximately 15% lower peak compression in team lifting for symmetric lifts, but no effect in asymmetric lifts.

The effect of the number of lifts (frequency times duration) performed on the probability of injury cannot be evaluated in the same way as the previous factors that all affect load magnitude. However, alternative models have been developed based on studies on repetitive compression until endplate failure [174]. These models predict that the probability of injury increases substantially, if the number of lifts increases from 1 up to 10 and no substantial recovery period in between lifts is allowed. However, the effect of an increase in number of lifts quickly levels off beyond 10 lifts and, in general, effects of the magnitude of the compressive force outweigh the effect of the number of lifts. Repetitive bending also increases the probability of damaging the annulus fibrosus or ligaments (see above) and depending on the degree of bending in a particular task, the number of lifts will thus codetermine the probability of these types of injury. Quantitative predictions of these effects are at present not feasible. Repetitive lifting can in addition cause considerable muscle fatigue, which as discussed, constitutes a risk in itself. Furthermore, with the development of fatigue, back loading increases due to a gradual increase in trunk bending and thus stresses in ligaments and annulus fibrosus [123,175], which moreover coincides with an increase in compression on the spine [176]. Fatigue development was found to be faster for lifting lighter objects with a high frequency (approximately 13 kg at 6 lifts per minute) than heavier objects at a low frequency (approximately 26 kg at 3 lifts per minute) [157]. The multiple effects of the number of lifts on back load suggest that reducing the number of lifts may have substantial efficacy.

In the preceding sections, the potential determinants of back load were discussed consecutively. Each of these determinants could be seen as a target for intervention. Addressing the determinants with the largest effects on back load can be expected to yield interventions with the highest efficacy. Obviously, the design of interventions is more complex. For example, it was shown that providing beds with adjustable work height does not lead to a reduced back load in nurses handling a patient in bed [177], probably due to the fact the height adjustments were not used correctly [178]. For many ergonomic interventions also, a change in behavior is needed, which is difficult to establish. This might explain some of the negative findings described in Section 12.7. For lifting specifically, it has been shown that the determinants of back load interact [152]. For example, at low vertical positions, horizontal distance may not have an effect on back load [179]. In addition, with changes in one determinant, behavioral changes may occur that affect other determinants and can amplify or attenuate the expected effects [179,180].

12.6.2 Determinants of Low Back Load in Awkward Trunk Postures

Trunk postures are determined by workplace layout. The position that the hands need to be in to perform a task and the position that the eyes need to be in to control task performance in relation to the standing or sitting position of the worker are the main determinants of trunk posture. However, also individual habits play an important role and most workplace layouts allow a wide variety of postures. Therefore, efficacy will be discussed here in terms of the magnitude of the effects of change in posture itself rather than in terms of determinants of posture. For a more detailed background of the findings described, the reader is referred to Ref. [128].

Forward inclination of the trunk often coincides with bending and vice versa, but not necessarily so. The effect of inclination on back load is sinusoidal. Back load is minimal in upright stance and increases to a maximum at 90° inclination. An important implication of this relationship is that the effect of a change in posture from say 20° inclination to 10° is much bigger than the effect of a change from 90° to 80°. For the effects of a change in bending angle on stresses in ligaments and annulus fibrosus, the opposite is true, due to the exponential relationship of tissue stress with bending angle, a change from 90° to 80° has a much larger effect than a change from 20° to 10°.

For sideward inclination and bending, a similar line of reasoning holds as for forward inclination, except that the range of sideward inclination is low because of which the relationship between inclination angle and mechanical load can be approximated as linear.

Twisting does not increase the load on the back due to gravity and therefore back load is determined only by the exponential relationship between the twisting angle and tissue stresses.

Comparing motions in the three planes, the compression forces during maximal forward inclination (and bending) are much higher than in maximal sideward inclination (and bending) and maximal twisting.

Mechanical loads due to awkward trunk postures can only cause adverse effects after sustained exposure; the load magnitudes in themselves are not high enough to immediately cause tissue damage. Therefore limiting the duration of exposure can have a high efficacy. However, in vitro and animal studies indicate that substantial rest periods (outlasting the loading period) may be required to recover from sustained loading of ligaments and annulus fibrosus [65,130]. Finally, it is important to note that the mechanical load imposed by posture can strongly interact with the exertion of external forces, as in manual lifting or pushing and pulling.

12.6.3   DETERMINANTS OF LOW BACK LOAD DUE TO WHOLE-BODY VIBRATION

The models that have been proposed to predict tissue damage due to whole-body vibration comprise two terms: the magnitude of the cyclic load imposed by the vibrations and the number of cycles [139]. For the number of cycles with regard to repetitive lifting, a logarithmic relationship was proposed, which implies that limiting the duration of exposure to whole-body vibration has only limited effects above a certain threshold. Thus, large reductions in exposure duration would generally be needed to attain a substantial effect. The magnitude of the cyclic load that is caused by vibration depends on the intensity of the vibrations as well as their characteristic frequency. Due to the resonance properties of the human body, vibrations around 4–5 Hz have a much more potent effect than vibrations with either a higher or lower frequency. Therefore, suspension systems, such as used in most modern cars, that reduce the frequency content of the vibration exposure of the driver to frequencies around 1.5 Hz are highly effective. For a seated operator, changing the frequency of the vibrations from 4 to 1 Hz would cause 60% reduction in the compression forces on the spine [141].

12.6.4 INDIVIDUAL CAPACITY

The load-bearing capacity of spinal tissues can be evaluated in vivo for compressional loading only. The compression strength of the spine is more or less linearly dependent on the product of the cross-sectional area of the vertebrae and their bone mineral density [89–91] and thus depends on age and gender. This product, also known as bone mineral content (BMC), can be determined using dual energy x-ray absorption (DEXA). Theoretically, this could be used to select workers with strong spines for physically exerting jobs in preemployment screening. However, x-ray exposure involves an obvious ethical problem. Moreover, the residual variance of the relationship between BMC and strength is such that prediction of spine strength at the individual level is insufficiently reliable. In general, it can be said that the lack of reliable predictors of the individual probability of developing LBP precludes selection through preemployment screening as a cost-effective intervention [181].

Given the fact that stability of the spine requires adequate control over and function of muscles, it is conceivable that training of muscle coordination, strength, and endurance all have their place in the prevention of LBP. From the perspective of tissue loading and injury, a word of caution should be given. Some strength training exercises cause very high spine loads [182]. In addition, adaptation of different tissues to training occurs at different rates. It is conceivable that a fast increase in muscle strength occurs, while, for example, BMC increases only slowly [183]. This may put the spine at an increased risk of compression injury [184].

12.7 EFFECTIVENESS OF PRIMARY PREVENTIVE MEASURES

In this section, we will give an overview of the evidence that can be found in the epidemiologic literature with regard to the effectiveness of interventions aiming at primary prevention of LBP. We will group the evidence according to the three intervention categories described in Section 12.3: (1) organizational ergonomics interventions, (2) physical ergonomics interventions, and (3) individual worker interventions.

This overview will mainly be based on systematic reviews of intervention studies. Apart from that, we will specifically make use of the recently published European guidelines for prevention of low back pain [185], since in this guideline-specific recommendations were given for workers based on all available systematic reviews and existing evidence-based guidelines.

12.7.1 ORGANIZATIONAL ERGONOMICS INTERVENTIONS

None of the interventions in the review by Westgaard and Winkel [186] covered "work organization" as main dimension, even though it is a component of many ergonomic intervention studies. Organizational ergonomics interventions were separately studied in the systematic review by Lotters and Burdof [151], but none of the four included studies evaluating this type of intervention focused on LBP. The conclusion of the European guidelines for prevention in LBP [185] was that there is inconsistent evidence that work organization interventions are successful for reduction of LBP. This conclusion is based on two studies: one positive study with a low methodological quality on the implementation of lift teams in hospitals [187] and one negative study with moderately high methodological quality on a reduction of daily working hours [188].

In the literature, positive statements can be found in favor of the formation of work groups. This means that work is changed from an extreme division of tasks and subtasks among workers according to Taylorism to a situation in which a small team of workers is responsible for a larger part of the production. It is considered that the resulting job enlargement is beneficial for workers from a psychosocial point of view, and that in most cases, harmful mechanical exposures are reduced as well.

For organizational measures, such as job rotation, a simple modeling approach shows that exposure to physical workload can be considerably reduced. However, a recent narrative review of the epidemiologic literature pointed out that the effectiveness of job rotation or more breaks is weakly supported by empirical evidence [189]. For instance, job rotation was found to be associated with an increased risk of LBP in a study in which two garbage collectors were rotating with the driver of the garbage truck [190].

Little information is available on the effectiveness of administrative interventions aimed at primary prevention performed by occupational health services. For instance, for periodic health examinations the question of whether this has any preventive result remains unanswered. More studies have been performed on preemployment selection and preplacement screening. The difference between these two activities is that the former might give reason for the employer to relinquish the offer of employment, while the latter occurs after an offer of employment has been given and certainly bares no selection element in it. Both preemployment selection and preplacement screening should be able to predict future work absenteeism and work disability, but research conducted on this topic has generally failed to show positive results. First, the interrater reliability is poor to moderate in these medical preplacement tests, which may result in severe bias in the final outcome of the selection or screening procedure [191,192]. Second and probably more important, the predictive validity of these outcomes is not sufficiently investigated and the few studies conducted on this particular aspect could not report encouraging conclusions at all [181,192]. As a result of general human rights legislation, as well as the serious indications regarding the poor predictive power of preemployment selection [191], this type of medical selection is not allowed in many industrialized countries. It can generally be concluded that the efficacy of preemployment selection or employee restriction is low for most job categories if the only goal is a reduction in LBP. Preemployment selection is probably only advantageous for the jobs with specific work demands, such as firefighters or aircraft pilots. In other words, fitting the worker to the job by selection of persons for their strength or ability to perform certain tasks is not legitimate except for specific jobs.

12.7.2 Physical Ergonomics Interventions

Primary prevention through workplace intervention is the most important playground of ergonomics/human factors, as it is the ultimate example of "fitting the job to the worker." The workplace should be (re)designed such that the risk of occurrence of LBP is minimized. A large number of ergonomic studies have been performed on workplace interventions. By far the most of these workplace interventions aim at the optimization of mechanical workload on (parts of) the worker's low back to thereby reduce the risk of LBP [151]. It is postulated that exposure to mechanical load is one of the most important risk factors for the occurrence of LBP, but it is rarely evaluated whether or not a decreased mechanical load indeed resulted in effects on LBP. In other words, in many studies, it was shown that a relatively simple ergonomic intervention, such as redesign of the workstation, established a decrease in exposure to risk factors. Unfortunately, however, the use of outcome measures regarding LBP has been sparse.

There are three systematic reviews on this topic. However, partly due to differences in the search strategy, inclusion criteria, and exclusion criteria, these systematic reviews had different conclusions. Westgaard and Winkel [186] found a general lack of success from mechanical exposure interventions, Linton and van Tulder [193] offered a negative conclusion about the primary preventive role of ergonomic interventions, while Lotters and Burdof [151] were somewhat more optimistic, although they did not draw firm conclusions. One subsequent good quality study [194] reported that physical ergonomics interventions might reduce the prevalence of LBP, whereas another subsequent good quality study did not report an improvement following changes intended to reduce exposure to physical risk factors [195]. There are indications that physical ergonomic interventions that include an organizational dimension, actively involving the workers and leading to substantial changes in exposure to the risk factors, might (in principle) be the most effective [196].

In conclusion, there is contradictory evidence from three systematic reviews [151,186,193] for physical ergonomics interventions in the primary prevention of LBP.

12.7.3 INDIVIDUAL WORKER INTERVENTIONS

Preventive programs aiming at individual, healthy workers most often consist of either (1) physical exercise to improve strength and/or working capacity, (2) advice, instruction, or education to give information about LBP or to improve work methods, such as lifting technique, or (3) lumbar supports or back belts. Of course, employers introduce combinations of these three programs in industry as well. However, the three programs will be separately discussed in this section.

First, physical exercise to improve muscle strength and/or working capacity of employees is often recommended to prevent LBP, since LBP might be caused by an imbalance in physical load and capacity. Seven systematic reviews indeed concluded that there is a preventive effect of physical exercise [193,197–202]. In one review [203], the authors concluded that there was contradictory evidence of effect of physical exercise on the prevention of LBP. In the two most recent reviews of the literature, it was concluded that there is limited evidence for the effectiveness of physical exercise as primary preventive approach [201,202]. Most beneficial results can be expected from specific exercises aiming at an increase of back muscle strength and endurance, but it might be advantageous to involve abdominal muscles in the exercises as well. It should be stressed, however, that relative strength, i.e., the ratio of task demands and worker capacity, is probably more important from a preventive point of view than absolute strength [32].

Second, educational programs and/or back schools are increasingly implemented in the industry to prevent LBP. The providers of these programs claim that their approach is capable of causing a decrease in LBP rates of up to 30%. In spite of extensive research efforts, however, the empirical proof of these claims has not been published so far. To the contrary, by far the majority of systematic reviews showed no beneficial effects of advice, instruction, or education in the prevention of LBP. In seven different systematic reviews and one review of occupational health guidelines, randomized controlled trials on educational interventions have been evaluated. One rather old review concluded that there was a modest relation between training of employees and a decrease in the occurrence of LBP [198]. However, seven reviews, including two recent ones, concluded that there is no effect of advice, instruction, or education for preventing LBP [193,197,199,200,202,203]. It should be noted that the educational programs vary widely in type and intensity, so that it is difficult to draw one solid conclusion for all of them. Furthermore, most programs also involve some kind of training. This training is mostly focused on working posture and/or lifting technique. A squat lift was considered to be a safe way of lifting as opposed to a stoop lift, but this has recently been debated in the literature (see Section 12.6.1). However, the most important drawback of this preventive approach is that a long-lasting change in behavior of people is extremely difficult to achieve, whether it is working posture or lifting technique. Possibly partly as a result of this, hardly any study was able to report positive effects on the occurrence of LBP.

Third, based on the consistently negative results of several high-quality studies there is no evidence for the effect of wearing a lumbar support or back belt to prevent LBP. Eight reviews evaluated the use of lumbar supports or back belts. Two early reviews concluded that there is insufficient evidence of the efficacy of lumbar supports [197,199]; three reviews concluded that there was strong evidence that lumbar support is not effective for the prevention of LBP [193,200,203]; one review concluded that there is moderate evidence that lumbar supports do not prevent LBP [204], and two recent others concluded that there is no evidence of effect of back belt for prevention of LBP [201,202]. Hence, all reviews basically report that lumbar supports or back belts are not effective for primary prevention of LBP. This is of great importance, because, particularly in the United States, many workers use a lumbar support and still are convinced that its primary preventive value is high.

In conclusion, primary prevention of LBP aiming at the individual worker is not effective except for physical exercises specific for back and abdominal muscles. However, it should be noted that the evidence for secondary and tertiary prevention of LBP is much more positive.

12.8   CONCLUSIONS

It is clear that a large gap exists between the literature on risk factors for LBP and effectiveness of interventions on one hand, and the literature on mechanisms behind LBP and efficacy of measures to intervene on these mechanisms on the other hand. In part, this is due to the fact that detailed measurements used in experimental studies on low back load and LBP cannot readily be applied in large-scale epidemiologic studies. This is regrettable as it may obscure the true relationships between exposure to certain physical factors and the incidence of LBP. For example, if in an epidemiologic study risk factors are measured at the level of activities, such as lifting and pushing/pulling, and a common factor in both activities causes LBP (e.g., a high compression force), then for none of these activities an association with LBP incidence may be found, because the compression forces are high in all groups compared. In other words, although external exposures differ, internal exposures can still be in the same order. However, we do not support the idea of only assessing internal exposure parameters, such as compression forces. To be of practical value, external exposure information is certainly needed at the level of activities or other determinants of physical exposure that can be recognized by the practitioner, which may be problematic for a parameter of internal exposure, such as compression force. Hence, we believe that it is important to relate these different levels of description of physical exposure to each other. Studies should be designed in which external exposures as well as internal exposures are assessed. This would not only increase our understanding of the origin of LBP, but also provide opportunities to design better interventions to achieve a reduction in physical exposure and ultimately reduce the incidence of LBP. For the time being, we believe that the knowledge on risk factors and on low back loading as summarized in this chapter may guide the design of preventive interventions. Effectiveness of such interventions of course remains to be shown. Again, it would be of great value if studies on effectiveness of interventions would also quantify effects on low back load, because this could be used to test such an approach [151].

The main targets for interventions to reduce LBP incidence would be manual lifting, awkward postures, and whole-body vibration. With respect to whole-body vibration, it should be mentioned that current design of cars, trucks, and other road vehicles has already reduced vibration exposure below levels at which LBP effects are expected. For the other two factors, the sections on efficacy provide some guidance. A wide range of interventions are generally possible to achieve the same reduction in exposure. For example, both workplace redesign and interventions aimed at individual behavior can have an effect on horizontal distances in manual lifting. When aiming for interventions with scientifically proven effectiveness, improvement of individual capacity should be addressed by means of physical exercises specific for back and abdominal muscles.

Although it seems plausible that targets for primary intervention should also be addressed in secondary and tertiary intervention, this does not mean that these should overlap completely. For example, it has been shown that prolonged sitting is not a risk factor for the incidence of LBP, but it is also known that prolonged sitting can provoke pain in patients with LBP [205]. Consequently, interventions aimed at sitting behavior or the duration of sitting may not be indicated in primary prevention of LBP, while the same interventions may have an important contribution to tertiary prevention of LBP.

REFERENCES

1. Andersson GBJ. Epidemiological features of chronic low-back pain. *The Lancet* 1999;354:581–585.
2. Biering-Sorensen F. A prospective study of low back pain in a general population. I: Occurrence, recurrence and aetiology. *Scandinavian Journal of Rehabilitation Medicine* 1983;15:71–79.

3. Riihimäki H. Back pain and heavy physical work: A comparative study of concrete reinforcement workers and maintenance house painters. *British Journal of Industrial Medicine* 1985;42:226–232.

4. Reisbord LS and Greenland S. Factors associated with self-reported back pain prevalence: A population based study. *Journal of Chronic Disease* 1985;38:691–702.

5. May C, Doyle H, and Chew-Graham C. Medical knowledge and the intractable patient: The case of chronic low back pain. *Social Science Medicine* 1999;48:523–534.

6. Nachemson A. Towards a better understanding of low back pain: A review of the mechanics of the lumbar disc. *Rheumatology and Rehabilitation* 1975;14:129–143.

7. Deyo RA. Low-back pain. *Science America* 1998;279:48–53.

8. Bigos SJ, Battie MC, Spengler DM, Fisher LD, Fordyce WE, Hansson T, Nachemson AL, and Zeh J. A longitudinal, prospective study of industrial back injury reporting. *Clinical Orthopedics and Related Research* 1992;279:21–34.

9. Volinn E, Spratt KF, Magnusson M, and Pope MH. The Boeing prospective study and beyond. *Spine* 2001;26:1613–1622.

10. Mannion AF, Dolan P, and Adams MA. Psychological questionnaires: Do "abnormal" scores precede or follow first-time low back pain? *Spine* 1996;21:2603–2611.

11. Hartvigsen J, Lings S, Leboeuf-Yde C, and Bakketeig L. Psychosocial factors at work in relation to low back pain and consequences of low back pain; a systematic, critical review of prospective cohort studies. *Occupational and Environmental Medicine* 2004;61:e2.

12. Barker ME. A classification of back pain in general practice. *Practitioner* 1987; 231:109–112.

13. Deyo RA, Rainville J, and Kent DL. What can the history and physical examination tell us about low back pain? *JAMA* 1992;268:760–765.

14. Waddell G. Low-back-pain—A 20th-century health-care enigma. *Spine* 1996; 21:2820–2825.

15. van den Hoogen JMM, Koes BW, Devillé W, van Eijk JTM, and Bouter LM. The prognosis of low back pain in general practice. *Spine* 1997;22:1515–1521.

16. Pengel LH, Herbert RD, Maher CG, and Refshauge KM. Acute low back pain: Systematic review of its prognosis. *BMJ* 2003;327:323.

17. Mason V. *The Prevalence of Back Pain in Great Britain*. London: Office of Population Censuses and Surveys, Social Survey Division (now Office of National Statistics) HSMO, 1994.

18. van Tulder MW, Koes BW, and Bouter LM. A cost-of-illness study of back pain in the Netherlands. *Pain* 1995;62:233–240.

19. Waddell G. *The Back Pain Revolutioned*. Edinburgh: Churchill-Livingstone, 1998.

20. OpdeBeeck R and Hermans V. *Research on Work-Related Low Back Disordered*. Luxembourg: Office for Official Publications of the European Communities, 2000.

21. Bernard BP. *Musculoskeletal Disorders and Workplace Factors. A Critical Review of Epidemiologic Evidence for Work-Related Musculoskeletal Disorders of the Neck, Upper Extremity, and Low Back*, 2nd edn. Cincinnati, OH: NIOSH, US Department of Health and Human Services, 1997.

22. Burdorf A and Sorock G. Positive and negative evidence of risk factors for back disorders. *Scandinavian Journal of Work, Environment and Health* 1997;23:243–256.

23. Hoogendoorn WE, van Poppel MNM, Bongers PM, Koes BW, and Bouter LM. Physical load during work and leisure time as risk factors for back pain. *Scandinavian Journal of Work, Environment and Health* 1999;25:387–403.

24. Kuiper J, Burdorf A, Verbeek JHAM, Frings-Dresen MHW, van der Beek AJ, and Viikari-Juntura ERA. Epidemiologic evidence on manual materials handling as a risk factor for back disorders: A systematic review. *International Journal of Industrial Ergonomics* 1999;24:389–404.

25. National Research Council and the Institute of Medicine. *Musculoskeletal Disorders and the Workplace: Low Back and Upper Extremities.* Washington, DC: National Academy Press, 2001.
26. Lotters F, Burdorf A, Kuiper J, and Miedema H. Model for the work-relatedness of low-back pain. *Scandinavian Journal of Work, Environment and Health* 2003;29:431–440.
27. Hartvigsen J, Leboeuf-Yde C, Lings S, and Corder EH. Is sitting-while-at-work associated with low back pain? A systematic, critical literature review. *Scandinavian Journal of Public Health* 2000;28:230–239.
28. Lis AM, Black KM, Korn H, and Nordin M. Association between sitting and occupational LBP. *European Spine Journal* 2006;16:283–298.
29. Hoogendoorn WE, van Poppel MNM, Bongers PM, Koes BW, and Bouter LM. Systematic review of psychosocial factors at work and private life as risk factors for back pain. *Spine* 2000;25:2114–2125.
30. Linton SJ. Occupational psychological factors increase the risk for back pain: A systematic review. *Journal of Occupation and Rehabilitation* 2001;11:53–66.
31. Frank JW, Kerr MS, Brooker AS, DeMaio SE, Maetzel A, Shannon HS, Sullivan TJ, Norman RW, and Wells RP. Disability resulting from low back pain. Part I: What do we know about primary prevention? A review of the scientific evidence on prevention before disability begins. *Spine* 1996;21:2908–2917.
32. Dempsey PG, Burdorf A, and Webster BS. The influence of personal variables on work-related low-back disorders and implications for future research. *Journal of Occupational and Environmental Medicine* 1997;39:748–759.
33. van Tulder M, Koes B, and Bombardier C. Low back pain. *Best Practice and Research Clinical Rheumatology* 2002;16:761–775.
34. Leboeuf-Yde C. Back pain—Individual and genetic factors. *Journal of Electromyography and Kinesiology* 2004;14:129–133.
35. van Tulder MW, Assendelft WJ, Koes BW, and Bouter LM. Spinal radiographic findings and nonspecific low back pain. A systematic review of observational studies. *Spine* 1997;22:427–434.
36. Vanharanta H, Sachs BL, Spivey MA, and Guyer RD. The relationship of pain provocation to lumbar disc deterioration as seen by CT/discography. *Spine* 1987;12:295–298.
37. Grubb SA, Lipscomb HJ, and Guilford WB. The relative value of lumbar roentgenogram, metrizamide, myelography and discogaphy in the assessment of patients with chronic low back syndrome. *Spine* 1987;12:282–286.
38. Walsh TR, Weinstein JN, Spratt KF, Lehmann TR, Aprill C, and Sayre H. Lumbar discography in normal subjects. A controlled prospective study. *Journal of Bone and Joint Surgery* 1990;72A:1081–1088.
39. Schwarzer AC, Aprill CN, Derby R, Fortin J, Kine G, and Bogduk N. The prevalence and clinical features of internal disc disruption in patients with chronic low back pain. *Spine* 1995;20:1878–1883.
40. Manchikanti L, Singh V, Pampati V, Damron KS, Barnhill RC, Beyer C, and Cash KA. Evaluation of the relative contributions of various structures in chronic low back pain. *Pain Physician* 2001;4:308–316.
41. Videman T, Nurminen M, and Troup JDG. Lumbar spinal pathology in cadaveric material in relation to history of back pain, occupation, and physical loading. *Spine* 1990;15:728–740.
42. Coventry MB, Ghormley RK, and Kernohan JW. The intervertebral disc: its microscopic anatomy and pathology. *Journal of Bone and Joint Surgery* 1945;27:460–474.
43. Hilton RC, Ball J, and Benn RT. Vertebral end-plate lesions (Schmorl's nodes) in the dorsolumbar spine. *Annals of the Rheumatic Diseases* 1976;35:127–132.
44. Vernon-Roberts B and Pirie C. Healing trabecular microfractures in the bodies of lumbar vertebrae. *Annals of the Rheumatology Diseases* 1973;32:406–412.

45. Vernon-Roberts B and Pirie CJ. Degenerative changes in the intervertebral discs of the lumbar spine and their sequelae. *Rheumatology and Rehabilitation* 1977;16:13–21.
46. Mullender M, Bonsen M, and van Dieën JH. Degeneration of the intervertebral disk is related to vertebral endplate fractures (abstract). *European Spine Journal* 2000;9:343.
47. Begg AC. Nuclear herniations of the intervertebral disc. *Journal of Bone and Joint Surgery—British Volume* 1954;36B:180–193.
48. Hansson T and Roos B. The relation between bone mineral content, experimental compression fractures and disc degeneration. *Spine* 1981;6:147–153.
49. Malmivaara A, Videman T, Kuosma E, and Troup JDG. Plain radiographic, discographic, direct observations of Schmorl's nodes in the thoracolumbar junctional region of the cadaveric spine. *Spine* 1987;12:453.
50. Takahashi K, Miyazaki T, Ohnari H, Takino T, and Tomita K. Schmorl's nodes and low-back pain. Analysis of magnetic resonance imaging findings in symptomatic and asymptomatic individuals. *European Spine Journal* 1995;4:56–59.
51. Yoganandan N, Larson SJ, Pintar FA, Gallageher M, Reinartz J, and Droese K. Intravertebral pressure changes caused by spinal microtrauma. *Neurosurgery* 1994;35:415–421.
52. Smith DM. Acute back pain associated with a calcified Schmorl's node. A case report. *Clinical Orthopaedics and Related Research* 1976;117:193–196.
53. McCall IW, Park WM, O'Brien JP, and Seal V. Acute traumatic intraosseous disc herniation. *Spine* 1985;10:134–137.
54. Hsu K, Zucherman JF, Dervy R, White AH, and Goldthwaite NGW. Painful lumbar end-plate disruptions: A significant discographic finding. *Spine* 1988;13:76–78.
55. Takahashi K and Takata K. A large painful Schmorl's node: A case report. *Journal of Spinal Disorders* 1994;7:77–81.
56. McNally DD, Shackleford IM, Goodship AE, and Mulholland RC. In vivo stress measurement can predict pain on discography. *Spine* 1996;21:2580–2587.
57. Lim CH, Jee WH, Son BC, Kim DH, Ha KY, and Park CK. Discogenic lumbar pain: Association with MR imaging and CT discography. *European Journal of Radiology* 2005;54:431–437.
58. Kuslich SD, Ulstrom CL, and Michael CJ. The tissue origin of low back pain and sciatica: A report of pain response to tissue stimulation during operations on the lumbar spine using local anesthesia. *Orthopaedic Clinics of North America* 1991;22:181–187.
59. Kuslich SD, Ahern JW, and Tarr DL. What tissues are responsible for low back pain and sciatica? Latest results of an ongoing investigation of tissue sensitivity in humans undergoing operations on the lumbar spine using local anesthesia. In Holm S, Pope M, and Szpalski M, eds. *The Lumbar Spine. A Basic Science Approach*. Brussels: International Society for the Study of the Lumbar Spine, 1994, p. 13.
60. Schwarzer AC, Wang SC, Bogduk N, McNaught PJ, and Laurent R. Prevalence and clinical features of lumbar zygapophysial joint pain: A study in an Australian population with chronic low back pain. *Annals of the Rheumatoid Diseases* 1995;54:100–106.
61. Schwarzer AC, Aprill CN, Derby R, Fortin J, Kine G, and Bogduk N. The relative contributions of the disc and zygapophyseal joint in chronic low-back-pain. *Spine* 1994;19:801–806.
62. Schwarzer AC, Aprill CN, Derby R, Fortin J, Kine G, and Bogduk N. Clinical-features of patients with pain stemming from the lumbar zygapophysial joints—Is the lumbar facet syndrome a clinical entity. *Spine* 1994;19:1132–1137.
63. Malmivaara A, Videman T, Kuosma E, and Troup JDG. Facet joint orientation, facet and costovertebral joint osteoarthrosis, disc degeneration, vertebral body osteophytosis, and Schmorl's nodes in the thoracolumbar junctional region of cadaveric spines. *Spine* 1987;12:458.
64. Taylor JR, Twomey LT, and Corker M. Bone and soft tissue injuries in post-mortem lumbar spines. *Paraplegia* 1990;28:119–129.

65. Solomonow M, Baratta RV, Zhou B-H, Burger E, Zieske A, and Gedalia A. Muscular dysfunction elicited by creep of lumbar viscoelastic tissues. *Journal of Electromyography and Kinesiology* 2003;13:381–396.
66. Panjabi MM. A hypothesis of chronic back pain: Ligament subfailure injuries lead to muscle control dysfunction. *European Spine Journal* 2006;15:668–676.
67. Rissanen PM. The surgical anatomy and pathology of the supraspinous and interspinous ligaments of the lumbar spine with special reference to ligament ruptures. *Acta Orthopaedica Scandinavica* 1960;Suppl. 46:1–100.
68. Bogduk N and Twomey LT. *Clinical Anatomy of the Lumbar Spine*, 1st edn. Melbourne: Churchill Livingstone, 1987.
69. Steindler A and Luck JV. Differential diagnosis of pain low in the back: Allocation of the source of pain by procain hydrocholride method. *Journal of the American Medical Association* 1938;110:106–112.
70. Wilk V. Pain arising from the intraspinous and supraspinous ligaments. *Australasian Musculoskeletal Medicine* 1995;1:21–31.
71. Panjabi MM. The stabilizing system of the spine. Part I. Function, dysfunction, adaptation, and enhancement. *Journal of Spinal Disorders* 1992;5:383–389; discussion 97.
72. Panjabi MM. The stabilizing system of the spine. Part II. Neutral zone and instability hypothesis. *Journal of Spinal Disorders* 1992;5:390–397.
73. Reeves NP, Narendra KS, and Cholewicki J. Spine stability: The six blind men and the elephant. *Clinical Biomechanics* 2007;22:266–274.
74. Posner I, White AA, Edwards WT, and Hayes WC. A biomechanical analysis of the clinical stability of the lumbar and lumbosacral spine. *Spine* 1982;7:374–389.
75. Kaigle AM, Holm SH, and Hansson TH. Experimental instability in the lumbar spine. *Spine* 1995;20:421–430.
76. Kaigle AM, Holm SH, and Hansson TH. Kinematic behavior of the porcine lumbar spine: A chronic lesion model. *Spine* 1997;22:2796–2806.
77. Fujiwara A, Lim TH, An HS, Tanaka N, Jeon CH, Andersson GB, and Haughton VM. The effect of disc degeneration and facet joint osteoarthritis on the segmental flexibility of the lumbar spine. *Spine* 2000;25:3036–3044.
78. White AA and Panjabi MM. *Clinical Biomechanics of the Spine*, 2nd edn. Philadelphia, PA: J.B. Lippincott Company, 1990.
79. Crisco JJ and Panjabi MM. Euler stability of the human ligamentous spine. Part II Experiment. *Clinical Biomechanics* 1992;7:27–32.
80. Johansson H, Arendt-Nielsen L, Bergenheim M, Djupsjöbacka M, Gold JE, Ljubisavljevic M, Mano T, Matre DA, Passatore M, Punnett L, Roatta S, van Dieën JH, and Windhorst U. Epilogue: An integrative model. In Johansson H, Windhorst U, Djupsjöbacka M, et al. eds. *Chronic Work-Related Myalgia. Neuromuscular Mechanisms Behind Work-Related Chronic Muscle Syndromes.* Gävle, Sweden: Gävle University Press, 2003, pp. 291–300.
81. Battie MC, Videman T, Gibbons LE, Fisher LD, Manninen H, and Gill K. Determinants of lumbar disc degeneration—A study relating lifetime exposures and magnetic-resonance-imaging findings in identical-twins. *Spine* 1995;20:2601–2612.
82. Norman R, Wells R, Neumann P, Frank J, Shannon H, and Kerr M. A comparison of peak vs cumulative physical work exposure risk factors for the reporting of low back pain in the automotive industry. *Clinical Biomechanics* 1998;13:561–573.
83. Porter RW, Adams MA, and Hutton WC. Physical activity and the strength of the lumbar spine. *Spine* 1989;14:201–203.
84. Granhed H, Jonson R, and Hansson T. The loads on the lumbar spine during extreme weight lifting. *Spine* 1987;12:146–149.
85. Oddsson LIE, Persson T, Cresswell AG, and Thorstensson A. Interaction between voluntary and postural motor commands during perturbed lifting. *Spine* 1999;24:545–552.

86. Adams MA, Freeman BJC, Morrison HP, Nelson IW, and Dolan P. Mechanical initiation of intervertebral disc degeneration. *Spine* 2000;25:1625–1636.

87. Brown T, Hansen RJ, and Yorra AJ. Some mechanical tests on the lumbo-sacral spine with particular reference to the intervertebral discs. *Journal of Bone and Joint Surgery* 1957;39A:1135–1164.

88. Perey O. Fracture of the vertebral endplate in the human spine. *Acta Orthopedica Scandinavica* 1957;Suppl. 25:1–101.

89. Bell GH, Dunbar O, Beck JS, and Gibb A. Variations in strength of vertebrae with age and their relation to osteoporosis. *Calcified Tissue Research* 1967;1:75–86.

90. Brinckmann P, Biggemann M, and Hilweg D. Prediction of the compressive strength of human lumbar vertebrae. *Spine* 1989;14:606–610.

91. Hansson TH, Roos B, and Nachemson A. The bone mineral content and ultimate compressive strength in lumbar vertebrae. *Spine* 1980;5:46–55.

92. Hansson TH, Keller TS, and Spengler DM. Mechanical behaviour of the human lumbar spine II. Fatigue strength during dynamic compressive loading. *Journal of Orthopaedic Research* 1987;5:479–487.

93. Brinckmann P, Biggemann M, and Hilweg D. Fatigue fracture of human lumbar vertebrae. *Clinical Biomechanics* 1988;Suppl. no.1:1–23.

94. Adams MA, McNally DS, Chinn H, and Dolan P. Posture and compressive strength of the lumbar spine. *Clinical Biomechanics* 1994;9:5–14.

95. Gunning JL, Callaghan JP, and McGill SM. Spinal posture and prior loading history modulate compressive strength and type of failure in the spine: A biomechanical study using a porcine cervical model. *Clinical Biomechanics* 2001;16:471–480.

96. van Dieën JH, Weinans H, and Toussaint HM. Fractures of the lumbar vertebral endplate in the etiology of low back pain. A hypothesis on the causative role of spinal compression in a-specific low back pain. *Medical Hypotheses* 1999;53:246–252.

97. Holm S, Holm AK, Ekstrom L, Karladani A, and Hansson T. Experimental disc degeneration due to endplate injury. *Journal of Spinal Disorders and Techniques* 2004;17:64–71.

98. Adams MA and Hutton WC. Prolapsed intervertebral disc: A hyperflexion injury. *Spine* 1982;7:184–191.

99. McNally DS, Adams MA, and Goodship AE. Can intervertebral disc prolapse be predicted by disc mechanics? *Spine* 1993;18:1525–1530.

100. Adams MA and Hutton WC. Gradual disc prolapse. *Spine* 1985;10:524–531.

101. Callaghan JP and McGill SM. Intervertebral disc herniation: Studies on a porcine model exposed to highly repetitive flexion/extension motion with compressive force. *Clinical Biomechanics (Bristol, Avon)* 2001;16:28–37.

102. Gordon SJ, Yang KH, Mayer PJ, Mace AH, Kish VL, and Radin EL. Mechanism of disc rupture: A preliminary report. *Spine* 1991;16:450–456.

103. Drake JD, Aultman CD, McGill SM, and Callaghan JP. The influence of static axial torque in combined loading on intervertebral joint failure mechanics using a porcine model. *Clinical Biomechanics (Bristol, Avon)* 2005;20:1038–1045.

104. Fazzalari NL, Costi JJ, Hearn TC, Fraser RD, Vernon-Roberts B, Hutchinson J, Manthey BA, and Parkinson IH. Mechanical and pathological consequences of induced concentric anular tears in an ovine model. *Spine* 2001;26:2572–2581.

105. Farfan HF, Cossette JW, Robertson GH, Wells RV, and Kraus H. The effect of torsion on the lumbar intervertebral joints: The role of torsion in the production of disc degeneration. *Journal of Bone and Joint Surgery* 1970;52-A:468–497.

106. Adams MA and Hutton WC. The relevance of torsion to the mechanical derangement of the lumbar spine. *Spine* 1981;6:241–248.

107. Liu YK, Goel VK, Dejong A, Njus G, Nishiyama K, and Buckwalter J. Torsional fatigue of the lumbar intervertebral joints. *Spine* 1985;10:894–900.

108. Cyron BM, Hutton WC, and Troup JDG. Spondylolytic fractures. *Journal of Bone and Joint Surgery—British Volume* 1976;58B:462–466.

109. Cyron BM and Hutton WC. The fatigue strength of the lumbar neural arch in spondylolysis. *Journal of Bone and Joint Surgery—British Volume* 1981;60B:234–238.
110. Lamy C, Bazergui A, Kraus H, and Farfan HF. The strength of the neural arch and the etiology of spondylolysis. *Orthopaedic Clinics of North America* 1975;6:215–231.
111. Yingling VR and McGill SM. Anterior shear of spinal motion segments—Kinematics, kinetics, and resultant injuries observed in a porcine model. *Spine* 1999;24: 1882–1889.
112. van Dieën JH, van der Veen A, van Royen BJ, and Kingma I. Fatigue failure in shear loading of porcine lumbar spine segments. *Spine* 2006;31:E494–E498.
113. Yano T, Miyagi S, and Ikari T. Studies of familial incidence of spondylolysis. *Singapore Medical Journal* 1967;8:203–206.
114. Jackson DW, Wiltse LL, and Cirincoine RJ. Spondylolysis in the female gymnast. *Clinical Orthopedics* 1976;117:68–73.
115. Pollintine P, Przybyla AS, Dolan P, and Adams MA. Neural arch load-bearing in old and degenerated spines. *Journal of Biomechanics* 2004;37:197–204.
116. Pollintine P, Dolan P, Tobias JH, and Adams MA. Intervertebral disc degeneration can lead to "stress-shielding" of the anterior vertebral body: A cause of osteoporotic vertebral fracture? *Spine* 2004;29:774–782.
117. van Dieën JH, Hoozemans MJM, and Toussaint HM. Stoop or squat: A review of biomechanical studies on lifting technique. *Clinical Biomechanics* 1999;14:685–696.
118. Davis KG and Marras WS. The effects of motion on trunk biomechanics. *Clinical Biomechanics* 2000;15:703–717.
119. van Dieën JHvan and Kingma I. Effects of antagonistic co-contraction on differences between electromyography based and optimization based estimates of spinal forces. *Ergonomics* 2005;48:411–426.
120. Adams MA and Hutton WC. Has the lumbar spine a margin of safety in forward bending? *Clinical Biomechanics* 1986;1:3–6.
121. Dolan P, Earley M, and Adams MA. Bending and compressive stresses acting on the lumbar spine during lifting activities. *Journal of Biomechanics* 1994;27:1237.
122. Green TP, Adams MA, and Dolan P. Tensile properties of the annulus fibrosus II. Ultimate tensile strength and fatigue life. *European Spine Journal* 1993;2:209–214.
123. Dolan P and Adams MA. Repetitive lifting tasks fatigue the back muscles and increase the bending moment acting on the lumbar spine. *Journal of Biomechanics* 1998;31:713–721.
124. Panjabi MM, Goel VK, and Takata K. Physiologic strains on the lumbar spinal ligaments. *Spine* 1982;7:192–203.
125. Brinckmann P, Frobin W, Biggermann M, Tillotson M, and Burton K. Quantification of overload injuries to thoracolumbar vertebrae and discs in persons exposed to heavy physical exertions or vibration at the workplace—Part II—Occurrence and magnitude of overload injury in exposed cohorts. *Clinical Biomechanics* 1998;13:S1–S36.
126. Kelsey JL, Githens PB, White AA, Holford TR, Walter SD, O'Connor T, Ostfeld AM, Weil U, Southwick WO, and Calogero JA. An epidemiological study of lifting and twisting on the job and risk for acute prolapsed lumbar intervertebral disc. *Journal of Orthopaedic Research* 1984;2:61–66.
127. ISO-11226. Ergonomics—Evaluation of static working postures, 1999.
128. van Dieën JH and Nussbaum MA. Trunk. In Delleman NJ, Haslegrave CM, and Chaffin DB, eds. *Working Postures and Movements: Tools for Evaluation and Engineering.* Boca Raton, FL: CRC Press, 2004, pp. 109–141.
129. Hoozemans MJM, Kingma I, de Vries WHK, and van Dieën JH. Effect of lifting height on low back loading. In Pikaar RN, Koningsveld EAP, and Settels P, eds. *XVIth Triennial Congress of the International Ergonomics Association.* Maastricht, the Netherlands: Elsevier, 2006.

130. Twomey LT and Taylor JF. Flexion creep deformation and hysteresis in the lumbar vertebral column. *Spine* 1982;7:116–122.

131. Little JS and Khalsa PS. Human lumbar spine creep during cyclic and static flexion: Creep rate, biomechanics, and facet joint capsule strain. *Annals of Biomedical Engineering* 2005;33:391–401.

132. McGill SM and Brown S. Creep response of the lumbar spine to prolonged full flexion. *Clinical Biomechanics* 1992;7:43–46.

133. Solomonow M, Baratta RV, Banks A, Freudenberger C, and Zhou BH. Flexion-relaxation response to static lumbar flexion in males and females. *Clinical Biomechanics (Bristol, Avon)* 2003;18:273–279.

134. Dickey JP, McNorton S, and Potvin JR. Repeated spinal flexion modulates the flexion-relaxation phenomenon. *Clinical Biomechanics (Bristol, Avon)* 2003;18:783–789.

135. Corlett EN and Manenica I. The effect and measurement of working postures. *Applied Ergonomics* 1980;11:7–16.

136. Boussenna M, Corlett EN, and Pheasant ST. The relation between discomfort and postural loading at the joints. *Ergonomics* 1982;25:315–322.

137. van Dieën JH. Asymmetry of erector spinae muscle-activity in twisted postures and consistency of muscle activation patterns across subjects. *Spine* 1996;21:2651–2661.

138. Dupuis H and Christ W. On the vibratory behavior of the stomach under the influence of sinusoidal and stochastic vibrations. *Interntationale Zeitschrift für Angewandte Physiologie* 1966;22:149–166.

139. Sandover J. Dynamic loading as a possible source of low-back disorders. *Spine* 1983;8:652–658.

140. Seidel H, Bluthner R, and Hinz B. Application of finite-element models to predict forces acting on the lumbar spine during whole-body vibration. *Clinical Biomechanics (Bristol, Avon)* 2001;16 Suppl. 1:S57–63.

141. Fritz M, Fischer S, and Brode P. Vibration induced low back disorders—Comparison of the vibration evaluation according to ISO 2631 with a force-related evaluation. *Applied Ergonomics* 2005;36:481–488.

142. Seidel H. Myoelectric reactions to ultra-low frequency and low-frequency whole body vibration. *European Journal of Applied Physiology and Occupational Physiology* 1988;57:558–562.

143. Seroussi RE, Wilder DG, and Pope MH. Trunk muscle electromyography and whole body vibration. *Journal of Biomechanics* 1989;22:219–229.

144. Brumagne S, Lysens R, Swinnen S, and Verschueren S. Effect of paraspinal muscle vibration on position sense of the lumbosacral spine. *Spine* 1999;24:1328–1331.

145. Martin BJ, Roll JP, and Gauthier GM. Spinal reflex alterations as a function of intensity and frequency of vibration applied to the feet of seated subjects. *Aviation Space Environmental Medicine* 1984;55:8–12.

146. de Oliveira CG, Simpson DM, and Nadal J. Lumbar back muscle activity of helicopter pilots and whole-body vibration. *Journal of Biomechanics* 2001;34:1309–1315.

147. Marras WS, Davis KG, Heaney CA, Maronitis AB, and Allread WG. The influence of psychosocial stress, gender, and personality on mechanical loading of the lumbar spine. *Spine* 2000;25:3045–3054.

148. Davis KG, Marras WS, Heaney CA, Waters TR, and Gupta P. The impact of mental processing and pacing on spine loading: 2002 Volvo Award in biomechanics. *Spine* 2002;27:2645–2653.

149. Davis KG and Marras WS. Partitioning the contributing role of biomechanical, psychosocial, and individual risk factors in the development of spine loads. *Spine Journal* 2003;3:331–338.

150. Bongers PM, Kremer AM, and ter Laak J. Are psychosocial factors, risk factors for symptoms and signs of the shoulder, elbow, or hand/wrist? A review of the epidemiomlogical literature. *American Journal of Industrial Medicine* 2002;41:315–342.

151. Lotters F and Burdof A. Are changes in mechanical exposure and musculoskeletal health good performance indicators for primary interventions? *International Archives of Occupational and Environmental Health* 2002;75:549–561.
152. Faber G, Kingma I, and van Dieën JH. Effects of ergonomic interventions on low back loading, a review of the literature. in preparation.
153. Gill KP, Bennett SJ, Savelsbergh GJ, and van Dieën JH. Regional changes in spine posture at lift onset with changes in lift distance and lift style. *Spine* 2007;32:1599–1604.
154. de Looze MP, Visser B, Houting I, van Rooy MAG, van Dieën JH, and Toussaint HM. Weight and frequency effects on spinal loading in a bricklaying task. *Journal of Biomechanics* 1996;29:1425–1433.
155. Kingma I, van Dieën JH, de Looze MP, Toussaint HM, Dolan P, and Baten CTM. Asymmetric low back loading in asymmetric lifting movements is not prevented by pelvic twist. *Journal of Biomechanics* 1998;31:527–534.
156. Marras WS and Davis KG. Spine loading during asymmetric lifting using one versus two hands. *Ergonomics* 1998;41:817–834.
157. Kim SH and Chung MK. Effects of posture, weight and frequency on trunk muscular activity and fatigue during repetitive lifting tasks. *Ergonomics* 1995;38:853–863.
158. Burgess-Limerick R, Abernathy B, and Neal RJ. Relative phase quantifies interjoint coordination. *Journal of Biomechanics* 1993;26:91–94.
159. Kingma I, Bosch T, Bruins L, and van Dieën JH. Foot positioning instruction, initial vertical load position and lifting technique: Effects on low back loading. *Ergonomics* 2004;47:1365–1385.
160. Kingma I, Faber GS, Bakker AJM, and van Dieën JH. Can low back loading during lifting be reduced by placing one leg beside the object to be lifted? *Physical Therapy* 2006;86:1091–1105.
161. Gagnon M. The efficacy of training for three manual handling strategies based on the observation of expert and novice workers. *Clinical Biomechanics (Bristol, Avon)* 2003;18:601–611.
162. van Poppel MNM, de Looze MP, Koes BW, Smid T, and Bouter LM. Mechanisms of action of lumbar supports. A systematic review. *Spine* 2000;25:2103–2113.
163. Cholewicki J, Juluru K, Radebold A, Panjabi MM, and McGill SM. Lumbar spine stability can be augmented with an abdominal belt and/or increased intra-abdominal pressure. *European Spine Journal* 1999;8:388–395.
164. Lavender SA, Shakeel K, Andersson GBJ, and Thomas JS. Effects of a lifting belt on spine movements and muscle recruitments after unexpected sudden loading. *Spine* 2000;25:1569–1578.
165. Marras WS, Jorgensen MJ, and Davis KG. Effect of foot movement and an elastic lumbar back support on spinal loading during free-dynamic symmetric and asymmetric lifting exertions. *Ergonomics* 2000;43:653–668.
166. Giorcelli RJ, Hughes RE, Wassell JT, and Hsiao H. The effect of wearing a back belt on spine kinematics during asymmetric lifting of large and small boxes. *Spine* 2001;26:1794–1798.
167. Kingma I, Faber GS, Suwarganda EK, Bruijnen TB, Peters RJ, and van Dieën JH. Effect of a stiff lifting belt on spine compression during lifting. *Spine* 2006;31:E833–E839.
168. Gagnon M. Box tilt and knee motions in manual lifting—Two differential factors in expert and novice workers. *Clinical Biomechanics* 1997;12:419–428.
169. Gagnon M, Larrivé A, and Desjardins P. Strategies of load tilts and shoulder positioning in asymmetrical lifting. A concomitant evaluation of the reference systems of axes. *Clinical Biomechanics* 2000;15:478–488.
170. Kingma I and van Dieën JH. Lifting over an obstacle: Effects of one-handed lifting and hand support on trunk kinematics and low back loading. *Journal of Biomechanics* 2004;37:249–255.

171. Dennis GJ and Barrett RS. Spinal loads during individual and team lifting. *Ergonomics* 2002;45:671–681.
172. Dennis GJ and Barrett RS. Spinal loads during two-person team lifting: Effect of matched versus unmatched standing height. *International Journal of Industrial Ergonomics* 2003;32:25–38.
173. Marras WS, Davis KG, Kirking BC, and Granata KP. Spine loading and trunk kinematics during team lifting. *Ergonomics* 1999;42:1258–1273.
174. van Dieën JH and Toussaint HM. Evaluation of the probability of spinal damage caused by sustained cyclic compression loading. *Human Factors* 1997;39:469–480.
175. van Dieën JH, van der Burg P, Raaijmakers TAJ, and Toussaint HM. Effects of repetitive lifting on the kinematics, inadequate anticipatory control or adaptive changes? *Journal of Motor Behavior* 1998;30:20–32.
176. van Dieën JH, Dekkers JJM, Groen V, Toussaint HM, and Meijer OG. Within-subject variability in low-back load in a repetitively performed, mildly constrained lifting task. *Spine* 2001;26:1799–1804.
177. de Looze MP, Zinzen E, Caboor D, Heyblom P, van Bree E, van Roy P, Toussaint HM, and Clarijs JP. Effect of individually chosen bed-height adjustments on the low-back stress of nurses. *Scandinavian Journal of Work, Environment and Health* 1994;20:427–434.
178. de Looze MP, Zinzen E, Caboor D, van Roy P, and Clarijs JP. Muscle strength, task performance and low back load in nurses. *Ergonomics* 1998;41:1095–1104.
179. Faber G, Kingma I, and van Dieën JH. The effects of ergonomic interventions on low back moments are attenuated by changes in lifting behaviour. *Ergonomics*, 2007;50:1377–1391.
180. Davis KG and Marras WS. Assessment of the relationship between box weight and trunk kinematics: Does a reduction in box weight necessarily correspond to a decrease in spinal loading? *Human Factors* 2000;42:195–208.
181. de Kort W and van Dijk F. Preventive effectiveness of pre-employment medical assessments. *Occupational Environmental Medicine* 1997;54:1–6.
182. McGill SM. Distribution of tissue loads in the low back during a variety of daily and rehabilitation tasks. *Journal of Rehabilitation Research & Development* 1997;34:448–458.
183. Sinaki M, Itoi E, Wahner HW, Wollan P, Gelzcer R, Mullan BP, Collins DA, and Hodgson SF. Stronger back muscles reduce the incidence of vertebral fractures: A prospective 10 year follow-up of postmenopausal women. *Bone* 2002;30:836–841.
184. Adams MA and Dolan P. Could sudden increases in physical activity cause degeneration of intervertebral discs? *The Lancet* 1997;350:734–735.
185. Burton AK, Balague F, Cardon G, Eriksen HR, Henrotin Y, Lahad A, Leclerc A, Muller G, and van der Beek AJ. Chapter 2. European guidelines for prevention in low back pain: November 2004. *European Spine Journal* 2006;15 Suppl 2:S136–68.
186. Westgaard RH and Winkel J. Ergonomic intervention research for improved musculoskeletal health: A critical review. *International Journal of Industrial Ergonomics* 1997;20:463–500.
187. Charney W. The lift team method for reducing back injuries. A 10 hospital study. *AAOHN Journal* 1997;45:300–304.
188. Wergeland EL, Veiersted B, Ingre M, Olsson B, Akerstedt T, Bjornskau T, and Varg N. A shorter workday as a means of reducing the occurrence of musculoskeletal disorders. *Scandinavian Journal of Work, Environment and Health* 2003;29:27–34.
189. Mathiassen SE. Diversity and variation in biomechanical exposure: What is it, and why would we like to know? *Applied Ergonomics* 2006;37:419–427.
190. Kuijer PPFM, van der Beek AJ, van Dieën JH, Visser B, and Frings-Dresen MHW. Effect of job rotation on need for recovery and (sick leave due to) musculoskeletal complaints: A prospective study among refuse collectors. *American Journal of Industrial Medicine* 2005;47:394–402.

191. Himmelstein JS and Andersson GB. Low back pain: Risk evaluation and preplacement screening. *Occupational Medicine* 1988;3:255–269.
192. Cohen JE, Goel V, Frank JW, and Gibson ES. Predicting risk of back injuries, work absenteeism, and chronic disability. The shortcomings of preplacement screening. *Journal of Occupational Medicine* 1994;36:1093–1099.
193. Linton SJ and van Tulder MW. Preventive interventions for back and neck pain problems: What is the evidence? *Spine* 2001;26:778–787.
194. Yassi A, Cooper JE, Tate RB, Gerlach S, Muir M, Trottier J, and Massey K. A randomized controlled trial to prevent patient lift and transfer injuries of health care workers. *Spine* 2001;26:1739–1746.
195. Smedley J, Trevelyan F, Inskip H, Buckle P, Cooper C, and Coggon D. Impact of ergonomic intervention on back pain among nurses. *Scandinavian Journal of Work, Environment and Health* 2003;29:117–123.
196. Evanoff BA, Bohr PC, and Wolf LD. Effects of a participatory ergonomics team among hospital orderlies. *American Journal of Industrial Medicine* 1999;35:358–365.
197. Lahad A, Malter AD, Berg AO, and Deyo RA. The effectiveness of four interventions for the prevention of low back pain. *JAMA* 1994;272:1286–1291.
198. Gebhardt WA. Effectiveness of training to prevent job-related back pain: A meta-analysis. *British Journal of Clinical Psychology* 1994;33 (Pt 4):571–574.
199. van Poppel MN, Koes BW, Smid T, and Bouter LM. A systematic review of controlled clinical trials on the prevention of back pain in industry. *Occupational Environmental Medicine* 1997;54:841–847.
200. Maher CG. A systematic review of workplace interventions to prevent low back pain. *Australian Journal of Physiotherapy* 2000;46:259–269.
201. Tveito TH, Hysing M, and Eriksen HR. Low back pain interventions at the workplace: A systematic literature review. *Occupational Medicine (London)* 2004;54:3–13.
202. van Poppel MN, Hooftman WE, and Koes BW. An update of a systematic review of controlled clinical trials on the primary prevention of back pain at the workplace. *Occupational Medicine (London)* 2004;54:345–352.
203. Waddell G and Burton AK. Occupational health guidelines for the management of low back pain at work: Evidence review. *Occupational Medicine (London)* 2001;51:124–135.
204. Jellema P, van Tulder MW, van Poppel MN, Nachemson AL, and Bouter LM. Lumbar supports for prevention and treatment of low back pain: A systematic review within the framework of the Cochrane Back Review Group. *Spine* 2001;26:377–386.
205. van Deursen LL, Snijders CJ, and Patijn J. Influence of daily life activities on pain in patients with low back pain. *Journal of Orthopaedic Medicine* 2002;24:74–76.

Section D

Ergonomics of Selected Interventions

13 A Critical Analysis of Therapeutic Exercise for Subacute Low Back Pain and Carpal Tunnel Syndrome

Anne Fenety and Katherine Harman

CONTENTS

13.1   INTRODUCTION

Humans are designed to move. Our movements are facilitated via a healthy musculoskeletal (MSK) system. When the MSK system is in dysfunction, restoring
movement is a primary rehabilitation goal—a goal that is generally achieved
through the prescription of therapeutic exercise. The American Physical Therapy
Association (2001) defines therapeutic exercise as the "systematic and planned
performance of bodily movements, postures or activities intended to provide a
client with the means to remediate or prevent impairments, improve, restore or
enhance physical function, prevent or reduce health-related risk factors, and optimize overall health status, fitness or sense of well being" (p. 682). Numerous
textbooks detail therapeutic exercise prescription linking varieties of impairment
(e.g., loss of endurance) to recommended therapeutic exercises (e.g., open or closed
kinetic chain), and descriptions of exercises by body part, by body region or specific population (e.g., postoperative) (Hall and Brody, 1999; Kisner and Colby,
2002). Despite the widespread use and excellent description of therapeutic exercise, a broad review of the literature has revealed that there is limited evidence of
its effectiveness.

Our goal in this chapter is not to reproduce the information existing in these
therapeutic exercise textbooks. Instead, we bring a critical analysis approach and
concentrate on two primary factors that we believe influence the effectiveness of
prescription of therapeutic exercise, namely pain and diagnostic accuracy. To further
focus this chapter, we chose two specific MSK conditions: low back pain (LBP) and
carpal tunnel syndrome (CTS). We consider nonspecific, mechanical LBP, that is,
LBP that does not include neurological signs and for which red flags (see Box 13.1)
have been cleared. CTS is a constellation of signs and symptoms that result from
irritation of the median nerve due to compression at the level of the carpal tunnel
(O'Connor et al., 2003). We chose these two conditions for a variety of reasons,
in part, because they differ in clinical presentation and diagnosis but also for the
numerous features these two conditions share. In the first place, LBP and CTS are
commonly related to ergonomic conditions at work and home. Second, health care
professionals are challenged with their treatment, particularly when they become
chronic conditions. And when LBP and CTS are chronic, they are two of the most
expensive MSK conditions to rehabilitate. Our final rationale for this selection relates

BOX 13.1 THE FOLLOWING SYMPTOMS ARE RED FLAGS AND THEY INDICATE THAT IMMEDIATE MEDICAL CARE IS NEEDED

- Severe unremitting pain
- Pain unaffected by medication or position
- Severe night pain
- Severe pain with no history of injury
- Severe spasm
- Swelling or redness in any joint without history of injury
- Psychological overlay
- Violent trauma, such as a fall from a height or a car accident
- Thoracic pain
- Previous history of carcinoma, systemic steroids, or drug abuse
- Persisting, severe restriction of lumbar flexion

to our overall concern: despite their prevalence and relative treatment costs, evidence for the effectiveness of therapeutic exercise prescription is particularly limited in LBP and CTS (O'Connor et al., 2003; Hayden et al., 2005) and we believe this merits a critical review.

In this chapter, we argue that the lack of evidence for therapeutic exercise effectiveness may not stem from the health care practitioner's ability to set out an exercise program per se, but rather the inability to set out a program that considers pain is based on an accurate diagnosis. The first foundation is pain. In recent years, we have become more aware of the complexity of pain presentation, especially when nervous tissue is involved. In dealing with persistent pain, taking a graded approach to the prescription of therapeutic exercise addresses the need of the client to confront the problem of movement associated pain. However, these considerations have not translated to the study of exercise effectiveness. The second foundation of therapeutic exercise prescription is the accuracy of diagnosis. As Graham et al. (2006) says "when the diagnosis is wrong, treatment will fail, no matter what it comprises" (pp. 1463–64). Nested within the issue of diagnosis is the determination of the stage of healing of the injury. Many would agree that the underlying formula for exercise prescription is *the right exercise, for the right reason, at the right time*. If this is true, then determining the stage of healing of the MSK dysfunction (i.e., the right time) is fundamental to success. As we will describe later, there is a considerable challenge to accurately determining the stage of healing in LBP and CTS (Waddell, 1998; MacDermid and Doherty, 2004; Wilder-Smith et al., 2006).

Therapeutic exercise is central to the rehabilitation of MSK conditions. Successful outcome depends on many factors. This chapter focuses on two important considerations: the impact of pain on how the client presents and responds to treatment and the importance and difficulty of having an accurate diagnosis to guide treatment. We discuss these factors as they apply to CTS and LBP as these conditions are commonly encountered in the workplace and evidence is sparse in regard to the effectiveness of therapeutic exercise. We believe that many lessons learned in LBP may be helpful to achieve better outcomes in CTS. We believe that with a better understanding of the complexity of the pain experience along with an improved diagnostic accuracy, therapeutic exercise effectiveness will also improve. In addition, applying a pathomechanic approach to the cervical/upper limb kinetic chain may be used to prevent progression when early symptoms are identified.

13.2 IMPACT OF PAIN AND PARESTHESIA ON THE INDIVIDUAL

The condition name, "low back pain" indicates undeniably that pain is the dominant symptom. However, the unpleasant sensations of CTS—numbness, paresthesia, tingling, and pain (Katz and Stirrat, 1990; Graham et al., 2003; Kamath and Stothard, 2003; Nora et al., 2005)—are a constellation of sensations that may be more precisely labeled peripheral neuropathic pain as defined by Merskey et al. (1994): "Pain initiated or caused by a primary lesion or dysfunction in the peripheral nervous system" (p. 210). Although the nature and quality of the sensations are different between the two conditions, they are both disabling and distressing for the individual and, for simplicity, we will generally refer to "pain" when discussing both LBP and CTS.

Health care professionals use pain reports as indicators of many things including how serious a problem is, which structure to focus treatment on, and if a problem is improving or getting worse. For the majority of MSK conditions, this biosensory approach is effective because the problem is straightforward, of relatively short duration, or not very disabling. However because LBP and CTS are complex, have a high prevalence of persistence (Waddell, 1998; Nathan et al., 2002; You et al., 2004), and are associated with significant lost work hours, effective treatment requires a broader, biopsychosocial approach. This will include the consideration of psychological interventions such as cognitive-behavioral strategies as well as screening tools that incorporate psychosocial factors to predict poor outcomes. To understand the impact of pain on an individual, one needs to consider, among other things, the combination of the neurophysiological response to a painful stimulus (sensitization), the psychological response (e.g., catastrophizing), and the behavioral response (e.g., avoidance).

When examining the impact of pain on progression from the preclinical to the symptomatic phase, health care practitioners must consider many factors, such as the difficulty of diagnosis and also external influences such as access to care, comorbid conditions, reinjury, or repeated painful experiences (Pengel et al., 2002). Predictability is a problem for the client and the health care provider because healing does not necessarily progress over a prescribed time frame due to reinjury; this can lead to a delay in healing and with repeated painful episodes there is an increased likelihood of persistence (Woolf and Salter, 2000). During the healing period, an individual will experience pain during activity and this may increase the possibility of negative psychological responses known to occur with painful conditions (Picavet et al., 2002; Sullivan et al., 2002; Vlaeyen, 2003).

In addition, the distraction of pain during activity has a negative effect on performance (Harman and Ruyak, 2005). These two findings put into question the old adage "No pain, no gain." When prescribing therapeutic exercise, it is therefore necessary to consider how the individual is responding to the pain experience. Linking the phase of healing to the neuroplasticity of pain perception may enhance the effectiveness of therapeutic exercise, because peripheral and central nervous pathways undergo modulation and modification in the presence of persistent or repeated pain, laying the foundation for chronicity (Woolf and Salter, 2000).

13.2.1 NEUROPLASTICITY

Neuroplasticity, the ability of elements of the nervous system to change (Cotman and Berchtold, 2002; Johansson, 2004), is the underlying mechanism attributed to the developmental organization of the nervous system (Constantine-Paton, 2000). This mutability, once believed to be lost at maturity, has been discovered in adult nervous systems and triggered not only by trauma, but also by day-to-day sensory and cognitive input (Arnstein, 1997; Constantine-Paton, 2000; Byl and Merzenich, 2001; Johansson, 2004).

As a result of a tremendous amount of research, it is now understood that the neurophysiology of pain involves neuroplastic changes. Injury or inflammation of nerve and innervated tissue results in long-term increased excitability (sensitization) of peripheral and central nervous system neurons (Campbell et al., 1988; Wright, 2002). The reflexive avoidance of a painful movement has a protective role and will in itself create neuroplastic changes in sensory and motor systems function. The result of these changes can be seen in decreased thresholds to painful stimuli (hyperalgesia) or to a stimulation that would not normally be considered painful (allodynia) (Woolf and Salter, 2000; Melzack et al., 2001). This sensitization can persist in the presence of repeated noxious stimulation through reinjury or tissue overloading (Wall, 1990; Coderre et al., 1993; Mao, 2002). Therefore as a condition progresses, the prescription of activity and exercise must be balanced between the encouragement of optimal physical functioning and avoidance of eliciting excessive unpleasant sensations because these may perpetuate the sensitization response and limit further progress (Coderre et al., 1993; Wright, 2002). In addition to sensitization, the experience of continuing symptoms and slowness of healing can lead individuals to develop known psychological barriers to recovery, such as fear of movement and maladaptive beliefs and attitudes (Picavet et al., 2002; Vlaeyen, 2003).

13.2.2 FEAR-AVOIDANCE THEORY

Among the many theories that attempt to explain the persistence of pain, the fear-avoidance theory (Lethem et al., 1983; Vlaeyen and Linton, 2000; Vlaeyen et al., 2002; Vlaeyen, 2003) is highly relevant to movement and exercise because it describes how an individual interprets and copes with their perception of pain and how that perception influences movement (Vlaeyen, 2003). The model (Figure 13.1) represents two extremes: one path leads to the positive outcome of achieving

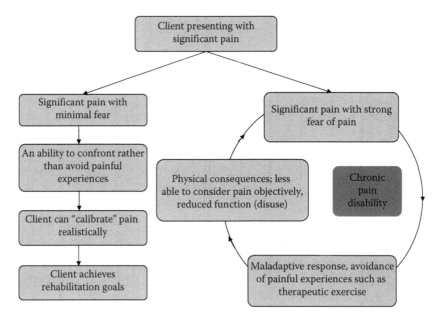

FIGURE 13.1 Diagrammatic representation of the fear-avoidance model. (Modified from Lethem et al., *Behav. Res. Ther.*, 21, 401, 1983; Vlaeyen, J. and Linton, S., *Pain*, 85, 317, 2000.)

rehabilitation goals where, the individual is not without pain, but the pain experienced is interpreted as something to be coped with or managed. The other side of the model depicts a cyclical pattern that leads to a negative outcome. It starts with the fear of pain, leads to the avoidance of movement (which, unfortunately does not usually lead to pain reduction), a reduced capacity to exercise, and chronic disability. This pattern is familiar to many health care providers. Although avoidance of pain-provoking movements offers a protection against further injury or hurt, this avoidance is maladaptive when the individual becomes caught in the cycle of chronic pain disability depicted in the model [adapted from Vlaeyen et al. (1995)]. Avoidance is a natural response to unpleasant events or symptoms and is observed with other conditions as well [e.g., dyspnea (Rose et al., 2002) and falling (Wijhuizen et al., 2006)].

13.2.3 MALADAPTIVE BELIEFS AND ATTITUDES

What people think and how they respond to the condition they are in has a strong influence on outcomes. There are key psychological responses to painful events that are important to understand. Catastrophizing is a form of coping that, instead of providing a positive outlook, is a dramatically negative response to the experience of pain (Sullivan et al., 1995). Catastrophizers have been found to experience pain to a greater extent than noncatastrophizers (Keefe et al., 1989) and catastrophizing is predictive of poor outcomes (Burton et al., 1995). These individuals do not deal well with pain and will avoid activity such as therapeutic exercise, which might elicit this extremely negative experience. In addition, those who catastrophize begin to feel that they cannot engage in any activity, impairing their self-efficacy, defined as the belief that one can accomplish or complete something (Turk and Okifuji, 1998). Self-efficacy is improved with the successful completion of a goal (such as exercising with minimal negative effect) and will help direct an individual toward the path to successful rehabilitation as opposed to the vicious cycle of pain and disability (Linton and Ryberg, 2001; Vlaeyen et al., 2002).

There are measures available that can help identify the presence of problematic psychological responses, referred to as "yellow flags" (Sullivan et al., 1995). In LBP, four key predictors of poor outcome have been identified (Watson and Kendall, 2000):

1. The presence of a belief that back pain is harmful or potentially severely disabling
2. Fear-avoidance behavior and reduced activity levels
3. Tendency to low mood and withdrawal from social interaction
4. An expectation that passive treatment rather than active participation will help (Waddell et al., 1993; Accident Compensation Corporation, 2004).

A similar risk assessment has not been identified with CTS. In fact, the relationships are unclear. The few studies on pain reports and psychological response in CTS present different views regarding outcomes. For example, when examining relations among measures of electrodiagnostic testing and psychosocial factors in CTS, the findings revealed no statistically significant relationship (Chan et al., 2007). Another study found that clients diagnosed with nonspecific hand pain (i.e., not CTS) had higher scores on measures indicative of psychological distress than those diagnosed with CTS (Crossman et al., 2001). These suggest that understanding the diagnosis of the symptoms may mitigate negative psychological response to symptoms. Another study found no relation between preoperative psychological distress and surgical outcomes (Hobby et al., 2005). Understanding how the neurophysiological response (sensitization), the psychological response (catastrophizing), and the behavioral response (avoidance) to painful stimuli all combine is important when considering the timing and intensity of therapeutic exercise. With CTS and LBP, it is important to understand their differences as well as their similarities.

13.2.4 IMPLICATIONS FOR THERAPEUTIC EXERCISE

When prescribing exercise, a common question is when to start? Later in this chapter, we discuss diagnosis and staging, and the timing of exercise prescription. So, here we consider the psychological response to a sensitized nervous system. During the preclinical phase of CTS, symptoms are mild and therefore a more aggressive approach could be taken with less risk of eliciting an avoidance response. Whereas, as the symptoms become stronger, the nervous system is being subjected to persistent noxious stimulation, thus making the individual's response more complex. Exercise prescription should consider the impact of triggering more symptoms, which may lead to the vicious cycling depicted in the fear-avoidance model (Figure 13.1).

In LBP, guidelines for the acute phase are clear: to maintain activity and palliate symptoms (Accident Compensation Corporation, 2004). As the individual moves into the subacute phase of healing, exercise prescription can progress. This subacute phase of LBP is somewhat challenging: those who have involvement of psychosocial factors are at higher risk to develop persistence, and therefore screening for these complicating issues is recommended at this stage (Watson and Kendall, 2000; Accident Compensation Corporation, 2004). If "yellow flags" are not identified by screening, then a steady, graded increase in exercises is recommended (Fritz and George, 2000; George et al., 2003; Staal et al., 2004). The chronic phase of LBP requires a multidisciplinary team (Hayden et al., 2005) and the chronic phase of CTS is mostly managed through surgical intervention (MacDermid and Doherty, 2004). In conclusion, considering pain when prescribing exercise is an important part of the intervention. The lack of consideration of the impact of pain on the individual may in part explain the limited evidence available of successful therapeutic exercise in both subacute LBP and CTS.

13.3 THERAPEUTIC EXERCISE PRESCRIPTION IN LBP: WHERE IS THE EVIDENCE?

In LBP, very often (but not always), there is a defining movement or injury when the back pain started. The acute phase that follows requires rest, maintenance of activity, and medication (Accident Compensation Corporation, 2004). However, it is the subacute phase of recovery where there is consensus that we should focus our rehabilitation efforts (Karjalainen et al., 2001; Philadelphia Panel, 2001; Pengel et al., 2002; Accident Compensation Corporation, 2004; Abenhaim et al., 2005). Health care practitioners generally follow the "educate and activate" approach with the following principles to guide therapeutic exercise prescription (p. 291) (Kisner and Colby, 2002):

- Educate
  Knowledge of the injury and participation in the plan will enhance compliance
- Promote healing
  Rest when necessary, but assure as much freedom of movement as possible
- Systematically pursue restoration of function
  Transition from passive to active exercises aimed at mobility
- Practice smooth, coordinated movement
  Using a variety of exercises, challenge flexibility, and coordination
- Increase strength
  Apply progressive resistance to strengthen key muscles according to ACSM guidelines (American College of Sports Medicine, 2006).

In searching for best practice and in the presence of a small number of high-quality research articles, we found that the largest amount of supporting evidence for treating LBP in the subacute phase was in the prescription of activity and therapeutic exercise. In the subacute phase, the recommendation is to keep active, but also to add exercise (Philadelphia Panel, 2001). We now consider studies in which the effectiveness of prescribing therapeutic exercise has been demonstrated during subacute LBP.

One difficulty in reviewing these studies involving activity and therapeutic exercise for LBP is that many interventions are combined or not described, making their individual contribution to the results difficult to determine (Abenhaim et al., 2005). In addition, studies often report a therapeutic intervention (which may or may not include exercise) in a vague manner, such as "as available" (Lindström et al., 1992a,b). A final challenge is the variability of nomenclature in therapeutic exercise. This led the International Task Force on Back Pain to outline common LBP exercises according to the following six criteria: direction of spinal movement (e.g., flexion), nature of exercise (e.g., aerobic, isokinetic), type of exercise (e.g., active, graded, passive), exercise parameters (e.g., duration, intensity), exercise evaluation techniques (e.g., lifting test, muscle strength), and specific exercise techniques (e.g., resisted trunk extension, yoga). Abenhaim et al. (2005) went on to recommend that researchers and clinicians implement classification schemes such as theirs to standardize the manner in which exercise is prescribed, named, and documented.

Despite the above criticisms, there are some findings in the literature that may be helpful to develop best practices for exercise prescription during the subacute phase of healing in LBP. This next section relies on five recent articles (Karjalainen et al., 2001; Philadelphia Panel, 2001; Pengel et al., 2002; Abenhaim et al., 2005; Hayden et al., 2005) that each provide a critical review of LBP management, with some attention to the subacute phase of healing. Each reported only on studies that met a standard of quality. Table 13.1 presents nine papers according to the type of exercise that was studied and the quality of evidence according to standards of the five review papers. They were rated as low, moderate, or high quality or as having demonstrated clinical effectiveness. From the five review papers, support was found for a graded approach, multidisciplinary or group interventions and some specific exercises. Next, we review each of these four approaches, in turn, beginning with graded activity.

13.3.1 Graded Activity

The concept of graded activity was first described during rehabilitation when having individuals walk on graded slopes increased the exercise challenge. Graded (or quota-based) exercise is a term that identifies a method of exercise progression based on predetermined targets and reinforcement strategies. This approach is based on the following ideas: (1) pain and pain behaviors are reinforced by favorable consequences (operant conditioning); (2) exercise and physical activity are not compatible with pain and pain behaviors; and therefore (3) if exercise increases, this should lead to a decrease in pain behaviors (Lindström et al., 1992b). Activity, per se, is not broadly prescribed in the rehabilitation of LBP, perhaps due to challenges of describing and measuring activity (Lindström et al.,

TABLE 13.1

**Available Evidence from Five Systematic Reviews to Support
Therapeutic Exercise Prescription in Subacute LBP**

Exercise Approach	Research Articles	Study Details: Exercise for Clients with Subacute LBP	Results	Quality of Evidence per Five Systematic Reviews
Graded	Staal et al. (2004)	—Randomized control trial (RCT): treatment (tx) for 4/52 P/O until return to work (RTW)	—Time off work in 6/12: GrEx < USUAL ($p < .01$)	—All: moderate quality Cited in:
		—GrEx (Graded Exs— aerobics, strength @ 75% max) ($n = 67$) vs USUAL (Occup MD) ($n = 67$)	—Functional Status & decreased pain: GrEx > USUAL @ 3, 6/12 (trend)	—Hayden et al. (2005), Abenhaim et al. (2001)
	Lindström et al. (1992a)	—RCT: tx for 6/52 post-onset until RTW	—RTW: GrAc < USUAL ($p = .03$)	
	Lindström et al. (1992b)	—GrAc (Graded Activity) ($n = 51$) vs USUAL care (MD/PT) ($n = 52$)	—Sick Leave (yr 2) GrAc < USUAL ($p = .03$) (males only)	
Specific	Cherkin et al. (1998)	—RCT: tx for 1/12; follow-up (F/U) for 2 yrs —McKenzie exs ($n = 133$) vs CHIROpractic manipulation ($n = 122$) vs MINimal physiotherapy (PT) tx ($n = 66$)	—McK, CHIRO marginally better outcomes compared to MIN	—Cherkin: low quality rating —Hansen: demonstrated effectiveness
	Hansen et al. (1993)	—RCT: tx for 4/52; maximum 8 visits, F/U @ 1, 6, & 12/12 —BckExt (Back Extension—3 exs × 100 reps/day) ($n=60$) vs StdPT (Standard PT—tx passive exercise, strength, flexibility, coordination) ($n = 59$) vs Ctrl (control —hot packs, traction)	—No signif diff in 3 gps: pain, Fx status —StdPT >er effect for males & heavy manual laborers —BckExt >er effect for females & sedentary workers	—Cited in: —Hayden et al. (2005), Abenhaim et al. (2001)
Group	Moffett et al. (1999)	—RCT: duration 4/52 —GpEx (Group Exs) ($n = 70$) (stretching, strengthening, aerobics vs USUAL ($n = 74$) (PT care + education)	—Distressing pain @ 6/52: GpEx < USUAL ($p = .03$) —ABPS & RDQ improvement:	—Moffett: low (Hayden et al., 2005) & high quality (Pengel et al., 2002) —Storheim et al. (2003): low quality

TABLE 13.1 (continued)
Available Evidence from Five Systematic Reviews to Support
Therapeutic Exercise Prescription in Subacute LBP

Exercise Approach	Research Articles	Study Details: Exercise for Clients with Subacute LBP	Results	Quality of Evidence per Five Systematic Reviews
		—Used Cognitive Behavioral Therapy (CBT)	GpEx > than USUAL ($p < .05$)	—Kellett et al. (1991): demonstrated effectiveness Cited in:
	Storheim et al. (2003)	—RCT: duration: 15/52 —GpEx (Group Exs —safe-to-move, fitness, Fx capacity) ($n = 30$); vs Cogn (Cognitive—re: education, reassurance, spinal stability exs)($n = 34$) vs USUAL ($n = 29$) (usual PT care)	—Pain intensity: GpEx < Cogn ($p = .04$) —Disability score: GpEx < Cogn ($p = .02$)	—Hayden et al. (2005), Philadelphia Panel (2001), Abenhaim et al. (2005), Pengel et al. (2002)
	Kellett et al. (1991)	—RCT with 1.5 yr F/U —GpEx (Group Exs—graded exs of increasing intensity to improve strength, flexibility & coordination) ($n = 58$) vs Ctrl (Control) ($n = 53$) (usual PT care)	—Sick days due to LBP: GpEx < Ctrl ($p < .02$) —# LBP episodes: GpEx < Ctrl ($p < .05$)	
Multi-disciplinary	Lindström et al. (1992a)	—As above (Lindström 1992a,b) —plus Fx capacity/work evaluations & F/U with social work, orthopedic surgeon	Sick leave, RTW results as above (Lindström 1992a,b)	—All: moderate quality Cited in: —Karjalainen et al. (2001)
	Loisel et al. (1997)	—RCT: 130 workers from 4/52 until RTW —USUAL MD care, CLINical tx (specialist, Back School, Functional rehabilitation, CBT, *therapeutic* RTW), OCCUPational tx (ergonomics, OCCUP MD), COMBined (CLIN + OCCUP)	—RTW: COMB < USUAL ($p = .01$) —Oswestry @ 1 yr: CLIN, OCCUP, COMB > USUAL ($p < .05$)	

ABPS, Aberdeen Pain Intensity Scale; RDQ, Roland Disability Questionnaire.

1992a; Staal et al., 2004). In response to these needs, the International Task Force on Back Pain (Abenhaim et al., 2005) created a graded scale of seven mobility-related activities most likely affected by LBP, that would help standardize the prescription of activity, prior to progressing to an exercise program. These activities include walking, sitting, standing, lying down/getting up, staying in bed, climbing stairs and transportation. For any of these activities (e.g., walking) the researchers encourage practitioners to quantify (e.g., distance walked in 20 min) or qualify (e.g., able to walk a short/long time) the activity in their exercise prescription and charting (Abenhaim et al., 2005).

As seen in Table 13.1, whether graded activity (Lindström et al., 1992a,b) or graded exercises (Staal et al., 2004) were prescribed by a health care practitioner, clients with subacute LBP returned to work earlier than controls. In some cases, workers also showed a trend toward improved functional status and reduced pain ratings (Lindström et al., 1992a,b). Staal et al. (2004) used a structured, incremental quota-based program where clients started at 75%–80% of maximal capacity (aerobic, strength) and finished at a target capacity—usually on a return to work date. What set this study apart was their incorporation of operant conditioning (Fordyce, 1974) into therapeutic exercise prescription. Here, early goals were easy to attain, subsequent goals were met (but not exceeded) and goal attainment was positively reinforced. These results have positive implications for therapeutic exercise prescription (Box 13.2). The graded approach is an appropriate transition during the acute/sub-acute phases of healing, as the health care practitioner assesses their client's response to exercise both psychologically and physically.

13.3.2 SPECIFIC EXERCISES

As it currently stands, there is no evidence that specific exercises alone are sufficient to produce improved global outcomes such as return to work for subacute LBP (Philadelphia Panel, 2001; Pengel et al., 2002; Abenhaim et al., 2005; Hayden et al., 2005). Nonetheless, there are many specific types of exercise prescribed by

---

BOX 13.2   GRADED ACTIVITY/EXERCISE: IMPLICATIONS FOR THERAPEUTIC EXERCISE PRESCRIPTION

1. Using an operant conditioning behavioral approach, graded activity/graded exercise prescription should include
   a. Setting realistic activity goals based on activity levels
   b. Positively reinforcing every success, appropriately pacing clients who move ahead too quickly and encouraging the slowly advancing clients with smaller increments success
2. Remember: the overall goal of graded activity/exercise is not to improve aerobic fitness or muscle strength per se, but to have the individual learn that it is safe to move and be active in the presence of pain.

health care practitioners. In the absence of supporting evidence for one particular exercise or technique, the International Paris Task Force on Back Pain concluded that the key to success is physical activity itself, activity of any form (*"Just Do It"*™). Reinforcing the idea that physical activity affords the greatest therapeutic value and this positive effect is widespread to most systems in the body (Cotman and Berchtold, 2002).

From two systematic reviews of research regarding effectiveness of specific exercise for LBP (Abenhaim et al., 2005; Hayden et al., 2005), only two types of exercise were identified. However, when evaluated further, neither McKenzie exercises (Cherkin et al., 1998) nor intensive back extension exercises resulted in any significant treatment effect when compared to a control group, an alternate treatment group (i.e., chiropractic manipulation) (Cherkin et al., 1998), or standard physiotherapy treatment consisting of passive and active (e.g., exercise for strength, flexibility, and coordination) components (Hansen et al., 1993).

In 2006, a systematic review of spinal stabilization exercises (SSE) for multifidus and transversus abdominus muscles found that SSE are better than general practitioner treatment when considering the outcomes of disability and pain, but it was unclear whether they are more effective than other physiotherapy interventions (Rackwitz et al., 2006). A recent RCT compared general to specific SSEs and found no between group differences after 8 weeks (Koumantakis et al., 2005). Although there are only a few studies that showed the effectiveness of specific exercises in this population, it is worthwhile to note that there is no evidence of an adverse effect either (Box 13.3). This is an area of growth and development and should be a large effort in research in the coming years.

13.3.3 GROUP EXERCISES

From four systematic reviews of group exercise for subacute LBP (Philadelphia Panel, 2001; Pengel et al., 2002; Abenhaim et al., 2005; Boersma and Linton, 2005), only three studies of moderate quality were found (Kellett et al., 1991; Moffett et al., 1999; Storheim et al., 2003). These studies found that group exercise was

---

BOX 13.3   SPECIFIC EXERCISE: IMPLICATIONS FOR THERAPEUTIC EXERCISE PRESCRIPTION

1. As part of the biopsychosocial model of health care delivery, consider prescription of specific exercises in conjunction with graded activity/ graded exercise.
2. Evidence of the effectiveness of specific exercises is limited and a considerable research effort is required to determine the relationship between specificity of the LBP diagnosis, the stage of healing and the need for specific exercises—type and parameters (e.g., repetitions, duration, etc.).

favorable in terms of improvements in disability, pain distress, and pain intensity ratings (Moffett et al., 1999; Storheim et al., 2003) and reductions in sick day listings and repeat episodes of LBP (Kellett et al., 1991). These studies examined the effect of group exercise prescription by health care practitioners and, although two studies (Kellett et al., 1991; Storheim et al., 2003) had sufficient durations (i.e., 15 weeks, 18 months, respectively) to cause tissue modification, little therapeutic effect on tissues could occur during the 4-week program (Moffett et al., 1999). A number of factors might explain that positive result. First, as with the other types of exercise, subjects would have learned that back pain can coexist with being active. Furthermore, as part of a group, these individuals would see that others were also active and managing. Finally, they might reap other benefits of exercising in groups such as the benefits of social interaction, the documented improvements in compliance with group exercise, and the message that exercise is important as evidenced by the number of subjects and the attitude of the group leader (Friedrich et al., 1998). In addition to the benefits noted above, group exercise programs are an excellent way to facilitate the continuation of exercise with supervision (Box 13.4).

13.3.4 MULTIDISCIPLINARY INTERVENTIONS

Multidisciplinary team interventions have been demonstrated to be effective in chronic LBP, but there are few studies upon which to determine effectiveness in subacute LBP. For example, a recent systematic review (Karjalainen et al., 2001) of over 1800 citations found only two papers (Lindström et al., 1995; Loisel et al., 1997) of moderate quality. These two RCTs considered a comprehensive range of outcomes, with interventions that were multidisciplinary. Physiotherapy was included in both studies, with at least two other professions including psychology represented in the team. The results of both studies indicate a positive effect of this approach in an occupational setting specifically with regard to return to work, sick leave, and subjective disability. Karjalainen et al. (2001) concluded that there is a considerable amount of work to be done in this area, with attention needed on the quality of the studies. This resource intensive intervention should be provided earlier, during the subacute phase for those

---

BOX 13.4   GROUP EXERCISE: IMPLICATIONS FOR THERAPEUTIC EXERCISE PRESCRIPTION

1. Group exercises should not be performed until the client understands their exercise limitations and has demonstrated their ability to perform standard exercises safely.
2. Health care practitioners should interact with fitness leaders to ensure that clients perform exercise in a group format in fitness facilities for 2–3 months after discharge from traditional treatment.
3. Consider the multiple nonphysical benefits of group exercise.

> **BOX 13.5   MULTIDISCIPLINARY APPROACH: IMPLICATIONS FOR THERAPEUTIC EXERCISE PRESCRIPTION**
>
> Identify high-risk individuals who may require the higher cost multidisciplinary intervention and those at lower risk directed to a graded exercise program.

who have been identified as high risk for persistence (Box 13.5) (Karjalainen et al., 2001). The Orebro questionnaire was designed for this purpose (Accident Compensation Corporation, 2004).

13.3.5   SUMMARY

Authors of the LBP exercise reviews consistently concluded that subacute LBP is distinct from acute or chronic LBP and that effective intervention at this phase should play an important role in preventing chronic LBP. This role includes therapeutic exercise. What is interesting about the four types of exercise intervention described above is that each type: graded, multidisciplinary, group, and specific exercises employs, to a greater or lesser extent, elements of psychological theory and this may be an important component to their success. That is, the delivery of the intervention is part of the intervention. Pain relief is an important factor for clients with subacute LBP, but treatments aimed at pain relief are often unsuccessful, while approaches aimed at reducing the impact of pain have better outcomes (Waddell, 1998). Based upon the preceding section on the impact of pain and results of our review of exercise effectiveness, we have included several "Implications for Therapeutic Exercise Prescription" text boxes throughout this section. In these we made several recommendations that may assist in improving practice and research design and reporting. Authors also agreed that existing research is limited and not of high quality. Among their concerns were: there is inadequate description of how activity and exercise are prescribed, there are inconsistencies in operational definitions and outcome measures used, that control over important study factors was poor, and that studies exhibited low reproducibility.

13.4   SUBACUTE LBP: DIAGNOSTIC CHALLENGE

Clients with subacute LBP represent a large part of primary health care, played out over a period of time anywhere from 4 weeks postinjury to approximately 12 weeks. The subacute phase of healing occurs in all people, and most recover without difficulty. Many of these shortcomings relate to concerns regarding the accuracy of naming and staging the diagnosis for LBP patients. Considering Graham et al. (2006) admonition that treatment will fail in the presence of the wrong diagnosis, next we turn to diagnostic challenges in LBP. In this section, we focus on the challenge of diagnosing subacute LBP by discussing the name of the diagnosis and the subacute stage of healing.

13.4.1 NAMING THE DIAGNOSIS

The treatment of LBP is hindered by the challenge of providing an accurate diagnosis (DeRosa and Porterfield, 1992). In many regions of the body, clinicians accurately identify the tissue that causes the symptoms in various MSK dysfunctions. In the lumbar spine, however, many health practitioners are wary of pathoanatomic or tissue-based diagnoses due to the difficulty of accurately identifying a pathoanatomic fault (e.g., facet capsule strain) as the primary source of pain (Abenhaim et al., 1995). One solution to these pathoanatomic challenges has been to classify (i.e., diagnose) LBP using a pathomechanic approach. According to Porterfield and DeRosa (1998), a pathomechanic diagnosis "emphasizes the analysis of function—the use of movement patterns with the application of specific stresses and overpressure to determine if familiar pain is elicited" (p. 169). Thus, from a pathomechanic perspective, LBP disorders are classified based on the reproduction of a patient's pain and symptoms elicited by a clinician using a logical, sequential application of stresses into the lumbopelvic region.

The various pathomechanic classification systems found in the rehabilitation literature include the Mackenzie-based (McKenzie, 1981), treatment-based (Delitto et al., 1995) and activity-based (DeRosa and Porterfield, 1992) classification systems, among others. While full descriptions of these systems are beyond the scope of this text, we can summarize their value in the prescription of therapeutic exercise. When no anatomic structure can be identified as of concern (e.g., not of diskogenic origin), then the value of the pathomechanic approach resides in the possible direct link to therapeutic exercise prescription as follows: First, pathomechanic tests identify postures (e.g., prolonged standing) and directions of spinal movement (e.g., extension with left side bending) that reproduce/aggravate (DeRosa and Porterfield, 1992) or reduce (McKenzie, 1981) a patient's symptoms. These aggravating postures and movements often replicate the patient's daily movement patterns and working postures. Thus, they are initially avoided. Second, with the aggravating/relieving postures in mind, therapeutic exercise programs are designed to enable clients to perform strengthening and stretching exercise without compensation or discomfort.

This pathomechanic approach is appealing and has some limited supporting research in LBP (Fritz and George, 2000). More research is needed to link pathomechanic diagnoses with the outcomes of specific therapeutic exercise protocols. Next we extend the concept of naming a diagnosis to include the issue of determining the stage of healing in LBP clients. As will be seen, clinicians and researchers are challenged beyond the issue of diagnostic accuracy in LBP.

13.4.2 STAGING SUBACUTE LOW BACK PAIN

Health care practitioners can now use best practice for treating acute LBP, given the publication of several clinical practice guidelines (CPGs) (Bigos et al., 1994;

Waddell et al., 1996; Philadelphia Panel, 2001; Abenhaim et al., 2005), including the most recent from the New Zealand Acute Low Back Pain Guidelines Group (Accident Compensation Corporation, 2004). Among these various guidelines, there is consensus that once the possibility of red flags has been eliminated, intervention for the acute phase should be limited to reassurance, palliation of symptoms, close monitoring, and encouragement to stay active for 2–4 weeks. This approach is consistent with the importance of a rest/activity balance combined with pain relief to promote healing of MSK tissues (Buckwalter, 1996; Abenhaim et al., 2005).

Despite the validity and utility of CPGs for acute and chronic stage LBP, gaps exist in both clinical and laboratory research with regard to effective treatment for subacute pain. Here, we argue that a major contributor to this knowledge gap is the inconsistency regarding an operational definition of subacute LBP. One operational approach is a time-based staging (i.e., time since injury), with subacute defined inconsistently as 4–12 weeks (Philadelphia Panel, 2001; Abenhaim et al., 2005), 6–12 weeks (Karjalainen et al., 2001; Hayden et al., 2005), or 6–8 weeks postinjury (Hansen et al., 1993). These subacute time frames are not very instructive for the practitioner, given their broad range. Further complicating this time-based approach is the fact that progression from acute to subacute can be influenced by many factors including availability of early access to primary care, reinjury, or repeated painful experiences (Pengel et al., 2002).

Many health care practitioners, such as physiotherapists and osteopaths use a tissue-based, rather than a time-based approach. They use signs such as pain-at-rest to denote the acute (i.e., hyperemic phase) versus pain-on-activity only to denote the subacute (i.e., reparative) phase (Hertling and Kessler, 1996). Alternatively, they may use the duration of postexercise discomfort to determine the stage (e.g., lasting more than 2 h) and guide further exercise interventions (Kellett et al., 1991). Others use function-based scales to stage LBP where, for example, patients in the subacute phase likely will have Modified Oswestry scores in the range of 20–40 (Delitto et al., 1995). The ability of the practitioner to correctly determine the stage of their client's LBP has a significant and profound influence on the prescription of therapeutic exercise. Basic scientists have demonstrated a relationship between the stages of healing and the type and amount of exercise load that can safely be applied to tissues such as cartilage (Salter et al., 1980). The translation of this basic science regarding healing stages into therapeutic exercise prescription has been slow. Finally, whether the clinician's basis for staging LBP is a tissue, time, or functional approach, there is little agreement among health care practitioners regarding an operational definition of subacute LBP (Box 13.6).

13.4.3 SUMMARY

What we know is that, while the diagnosis of nonspecific LBP is challenging, it can be better linked to therapeutic exercises if a pathomechanic approach is used. We also know that, while staging LBP is difficult, the health practitioner should assume that most LBP patients will be in the subacute phase between 4 and 6 weeks

---

**BOX 13.6   STAGING SUBACUTE LBP: IMPLICATIONS
FOR THERAPEUTIC EXERCISE PRESCRIPTION**

1. Recommended type of exercises: stretching (for flexibility), resistance exercises for strength, then endurance, followed by exercises to increase aerobic capacity (e.g., cycling, swimming, etc.). The reader is further advised to consult the 2006 ACSM Guidelines of Exercise Testing and Prescription for specifics regarding strength and endurance prescription.
2. Indications to begin therapeutic exercise:
   - Can perform active range of motion (ROM) in required ROM
   - Have reliable subjective/objective outcome measures to guide success
   - Patient understands when & why to stop the exercises
3. Indications of too much activity or exercise:
   - Excessive discomfort during exercise
   - Postexercise resting pain than lasts more than two hours
   - Increased weakness
   - Muscle spasm

---

postonset. Practitioners should be guided in their prescription of therapeutic exercise by the variety of subjective and objective signs found in their clinical examination. In the absence of strong evidence on specific parameters for therapeutic exercise prescription in LBP, we present a best practice approach (see Box 13.6) regarding exercise types and indications to begin and indications of excessive activity/exercise. Next we will explore the evidence supporting therapeutic exercise and the challenge of diagnosis in CTS.

13.5   THERAPEUTIC EXERCISE PRESCRIPTION IN CTS: WHERE IS THE EVIDENCE?

It is difficult to tell clinically when or where CTS starts. In the "preclinical" stage, the individual has symptoms of paresthesia with activity or prolonged positioning and some resulting restriction of hand function, but other symptoms are not yet present (MacDermid and Doherty, 2004). Because pain symptoms are low, and function is relatively unchanged, aggressive intervention is a logical and likely a cost-saving preventive measure. Therapeutic exercise prescription can be carried out with less of a caution in the preclinical stage compared to later stages when moderate or severe symptoms are present (MacDermid and Doherty, 2004). In these later stages, the experience of strong unpleasant symptoms may reinforce sensitization of the nervous system. In the preclinical stage starting with nonpainful activity and gradually increasing the intensity and frequency of the exercise would create less swelling, be more encouraging to the client, and therefore attenuate pathological responses.

In searching for best practice regarding therapeutic exercise prescription in CTS, we once again turned to recent systematic reviews. The reviewers used strict criteria that included electrodiagnostic confirmation of the CTS diagnosis, and few studies of nonsurgery, nonsteroidal CTS therapy were included (Muller et al., 2004; O'Connor et al., 2003). For example, Muller et al. (2004) accepted only 24 of the original 2027 articles. Regarding therapeutic exercise in CTS, the number of studies dropped from there. Only three exercise-based studies in CTS had sufficient quality (see Table 13.2) and provide generally "limited" or "moderate" evidence of the effectiveness of therapeutic exercise in treating CTS. The usefulness of these studies is further weakened due to the short-term nature of both the interventions and the follow-up. On a positive note, all three studies received an "A" rating for the quality of their diagnostic criteria due to their combined use of positive clinical and electrodiagnostic findings in screening for CTS subjects.

The review authors suggested a variety of reasons for the limited number of acceptable research articles. A primary issue was that therapeutic exercise studies were disadvantaged by the Cochrane scoring system (O'Connor et al., 2003), which resulted in lower quality scores because the studies did not readily lend themselves to double blinding. Another concern relates to multiple interventions—a common clinical approach. While many studies used combined therapies, none did so in a systematic, additive manner that would allow the researcher to draw specific conclusions about each individual therapy (O'Connor et al., 2003). A final concern is that, the use of "no treatment" in control groups prevented the researchers from making inferences about relative benefits of the differing therapies (Muller et al., 2004). Despite these challenges, the two systematic review papers supported the use of nerve gliding (or neuromobilizations), combined nerve and flexor tendon gliding, and yoga (Table 13.2). Next, we review each of these three approaches, in turn, beginning with nerve gliding exercises or nerve mobilizations (Shacklock, 2005).

13.5.1 NERVE MOBILIZATIONS

The concept of mobilizing the median nerves in CTS relates to its tendency to become tethered in the carpal tunnel, thereby increasing nerve tension during everyday motions that place the median nerve on stretch. Butler (1991) introduced a specific upper limb nerve tension test (ULNTT) with a median nerve bias (ULNTT2a), designed to reproduce or change the intensity/quality of existing symptoms. The ULNTT2a has been used to mobilize the median nerve in subjects with confirmed CTS and compared treatment outcomes to a control group (no treatment) and to another intervention (carpal bone mobilizations) (Tal-Akabi and Rushton, 2000). The two reviewers drew differing conclusions about Tal-Akabi and Rushton's study. O'Connor et al. (2003) stated the nerve mobilizations had no effect on symptom ratings, pain, hand function, wrist movement, ULNTT results, or the need for surgery.

TABLE 13.2

Available Evidence from Two Systematic Reviews to Support Therapeutic Exercise Prescription in CTS

CTS Exercise Approach	Research Articles	Study Details	Reviewer's Conclusions	Quality of Evidence per Two Systematic Reviews
Nerve gliding or Neuromobilization	Tal-Akabi et al. (2000)	—RCT; 3 groups: 1. Control (Ctrl) ($n = 7$) 2. Neurodynamic mobilizations—median nerve via ULNTT (Neuro-Mo) ($n = 7$) 3. Carpal bone mobilizations (Carp—Mo) ($n = 7$) —duration: 3/52 Note: ULNTT = Upper Limb Nerve Tension Test	O'Connor et al. (2003): Neuro-Mo: no significant effect on symptoms, pain, hand function, wrist active range of motion (AROM), ULNTT, or need for surgery Muller et al. (2004): Neuro-Mo had decreased pain & increased wrist AROM compared to Ctrl	O'Connor et al. (2003): —Quality: C —Bias: High —Diagnostic quality: A Muller et al. (2004) —Recommended Grade: B
Nerve & tendon gliding	Akalin et al. (2002)	—RCT; 2 groups: 1. Tendon and nerve glides (Totten and Hunter, 1991) plus splint (T&N Glide) ($n = 14$) 2. Splint only ($n = 14$) —Duration: 4/52	O'Connor et al. (2003): T&N Glide increased 2 pt discrimination > Splint (not clinically significant) Muller et al. (2004): T&N Glide increased pinch (moderate quality evidence)	O'Connor et al. (2003): —Quality: C —Bias: High —Diagnostic quality: A Muller et al. (2004) —Recommended Grade: B
Yoga	Garfinkel et al. (1998)	—RCT; 2 groups: 1. Yoga (11 yoga postures for strength, flexibility, balancing) ($n = 22$) 2. Ctrl (wrist splint only) ($n = 20$) Duration: 8/52	O'Connor et al. (2003): significant decrease in pain and Phalen's vs Ctrl Muller et al. (2004): decreased Phalen's vs Ctrl ($p < .01$)	O'Connor et al. (2003): —Quality: C —Bias: High —Diagnostic quality: A Muller et al. (2004) —Recommended Grade: B

On the other hand, Muller et al. (2004) performed a post-hoc analysis of results of Tal-Akabi and Rushton (2000) and reported that there was moderate evidence that nerve gliding had positive effects on pain and active wrist range of motion. Although pathoanatomic reasoning would support this specific therapy, more research is required to demonstrate clinical effectiveness.

13.5.2   COMBINED NERVE AND FLEXOR TENDON GLIDING

The treatment concept of mobilizing both the median nerve and the underlying finger flexor tendons (profundus and superficialis) similarly relates to their tendency to become tethered in the carpal tunnel. In this case, the nerve and tendons fail to glide differentially on each other. The pathological mechanism of tethering that includes increased intracarpal canal pressure (ICCP), friction, edema, and scarring (i.e., tethering) (Sunderland, 1991) is covered later in Section 13.6.1. In a recent randomized controlled trail (RCT), Akalin et al. (2002) compared splinting alone to a treatment of combined splinting and nerve/tendon gliding. The exercises, designed by Totten and Hunter (1991), consisted of five tendon gliding exercises (i.e., hand/wrist stretch positions) and six median nerve gliding exercises (i.e., hand/thumb/wrist stretch positions held for 5 s each). Of note, these nerve gliding exercises did not attempt to include the entire path of the median nerve (Butler, 1991). The use of a wrist splint combined with flexor tendon and median nerve mobilizations was reported to be superior to a wrist splint alone in terms of improving 2-point discrimination (O'Connor et al., 2003) and pinch grip (Muller et al., 2004). Neither reviewer found evidence to support the treatment combination regarding improved hand function or grip strength, or a decreased response to CTS provocation tests (e.g., Tinel's or Phalen's signs).

13.5.3   YOGA

In a single blind RCT, a Hatha yoga program was compared to a control group (wrist splint) over an 8-week trial. The yoga postures/positions were selected because they reportedly increased general flexibility, strength, and blood flow (Garfinkel et al., 1998). Of all the CTS exercise-based interventions, yoga received the highest ratings in the two reviews. There is Grade B evidence that yoga reduces wrist and hand pain and decreases the response to the Phalen's CTS provocation test (Muller et al., 2004; O'Connor et al., 2003).

13.5.4   SUMMARY

The evidence regarding therapeutic exercise is limited for symptom improvement with CTS (Box 13.7) (O'Connor et al., 2003). This is most likely due to the fact that studies are restricted regarding research quality (three acceptable studies) and treatment diversity (three types of therapeutic exercise). These results are also

BOX 13.7   IMPLICATIONS FOR THERAPEUTIC EXERCISE IN CTS

1. Nerve gliding using the upper limb nerve tension test with a median nerve bias (ULNTT2a) can be performed using a two-stage approach, first by a qualified health care practitioner for at least 3 weeks, then as a home self-mobilization exercise.
2. Combined nerve and flexor tendon gliding of the median nerve and flexor digitorum profundus and superficialis can be performed using the five tendon gliding and six nerve gliding exercises for at least 1 month.
3. Hatha yoga is recommended twice per week for a minimum of 8 weeks to improve general flexibility, strength, and blood flow.
4. Health care practitioners should use a broad variety of tools to measure outcomes of these exercises, including subjective signs (pain, paresthesia), hand function tests, objective tests (2-point discrimination, pinch grip, grip strength), and response to CTS provocation tests, such as Tinel's or Phalen's signs.

disappointing from a functional perspective: there is little evidence that any of the three exercise regimes that were reviewed, resulted in an improvement in function, such as gripping a tool or increasing typing endurance. We also note that other common therapeutic exercise approaches were absent. For example, is there a role for strengthening exercises in CTS? Considering the role of repetitiveness in CTS risk, is there a role for muscle imbalance interventions in CTS? We raise this point in reference to typists whose work requires a single, fixed posture of forearm pronation, wrist extension, and repetitive finger flexor work. Would stretching shortened muscles and strengthening lengthened muscles decrease typists' risk of developing CTS? Later in this chapter, we attempt to answer another question: Should CTS be treated more holistically by treating the entire kinetic chain—rather than just the wrist and hand?

In all three reviewed studies, CTS was confirmed in the subjects with electrodiagnostic testing of the median nerve. According to Wilder-Smith et al. (2006), electrodiagnostic procedures are most accurate when CTS is in the later stages. Thus, all clients in the three studies (Akalin et al., 2002; Garfinkel et al., 1998; Tal-Akabi and Ruston, 2000) likely had late stage CTS. Based on CTS neuropathology, therapeutic exercise in CTS would have been most effective in early, rather than late stage CTS (MacDermid and Doherty, 2004). As seen, however, this assertion has not been tested due to difficulties of making an early stage diagnosis for CTS. In the next section, we will present the current understanding of staging and diagnosis of CTS, making the point that the earlier in the process exercise is begun, the more likely there will be a positive impact.

13.6   CTS: DIAGNOSTIC CHALLENGE

Predisposition to CTS is associated with numerous non-MSK conditions including tumors, pregnancy, or endocrine and inflammatory conditions. Electrodiagnostic testing (nerve conduction velocity) is commonly used, however, it does not have demonstrated reliability and cannot detect the early stages of nerve compression (MacDermid and Doherty, 2004; Graham et al., 2006). Currently, there is no single test that will provide an accurate diagnosis, however a history identifying risk factors and clearly defined type and distribution of symptoms are the main elements that have contributed to an approach of clinical staging (Graham et al., 2003; MacDermid and Doherty, 2004). It is the early detection, when therapeutic exercise may be most valuable that appears to be the biggest challenge (Wilder-Smith et al., 2006).

13.6.1   NEUROPATHOLOGY OF INCREASED INTRACARPAL CANAL PRESSURE

The focus of much of the research into CTS is in regard to the local impact of increased ICCP on the median nerve. Causes of ICCP include mechanical (e.g., repetitive or forceful motions) (Werner and Armstrong, 1997; Seradge et al., 2000) or chemical (e.g., by-products of synovial inflammation) irritants (Rydevik et al., and Myers, 2001). Ischemia and intraneural edema can result from brief periods of elevated pressures (20–30 mm Hg as compared to the norm of 2.5 mm Hg (Gelberman et al., 1981; Kervin et al., 1996; Rydevik et al., 2001). When movement is added in the presence of increased ICCP, the gliding of tendons and the median nerve produce frictional or shear forces that can cause more ischemia and edema (see Box 13.8). The end result of this process is scar formation and resultant local tethering of the nerve and tendons (Rozmaryn et al., 1998).

When nerves are repeatedly subjected to pressure, cyclic ischemia and, reperfusion, they undergo oxidative injury, edema, and fiber degeneration (Nagamatsu et al., 1996; Anderson et al., 1997). Given the absence of lymphatics within a nerve bundle, the prolonged presence of edema fosters fibroblast proliferation and intraneural fibrosis (Sunderland, 1991). A worsening cycle continues as this scarring produces an irritant on its own, further reducing the size of the canal, precipitating repeated blood flow compromise, and resulting in a further reduction of nerve mobility (tethering) in the carpal tunnel. These responses to pressure are associated with the clinical presentation of CTS. The distinctive nature of this pressure → ischemia → edema → tethering cycle points to the need for an early diagnosis in CTS.

BOX 13.8.   INCREASED ICCP: IMPLICATIONS FOR THERAPEUTIC EXERCISE PRESCRIPTION

Given that ICCP will increase with repetitive flexion and extension exercises through full range when increased ICCP is suspected or known, then differential tendon and nerve gliding exercises are most appropriate.

13.6.2 Nerve Damage and Early Diagnosis

Despite considerable research, a single test to establish a clinical diagnosis of CTS remains elusive (Graham et al., 2003; MacDermid and Doherty, 2004). Current best practice suggests administering a battery of tests (Graham et al., 2003; MacDermid and Doherty, 2004) that combine local and kinetic chain tests, in conjunction with the assessment of risk factors. Local CTS tests are based on the premise that the affected sensory and motor functions of the median nerve will be detected in the hand and wrist region. The kinetic chain approach includes the application of median nerve provocation tests, such as the ULNTT (Butler, 1991; Shacklock, 2005). The weakness in using currently available test batteries, such as the CTS-7 (Graham et al., 2003), is the lack of rigorous testing regarding their sensitivity, specificity, and reliability. Regardless of which type of clinical or electrodiagnostic test is used, the major problem is that diagnosis is most accurate when CTS is at an advanced stage (Graham et al., 2003; MacDermid and Doherty, 2004; Wilder-Smith et al., 2006). By this time, CTS may not be reversible (Mackinnon, 2002) and, more importantly, clients in the late stage CTS may be less likely respond to therapeutic exercise interventions. Consequently, health care practitioners need to recognize the early stages of CTS to plan timely interventions. In looking for these early signs, we next examine the grades of peripheral nerve injury and link them to the clinical signs.

There are three grades of peripheral nerve injury, which are described in terms of progressive pathological nerve changes; each grade is associated with clinical signs and symptoms of CTS (Butler, 1996; Mackinnon, 2002; MacDermid and Doherty, 2004). As seen below, a client's chances of recovery is greatest when they are treated in the early (i.e., grade 1) stage and are reduced as the severity progresses to grade 2 and grade 3. Based on this staging process, we have set out some key clinical signs and symptoms that may assist in detecting early CTS and distinguishing it from moderate stage CTS (MacDermid and Doherty, 2004).

1. With a grade 1 injury (neuropraxia), there is nerve conduction block without axonal damage. Grade 1 corresponds to MacDermid and Doherty (2004) early (i.e., preclinical and mild) clinical stages of CTS and has excellent potential for full recovery. *Key clinical signs and symptoms*: (i) clients report altered touch and vibration thresholds or paresthesia (numbness and tingling in the median nerve distribution of the hand) that are either activity-related or in response to provocation tests (e.g., Phalen's test) (Omura et al., 2004), and wakening at night with paresthesia as symptoms progress and (ii) subtle strength and endurance deficits of thenar muscles (i.e., abductor pollicis brevis [ABP]) that may be difficult to detect.

2. With a grade 2 injury (axonotmesis), there is some axonal damage. Grade 2 corresponds to a moderate clinical stage of CTS and clients have good potential for full recovery if they reduce prolonged, repetitive hand activities (MacDermid and Doherty, 2004). *Key clinical signs and symptoms*: (i) paresthesia (numbness and tingling) that now persists beyond activities, (ii) night wakening that is a constant feature, (iii) 2-point discrimination

   is altered (i.e., increased to 5–7 mm), (iv) the likelihood of a positive Tinel's and Phalen's test is high, and (v) thenar muscle weakness (i.e., APB) is easily detected.

3. A grade 3 nerve injury features endoneurial scarring and more extensive loss of axons. Grade 3 corresponds to a severe clinical stage of CTS and has a poor chance of full recovery (MacDermid and Doherty, 2004). *Key clinical signs and symptoms*: Patients present with (i) thenar atrophy, (ii) near constant numbness, and (iii) 2-point discrimination that is further increased (i.e., >7 mm).

We know that it is too long to wait for a definitive diagnosis of CTS, so we need to look for early signs and symptoms and treat as though the client is going on to develop moderate to severe CTS. What we do not know is the direct impact of physical factors on the entire kinetic chain. We would like to suggest that looking up the kinetic chain may provide answers for early intervention.

13.7   KINETIC CHAIN APPROACH

The preceding discussion is focused on pathological changes to the median nerve from the localized perspective in the carpal tunnel. However, if we were to look beyond the local problem and explore the kinetic chain above for other potential adverse influences along the path of the median nerve, a kinetic chain approach may illuminate other therapeutic exercise options.

   To begin with, consider that the median nerve begins its descent into the upper extremity at the neck, formed by the lateral and medial cords of the brachial plexus, travels through the thoracic outlet and the upper arm, around the elbow, through the two heads of pronator teres muscle and under the transverse carpal ligament into the hand (Dutton, 2004). Normal nerve mobility in the form of longitudinal nerve sliding and elongation allows for the large varieties of movement and postures of the upper extremities and neck without impairment of nerve function (Butler, 1991; Shacklock, 2005). For example, in 90° shoulder abduction, wrist and elbow movements result in 20% elongation of the median nerve (Millesi, 1986). There are several physical factors (see Box 13.9) that can negatively influence this normal mobility. If these factors are present, they can incrementally affect nerve function and may contribute to the signs and symptoms of CTS.

13.7.1   TETHERING

The presence of these additional forces has been demonstrated in clinical studies, as well as the presence of multiple sites of compression along the median nerve. As mentioned above, tethering restricts movement, and as a nerve elongates (sometimes as little as 8%), blood flow in nerve capillaries becomes restricted (Rydevik et al., 2001). In a study of CTS clients, their median nerves exhibited up to 50% reduction in mobility. Authors have reported the coexistence of CTS with cervical radiculopathy and thoracic outlet (Massey et al., 1981; Valls-Solé et al., 1995).

> **BOX 13.9   PHYSICAL STRESSORS ON THE MEDIAN
> NERVE THAT CAN INFLUENCE NERVE MOBILITY**
>
> 1. Although the median nerve is anchored at each end, the flexibility necessary for normal movement is decreased when there is restricted movement at one point on the nerve (e.g., tethering at carpal tunnel).
> 2. Nonneutral postures (i.e., forward head posture with rounded shoulders) increase the tension of the entire nerve path by increasing the distance it must cover.
> 3. Especially in the presence of increased tension over the entire nerve, when there is additional local compression (e.g., sustained pronator teres contraction) this causes further increases in tension (rationale behind provocation tests to elicit clinical signs).

A retrospective review of 43 clients with confirmed CTS found that most had three levels of nerve compression: carpal tunnel, forearm, and thoracic outlet (Omurtag et al., 1996). On the basis of their electrodiagnostic findings, Omurtag et al. (1996) reported that in most cases, provocative compression of a single site was not sufficient to reproduce the client's symptoms. This concurs with an earlier animal study of sciatic nerve where Dellon and MacKinnon (1991) found that neurological function of sciatic nerve deteriorated rapidly when a second site of low-level compression was added proximal or distal to the primary compression site. Combining compression and tension enhances the potential for damage. These findings support the idea of the double crush (Upton and McComas, 1973) that a proximal site of median nerve compression in the neck would increase the median nerve's susceptibility to injury at a distal site, such as the carpal tunnel (Mackinnon, 1992).

These findings also support a kinetic chain framework and next we consider where and how adverse conditions are created along the median nerve that might result in CTS. By taking into account the entire nerve path, there are additional indirect ways to decrease tension on the median nerve. In doing so, we will present a two-stage kinetic chain approach to therapeutic exercise prescription for CTS. The first is to free the nerve at four anatomic sites along the kinetic chain where its mobility may be compromised. This leads to the second approach which is to then move the nerve, via nerve mobilizations.

13.7.2   Free the Nerve

In this section, we examine the four sites along the path of the median nerve where there is the highest potential for compression and or tension on the median nerve. These anatomical sites are spaces where the potential exists for compression or traction of the median nerve. We begin with the cervical intervertebral foramen (IVF) and end with the carpal tunnel itself.

13.7.2.1 Cervical Intervertebral Foramen

The five cervical nerve roots that contribute to the median nerve (C5, C6, C7, C8, and T1) exit through their respective IVF. These roots are vulnerable to compression forces, if the IVFs are decreased in size, as naturally occurs when the neck is extended (Porterfield and DeRosa, 1995). These same roots are vulnerable to tension (i.e., traction forces) when the nerve roots are drawn out of the IVFs during normal cervical flexion movements (Porterfield and DeRosa, 1995). In rehabilitation ergonomics, a situation exists where regions of the neck are differentially and simultaneously flexed and extended. We refer here to forward head posture (FHP). FHP is a head-on-trunk misalignment and is described (in sitting or standing) as the excessive anterior positioning of the head in relation to a vertical reference line, accompanied by increased lower cervical spine flexion, increased middle cervical spine extension, and rounded shoulders with thoracic kyphosis (McKenzie, 1983; Cailliet, 1988; Braun and Amundson, 1989). Thus, the implications for the median nerve are that its upper roots may experience compression (in extension) and its lower roots may experience traction (in flexion)—beyond what the roots would experience in a neutral upright posture (Shacklock, 2005). Adding to this issue is the fact that during many seated work tasks, FHPs are maintained for prolonged periods (Harman et al., 2003)—thus adding to the risk of nerve irritation.

FHP is associated with weakness in the deep cervical short flexor muscles and mid-thoracic scapular retractors (i.e., rhomboids, serratus anterior, middle and lower fibers of the trapezius) and shortening of the opposing cervical extensors and pectoralis muscles (known as the upper crossed postural syndrome) (McKenzie, 1983; Darling et al., 1984; Cailliet, 1988; Kendall et al., 1993; Janda, 1994; Magee, 1997). Health care practitioners target this head-on-trunk misalignment with corrective exercises to stretch short muscles and strengthen lengthened muscles (Darling et al., 1984; Abdulwahab and Sabbahi, 2000; Wright et al., 2000). A recent study demonstrated that a simple, targeted exercise program in asymptomatic subjects with FHP can modify postural alignment (Harman et al., 2005). The program consisted of two strengthening (deep cervical flexors and shoulder retractors) and two stretching (cervical extensors and pectoral muscles) exercises. Asymptomatic subjects who performed these four exercises for 10 weeks, demonstrated improvements in their postural alignment, such that—among other things—upper cervical extension and lower cervical flexion were reduced (Harman et al., 2005). In closing, we see that the kinetic chain approach of freeing the median nerve starts by moving the client to a more neutral, upright head and neck posture with the following two postural alignment goals in mind. The first is to potentially decrease compression on the upper median nerve roots by opening the upper IVFs through decreased extension in the upper cervical spine. The second is to potentially decrease tension in the lower median nerve roots by decreasing traction on the roots through decreased flexion in the lower cervical spine.

13.7.2.2 Thoracic Outlet

Next down the kinetic chain is the thoracic outlet, bound by the first rib, clavicle, the superior border of the scapula and the scalene muscles. As the brachial plexus passes through this outlet, the medial and lateral cords of the median nerve may become compressed when the outlet size is mechanically reduced by either a dynamic or a static force. Dynamic (i.e., muscular) reduction in the outlet size can occur with increased tone in muscles that the plexus cords pass between (i.e., anterior and posterior scalenes) or under (e.g., pectoralis minor). These hypertonic muscles can be treated with myofascial release techniques and stretching (Hall and Brody, 1999). Static reduction in the outlet can occur with postural adaptations that result in forward (i.e., rounded) shoulders, often accompanied by FHP (Dutton, 2004; Pecina et al., 1997). Prolonged exposure to these static postural adaptations "closes" the thoracic outlet by decreasing the available space between the clavicle and the first rib. These forward head and forward shoulder adaptations are the result of muscle imbalances, such that several muscles are adaptively shortened and require stretching (i.e., scalenes, subclavius, pectoralis major and minor, sternocleidomastoid), while some muscles that "open" the thoracic outlet are found to be weak (e.g., middle and upper trapezius, serratus anterior) (Dutton, 2004). These muscle imbalances are treated by lengthening the shortened muscles and strengthening the weak muscles. Finally, since forward head and forward shoulder postures frequently co-occur in seated typing tasks (Harman et al., 2003), the kinetic chain approach to freeing the median nerve should also include ergonomic interventions to improve working postures to avoid those postural mal-adaptations that "close" the outlet.

13.7.2.3 Two Heads of Pronator Teres Muscle

At the elbow, the median nerve passes between the humeral and ulnar heads of the pronator teres muscle. Here, the nerve is vulnerable to static pressure from tethering due to fibrous connective tissue bands from the lacertus fibrosus (Spinner, 1978). Treatment would include median nerve mobilizations via the ULNTT (Butler, 1991). The median nerve is also vulnerable in this interval via dynamic (i.e., muscular) compression. This could occur during repeated forearm supination and pronation movements or during sustained work with the forearm held in pronation by pronator teres muscle activity (Pecina et al., 1997). Researchers have recently demonstrated that during wrist extension activities, pronator teres must cocontract with the wrist extensor muscles to counteract forearm supination (Fujii et al., 2007). As such, typing—a very common work task—would require constant low-level contraction of pronator teres. This dynamic compression of pronator teres can be treated by stretching the muscle and reducing the aggravating work postures (Dutton, 2004).

13.7.2.4 Carpal Tunnel

The carpal tunnel—created by the carpal bones on three sides—has the flexor retinaculum for a roof and the palmar carpal ligament for a floor. In addition to activating pronator teres, wrist extension physically "closes" the carpal tunnel (Werner and Armstrong, 1997). The carpal bones glide in a palmar direction, move into the carpal tunnel, and cause the tunnel contents to be compressed between the flexor retinaculum and the carpal bones (Werner and Armstrong, 1997). In normal (i.e., healthy) wrists, this palmar glide with tunnel compression results in a transient increase in ICCP and a transient increase in pressure on the median nerve. Mechanically, ICCP pressure could be reduced by two treatment approaches: reducing the palmar carpal glide or increasing the extensibility of the flexor retinaculum (Tal-Akabi and Rushton, 2000). Reducing the palmar glide is accomplished by changing movement patterns in other carpal bones. In multijoint complexes like the wrist, excessive movement in one (or more) joints is often due to reduced movement in one or more other joints. Thus, if the palmar carpal glide is excessive, treatment may consist of increasing the movement of other wrist articulations with anterior–posterior joint mobilizations (Tal-Akabi and Rushton, 2000). In terms of the flexor retinaculum, ICCP may be reduced by stretching the ligament using a 3-point opposing pressure maneuver (Sucher and Glassman, 1996). There is moderate evidence that carpal mobilizations combined with 3-point flexor retinaculum stretches reduce CTS symptoms (Tal-Akabi and Rushton, 2000; O'Connor et al., 2003). Assuming the physical barriers/constraints that reduce nerve movement are treated, the nerve is now ready to be mobilized (i.e., moved).

13.7.3   MOVE THE NERVE

Here we assume that the four sites of neural tension mentioned above have been addressed through stretching, strengthening, and posture correction. In conjunction with those therapeutic exercises, the health care practitioner can address the issue of nerve mobility. Alterations in neural tension of the median nerve can be detected using the ULNTT (Butler, 1991). This test has also been described in the context of a treatment. To perform the ULNTT, the examiner puts tensile stresses on specific nerve roots and peripheral nerves (e.g., median nerve) by moving the upper extremity joints in a logical, sequential pattern for the purpose of reproducing the patient's symptoms and signs (Shacklock, 2005). In an extensive review of the ULNTT, Walsh (2005) reported support for its scientific validity and intrarater reliability, but cautioned that the inter-rater reliability was essentially untested. Length/tension alterations in the median nerve can also be treated using the ULNTT as a technique to mobilize the tethered median nerve by repeating the specific movements of the ULNTT that reproduced the client's signs and symptoms. Results are promising for CTS. In a randomized control study, Rozmaryn et al. (1998) found that patients treated with standard CTS care plus ULNTT procedures specific to the carpal tunnel ($n = 93$) had a significantly reduced need for surgical decompression compared to the standard CTS care control group ($n = 104$). A variant of the ULNTT has also been successfully used as a preventative measure for CTS in production line workers ($n = 286$). In the first year following the inception of the prevention program, Seradge et al. (2000) reported a 45.4% reduction in the incidence of CTS.

13.8 SUMMARY AND CONCLUSIONS

Therapeutic exercise is the foundation for the successful rehabilitation of MSK dysfunction. Despite that, in LBP and CTS—the two MSK conditions most prone to chronicity—there is limited evidence of the effectiveness of therapeutic exercise. The many reviewers cited in this chapter acknowledge numerous reasons for this finding and most related to poor study quality. We argued that two other reasons may have contributed to these limited results regarding therapeutic exercise. The first relates to pain. Here we suggest that the challenge for health care practitioners in prescribing therapeutic exercises was to consider, among other things, the combination of the neurophysiological response to a painful stimulus (sensitization), the psychological response (catastrophizing), and the behavioral response (avoidance). The second reason relates to the diagnosis and staging of LBP and CTS. Here we suggest that traditional pathomechanic diagnosis of LBP is not very instructive for therapeutic exercise prescription and should be replaced with a pathomechanic approach. We further note that exercise prescription in CTS could be enhanced by taking a kinetic chain approach to the entire median nerve, rather than focusing on the carpal tunnel. In terms of staging, we found evidence that tissue-based and function-based methods of staging LBP and CTS are more instructive than time-based methods when prescribing therapeutic exercises in these conditions. We further suggest that the subacute phase of LBP and the preclinical stage of CTS are the optimal time to prescribe therapeutic exercises.

In the LBP literature, there was moderate evidence to support the use of a graded approach, some specific exercises, group exercises in the later stages of the subacute phase and for multidisciplinary approaches (including exercises) for clients who have been identified as high risk for persistence. Interestingly, each of these four types of exercise interventions used elements of psychological theory, further strengthening our hypothesis regarding the role of pain psychology in therapeutic exercise prescription. In the CTS literature, only three studies met review standards and in these, reviewers found limited to moderate evidence to support only three types of therapeutic exercise: nerve mobilizations, combined nerve and tendon gliding, and yoga. Interestingly, these three types of exercises are based on a kinetic chain approach.

In closing, we acknowledge that our recommendations are somewhat limited in generalizabilty because we focused exclusively on two MSK conditions. However, by opting to focus on LBP and CTS, we chose the two MSK conditions that were the most difficult and expensive to treat. We would urge health practitioners to use this model and take a critical analysis approach toward therapeutic exercise prescription in other MSK conditions, injuries, and dysfunctions.

REFERENCES

Abdulwahab, S. and Sabbahi, M. 2000. Neck retractions, cervical root decompression, and radicular pain. *Journal of Orthopaedic and Sports Physical Therapy*, 30, 4–9.
Abenhaim, L., Rossignol, M., Gobeille, D., Bonvalot, Y., Fines, P., and Scott, S. 1995. The prognostic consequences in the making of the initial medical diagnosis of work-related back injuries. *Spine*, 20, 791–795.

Abenhaim, L., Rossignol, M., Valat, J. -P., Nordin, M., Avouac, B., Blotman, F., Charlot, J., Dreiser, R. L., Legrand, E., Rozenberg, S., and Vautravers, P. 2005. The role of activity in the therapeutic management of back pain: Report of the International Paris Task Force on Back Pain. *Spine*, 25, 1S–31S.

Accident Compensation Corporation 2004. *New Zealand Acute Low Back Pain Guide; Incorporating the Guide to Assessing Psychosocial Yellow Flags in Acute Low Back Pain* (http://www.acc.no.nz/DIS_EXT_CSMP/groups/external_ip/documents/internet/wcm002131.pdf). Wellington, New Zealand: Accident Compensation Corporation.

Akalin, L., El, O., Senocak, O., Tamci, S., Gulbahar, S., Cakmur, R., and Oncel, S. 2002. Treatment of carpal tunnel syndrome with nerve and tendon gliding exercises. *American Journal of Physical Medicine*, 81, 108–113.

American College of Sports Medicine 2006. *ACSM's Guidelines for Exercise Testing and Prescription* (7th ed.). Philadelphia, PA: Lippincott Williams & Wilkins.

American Physical Therapy Association 2001. Guide to physical therapist practice. *Physical Therapy*, 81, 9–744.

Anderson, G., Nukada, H., and McMorran, P. 1997. Carbonyl histochemistry in rat reperfusion nerve injury. *Brain Research*, 772, 156–160.

Arnstein, P. M. 1997. The neuroplastic phenomenon: A physiologic link between chronic pain and learning. *Journal of Neuroscience Nursing*, 29, 179–186.

Bigos, S., Bowyer, O., and Braen, G. 1994. *Acute Low Back Problems in Adults (Rep. No. 95–0643)*. Rockville, MD: U.S. Department of Health and Human Services, Public Health Service, Agency for Health Care Policy and Research.

Boersma, K. and Linton, S. 2006. Expectancy, fear and pain in the prediction of chronic pain and disability: A prospective analysis. *European Journal of Pain*, 10, 551–557.

Braun, B. and Amundson, L. 1989. Quantitative assessment of head and shoulder posture. *Archives of Physical Medicine & Rehabilitation*, 70, 322–329.

Buckwalter, J. A. 1996. Effects of early motion on healing of musculoskeletal tissues. *Hand Clinics*, 12, 13–24.

Burton, A. K., Tillotson, K. M., Main, C. J., and Hollis, S. 1995. Psychosocial predictors of outcome in acute and subchronic low back trouble. *Spine*, 20, 722–728.

Butler, D. S. 1991. *Mobilisation of the Nervous System*. Melbourne: Churchill Livingstone.

Butler, D. S. 1996. Nerve: Structure, function and physiology. In J. Zachazewski, D. Magee, and W. Quillen (Eds.), *Athletic Injuries and Rehabilitation* (pp. 170–185). Philadelphia, PA: WB Saunders Co.

Byl, N. and Merzenich, M. (2001). Principles of neuroplasticity: Implications for neurorehabilitation and learning. In E. Gonzalez, S. Myers, J. Edelstein, J. Lieberman, and J. Downey (Eds.), *Downey and Darling's Physiological Basis of Rehabilitation Medicine* (3rd ed., pp. 609–628). Boston, MA: Butterworth Heinemann.

Cailliet, R. 1988. *Neck and Arm Pain. In Soft Tissue Pain and Disability* (2nd ed., pp. 123–169). Philadelphia, PA: F.A. Davis Company.

Campbell, J., Raja, S., Meyer, R., and Mackinnon, S. 1988. Myelinated afferents signal the hyperalgesia associated with nerve injury. *Pain*, 32, 89–94.

Chan, L., Turner, J. A., Comstock, B., Levenson, L., Hollingworth, W., Heagerty, P., Kliot, M., and Jarvik, J. 2007. The relationship between electrodiagnostic findings and patient symptoms and function in carpal tunnel syndrome. *Archives of Physical Medicine & Rehabilitation*, 88, 19–24.

Cherkin, D., Deyo, R. A., Battié, M. C., Street, J., and Barlow, W. 1998. A comparison of physical therapy, chiropractic manipulation, and provision of an educational booklet for the treatment of patients with low back pain. *New England Journal of Medicine*, 339, 1021–1030.

Coderre, T. J., Katz, J., Vaccarino, A. L., and Melzack, R. 1993. Contribution of central neuroplasticity to pathological pain: Review of clinical and experimental evidence. *[Review]. Pain*, 52, 259–285.

Constantine-Paton, M. 2000. The plastic brain. *Neurobiology of Disease*, 7, 515–519.

Cotman, C. W. and Berchtold, N. 2002. Exercise: A behavioural intervention to enhance brain health and plasticity. *Trends in Neuroscience*, 25, 295–301.

Crossman, M., Gilbert, C., Travlos, A., Craig, K. D., and Eisen, A. 2001. Nonneurologic hand pain versus carpal tunnel syndrome: Do psychological measures differentiate? *American Journal of Medicine and Rehabilitation*, 80, 100–107.

Darling, D., Kraus, S., and Glasheen-Wray, M. 1984. Relationship of head posture and rest position of mandible. *The Journal of Prosthetic Dentistry*, 52, 111–115.

Delitto, A., Erhard, R., and Bowling, R. 1995. A treatment-based classification approach to low back pain syndrome: Identifying and staging patients for conservative treatment. *Physical Therapy*, 75, 470–489.

Dellon, A. and Mackinnon, S. 1991. Chronic nerve compressions model for the double crush hypothesis. *Annals of Plastic Surgery*, 26, 259–264.

DeRosa, C. P. and Porterfield, J. A. 1992. A physical therapy model for the treatment of low back pain. *Physical Therapy*, 72, 21–32.

Dutton, M. (2004). Manual techniques. In M. Brown and K. Davis (Eds.), *Orthopedic Examination, Evaluation, and Intervention* (pp. 322–356). New York: McGraw-Hill.

Fordyce, W. E. 1974. Pain viewed as a learned behaviour. *Advances in Neurology*, 4, 415–422.

Friedrich, M., Gittler, G., Halberstadt, Y., Cermak, T., and Heiller, I. 1998. Combined exercise and motivation program: Effect on the compliance and level of disability of patients with chronic low back pain: A randomized controlled trial. *Archives of Physical Medicine & Rehabilitation*, 79, 475–487.

Fritz, J. and George, S. 2000. The use of a classification approach to identify subgroups of patients with acute low back pain. *Spine*, 25, 106–114.

Fujii, H., Kobayashi, S., Sato, T., Shinozaki, K., and Naito, A. 2007. Co-contraction of the pronator teres and extensor carpi radialis during wrist extension movements in humans. *Journal of Electromyography and Kinesiology*, 17, 80–89.

Garfinkel, M., Singhal, A., Katz, W., Allan, D., Reshetar, R., and Schumacher, R. 1998. Yoga-based intervention for carpal tunnel syndrome: A randomized trial. *Journal of the American Medical Association*, 280, 1601–1608.

Gelberman, R., Hergenroeder, P., and Hargens, A. 1981. The carpal tunnel syndrome. A study of caarpal canal pressures. *Journal of Bone and Joint Surgery (American)*, 63, 380–383.

George, S., Fritz, J., Bialosky, J., and Donald, D. 2003. The effect of a fear-avoidance-based physical therapy intervention for patients with acute low back pain: Results of a randomized clinical trial. *Spine*, 28, 2551–2560.

Graham, B., Regehr, G., Naglie, G., and Wright, J. 2006. Development and validation of diagnostic criteria for carpal tunnel syndrome. *Journal of Hand Surgery*, 31A, 919. e1–919.e7.

Graham, B., Regehr, G., and Wright, J. 2003. Delphi as a method to establish consensus for diagnostic criteria. *Journal of Clinical Epidemiology*, 56, 1150–1156.

Hall, C. and Brody, L. 1999. *Therapeutic Exercise: Moving Toward Function*. Philadelphia, PA: Lippincott Williams & Wilkins.

Hansen, F. R., Bendix, T., Skov, P., Jensen, C. V., Dristensen, J. H., Krohn, L., and Schioeler, H. 1993. Intensive, dynamic back-muscle exercises, conventional physiotherapy, or placebo-control treatment of low-back pain: A randomized, observer-blind trial. *Spine*, 18, 98–108.

Harman, K., Hubley-Kozey, C., and Butler, H. 2005. Effectiveness of an exercise program to improve forward head posture in normal adults: A randomized, controlled 10-week trial. *The Journal of Manual & Manipulative Therapy*, 13, 163–176.

Harman, K., Putnam, C., Fenety, A., Tingley, M., McClellan, A., and Crouse, J. 2003. A new dynamic method to measure sitting behaviour: The effect of a stressful typing task on head, neck and shoulder angles. In *IEA Conference*, Seoul, Korea.

Harman, K. and Ruyak, P. 2005. Working through the pain: A controlled study of the impact of chronic pain on performing a computer task. *Clinical Journal of Pain* 21(3):216–222.

Hayden, J., van Tulder, M., Malmivaara, A., and Koes, B. 2005. Meta-analysis: Exercise therapy for nonspecific low back pain. *Annals of Internal Medicine*, 142, 765–775.

Hertling, D. and Kessler, R. (1996). Assessment of musculoskeletal disorders and concepts of management. In D. Hertling and R. Kessler (Eds.), *Management of Common Musculoskeletal Disorders: Physical Therapy Principles and Methods* (3rd ed., pp. 69–111). Philadelphia, PA: Lippincott.

Hobby, J., Venkatesh, R., and Motkur, P. 2005. The effect of psychological disturbance on symptoms, self-reported disability and surgical outcome in carpal tunnel syndrome. *The Journal of Bone and Joint Surgery*, 87-B, 196–200.

Janda, V. 1994. Muscles and motor control in cervicogenic disorders: Assessment and management. In R. Grant (Ed.), *Physical Therapy of the Cervical and Thoracic Spine,* New York: Churchill Livingstone.

Johansson, B. 2004. Brain plasticity in health and disease. *Keio Journal of Medicine*, 53, 231–246.

Kamath, V. and Stothard, J. 2003. A clinical questionnaire for the diagnosis of carpal tunnel syndrome. *Journal of Hand Surgery*, 28, 455–459.

Karjalainen, K., Malmivaara, A., van Tulder, M., Roine, R., Jauhiainen, M., Hurri, H., and Koes, B. 2001. Multidisciplinary biopsychosocial rehabilitation for subacute low back pain in working-age adults: A systematic review within the framework of the Cochrane Collaboration Back Review Group. *Spine*, 26, 262–269.

Katz, J. N. and Stirrat, C. 1990. A self-administered hand diagram for the diagnosis of carpal tunnel syndrome. *Journal of Hand Surgery*, 15, 360–363.

Keefe, F., Brown, G. K., Wallston, K. A., and Caldwell, D. 1989. Coping with rheumatoid arthritis pain: Catastrophizing as a maladaptive strategy. *Pain*, 37, 51–56.

Kellett, K., Kellett, D., and Nordholm, L. 1991. Effects of an exercise program on sick leave due to back pain. *Physical Therapy*, 71, 283–293.

Kendall, F., Kendall McCreary, E., and Provance, P. 1993. *Muscles: Testing and Function* (4th ed.). Baltimore, MD: Williams & Wilkins.

Kervin, G., Williams, C., and Seiller, J. I. 1996. The pathophysiology of carpal tunnel syndrome. *Hand Clinics*, 12, 243–251.

Kisner, C. and Colby, L. 2002. *Therapeutic Exercise: Foundations and Techniques* (4th ed.). Philadelphia, PA: F.A. Davis Company.

Koumantakis, G., Watson, P., and Oldham, J. 2005. Trunk muscle stabilization training plus general exercise versus general exercise only: Randomized controlled trial of patients with recurrent low back pain. *Physical Therapy*, 85, 209–225.

Lethem, J., Slade, P. D., Troup, J. D., and Bentley, G. 1983. Outline of a fear-avoidance model of exaggerated pain perception. *Behaviour Research & Therapy*, 21, 401–408.

Lindström, I., Öhlund, C., Eek, C., Wallin, L., Peterson, L., Fordyce, W. E., and Nachemson, A. 1992a. The effect of graded activity on patients with subacute low back pain: A randomized prospective clinical study with an operant-conditioning behavioural approach. *Physical Therapy*, 72, 279–293.

Lindström, I., Öhlund, C., Eek, C., Wallin, L., Peterson, L., and Nachemson, A. 1992b. Mobility, strength and fitness after a graded activity program for patients with subacute low back pain: A randomized prospective clinical study with a behavioural therapy approach. *Spine*, 17, 641–652.

Lindström, I., Öhlund, C., and Nachemson, A. 1995. Physical performance, pain, pain behaviour and subjective disability in patients with subacute low back pain. *Scandinavian Journal of Rehabilitation Medicine*, 27, 153–160.

Linton, S. and Ryberg, M. 2001. A cognitive-behavioral group intervention as prevention for persistent neck and back pain in a non-patient population: A randomized controlled trial. *Pain*, 90, 83–90.

Loisel, P., Abenhaim, L., Durand, P., Esdaile, J. M., Suissa, S., Gosselin, L., Simard, R., Turcotte, J., and Lemaire, J. 1997. A population-based, randomized clinical trial on back pain management. *Spine*, 22, 2911–2918.

MacDermid, J. and Doherty, T. 2004. Clinical and electrodiagnostic testing of carpal tunnel syndrome: A narrative review. *Journal of Orthopaedic and Sports Physical Therapy*, 34, 565–588.

Mackinnon, S. 1992. Double and multiple "crush" syndromes: Double and multiple entrapment neuropathies. *Hand Clinics*, 8, 369–390.

Mackinnon, S. 2002. Pathophysiology of nerve compression. *Hand Clinics*, 18, 231–241.

Magee, D. 1997. *Orthopedic Physical Assessment* (3rd ed.). Philadelphia, PA: W.B. Saunders Company.

Mao, J. 2002. Translational pain research: Bridging the gap between basic and clinical research. *Pain*, 97, 183–187.

Massey, E., Riley, T., and Pleet, B. 1981. Coexistent carpal tunnel syndrome and cervical radiculopathy (double crush syndrome). *Southern Medical Journal*, 74, 957–959.

McKenzie, R. 1981. *The Lumbar Spine: Mechnical Diagnosis and Therapy*. Waikanae: Spinal Publications Limited.

McKenzie, R. 1983. *Treat Your Own Neck*. Waikanae: Spinal Publications New Zealand, Ltd.

Melzack, R., Coderre, T. J., Katz, J., and Vaccarino, A. L. 2001. Central neuroplasticity and pathological pain. *Annals of the New York Academy of Sciences*, 933, 157–174.

Merskey, H., Bond, M. R., and Boyd, D. 1994. *Classification of Chronic Pain: Descriptions of Chronic Pain Syndrome and Definitions of Pain Terms*. H. Merskey and N. Bogduk (Eds.) (2nd ed., pp. 1–215). Seattle, WA: IASP Press.

Millesi, H. 1986. The nerve gap: Theory and clinical practice. *Hand Clinics*, 4, 651–663.

Moffett, J., Togerson, D., Vell-Syer, S., Jackson, D., Llewlyn-Phillips, H., Farrin, A., and Barber, J. 1999. Randomised controlled trial of exercise for low back pain: Clinical outcomes, costs, and preferences. *British Medical Journal*, 319, 279–283.

Muller, M., Tsui, D., Schnurr, R., Biddulph-Deisroth, L., and Hard, J. 2004. Effectiveness of hand therapy interventions in primary management of carpal tunnel syndrome: A systematic review. *Journal of Hand Therapy*, 17, 210–228.

Nagamatsu, M., Schmelzer, J., Zollman, P., Smithson, I., Nickander, K., and Low, P. A. 1996. Ischemic reperfusion causes lipid peroxidation and fiber degeneration. *Muscle & Nerve*, 19, 37–47.

Nathan, P., Meadows, K., and Istvan, J. 2002. Predictors of carpal tunnel syndrome: An 11-year study of industrial workers. *The Journal of Hand Surgery*, 27A, 644–651.

Nora, D., Becker, J., Ehlers, J., and Gomes, I. 2005. What symptoms are truly caused by median nerve compression in carpal tunnel syndrome? *Clinical Neurophysiology*, 116, 275–283.

O'Connor, D., Marshall, S., and Massey-Westropp, N. 2003. Non-surgical treatment (other than steroid injection) for carpal tunnel syndrome (Review). *The Cochrane Library*, 7.

Omura, T., Sano, M., Omura, K., Haseqawa, T., and Naqano, A. 2004. A mild acute compressions induces neuraprazia in rat sciatic nerve. *International Journal of Neuroscience*, 114, 1561–1572.

Omurtag, M., Novak, C., and Mackinnon, S. 1996. Multiple level nerve compression is frequently unrecognized. *Canadian Journal of Plastic Surgery*, 4, 165–167.

Pecina, M., Krmpotic-Nemnic, J., and Markiewitz, A. 1997. *Tunnel Syndromes: Peripheral Nerve Compression Syndromes* (2nd ed.). Boca Raton, FL: CRC Press.

Pengel, H., Maher, C., and Refshauge, K. 2002a. Systematic review of conservative interventions for subacute low back pain. *Pain Reviews*, 9, 153–163.

Pengel, H., Maher, C., and Refshauge, K. 2002b. Systematic review of conservative interventions for subacute low back pain. *Clinical Rehabilitation*, 16, 811–820.

Philadelphia Panel 2001. Philadelphia panel evidence-based clinical practice guidelines on selected rehabilitation interventions for low back pain. *Physical Therapy*, 81, 1641–1674.

Picavet, S., Vlaeyen, J., and Schouten, J. 2002. Pain catastrophizing and kinesiophobia: Predictors of chronic low back pain. *American Journal of Epidemiology*, 156, 1028–1034.

Porterfield, J. A. and DeRosa, C. P. 1995. Neurophysiological implications of mechanical neck pain. In *Mechanical Neck Pain: Perspectives in Functional Anatomy* (pp. 21–46). Philadelphia, PA: W.B. Saunders.

Porterfield, J. A. and DeRosa, C. P. 1998. *Mechanical Low Back Pain: Perspectives in Functional Anatomy* (2nd ed.). Philadelphia, PA: W.B. Saunders.

Rackwitz, B., de Bie, R., Ewert, T., and Stucki, G. 2006. Segmental stabilizing exercises and low back pain. What is the evidence? A systematic review of randomized controlled trials. *Clinical Rehabilitation*, 20, 553–567.

Rose, C., Wallace, L., Dickson, R., Ayres, J., Lehman, R., Searle, Y., and Burge, P. 2002. The most effective psychologically-based treatments to reduce anxiety and panic in patients with chronic obstructive pulmonary disease (COPD): A systematic review. *Patient Education and Counseling*, 47, 311–318.

Rozmaryn, L., Dovelle, S., Rothman, E., Gorman, K., Olvey, K., and Bartko, J. 1998. Nerve and tendon gliding exercises and the conservative management of carpal tunnel syndrome. *Journal of Hand Therapy*, 11, 171–179.

Rydevik, B., Lundborg, G., Olmarker, K., and Myers, R. (2001). Biomechanics of peripheral nerves and spinal nerve roots. In M. Nordin and V. Frankel (Eds.), *Basic Biomechanics of the Musculoskeletal System* (3rd ed., pp. 126–146). Philadelphia, PA: Lippincott Williams & Wilkins.

Salter, R., Simmonds, D., Malcolm, B., Rumble, E., Macmichael, D., and Clements, N. 1980. The biological effects of continuous passive motion on the healing of full thickness defects in articular cartilage: An experimental investigation in the rabbit. *Journal of Bone and Joint Surgery*, 62A, 1232–1251.

Seradge, H., Bear, C., and Bithell, D. 2000. Preventing carpal tunnel syndrome and cumulative trauma disorder: Effect of carpal tunnel decompression exercises—an Oklahoma experience. *Journal of Oklahoma State Medical Association*, 93, 150–153.

Shacklock, M. 2005. *Clinical Neurodynamics: A New System of Musculoskeletal Treatment*. Edinburgh: Elsevier.

Spinner, M. 1978. *Injuries to the Major Branches of Peripheral Nerves of the Forearm* (2nd ed.). Philadelphia, PA: W.B. Saunders.

Staal, J., Hlobil, H., Twisk, J., Smid, T., Köke, A., and van Mechelen, W. 2004. Graded activity for low back pain in occupational health care: A randomized, controlled trial. *Annals of Internal Medicine*, 140, 77–84.

Storheim, K., Brox, J., Holm, I., Koller, A., and Bo, K. 2003. Intensive group training versus cognitive intervention in sub-acute low back pain: Short-term results of a single-blind randomized controlled trial. *Journal of Rehabilitation Medicine*, 35, 132–140.

Sucher, B. and Glassman, J. 1996. Upper extremity syndromes. *Physical Medicine and Rehabilitation Clinics of North America*, 7, 787–810.

Sullivan, M., Bishop, S., and Pivik, J. 1995. The pain catastrophizing scale: Development and validation. *Psychological Assessment*, 7, 524–532.

Sullivan, M., Rodgers, W., Wilson, P., Bell, G., Murray, T., and Fraser, S. 2002. An experimental investigation of the relation between catastrophizing and activity intolerance. *Pain*, 100, 47–53.

Sunderland, S. 1991. *Nerve Injuries and their Repair: A Critical Appraisal*. Edinburgh: Churchill-Livingston.

Tal-Akabi, A. and Rushton, A. 2000. An investigation to compare the effectiveness of carpal bone mobilization and neurodynamic mobilization as methods of treatment for carpal tunel syndrome. *Manual Therapy*, 5, 214–222.

Totten, P. and Hunter, J. 1991. Therapeutic techniques to enhance nerve gliding in thoracic outlet syndrome and carpal tunnel syndrome. *Hand Clinics*, 11, 171–179.

Turk, D. and Okifuji, A. (1998). Behavioural management of patients with pain. In G.M. Aronoff (Ed.), *Evaluation and Treatment of Chronic Pain Patients* (2nd ed., pp. 323–333). Baltimore, MD: Williams and Wilkins.

Upton, A. and McComas, A. 1973. The double crush in nerve entrapment syndromes. *Lancet*, 2, 359–362.

Valls-Solé, J., Alvarez, R., and Nunez, M. 1995. Limited longitudinal sliding of the median nerve in patients with carpal tunnel syndrome. *Muscle & Nerve*, 18, 761–767.

Vlaeyen, J. (2003). Fear in musculoskeletal pain. In J. O. Dostrovsky, D. Carr, and M. Koltzenburg (Eds.), *Progress in Pain Research and Management* (pp. 631–650). Seattle, WA: IASP Press.

Vlaeyen, J., de Jong, J., Geilen, M., Heuts, P., and van Breukelen, F. 2002. The treatment of fear of movement/(re)injury in chronic low back pain: Further evidence on the effectiveness of exposure in vivo. *Clinical Journal of Pain*, 18, 251–261.

Vlaeyen, J., de Jong, J., Onghena, P., Kerckhoffs-Hanssen, M., and Kole-Snijders, A. 2002. Can pain-related fear be reduced? The application of cognitive-behavioural exposure in vivo. *Pain Research & Management*, 7, 144–153.

Vlaeyen, J., Kole-Snijders, A., Boeren, R., and Van Eck, H. 1995. Fear of movement/(re) injury in chronic low back pain and its relation to behavioural performance. *Pain*, 62, 363–372.

Vlaeyen, J. and Linton, S. 2000. Fear-avoidance and its consequences in chronic musculoskeletal pain: A state of the art. *Pain*, 85, 317–332.

Waddell, G. 1998. *The Back Pain Revolution*. Toronto: Churchill Livingstone.

Waddell, G., Feder, G., McIntosh, A., Lewis, M., and Hutchinson, A. 1996. *Low Back Pain Evidence Review*. London: Royal College of General Practitioners.

Waddell, G., Newton, M., Henderson, I., Somerville, D., and Main, C. J. 1993. A Fear-Avoidance Beliefs Questionnaire (FABQ) and the role of fear-avoidance beliefs in chronic low back pain and disability. *Pain*, 52, 157–168.

Wall, P. D. 1990. [Editorial] Neuropathic pain. *Pain*, 43, 267–268.

Walsh, M. 2005. Upper limb neural tension testing and mobilization: Fact, fiction and a practical approach. *Muscle & Nerve*, 18, 761–767.

Watson, P. and Kendall, N. (2000). Assessing psychosocial yellow flags. In L.S. Gifford (Ed.), *Biopsychosocial Assessment and Management; Relationships and Pain* (pp. 111–130). Cornwall, UK: Rowe the Printers.

Werner, R. and Armstrong, T. 1997. Carpal tunnel syndrome: Ergonomic risk factors and intracarpal canal pressure. *Physical Medicine and Rehabilitation Clinics of North America*, 8, 555–569.

Wijhuizen, G., de Jong, R., and Hopman-Rock, M. 2006. Older persons afraid of falling reduce physical activity to prevent outdoor falls. *Preventive Medicine* 44(3): 260–264.

Wilder-Smith, E., Seet, R., and Lim, E. 2006. Diagnosing carpal tunnel syndrome—clinical criteria and ancillary tests. *National Clinical Practice in Neurology*, 2, 366–374.

Woolf, C. J. and Salter, M. 2000. Neuronal plasticity: Increasing the gain in pain. *Science*, 288, 1765–1768.

Wright, A. (2002). Neurophysiology of pain and pain modulation. In J. Strong, A. Unruh, A. Wright, and G. Baxter (Eds.), *Pain: A Textbook for Therapists* (pp. 43–64). Edinburgh: Churchill Livingstone.

Wright, E., Domenech, M., and Fischer, J. 2000. Usefulness of posture training for patients with temporomandibular disorders. *Journal of American Dental Association*, 131, 202–210.

You, H., Simmons, Z., Freivalds, A., Kothari, M., Naidu, S., and Young, R. 2004. The development of risk assessment models for carpal tunnel syndrome: A case-referent study. *Ergonomics*, 47, 688–709.

14 Effective Utilization of Assistive Devices in the Workplace

Desleigh de Jonge and Libby Gibson

CONTENTS

14.1 WORKPLACE ACCOMMODATION

One of the essential requirements of the American Disabilities Act (ADA) is that employers make reasonable accommodations for the employees with a disability or injury. A reasonable accommodation is described as "a modification or adjustment to a job, the work environment, or the way things usually are done that enables a qualified individual with a disability to enjoy an equal employment opportunity" [1]. Workplaces that employ more than 15 people are obliged to provide such accommodations unless undue hardship is likely to result. "Undue hardship" may be declared when actions are "excessively costly, extensive, substantial or disruptive" (p. 194) [2]. People with disabilities have the right of appeal if a reasonable accommodation is denied. Data collected by the Job Accommodation Network (JAN) suggests that over half of all accommodations cost less than $500. Most employers report that providing accommodations results in financial benefits due to an increase in worker productivity and a reduction in the cost of insurance and training new employees. However, it can be difficult to determine the real cost of accommodations [3]. Costs can sometimes exceed $10,000–$15,000 when employees have a significant injury or impairment [3,4].

Workplace accommodation is commonly used to enable a person with a disability to enter and remain in the workforce and for a worker with an injury to return to work [5,6]. A range of strategies are typically used in workplace accommodations namely, job restructuring, suitable duties programs, flex time, shared duties, job or task modification, workplace modification, and case management [3,7]. Assistive devices or technologies are also a common accommodation strategy [5,6] and are frequently used in combination with other strategies, to improve the match between the worker and the workplace [8]. Assistive technology (AT) is often central to the successful integration of people with physical disabilities into the workplace [9]. Assistive devices, such as alternative input devices, augmentative communication systems, reading and writing software, and assistive listening devices are often recommended to assist workers with a range of disabilities gain or remain in employment [10]. The comfort and performance of workers with injuries such as low back pain is commonly addressed using equipment such as special seating and desks and lifting devices [5]. Use of assistive devices such as arm supports, ergonomic seating, and mechanical lifting devices is also commonplace for preventing injuries at work, especially musculoskeletal disorders [11,12].

Although the evidence for the benefit of work accommodation in general for workers who have an injury or disability appears strong [13], there is less evidence about the use of assistive devices specifically. This is the case for assistive devices used for both rehabilitation and prevention purposes. A comprehensive study conducted by the National Council on Disability (NCD) in 1993 identified the benefits of AT in the workplace. People with disabilities reported that AT assisted them to obtain employment (67%), work faster (92%), and earn more money (83%) [14]. More recently, a systematic review of workplace interventions to prevent musculoskeletal and visual symptoms and disorders among computer users found a mixed level of evidence for the effects of a variety of these interventions, including some assistive devices [11]. However, the authors cautioned that there was limited high-quality evidence available for review and called for more high-quality research in the area to inform practice. Although the evidence is limited and mixed at present, assistive devices are commonly used for optimizing performance at work, both by the person with a disability or injury and by workers who may be at risk of injury or disability.

Section 14.2 explores the range of assistive devices that is available for optimizing such performance at work.

14.2   ASSISTIVE DEVICES

Assistive devices are generally referred to as AT, which refers to "any item, piece of equipment, or product system, whether acquired commercially off the shelf, modified, or customized, that is used to increase, maintain, or improve the functional capacities of an individual with a disability" (U.S. PL Section 3.1. Public Law 100-407). AT range from simple low-tech options to sophisticated, high-tech devices [15]. Low-tech options are generally inexpensive and can be equipment or software that improves a person's ability to carry out a work task. These include antifatigue standing mats to improve standing tolerance [16–18] footrests, wrist supports, padded grips, magnifiers, alternative keyboards as well as the accessibility software provided standard on computers. Low-tech devices have been found to contribute to the successful employment of people with disabilities [10].

High-tech options include expensive, sophisticated, dedicated technologies, such as remote-controlled devices, specialized hoists [12], voice recognition and screen reading technologies, voice output communication devices, closed-circuit television (CCTV), and robotics. These technologies have been found to be invaluable in the successful employment of people with significant impairments [19].

Many devices used to accommodate people with injuries or impairments in the workplace are mainstream commercial devices that are often not considered to be specialized [10]. Computer technologies in general have been instrumental in increasing employment opportunities for people with injuries or impairments [19,20]. Information technologies have changed the work environment, making it less physically demanding and affording people many efficiencies and conveniences previously unimaginable. Networks, the Internet, e-mail, and mobile phones have increased connectivity and communication such that work can be undertaken any where, any time [19]. Readily available mainstream technologies also offer improved flexibility and productivity that enables individuals to customize workstations to their specific requirements and maintain their output. Mainstream technologies can also be extended to optimize performance by using existing features to their full potential. For example, the autocorrect function in Microsoft Word® can be used to expand abbreviations and reduce the number of keystrokes required [19]. Many workers also have access to mainstream office equipment such as electric staplers, document holders, and footrests [21] that can improve comfort and efficiency and reduce musculoskeletal strain.

There are also a number of alternative mainstream technologies, which some people find easier to use or accommodate their specific requirements more effectively. Standard seating can be replaced with an alternative design such as a sit-stand stool [17] or saddle seat [22]. Computer access may be easier or more efficient using an ergonomic keyboard and trackball or voice recognition in place of a standard keyboard and mouse. Sometimes people make adaptations to standard technology (e.g., use a wrist support, back cushions on existing seating, padded handles on equipment or a mount for a telephone handset) to position the equipment or assist in using

TABLE 14.1

Examples of Different Types of Devices for the Same Tasks

Mainstream	Alternative	Adapted	Dedicated/Specialized
Sitting			
Adjustable ergonomic seating footrests	Saddle seat	Lumbar cushion in existing seating	Adjustable height desk
Keyboarding			
Keyboard with integrated mouse autocorrect	Ergonomic Keyboard Trackball Voice recognition	Typing splints	Onscreen keyboard

standard technologies more effectively. Once standard technologies have been fully exploited, specialized or dedicated technologies are often explored. An expanding range of devices are available, which have been designed with a specific purpose in mind. For example, CCTVs designed to assist people with vision impairments to read documents and books. Table 14.1 provides an overview of different types of devices that can be used to address sitting and keyboarding issues.

Exploration of possible mainstream, alternative, adaptations, and specialized or dedicated devices may follow a progression in a hierarchical order or be undertaken simultaneously. It is sometimes recommended that mainstream options be exhausted before alternative or specialized devices are considered, with the proviso that the best fit should be the main priority [23]. Mainstream products often have proven reliability and are supplied with product warranties [23]. They may be regarded as more socially acceptable, allow more flexibility and mobility in the workplace, and be less expensive due to economies of scale. However, mainstream products may have only a limited number of features or capacity to adjust or be customized to the user-specific requirements. Specialized or dedicated products are designed for a targeted market. While this can mean that they are more expensive than they would otherwise be, they can often provide users with greater ease, comfort, and efficiencies that offset the initial outlay. A hierarchical approach to assistive devices within the work accommodation process may limit the possibilities for the worker with a disability or injury and force a solution that may not necessarily optimally improve the match between the worker, work, and workplace environment. It is therefore preferable that the relative merits of each device are considered taking into account a range of factors such as cost, aesthetics, comfort, and function.

14.3 PROCESS OF SELECTING AND UTILIZING ASSISTIVE TECHNOLOGIES

At first, providing people with ATs seems straightforward [24]. However, the ever-increasing range of devices and scattered resources make this a complex process. Without experience of assistive devices, it is difficult to identify suitable options and locate useful information and expertise. People can quickly feel overwhelmed and ill equipped to navigate the process and make informed decisions. Traditionally, service providers have tended to be prescriptive with devices being selected based on the nature of the person's disability or injury rather than the specific requirements of the person, the work tasks to be undertaken, and the work environment. However, abandonment and nonuse of devices continues to be of concern [4,25–29]. While a number of factors have been identified as influencing continued device use such as change in the priorities or needs of the user, motivation to use the device or do the task, environmental obstacles, and whether the device was seen as effective, reliable, durable, comfortable, and easy to use [29–34], consumer involvement in device selection has been found to positively influence device use [35].

The degree to which consumers are involved in device selection depends on their understanding of the process, the approach or process used to determine the best device, and the opportunities afforded them by service providers to contribute to or direct the process. In order to be meaningfully involved in the process, consumers or AT users need to understand what is technically possible, what the process involves, the range of resources available, and how they can utilize these effectively to identify the best option. The following section examines the process of selecting and using technology from the perspective of the consumer or AT user. It describes the steps required to select and use technology effectively from envisaging the technological possibilities to ongoing use of the technology in the changing work environment. Each step of the process will be discussed in turn with view to understanding each from the AT user's position. The resources required at each of these stages will also be discussed.

14.4 CONSUMER-CENTERED APPROACH TO SELECTING AND USING TECHNOLOGY

Few people who use ATs talk about the process of selecting and using them, or how to best go about identifying their needs and evaluating effectiveness. The process they use to select and utilize devices is not dissimilar to the way many of us choose a new car or computer, except that the choices may be unfamiliar or limited and resources are more fragmented [36]. While each of us might have our own unique approach to decision making, we essentially go through a similar process when embarking on a new purchase. The quality of the outcome relies on having a clear idea of requirements, knowledge of the options available (or the availability of suitable expertise to assist in identifying what is available), and taking care to match requirements with the available options.

If you were to reflect on a recent technology purchase, there would be a number of things you might have found useful in the process. First, your decision would be assisted by previous experience with the product and an understanding of what it could be used for. You possibly used a range of resources, e.g., talking with others, reading reviews, and seeking the opinions of a range of sales people, to gather information on the options available, and understand the features each offered. It is likely that there were many competing factors to consider and compromises to be made when weighing up the relative benefits of various options. You may have had to consider the preferences and needs of other people, facilities in the environment, and your future needs, in order to ensure the purchase had good long-term potential. Once you had obtained the device, you would have familiarized yourself with its features, adjusted it to your preferences, developed your skills in using it and established what was required to keep it in good working order. It is likely that you had to source and utilize a range of resources and supports throughout this process. The steps you undertook and the resources you used are likely to be similar to those outlined in Table 14.2.

The 16 steps outlined in the process of device selection and use have been drawn from the literature and the experiences of 26 people with disabilities who are successfully employed and shared their experiences of selecting and using technology in the workplace [19]. The first eight steps contribute to the selection of a device while the following eight steps support the effective implementation of the technology.

TABLE 14.2
Steps in the Process of Selecting and Using Technology and Resources Required

Steps in the Process	Resources Used
Visioning possibilities	General media, seeing what others use, talking with people with similar goals/experience
Establishing goals/expectations	Talking things over with friends or people with experience or expertise
Identifying specific requirements	Examining and appraising personal skills and experience through self-reflection or testing or seeking expert advice
Defining required features	Expert advice, talking with friend, reflecting on personal goals and experience
Information on potential technologies and resources	Information systems (formal and informal)– experts, Internet, Directories, reading relevant literature, friends and advertisements
Locate local resources and supports	Seek recommendations from experts and friends
Develop a funding strategy	Search local directories
Trialing and evaluating options	Display rooms, demonstration models with access to friends and experts to weight up relative benefits
Purchase of device	Manufacturer and Supplier
Integrate with other technologies	Supplier, expert, or friend
Customize device to personal requirements	Supplier, expert, or friends
Learn to use device	Attend a course, read manual, ask a friend with experience, experiment
Maintenance and repair	Maintenance and repair services
Insurance	Supplier, expert, or friend
Review ongoing suitability	Expert, friend, self-reflection
Upgrading the technology as the need arises	Information on new technologies and recent advances in current technologies

Source: de Jonge, D.M., et al., *Assistive Technology in the Workplace*, Mosby, St. Louis, MO, 2007. With permission.

Traditionally, the process of device selection has been described from a clinical or service provider's perspective, outlining procedures for service provision. As such, services have not been delivered in a way that acknowledges the challenges that people experience when choosing and using equipment in the workplace or empowers them to be active in the process. Furthermore, traditional processes do not acknowledge that people begin the process of recognizing needs and exploring possibilities long before encountering a service provider and continue to update their technology in response to changing needs long after their contact with services.

14.4.1 VISIONING POSSIBILITIES

For most people, the process of exploration begins with a vision of what is possible [37]. Some people come to the process of exploring options with a clear vision of what they want to achieve. They may also have some understanding of what technology can offer them, even if they are unfamiliar with the range of products available. Others may be unaware of how technologies can assist them perform tasks more effectively and may not even seek out possibilities. Consequently, they tend to persist using ineffective strategies or technologies to complete work tasks, which often results in persistent discomfort, chronic pain, poor job performance, or potential job loss [19]. Before embarking on a process of exploring options, people need to first understand what is possible. This can often be achieved by talking with others who have expertise in workplace ATs, especially people who are already using these devices effectively in the workplace [38]. Employers can also benefit from an understanding of what ATs can offer so that they can better promote employee productivity. Frequently, once the benefits of a device put in place to enable a worker with an injury or disability become evident, it is often subsequently employed to improve the health and efficiency of other employees.

Visioning possibilities also relies on having a good perception of yourself and your capabilities, hope for a better future, and an awareness of what others have achieved. Traditionally, the focus of many service providers throughout the process of device selection has been on developing a "realistic" understanding of the worker's capabilities. This is often achieved by assessing the person's "naked" abilities that is, what they are currently able to do without devices or assistance. This may provide the service provider with a baseline of capacities but can undermine the worker's confidence and contribute little to their understanding of future possibilities. A focus on deficits or problems can obscure the person's capabilities and divert attention from envisaging new ways of participating successfully in the workplace. Many people have extended themselves through creativity and determination to exceed the expectations of "professionals" and provide motivation to others. Often these role models and success stories inspire others to create a new vision for themselves. It is therefore important that service providers work collaboratively with workers and enable them to think freely about what they want to be able to do [37].

With the constant evolution of technology, each day presents new possibilities. Even with a good knowledge of computer technology, it is often difficult to keep up with developments or to understand what specialized technologies can offer. Without a sound understanding of the potential of technology, many hesitate to invest time and money in exploring the possibilities. However, the constant development of technologies and ever-expanding range of new products also provides inspiration for new ways of doing things. For workers with an injury or disability, technological developments can not only make work more manageable but it can also extend the vision of potential work opportunities.

14.4.2 ESTABLISHING GOALS AND EXPECTATIONS

Once someone has an understanding that things could be improved, it is important to examine the person's need, preferences, past experiences, and expectations [39]. It is important to note that the selection of a suitable device is dependent on *how well* goals, preferences, and requirements are established in the first instance [40]. In this stage of the process, information is gathered about the employee to determine if they are open to the use of AT and able to manage it. In addition, the capacity of the work environment to accept and support the device is also considered [39]. As noted earlier, some consumers are likely to have a very clear and specific purpose in mind when exploring options [41], while others require assistance to develop and articulate their goals [29]. Service providers, with an understanding of ATs and their features, can often assist people in developing manageable goals and expectations [41]. It is also useful to collaborate with other stakeholders (e.g., the employer) when developing goals and expectations of the technology [15,39,41,42].

A number of strategies are available to assist in goal development. First, an informal interview with the worker and other stakeholders can assist service providers in developing an understanding of work demands, current strengths, and difficulties in carrying out work tasks. A number of tools have also been developed, which not only provide a structure for developing goals and identifying preferences and requirements but also provide a means of evaluating how well devices meet these. The Canadian Occupational Performance Measure (COPM) [43] is an individualized tool, which uses a semistructured interview to assist in identifying specific problems in areas such as self-care, productivity, and leisure [44]. Goal Attainment Scaling (GAS) [45], originally designed for use in community mental health settings, allows individualized goals to be established and outcomes to be defined in clear behavioral terms [46]. The instruments from the matching person and technology (MPT) process [29] enable the service provider and consumer to work together to identify the most appropriate technology in light of the person's perceptions of strengths and capabilities, needs/goals, preferences, and psychosocial characteristics as well as expectations regarding the benefits of technology. Specifically, the Workplace Technology Predisposition Assessment (WT PA) [47] examines the worker's and employer's preferences, expectations of technology and barriers to optimal technology use. It is vital that goals are established with due consideration of both the short- and long-term aspirations of the person. This ensures that that the solution does not limit the worker's long-term productivity or work options. In addition, it is important to recognize that goals may evolve and refine as the person develops a deeper understanding of what is possible during the process of exploring the technology. Goals will need to be periodically revisited to ensure they reflect the current expectations and aspirations of the worker as well as the demands and constraints of the work tasks and environment.

14.4.3 IDENTIFYING SPECIFIC REQUIREMENTS

This stage of the process centers on establishing the user's specific requirements [15,41,48,49]. A good definition of the user's requirements is necessary in order to identify the most suitable device [41]. Without a clear understanding of their specific needs, people tend to rely on ad hoc methods, trial and error, and suggestions from people they randomly encounter to identify potential options [19]. Traditionally, formal assessment has focused on specific skills and abilities, especially when investigating sophisticated technology options [15,39,41,42,48–51]. However, as noted previously, a detailed analysis of the user's "naked" abilities is not always the best approach when determining technology requirements.

A more holistic analysis of the person, the tasks to be undertaken, and the work environment and the interplay between these is needed in order to understand what is required of the technology. The human activities and assistive technology (HAAT) model [15] provides a useful foundation for analyzing the potential of technology to enable participation in the workplace. This model is concerned with using technology to enable "*someone* (a person with a disability) to do *something* (an activity) *somewhere* (in the environment)" p. 35 [15]. In Figure 14.1, Cook and Hussey [15] illustrate the interrelationship between the activity, the user, the technology, and the environment, which they describe as elements of the AT system. The AT system is seen as an open system, which is dynamic and interacts with the environment. In this model, AT is seen as a means of enabling the person, who is unable to complete a task using existing resources. The activity is described as the goal of the system, which, in combination with the environment, defines the requirements for task completion. Cook and Hussey [15] highlight the importance of the interplay between these factors throughout the whole process of acquiring and integrating the AT. In addition, they acknowledge that changes inevitably occur over time in the

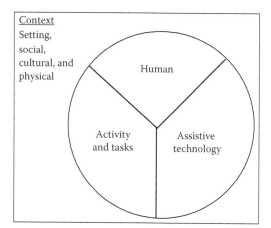

FIGURE 14.1 The human activity assistive technology (HAAT) model. (Adapted from Cook, A.M. and Hussey, S.M., *Assistive Technology: Principles and Practice*, 2nd ed., Mosby, St. Louis, MO, 2002. With permission.)

person, activity, technology, or context, which alter the way functions are allocated within the system. For example, the person may loose capacities or develop additional skills, which changes the way they utilize equipment. Alternatively, a change in the activity or environment may place additional demands on the system. Further, advances in technology may mean that more sophisticated functions are available to the user or incompatibilities may arise with workplace technologies. By detailing the elements in the AT system and establishing a good fit between the activities, user, technology, and environment, the HAAT model proposes that the user's goals can be effectively achieved.

14.4.3.1 Understanding the Person's Abilities and Experience

Information on the person's goals, preferences, experience with technology, injury or impairments, and skills and abilities [15] provide an essential foundation for understanding the person's specific requirements. Workers with established impairments and prior work experience are likely to be able to provide a reliable report of their preferences, skills, and abilities related to work tasks sufficient to identify the type of technology options to explore without the need for targeted assessment. Those without previous experience may benefit from more detailed discussions and assessments to determine their specific goals, preferences, and capacities. Cook and Hussey [15] advocate that assessments focus on the strengths and abilities of the user using both qualitative and quantitative measures in the form of interviews, functional evaluations, observations, and criterion-referenced performance measures. However, it is not always possible to anticipate how well technology will work for someone from this information alone. It is also important to observe the person carrying out tasks in the workplace in order to accurately define their requirements [41].

14.4.3.2 Defining Task Requirements

While the goal of the AT system may be to participate equitably in the workplace, it is essential to detail the specific tasks to be undertaken within the job. For example, a job may require a worker to communicate over the phone, make appointments, read documents, enter data, and dispatch letters. Understanding the range of tasks to be undertaken ensures that the various functions of system are identified and consideration given to how technology might be integrated to enable these activities to be performed effectively. In addition, the specific requirements of each activity also need to be defined so that barriers to activity engagement or task performance can be closely examined. For example, a user may need to do word processing, data entry, navigate the Internet, and draw, all of which require software and a computer with defined specifications. Each of these tasks also requires a different style on input, which varies in terms of the mode, speed, and control required. By determining the requirements of each task, a range of input devices can be explored to determine which are best suited to each task. While keyboard command alternatives, mouse keys, or voice commands may be sufficient to move about in a database file, they can prove to be tedious and unreliable when navigating Web pages or drawing documents.

A commonly used framework for further analyzing the requirements of tasks in a job is to analyze the presence, frequency, and nature of 22 physical demands from the *Dictionary of Occupational Titles* [52], defined in the *Handbook for Analysing Jobs* [53] (see Table 14.3). These physical demands provide a framework for considering and describing the activities performed on the job [54,55]. Once the essential job tasks are identified, each task can be observed and analyzed in terms of which physical demands are required for that task, how frequently the physical demand is performed during the task, and the nature of how the physical demand is performed in the environment. For example, a task may require standing all day (constantly) on a concrete floor at a bench that is at elbow height, handling vibrating tools. This provides a brief analysis of the task that can then be further analyzed, for example, the posture and specific ranges of movement required for the different or relevant body parts, the repetitions of movements to operate the tools, the environmental conditions etc. By looking at each task in detail, the potential requirements for an assistive device to minimize exposure to any hazardous factors or aggravating

---

TABLE 14.3
Physical Demands from the Dictionary of Occupational Titles

1	Standing
2	Walking
3	Sitting
4	Lifting
5	Carrying
6	Pushing
7	Pulling
8	Controls: Hand-Arm and Foot-Leg
9	Climbing
10	Balancing
11	Stooping
12	Kneeling
13	Crouching
14	Crawling
15	Reaching
16	Handling
17	Fingering
18	Feeling
19	Talking
20	Hearing
21	Tasting/smelling
22	Seeing (near acuity, far acuity, depth perception, accommodation, color vision, field of vision)

Source: United States Department of Labor, *Dictionary of Occupational Titles*, 4th ed., U.S. Government Printing Office, Washington, DC, 1991.

---

activities for the person with existing injury can be considered. In the case of the person with a disability, who has limited capacity to perform apparently essential job functions, the potential for an assistive device to assist with performance of these functions can be better considered based on a thorough job analysis.

Table 14.3 lists the physical demands from the *Dictionary of Occupational Titles*. It is important to acknowledge that the DOT approach to job analysis has limitations [56] and that a replacement taxonomy, O*NET, is available online [57] and provides an alternative detailed approach to job analysis. However, the physical demands framework can still be useful in prevention and rehabilitation as a starting point for considering task requirements.

14.4.3.3   Review of the Application Environments

In recent times, there has been a growing awareness of the environment and how it can enable or limit participation. Consequently, there has been greater emphasis on examining the settings in which activities are to be performed [15,48], acknowledging the physical as well as the psychological, social, and cultural aspects of the application environment. In particular, it is important to evaluate the needs of the employee with an injury or impairment within the actual workplace [3,58] and to gain an understanding of the employer's or supervisor's perspective of the job requirements [3]. It is important to understand the topography, temperature, climate, sound and lighting conditions and existing systems in the application environments [15,48], how these interact with the person and work activities, and how well they support current or potential devices. It is also essential that the expectations and attitudes of others in the workplace be understood so that the system can be appropriately designed and supported. When examining the environment, the success of technology accommodation is also dependent on identifying barriers and enablers in current as well as future work environments [48]. Due consideration to career planning and potential work opportunities will ensure that the technology does not limit prospective employment opportunities. Consideration should also be given to other environments the user operates in, especially if the technologies are likely to move within and across application environments. For example, it is likely that the person will require similar access technologies on their home computer to either complete work at home or to undertake recreational activities. Careful planning can ensure that performance in not constrained to one environment.

14.4.4   ESTABLISHING DEVICE CRITERIA

A good technology match relies on an understanding of the difficulties workers experience in performing tasks [15,59] and matching the features of the potential devices to the specific needs and skills of the individual, demands of the job and the work environment [15,41,42,48]. Once the requirements of the person, activities, and environment have been determined [15,41], device criteria/characteristics can be established [37,48,49]. Tables 14.4 through 14.6 detail the specific requirements of the person, work activities, and the environment and the corresponding characteristics, features, and function required of the technology.

First, the type of device is determined by the user's goals whilst the style of device is shaped by their preferences. It is vital to acknowledge individual preferences

TABLE 14.4

Technology Criteria Based on the Person's Requirements

Person	Technology Criteria
Goal: To return to office work	Computer Technology—with modern office software
Preference: Sleek modern look	Black casing and flat screen
Experience: Word processing experience in Word 95	Consider Microsoft family of software
Skills and Abilities:	
Limited vision	Standard keyboard layout
Limited ROM, strength and endurance in upper limb	Enlarged visual output
Mobilizes in power wheelchair	Light touch keyboard/voice input /reduced keyboard size/ trackball word prediction capabilities able to be positioned easily e.g., monitor arm and adjustable workstation

Source: de Jonge, D.M., et al., *Assistive Technology in the Workplace*, Mosby, St. Louis, MO, 2007. With permission.

TABLE 14.5

Technology Criteria Based on the Requirements of the Activities to be Undertaken

Activity	Technology Criteria
Word processing	Keyboard voice entry (additional RAM)
Data entry—numbers	Separate numeric keypad
Navigating desktop and Internet environment	Mouse or alternative
Answer the phone	Headset, computer-based phone answering software
Need to man the reception area for 2 h a day	Duplicate or portable system for reception area
E-mailing and managing household finances at home	Compatible/duplicate system at home

Source: de Jonge, D.M., et al., *Assistive Technology in the Workplace*, Mosby, St. Louis, MO, 2007. With permission.

when exploring technology options [60] and even more importantly, the way in which devices contribute to the visibility of disability [61]. Working collaboratively with the user is the best way to ensure that the experience and preferences of the user are recognized and considered when identifying the best device [62,63]. The level of sophistication of the technology should reflect the user's level of experience while the interfaces and programming requirements will be determined by the user's

TABLE 14.6
Technology Criteria as Defined By the Application Environments

Environment	Technology Criteria
Open office environment	Quiet operation
Floor-to-ceiling glass windows	Discrete device
Strips of fluoro lights with diffusers run length of ceiling	Glare screen for enlarged monitor
Networked environment running on Windows environment	Windows compatible software and devices
High output expected	Efficient system
Funding limited	Cost-effective solution
Funding dedicated for workplace accommodation	Devices to meet workplace requirements

Source: de Jonge, D.M., et al., *Assistive Technology in the Workplace*, Mosby, St. Louis, MO, 2007. With permission.

skills and abilities. Care should be taken to acknowledge that not everyone relates to technology easily [29]. It is therefore important that a range of options is explored and that people are afforded the opportunity to explore less sophisticated solutions if that is their preference [29]. Table 14.4 provides an analysis of the technology characteristics based on a person's specific requirements.

The specific features and functions required of the system is derived from an analysis of the range of activities and tasks to be undertaken (both now and in the near future) will assist in determining. Table 14.5 provides an overview of the technology characteristics dictated by the nature of the activities to be undertaken. This may indicate that a number of devices are required to address each function or that one device needs to be configured to meet the range of demands. In computer technologies, input, storage, programming, and output specifications of the technology must also meet the demands of the tasks to be undertaken with associated software and hardware.

An analysis of the range of environments in which the technology is to be used and the nature of these environments will also provide valuable information about the characteristics required by the technology (see Table 14.6). Considerations include (1) the potential impact of the environment on the technology, (2) the effect of the technology on the environment, (3) existing or proposed technology the devices need to work with, and (4) the support available or required to support the technology.

As each aspect of the AT system in considered, it becomes apparent that some characteristics or features are compatible with requirements in other areas whereas some may contradict other requirements. At this point it is important to discuss priorities with the employee and other stakeholders so that these can be appropriately weighted when evaluating the usefulness of potential options.

14.4.5 Identifying Potential Devices

With an ever-expanding range of mainstream and specialized technologies, it has become increasingly difficult to develop a thorough understanding of the range of products available and to distinguish between them [37]. Many people seem to encounter options by accident [19]. Because of the specialist nature of the assistive devices, it is often difficult to obtain information, however increasingly the Internet provides people with easy access to extensive amounts of information. Supplier catalogs, gateway sites, and online databases enable users and service providers to investigate the range of devices available. However, for the inexperienced, the amount of information is often overwhelming and the lack of detail makes it difficult to determine which devices are worthy of further exploration. At this stage of the process, it is useful to develop a "circle of support" [37] to assist in locating and navigating the diverse information systems and identifying potential options. Resource people can include other AT users, people with mainstream technology expertise, AT service providers and information services, suppliers, and friends. Each of these can bring a different perspective and understanding and assist in developing a broader understanding of the possibilities. For many, this is a complex field, which not only needs knowledge of a broad range of products and services, but also requires an understanding of how to match people with the "right" technologies [64]. The quality of support provided can impact significantly on the outcome for the individual [34]. For many professionals, equipment catalogs, fixed and searchable databases, selection hierarchies [3,60], equipment-based decision trees [65], and selection matrices [41] provide a concrete way of dealing with their lack of familiarity with devices, the problem of over choice and the complexity of the decisions that have to be made. However, these strategies can distract from using observation and clinical reasoning, which is essential in addressing specific requirements of the individual, work tasks, and the application environment [20].

14.4.6 IDENTIFYING AND UTILIZING RESOURCES

The process of device selection and implementation is seen by many as beginning at the point of referral to a service provider. For the employee with an injury or disability however, the journey begins well before the initial contact with a professional and is likely to extend well beyond their encounter with any particular service. However, once it is recognized that things can be improved and that potential solutions exist, they require access to resources that can assist them in selecting and implementing technology that can be invaluable. It is often assumed that people are well informed about technological possibilities and existing resources and can actively utilize these [37,39]. However, many who could benefit from technology are not aware of the possibilities or how to access information or expertise [19]. People who access information and resources on ATs generally self-refer or alternatively are referred by other sources such as friends, other service providers, employers, or third-party payers [42]. They often have very little understanding of the overall process and what the various services contribute to the process. Consequently, it is important that service providers assist the worker and other stakeholders to understand what the process of selecting and implementing technology involves, identify which aspects of the process they can competently address, and provide information on other suitable resources and services. While some services are primarily skilled in determining workplace requirements, others have expertise in identifying potential technology options, securing appropriate funding, providing training, or setting up or maintaining the technology. It is important that people are aware of all these resources so that they are adequately supported throughout the process.

Many people are either not aware that specialist resources exist or only find out about them during the process or through accidental encounters [19]. Even when people know about resources they sometimes do not make good use of them [19]. It could be that there is a lack of information about these resources or that the services are difficult or costly to access [66]. Alternatively, consumers may not understand what the services offer or be unaware of how to access these resources. They may also be wary that they do not know enough about options to ask the right questions [67]. Those who have accessed expertise about assistive devices have found the advice and information they provided invaluable [19]. With the bewildering array of devices available, it is important that people have access to accurate up-to-date information on the range of technologies available [24]. This assists with decision making and decreases the likelihood of technology abandonment [33]. Many people also value the support service providers can offer [19]. This support reduces the stress of having to locate resources and potential devices and the time required to navigate these alone [19,42,68–70]. In addition, people who access professional expertise have been found to develop more positive attitudes to information and devices than those relying on informal contacts [64]. As information about technologies becomes even more readily available on the Internet, it is important to ensure that people continue to have access to service providers who can assist them to negotiate the matrix of information and resources.

While having access to service providers with expertise is advantageous, users also need to be empowered to be their own "long-term technologist" [36]. Rather than being reliant on service providers, users need to develop "self determination" [71] so that they can address their ongoing needs. With a sound knowledge of technology possibilities and the resources available to them, users are better able to navigate the process, set goals, make decisions, and take action when the need arises [72].

14.4.7 Developing a Funding Strategy

The next step in the process is to develop a funding strategy [37,48,49]. While the prices of many mainstream technologies continue to decrease, ATs often remain expensive. The cost of specialized technologies continues to be a major obstacle for people with disabilities [67,73,74]. Even when there are designated funding sources, it is often necessary to be resourceful and persistent to secure adequate funds for AT [37]. It is important to develop an understanding of the potential funding schemes and their criteria and access people with experience and skills in navigating administrative processes and bureaucratic obstacles to achieve a good outcome. There may be a number of costs associated with workplace technologies, which may not have been anticipated. These can include the expense of upgrading of the computer or workstation to accommodate the new technologies, as well as the cost of training; ongoing maintenance and repairs and future upgrades [49]. Experienced users and service providers can assist in identifying additional expenses associated with specific purchases [49]. Ongoing funding sources may also need to be identified, as employees with injuries and disabilities often need to upgrade their technology regularly in order to stay competitive in the workforce [19].

14.4.8 Trialing and Evaluating the Suitability of Technologies

The best way to determine the suitability of any device is to trial it. The time required to trial equipment ranges from a few minutes for a simple device to weeks for a complex technology. Trialing allows the devices to be evaluated against the technology requirements determined earlier in the process [15,37,39,41,48]. It also enables the user to assess the aesthetics, comfort, and usability of the device and the service provider to examine the fit. Together they can discuss the relative merits of each option and acceptable compromises and trade-offs. Where possible, it is preferable for the trial to occur in the workplace so that the device can be evaluated with respect to its suitability to the application environment [49,58]. Trials extended over a number of days for example, 2–5 days [58], may also reveal discomfort that may not be evident in a brief trial. Extended on-site trials may also highlight obstacles to optimal use that can then be addressed prior to purchase thus reducing the likelihood of abandonment [75]. The effectiveness of the trial may also be improved if the user learns how to use and adjust the device prior to trialing [59,76] or is provided with assistance in adjusting and operating the device by someone familiar with its features and functions. It is important that the device is fitted and adjusted to the specific requirements of the user in order to optimize the effectiveness of the trial [59].

14.4.9 Purchasing the Technology

It is imperative that the employer and worker are actively involved in deciding on the best device. This not only ensures the immediate success of the intervention [9], but also provides them with an understanding of the process and the trade-offs required in making in the final selection. Collaborative approaches such as that used in the MPT model [29] can assist service providers, workers, and employers to work together to gain a mutual understanding of each other's perspective and determine the best option.

Once the most suitable device has been selected, it can then be purchased [15]. Prior to purchase, it is also useful to inquire whether the vendor provides ongoing maintenance, training, installation, or upgrade support and the cost of these services [37]. For sophisticated devices, ongoing technical assistance is critical [37] so it is important to consider the experience and reliability of the supplier when deciding where to purchase the technology. Valuable information about the experience and reliability of suppliers can also be sought from other users and service providers. It is also useful where possible to purchase all required equipment and accessories from the one vendor. This ensures that there is no confusion as to who holds the responsibility for attending to issues.

14.4.10 Setting Up the Technology

Once the technology has been purchased, it is vital that it is set up appropriately in the workplace to enable the worker to function effectively and independently.

In this stage of the process, the technology needs to be set up in the workplace without disrupting the productivity of the employee with an injury or disability or their coworkers. ATs need to be set up by someone with appropriate expertise with ATs [15,39] to ensure they are operating as intended. Some devices need to be installed and integrated with existing workplace equipment and technologies. In these cases, expertise in mainstream technologies is required to ensure the ATs are appropriately integrated with the workplace technologies [42].

14.4.11 CUSTOMIZING THE TECHNOLOGY

Once in place, devices need to be customized to meet the specific requirements and preferences of the user. Despite new technologies presenting many new challenges to the user, little attention has been paid to date to customizing technology after purchase to optimize use. Frequently, new devices may result in the user assuming new positions or using different actions [77]. This can result in discomfort or strain, which could be difficult to relieve as employees with injuries or a disability cannot easily adjust their position or vary their actions. If devices are not "fine tuned" to meet the individual's preferences and requirements, difficulties encountered in the early stages may ultimately lead to bad habits or abandonment [36]. Recent research has raised concern about the amount of pain and discomfort experienced by AT users and the long-term implications of this [67,78]. However, it is not always possible to predict the impact of a new technology during an initial assessment or limited trial. It is therefore important that they are adjusted and refined after installation to ensure ongoing comfort and productivity [15,39,41,42,48,49,75,79]. At the very least, technology accommodations should be adjusted to minimize discomfort and strain with ongoing use [75]. Ideally, careful adjustment and appropriate instruction optimize technology use [80] and secure a future for the user in the workforce.

First, it is important to ensure that users are positioned ergonomically and using equipment in a sustainable way. Since devices are often designed with the broadest possible application in mind, many workers with injuries and disabilities do not interact with equipment in a way anticipated by the designers [81]. Mainstream employment or occupational health and safety systems are not always able to address the specific requirements and risks of workers with injuries or disabilities, as they are not familiar with their unique needs. An assessment of the presence of risk factors for musculoskeletal disorders, e.g., awkward postures, static load and repetition, is needed to ensure preventative measures are put in place [82]. The worker needs to be educated about the risks associated with such risk factors so that they can take action and continue to function at an optimum. Users need to understand the long-term implications of working with awkward or prolonged static postures or repetitive and forceful movements and how maintaining neutral positions, varying postures, and taking frequent rest breaks can optimize their health and productivity. The user, equipment, and workstation need to be positioned ergonomically to reduce strain and promote productivity.

It is also essential that AT users understand the features and functions of their technology so that they can customize these to their individual requirements. Those who do not understand the adjustable features of their technology often struggle with tasks that could otherwise be completed effortlessly. Complex and unintuitive design can also make it difficult for users to utilize their technology effectively. When well informed of the capabilities of their technology, users are able to adjust for comfort and to improve their effectiveness. The user's ability to customize and use technology effectively can be promoted by providing information and training about features and ensuring time is available for adjustments to be undertaken regularly.

14.4.12   MASTERING THE USE OF THE DEVICE

Training is essential to effective use of technologies [15,42,49]. Inadequate training can result in poor device use and in some cases, abandonment [15]. Many device users continue to have individual training needs that remain unmet despite having had their technology for some time [19]. When devices require specialist training, the cost of this training needs to be included in the funding application so that the user is equipped with the skills and knowledge required to operate the technology in the work environment [15]. However, frequently training needs are not anticipated in funding packages and the user is left to rely on their own resources, trial and error, or consulting friends to understand the technology. Many teach themselves through experimentation, wading through complex manuals, or completing online tutorials [19]. However, this often results in them understanding only the basic aspects of their technology and being unable to extend their technology beyond essential functions [19]. Workers with injuries or disabilities are often isolated from others using similar AT and, therefore, have limited opportunities to benefit from their experience. In the absence of this incidental learning, they are forced to seek the informal support of friends and colleagues, many of whom are unfamiliar with the technology and how it can be used efficiently to complete work tasks. Skill development that relies on "miscellaneous sources cannot be said to provide a secure foundation for planning, development or long-term viability" (p. 30) [83].

Training is most effective if well-defined objectives are established [15]. Users need to develop "operational competence" [15], which is to be able to turn the device on and off, know how to adjust the various features of the device, understand the maintenance requirements, and troubleshoot problems they are likely to encounter in using the device. In addition, they require "strategies competence" [15], which enable them to use the device to perform specific tasks. Operational training is best provided soon after delivery of the device while strategic training is most effective when the user is "on-the-job" [42] and familiar with the range of tasks they will be using the device for. It is important to be aware that it can be challenging for users to develop the skills required to carry out work tasks while developing skills in using their new device [42]. It is therefore important in the initial stages that time is allocated for the user to become familiar with their technology. Access to ongoing training support is also required so that they can continue to develop skills once they have established basic competencies.

14.4.13   MAINTENANCE AND REPAIR FOLLOW-UP

It is often tempting to think that the process is complete once the technologies are in place; however, this marks the beginning of the implementation process for the user [15]. Many are left to fend for themselves or with limited resources to deal with ongoing technological difficulties [19]. While some are resourceful and find ways of accessing suitable support, others find this more difficult [19]. Despite the ongoing difficulties users experience using their technology in the workplace, little attention has been given to ensuring the AT user is provided with ongoing maintenance and repair support. Technologies need to be maintained regularly if they are to remain effective [42]. Users therefore need to know how to carry out basic maintenance of their technology and who to contact when they have more complex maintenance or repair needs [49]. Costs associated with this support also need to be considered when costing the technology [42].

14.4.14 Insuring the Device

Another important consideration, particularly when using expensive and sophisticated devices is insurance [49]. As AT users are often reliant on their technology to remain productive in the workplace, it is important that faulty, damaged, or lost devices are replaced quickly. This ensures that the user remains productive in the workplace and does not need to navigate workplace or external funding processes to replace or repair the device. Some users have also found it useful to have a backup technology to use when their specialized technology is inactive, being repaired, or if it temporarily "crashes" [19]. In addition, alternative options can also provide users with an opportunity to vary their actions. It is clear that further consideration needs to be given to strategies to prevent the loss of productivity that results from technology failure or fatigue.

14.4.15 Monitoring and Evaluation

Monitoring and evaluation is a crucial stage in the process, and is often overlooked. Ongoing monitoring and periodic reevaluation allows changes and issues to be identified and resolved quickly, which promotes the continued productivity of the worker. As noted earlier, there are likely to be many changes in the AT system over time [15]. First, the worker's skills are likely to continue to develop or their injury or impairment may change. These may require the technology to be adjusted or replaced. Second, work responsibilities may change necessitating changes to the system. Third, developments in technology may result in advances, which may afford greater comfort, efficiency, or productivity. Finally, there may be changes in the workplace that place additional demands on the system. In order to empower workers with an injury or disability in the long term, they need to be provided with information on resources available to meet their ongoing and changing needs and how to use these effectively. This ensures that they are "informed, demanding and responsible consumers of AT service and devices" (p. 152) [72]. It is generally assumed that workers will initiate requests for changes to their technology when they feel it is no longer meeting their needs. However many workers are hesitant to request a review of their technology as they are reluctant to draw attention to themselves, uncertain how their situation could be improved or anxious that their request could have a negative impact on their employment [19]. It is therefore important that a process is established in the workplace to ensure that regular reviews are undertaken to optimize the worker's health, safety, and productivity.

14.4.16 UPGRADING

Finally, employees with an injury or disability find that keeping abreast of technology advancements enables them to remain competitive in the workplace [19]. The productivity of AT users in the workplace can be assured if their technologies are regularly updated, as new developments become available. Many users may find it useful to keep up with technological developments so that they can identify useful advancements and ensure that they are using the best technology [19]. A range of resources can be used to monitor development namely, computer magazines, computer literate friends, specialist information services, occupational therapists, or disability organizations and increasingly the Internet. With the rapid development of technology, it is essential that users have access to independent information about developments in technology. Specialist information services with their extensive databases and specialist professionals can provide advice and reliable, quality information on upcoming technologic developments.

14.5 SUMMARY

This chapter has identified the role assistive devices play in workplace accommodations and highlighted the importance of using a consumer-centered process when selecting and using technology in the workplace. Assistive devices range from low-tech devices such as a standing mat to highly sophisticated technologies such as screen reading technologies. While mainstream technologies may be extended to optimize the work performance of an employee with an injury or disability, there is an ever-expanding range of alternative and specialized technologies designed to address specific purposes.

Traditional approaches to device selection have favored a prescriptive approach, which focuses on the person's specific injury or disability rather than the preferences, experience and skills of the person, the full range of work tasks to be undertaken and the constraints and demands of the work environment. The process detailed in this chapter describes the experience of device selection and use from the perspective of an employee with an injury or disability. It begins with a vision of possibilities, which then inspires people to explore options, to improve their health, safety, and productivity in the workplace. The quality of the outcome is then dependent on how well the goals, preferences, and expectations are articulated with due attention being given to both the short- and long-term aspirations of the employee.

Next, detailing the specific requirements of the person, work tasks, and environment assists in understanding the requirements of the AT system and establishing device criteria. Once the device criteria are specified, priorities and potential trade-offs can be discussed. A range of resources can then be accessed to identify the potential options. With the bewildering range of options available, this is often an overwhelming experience. Consequently, accessing quality information and support at this stage of the process can impact significantly on the outcome. Many find it useful to develop a "circle of support" to assist in locating and navigating the diverse information systems and identifying potential options. Resource people include other AT users, people with mainstream technology expertise, AT service providers and information services, suppliers, and friends. Each of whom bring a different perspective and understanding of the range of options.

A funding strategy is very important in the process and suitable expertise can assist in understanding the funding options and successfully navigating administrative processes. Consideration also needs to be given to anticipating additional costs associated with technology accommodations. Trialing options in the workplace is fundamental to determining its suitability for the workplace and work tasks as well as the ongoing comfort and productivity of the user. Once the most suitable option is selected it is advisable to purchase it from a vendor who can provide ongoing maintenance, training, installation and upgrade support as required. Care should then be taken to ensure that the device is appropriately installed and adjusted to meet the specific requirements of the user.

Training is then required to promote effective use of the technology. AT users also benefit from allocating additional time to become familiar with their technology to perform work tasks. Over reliance on trail and error and informal training supports can limit both operational and strategic competence. The ongoing effectiveness of AT relies on the device being in good working order. Consequently, maintenance and repair follow-up is an essential aspect of ongoing AT support. For expensive and sophisticated technologies, insurance can assist users who are reliant on devices to remain productive in the workplace when their equipment is lost, damaged, or faulty. Backup devices can also be useful in maintaining productivity when technologies are unavailable or fatigue develops. Ongoing maintenance and periodic evaluation of the AT system ensures that changes in the person's skills, capacities and priorities, the nature of the work tasks, or the demands of the work environment are identified and addressed quickly. Since employees are often reluctant to declare their difficulties to their supervisors, it is important that processes are established in the workplace for regular review. Finally, employees with an injury or disability can ensure their competitiveness in the workplace by keeping abreast of technology advancements. Once again, up-to-date, quality information, and support resources can provide invaluable information on technology developments.

In the long term, employees with an injury or disability need to understand the process of selecting and using ATs so that they can effectively address their ongoing needs. Consequently it is important that they not only understand what is involved in the process but that they also develop a sound knowledge of the resources available and how to utilize these effectively.

REFERENCES

1. Job Accommodation Network, *Employer's Practical Guide to Reasonable Accommodation under the Americans with Disabilities Act (ADA).* Job Accommodation Network, 2006 [cited 23 February 2007], Available from: www.jan.wvu.edu/Erguide/One.htm#D.
2. Schall, C.M., The American Disabilities Act—are we keeping our promise? An analysis of the effect of the ADA on the employment of persons with disabilities. *J. Voc. Rehabil.*, 10, 191–203, 1998.
3. Langton, A.J. and Ramseur, H., Enhancing employment outcomes through job accommodation and assistive technology resources and services. *J. Voc. Rehabil.*, 16, 27–37, 2001.

4. Phillips, B., Technology abandonment from the consumer point of view. *NARIC Quart.*, 3, 4–91, 1993.
5. Anema, J.R. et al., The effectiveness of ergonomic interventions on return-to-work after low back pain; a prospective two year cohort study in six countries on low back patients sicklisted for 3–4 months. *Occup. Environ. Med.*, 61, 289–294, 2004.
6. Smith, R.O. and Ellingson, E.F. Job modification/accommodation and assistive technology, in: King P.M., editor. *Sourcebook of Occupational Rehabilitation*. Plenum Press, New York, 1998, p. 287–323.
7. Deen, M., Gibson, L., and Strong, J., A survey of occupational therapy in Australian work practice. *Work*, 19, 219–230, 2002.
8. Gibson, L., Allen, M., and Strong, J. Re-integration into work, in: Strong J., Unruh A., Wright A., and Baxter G.D., editors. *Pain: A Textbook for Therapists*. Harcourt, Edinburgh, 2002, p. 267–287.
9. Steinfeld, E. and Angelo, J., Adaptive work placement: A "horizontal" model. *Technol. Disabil.*, 1, 1–10, 1992.
10. Gamble, M., Dowler, D.L., and Orslene, L.E., Assistive technology: Choosing the right tool for the right job. *J. Voc. Rehabil.*, 24, 73–80, 2006.
11. Brewer, S. et al., Workplace interventions to prevent musculoskeletal and visual symptoms and disorders among computer users: A systematic review. *J. Occup. Rehabil.*, 16, 325–358, 2006.
12. van der Molen, H. et al., Effectiveness of measures and implementation strategies in reducing physical work demands due to manual handling at work. *Scand. J. Work Environ. Health*, 31, 75–87, 2005.
13. Franche, R.-L. et al., Workplace-based return-to-work interventions: A systematic review of the quantitative literature. *J. Occup. Rehabil.*, 15, 607–631, 2005.
14. National Council of Disability, *Study on the Financing of Assistive Technology Devices and Services for Individuals with Disabilities,* Washington, DC, 1993.
15. Cook, A. and Hussey, S., *Assistive Technologies: Principles and Practice*, 2nd ed, Mosby, St. Louis, 2002.
16. Cham, R. and Redfern, M.S., Effect of flooring on standing comfort and fatigue. *Hum. Factors*, 43, 381–391, 2001.
17. Konz, S.A. and Rys, M.J., An ergonomics approach to standing aids. *Occup. Ergonom.*, 3, 165–172, 2003.
18. Krumwiede, D., Konz, S., and Hinnen, P., Standing comfort on floor mats. *Occup. Ergonom.*, 1, 135–143, 1998.
19. de Jonge, D.M., Scherer, M., and Rodger, S., *Assistive Technology in the Workplace*, Mosby, St. Louis, MO, 2007.
20. Sowers, J.A., Employment for persons with physical disabilities and related technology. *Voc. Rehabil.*, 55–64, 1991.
21. Lincoln, A.E. et al., Impact of case manager training on worksite accommodations in workers' compensation claimants with upper extremity disorders. *J. Occup. Environ. Med.*, 44, 237–245, 2002.
22. Gadge, K. and Innes, E., An investigation into the immediate effects on comfort, productivity and posture of the Bambach™ saddle seat and a standard office chair. *Work*, 29, 189–203, 2007.
23. McQuistion, L. Ergonomics-for-one: An introduction, in: Rice V.J.B., editor. *Ergonomics in Health Care and Rehabilitation*. Butterworth-Heinemann, Boston, MA, 1998, p. 43–63.
24. Galvin, J.C., Assistive technology: Federal policy and practice since 1982. *Technol. Disabil.*, 6, 3–15, 1997.
25. Batavia, A.I. and Hammer, G.S., Toward the development of consumer-based criteria for the evaluation of assistive devices. *J. Rehabil. Res. Dev.*, 27, 425–436, 1990.

26. Hocking, C., Function or feelings: Factors in abandonment of assistive devices. *Technol. Disabil.*, 11, 3–11, 1999.

27. Mann, W.C. and Lane, J.P., *Assistive Technology for Persons with Disabilities*, 2nd ed, The American Occupational Therapy Association, Bethesda, MD, 1995.

28. Mann, W.C. and Tomita, M., Perspectives on assistive devices among elderly persons with disabilities. *Technol. Disabil.*, 9, 119–148, 1998.

29. Scherer, M.J., *Living in a State of Stuck: How Technology Impacts the Lives of People with Disabilities*, 2nd ed, Brookline Books, Cambridge, MA, 2005.

30. Cushman, L.A. and Scherer, M., Measuring the relationship of assistive technology use, functional status over time, and consumer-therapist perceptions of ATs. *Assist. Technol.*, 8, 103–109, 1996.

31. Garber, S. and Gregorio, T., Upper extremity assistive devices: Assessment of use by spinal cord injured patients with quadriplegia. *Am. J. Occup. Ther.*, 44, 126–131, 1990.

32. Mann, W.C., Hurren, D., and Tomita, M., Comparison of assistive device use and needs of home-based older persons with different impairments. *Am. J. Occup. Ther.*, 47, 980–987, 1993.

33. Phillips, B. and Zhao, H., Predictors of assistive technology abandonment. *Assist. Technol.*, 5, 36–45, 1993.

34. Rogers, J.C. and Holm, M.B., Assistive technology device use in patients with rheumatic disease: A literature review. *Am. J. Occup. Ther.*, 46, 120–127, 1992.

35. Wielandt, P.M. et al., Post discharge use of bathing equipment prescribed by occupational therapists: What lessons to be learned? *Phys. Occup. Ther. Geriatrics*, 19, 49–65, 2001.

36. Gradel, K., Customer Service: What is its place in assistive technology and employment services? *Voc. Rehabil.*, 41–54, 1991.

37. Alliance for Technology Access, *Computer and Web Resources for People with Disabilities*, Hunter House, Berkeley, CA, 2005.

38. Baum, C.M. Achieving effectiveness with a Client Centred Approach: A person-environment Interaction, in: Gray D.B., Quatrano L.A., and Lieberman M.L., editors. *Designing and Using Assistive Technology: The Human Perspective.* Paul H. Brookes, Baltimore, MD, 1998, p. 137–147.

39. Scherer, M.J. and Galvin, J.C. An outcomes perspective to quality pathways to the most appropriate technology, in: Galvin J.C., and Scherer M., editors. *Evaluating, Selecting, and Using Appropriate Assistive Technology.* An Aspen Publication, Gaithersburg, MD, 1996, p. 1–26.

40. Scherer, M.J. et al., Predictors of assistive technology use: The importance of personal and psychosocial factors. *Disabil. Rehabil.*, 27, 1321–1331, 2005.

41. Sprigle, S. and Abdelhamied, A. The relationship between ability measures and assistive technology selection, design and use, in: Gray D.B., Quatrano L.A., and Lieberman M.L., editors. *Designing and Using Assistive Technology: The Human Perspective.* Paul H. Brookes, Baltimore, MD, 1998, p. 229–248.

42. Nochajski, S.M. and Oddo, C.R. Technology in the Workplace, in: Mann W.C. and Lane J.P., editors. *Assistive Technology for People with Disabilities.* 2nd ed. AOTA, Bethesda, MD, 1995, p. 197–260.

43. Law, M. et al., Canadian Occupational Performance Measure, Canadian Association of Occupational Therapy, Toronto, 1994.

44. Dedding, C. et al., Validity of the Canadian Occupational Performance Measure: A client-centred outcome measurement. *Clin. Rehabil.*, 18, 660–667, 2004.

45. Malec, J.F., Goal attainment scaling in rehabilitation. *Neuropsychol. Rehabil.*, 9, 253–275, 1999.

46. Donnelly, C. and Carswell, A., Individualized outcome measures: A review of the literature. *Can. J. Occup. Ther.*, 69, 84–94, 2002.
47. Scherer, M.J., *The Matching Person & Technology (MPT) Model Manual and Assessment 5th edition*, The Institute for Matching Person & Technology, Inc., Webster, New York, 2005.
48. Bain, B.K. and Leger, D., *Assistive Technology: An Interdisciplinary Approach*, Churchill Livingstone, New York, 1997.
49. Kelker, K.A. and Holt, R., *Family Guide to Assistive Technology*, Brookline Books, Cambridge, MA, 2000.
50. Hawley, M.S. et al., A provision framework and data logging tool to aid the prescription of electronic assistive technology. *Technol. Disabil.*, 14, 43–52, 2002.
51. Turner, E. et al., Overcoming obstacles to community re-entry for persons with spinal cord injury: assistive technology, ADA and self advocacy. *J. Prevention Assess Rehabil.*, 9, 171–186, 1997.
52. United States Department of Labor, *Dictionary of Occupational Titles*, 4th ed, U.S. Government Printing Office, Washington, DC, 1991.
53. United States Department of Labor, *The Revised Handbook for Analyzing Jobs*, JIST Works, Indianapolis, IN, 1991.
54. Ellexson, M.T. Job analysis and worksite assessment, in: Sanders M.J., editor. *Ergonomics and the Management of Musculoskeletal Disorders*. 2nd ed. Butterworth Heinemann, St Louis, MO, 2004, p. 283–295.
55. Jacobs, K. and Wyrick, J. Use of Department of Labor references and job analysis, In S. Hertfelder, and Gwin C., editors. *Work in Progress*. American Occupational Therapy Association, Rockville MD, 1989, p. 23–65.
56. Lysaght, R., Job analysis in occupational therapy: Stepping into the complex world of business and industry. *Am. J. Occup. Ther.*, 51, 569–575, 1997.
57. U.S. Department of Labor Employment and Training Administration, *O*NET 9.0 Database, [Online]*. National O*NET Consortium, North Carolina Employment Security Commission., 2006, Available from: http://www. onetcenter. org.
58. Hammel, J.M. and Symons, J., Evaluating for reasonable accommodation: A team approach. *J. Prevention Assess Rehabil.*, 3, 12–21, 1993.
59. Bazinet, G. Assistive Technology, in: Karan O.C. and Greenspan S., editors. *Community Rehabilitation Services for People with Disabilities*. Butterworth-Heinemann, Boston, MA, 1995, p. 321–331.
60. Struck, M., Technology solutions for ADA compliance. *Occup. Ther. Health Care*, 11, 23–28, 1999.
61. Covington, G.A. Cultural and environmental barriers to assistive technology, in: Gray D.B., Quatrano L.A., and Lieberman M.L., editors. *Designing and Using Assistive Technology: The Human Perspective*. Paul H. Brookes, Baltimore, MD, 1998, p. 77–88.
62. Law, M., *Client-Centred Occupational Therapy*, SLACK Inc, Thorofare, NJ, 1998.
63. Scherer, M.J. and Craddock, G., Matching Person & Technology (MPT) assessment process. *Technol. Disabil.*, 14, 125–131, 2002.
64. Ehrlich, N.J., Carlson, D., and Bailey, N., Sources of information about how to obtain assistive technology: Findings from a national survey of persons with disabilities. *Assist. Technol.*, 15, 28–38, 2003.
65. Anson, D.K., *Alternative Computer Access: A Guide to Selection*, F. A. Davis, Philadelphia, PA, 1997.
66. Turner, E. et al., The user's perspective of assistive technology, in: Flippo K.F., Inge K.J., and Barcus J.M., editors. *Assistive Technology: A Resource for School, Work and Community*. 1st ed. Paul H. Brookes, Baltimore, MD, 1995, p. 283–290.

67. Cowan, D.M. and Turner-Smith, A.R., The user's perspective on the provision of electronic assistive technology: Equipped for life? *Brit. J. Occup. Ther.*, 62, 2–6, 1999a.

68. Inge, K.J. et al., Supported employment and assistive technology for persons with spinal cord injury: Three illustrations of successful work supports. *J. Voc. Rehabil.*, 10, 141–152, 1998.

69. Lash, M. and Licenziato, V., Career transitions for people with severe physical disabilities; integrating technology and psychosocial skills and accommodations. *Work*, 5, 85–98, 1995.

70. Rumrill, P.D. and Garnette, M.R., Career adjustment via reasonable accommodations: The effects of an employee-empowerment intervention for people with disabilities. *J. Prevent. Assess. Rehabil.*, 9, 57–64, 1997.

71. Wallace, J.F. and Gilson, B.B., Disabled and non-disabled: Allied together to change the system. *J. Prevention Assess. Rehabil.*, 9, 73–80, 1997.

72. Andrich, R. and Besio, S., Being informed, demanding and responsible consumers of assistive technology: An educational issue. *Disabil. Rehabil.*, 24, 152–159, 2002.

73. Lupton, D. and Seymour, W., Technology, selfhood and physical disability. *Soc. Sci. Med.*, 50, 1851–1862, 2000.

74. Wallace, J.F. Creative financing of Assistive Technology, in: Flippo K.F., Inge K.J., and Barcus J.M., editors. *Assistive Technology: A Resource for School, Work and Community.* Paul H. Brookes, Baltimore, MD, 1995, p. 245–268.

75. Scherer, M.J. and Vitaliti, L.T. Functional approach to technological factors and their assessment in rehabilitation, in: Dittmar S.S. and Gresham G.E., editors. *Functional Assessment and Outcome Measures for the Health Rehabilitation Professional.* Aspen, Gaithersburg, MD, 1997, p. 69–88.

76. Behrman, M.M. Assistive Technology Training, in: Flippo K.F., Inge K.J., and Barcus J.M., editors. *Assistive Technology: A Resource for School, Work and Community.* Paul H. Brookes, Baltimore, MD, 1995, p. 211–222.

77. Burwell, C.M. Ergonomics, in: Bain B.K., and Leger D., editors. *Assistive Technology: An Interdisciplinary Approach.* Churchill Livingston Inc, New York, 1997, p. 229–239.

78. Patterson, D.R., Jensen, M., and Engel-Knowles, J. Pain and its influence on assistive technology use, in: Scherer M.J., editor. *Assistive Technology: Matching Device and Consumer for Successful Rehabilitation.* American Psychological Association, Washington, DC, 2002, p. 59–76.

79. Sowers, J.A. Adaptive Environments in the Workplace, in: Flippo K.F., Inge K.J., and Barcus J.M., editors. *Assistive Technology: A Resource for School, Work and Community.* Paul H. Brookes, Baltimore, MD, 1995, p. 167–186.

80. Wessels, R.D. et al., Non-use of provided assistive technology devices, a literature overview. *Technol. Disabil.*, 15, 231–238, 2003.

81. King, T.W., *Assistive Technology: Essential Human Factors*, Allyn & Bacon, Needham Heights, MA, 1999.

82. Department of Employment Training and Industrial Relations, *Risk Management Advisory Standard 2000.* Department of Employment Training and Industrial Relations, 2000, Available from: http://www.dir.qld.gov.au/workplace/law/codes/riskman/.

83. Hunt, H.A. and Berkowitz, M. The background and setting, in: Hunt H.A. and Berkowitz M., editors. *New Technologies and the Employment of Disabled People.* International Labour Office, Geneva, 1992, p. 7–13.

15 Current Designs in Assistive Technology

Donald S. Bloswick and Bryan Howard

CONTENTS

15.1 INTRODUCTION/BACKGROUND

Assistive technology has been a part of our everyday lives for centuries. The earliest eye glasses were developed around the early 1300s. Since then, eye glasses and other assistive devices have been developed and evolved into more useful and more sophisticated technologies. Today, assistive technologies are designed to aid those with a host of disabilities ranging from visual impairments to learning disabilities; from hearing impairments to physical handicaps. Engineers from a variety of disciplines are continuously working together to develop new and better devices that will help to enhance the lives of impaired individuals by facilitating their participation in activities found in all aspects of modern life.

Currently, the emphasis is generally placed on the research and design of new devices that (1) aid impaired children, (2) aid elderly population, (3) aid persons with spinal cord injury, and (4) facilitate brain–computer interface. This chapter presents new assistive technology devices developed in the Ergonomics and Safety Laboratory at the University of Utah focusing on the first and second emphasized areas. These devices were designed and fabricated by undergraduate and graduate students in mechanical engineering in collaboration with faculty and students in the Department of Family and Preventive Medicine, Department of Physical Medicine and Rehabilitation, Division of Physical Therapy, and Division of Occupational Therapy.

Devices developed for use by children address rehabilitation/mobility issues for young children with cerebral palsy (CP) and include (1) a tricycle powered by hip extension that both increases mobility and helps to improve the child's gait, (2) an all-terrain walker (ATW) that increases the child's mobility and facilitates participation in family camping and hiking activities, and (3) a one-arm kayak/canoe paddle that helps facilitate the child's participation in family kayak/canoeing activities.

Devices developed for use by adults address wheelchair designs/modifications that increase the mobility in adults with disabilities or seniors with reduced capabilities due to normal aging. These designs include (1) a wheelchair with a spring powered lift-seat to facilitate movement from the seated to standing position; (2) foot extension propelled wheelchairs to allow forward wheelchair movement with knee extension; (3) hand-crank propelled wheelchair carriages to allow users of wheelchairs to mount the carriage, attach their wheelchair, and propel themselves over snow or sand; and (4) a hand-lever propelled wheelchair that reduces muscle fatigue and provides for proportional braking.

15.2 ASSISTIVE TECHNOLOGY DEVICES FOR CHILDREN WITH CEREBRAL PALSY

15.2.1 Hip Extensor Tricycle

Children with CP often have weak hip extensor muscles (Figure 15.1), a condition that often manifests itself in poor gait. Traditionally therapists have used calisthenics

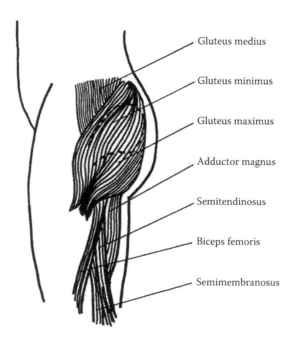

Gluteus medius

Gluteus minimus

Gluteus maximus

Adductor magnus

Semitendinosus

Biceps femoris

Semimembranosus

FIGURE 15.1 Hip extensor muscles.

and the use of a traditional tricycle in a program to strengthen the leg muscles. The biomechanics of traditional tricycle use, however, are not effective in exercising the hip extensor muscles. Other means of exercising the hip extensors, such as standing hip extension against the resistance generated from an elastic cord at the ankle, were disliked by the children. The challenge to develop a therapeutic device that would exercise the hip extensor muscles and be enjoyable for children was posed to engineers by physicians working with such children in the Department of Physical Medicine and Rehabilitation.

In the interest of simplicity, the first attempt was simply a tricycle modified to suspend the child in a flexible saddle so that the feet could just touch the ground, requiring the user to use a walking type motion to propel the tricycle. This device, however, did not result in the desired use of the hip extensor muscles. It was determined that, to be effective, the device must more directly require the use of these muscles for movement. A four-bar linkage connecting the pedals to the drive wheels was designed and configured in such a way that it allowed the user to effectively stand up on the pedals and use hip extension to propel the tricycle. This design was designated the hip extensor tricycle (HET) and is shown in Figure 15.2.

An initial test of the system indicated that the electromyographic (EMG) activity in the hip extensor muscles while using the HET was greater than that while using a normal tricycle (Figure 15.3). Further, the EMG followed the approximate temporal pattern and magnitude levels as during walking [1].

In subsequent testing (Figure 15.4), four of five children with CP had observable improvement in their gait patterns as determined by four rehabilitation physical therapists and one rehabilitation medicine physician. In a subsequent physical examination, it was found that the one test subject who did not demonstrate gait improvement had a degenerative hip disorder that prevented therapeutic progress.

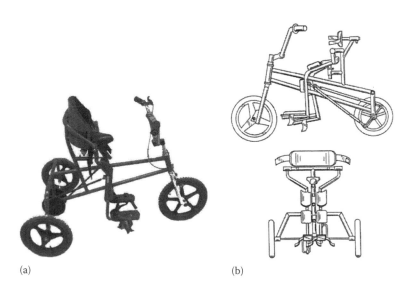

(a)   (b)

FIGURE 15.2   HET photograph and schematics. (From Howell, G. et al., *RESNA J. Assist. Technol.*, 5, 119, 1993. With permission.)

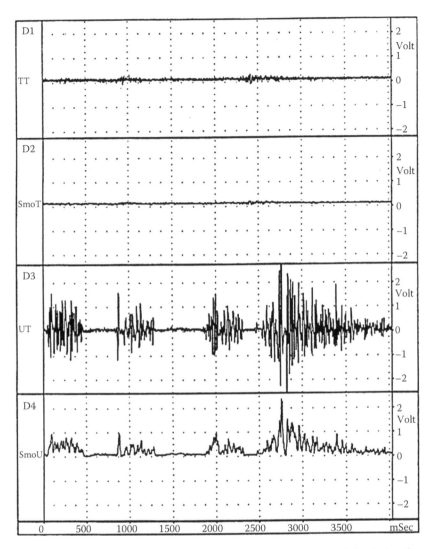

FIGURE 15.3 EMG patterns. The top two signals represent muscle activity during the use of a normal tricycle. The bottom two signals represent the hip extensor muscle activity during HET use.

A serendipitous benefit for the children was the enhanced self-esteem reported by the parents due to the children's greater independent mobility and enhanced involvement with neighborhood playmates. For some of the children with CP it was their first experience riding a tricycle and in one case the test subject became somewhat of a neighborhood celebrity because of the unique nature of his tricycle [2–4]. The HET has been patented (in both mobile and stationary configurations) and licensed to a local company. Currently the HET is being fabricated and distributed worldwide.

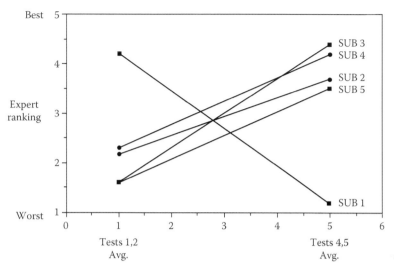

FIGURE 15.4   Expert ranking of gait improvement in children using the HET.

15.2.2   ALL-TERRAIN WALKER

In many cases children with CP use a walker to facilitate mobility. Their use of walkers, however, may limit their ability to maneuver over uneven terrain or sandy surfaces. At the request of the parents of one child with CP, an ATW was designed and fabricated by a team of three undergraduate mechanical engineering students as part of their senior design project. The major performance criteria for the design were that the walker have tires large enough to traverse obstacles up to approximately 3 in. and that some type of shock absorption be an integral part of the design. The need to traverse obstacles was addressed by the inclusion of pneumatic tires of 12 and 16 in. diameter on the front and rear, respectively. The tires were selected to have 2 in. width to allow the walker to "float" over uneven terrain. The need for shock absorption was addressed through the use of an innovative torsion "spring" where the rear wheels connect to the frame. The ATW is illustrated in Figure 15.5.

The ATW has been used extensively by a local family and has allowed the user much greater mobility during camping and hiking trips. A provisional patent has been requested and the torsion spring is being used as the basis for an extension of this design to a "ski-walker" for children with disabilities.

15.2.3   ONE-ARM KAYAK PADDLE

A normal kayak paddle stroke requires three major physical capabilities. First, the user must be capable of grasping the paddle with both hands, using one hand to pull the paddle through the water and the other to stabilize the opposite end of the paddle. Second, the user must be able to rotate their torso around the all three axes to keep the paddle blade in the water through the duration of the stroke. Third, the user must be able to extend and flex their wrists and lower and upper arms. Children with CP,

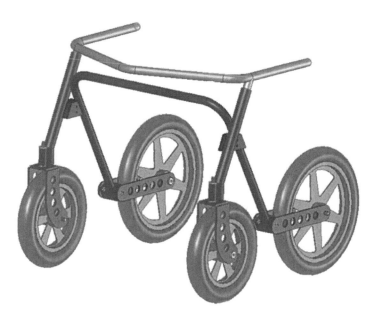

FIGURE 15.5   All-terrain walker (ATW).

however, cannot completely control the movements of their hand and arms and have difficulty controlling the movement of their torsos.

The primary purpose of this paddle is to improve the ability of children with CP to participate in family kayaking/canoeing activities by reducing the physical paddling requirements mentioned above, reduce the occurrence of blisters and other wear injuries, and enable the children to better maintain their balance while paddling. This paddle design eliminates the requirements to twist the torso about all three axes, reduces digital control requirements needed to independently grasp the paddle handle, and eliminates the requirement to use one's second arm as a fulcrum on which to base the paddles rotation. The design allows for adjustable length and paddle angle about two axes. Further the design incorporates a quick release pin on the chest harness to free the child from the paddle if the need arises. Paddle is shown in Figure 15.6.

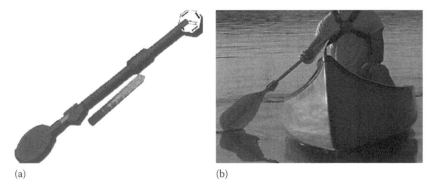

(a)   (b)

FIGURE 15.6   (a) One-arm kayak and (b) canoe paddle for use by children with CP and other upper body disabilities.

By facilitating the children's participation and contribution to the canoeing/ kayak activity, children will gain the physical benefits of the exercise while also improving their confidence and self-esteem by allowing them to accomplish the task of paddling on their own.

15.3 ASSISTIVE TECHNOLOGY FOR SENIORS USING WHEELCHAIRS

15.3.1 WHEELCHAIR WITH LIFT SEAT

Many people, particularly seniors, require assistance to move from a seated to a standing position and from a standing to a seated position. In general, devices designed to assist in this maneuver are complex and expensive. This led to the design and fabrication of the sit-to-stand (STS) wheelchair. The STS wheelchair fulfills the need for an inexpensive system that helps the user move from the seated to the standing position. The STS was designed with the following parameters in mind:

1. The lifting force must be higher at the beginning of the lift and decrease as the seat lifts the user. (This is required to allow the user to "back into" the wheelchair when going from the standing to the sitting position.)
2. The lifting velocity and force must be independent and adjustable.
3. All components must fit within the footprint of a normal wheelchair.
4. No external power sources are required.

Two versions of the STS wheelchair were developed [5]. The first uses a coil spring, the force of which is transmitted through a cam, which increases the moment arm (and lifting moment) of the seat when it is close to the horizontal position. The second uses a torsion spring, which by its nature, develops more lifting "torque" at the beginning of the lift. In both cases the spring tension is generated when the user moves into the seated position. The spring force is adjustable and the velocity is controlled through a hydraulic cylinder/circuit in parallel with (and independent of) the spring. Figure 15.7 illustrates the operation of the first of these two designs.

Comparisons of required muscle activity to achieve a standing position from a sitting position found that a standard wheelchair required the greatest muscle activity, the tension spring design require a reduced level of muscle activity, and the torsion spring design required the least amount of muscle activity (Table 15.1).

These wheelchairs were tested in an extended care facility with good results. Facility residents were able to move unassisted from the seated wheelchair and grasp the handles of a walker after movement into the standing position. These devices have been patented and licensed to a potential manufacturer.

15.3.2 KNEE EXTENSION PROPELLED WHEELCHAIRS

Older wheelchair users and people without adequate hand strength sometimes use knee extension to propel their wheelchair backward. These same users of wheelchairs may have limited neck mobility and find it difficult to see exactly where they are going, possibly putting themselves or other persons in danger of unintended

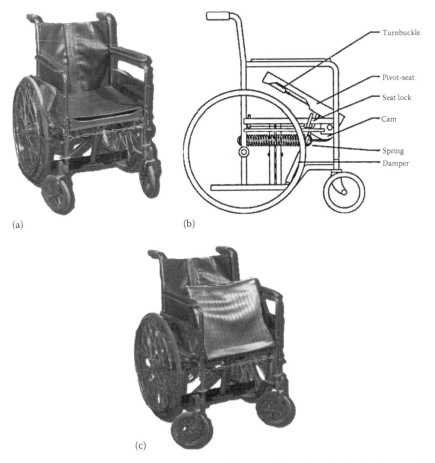

FIGURE 15.7 STS wheelchair. This device allows individuals with limited strength to move from a sitting to a standing position and vice versa without assistance.

contact. Collaboration between faculty in the Department of Family and Preventive Medicine and faculty and students in the Department of Mechanical Engineering resulted in the development of three different knee extension propelled wheelchairs

TABLE 15.1

Required Muscle Activity to Achieve a Standing Position from a Sitting Position for the Lift-Seat Wheelchairs as a Percentage of the Standard Wheelchair

Wheelchair	Total Expenditure (%)		Maximum Exertion (%)	
	Up	Down	Up	Down
Standard	100	100	100	100
Tension spring	78.13	71.56	74.14	57.85
Torsion spring	58.80	69.51	55.76	57.20

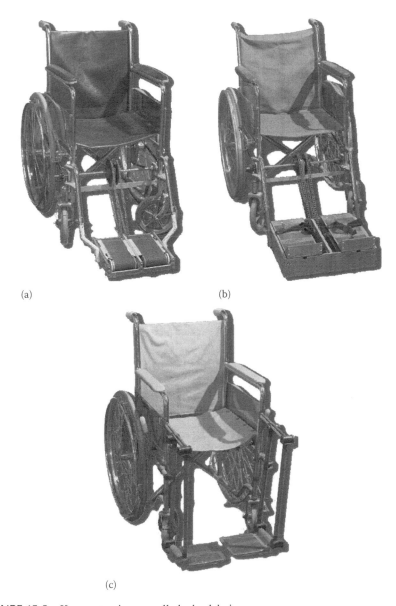

(a)   (b)

(c)

FIGURE 15.8   Knee extension propelled wheelchairs.

to address this need: (1) belt design, (2) slide design, and (3) four-bar linkage design
[5]. These are illustrated in Figure 15.8.

The first of these designs, the belt-driven wheelchair, allows the user to slide
either the left or right belt forward with the sole of the foot. The top surface of the
belt has a high coefficient of friction. The left and right belts are directly linked to
the left and right wheel respectively, which allows the user to turn by moving only
one foot forward. However, belt slippage and power loss through the series of chains
and sprockets made this design impractical.

To eliminate belt slip, the chair was redesigned to incorporate plates in place of the belts. Using the same movement as in the belt design, the user slides the plates back and forth to generate forward movement. As with the belt design, the user slides either the left or right foot forward with the sole of the foot and the left and right slide mechanisms are directly linked to the left and right wheel respectively, which allows the user to turn by moving only one foot forward. Unfortunately, as with the belt design, the power loss through the series of chains and sprockets made the design impractical.

The four-bar linkage design eliminates the need for the series of chains and sprockets. This design allows the user to propel the wheelchair through two four-bar linkages that can be activated independently by each foot. As the four-bar linkage swings forward, a cable attached to the footrest and to a ratcheting cam mechanism on the rear wheel rotates the wheel. When the footrest is rotated backward with the lower leg (knee flexion) the brake on that side is activated. This allows the user to turn by extending one leg and flexing the other leg. The power loss experienced in the two earlier designs was minimized in this design. A test of maneuverability indicated that the belt design and four-bar linkage design were the most maneuverable [6].

15.3.3 TRACK-BALL WHEELCHAIR

The concept for this design arose from the same need for as for the knee extension propelled wheelchairs just discussed. A new approach was utilized, resulting in the "track-ball" wheelchair shown in Figure 15.9. This design allows the user to move

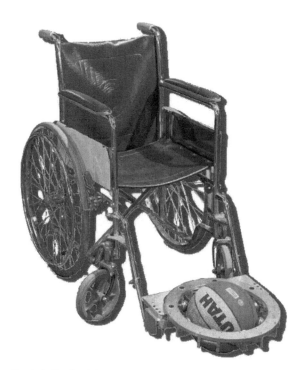

FIGURE 15.9   Track-ball wheelchair.

the wheelchair in any direction simply by rolling the "track-ball" (a basketball with high coefficient of friction surface) with the feet. This design was preferred by the residents of the extended care facility in which the different devices were tested. A provisional patent has been requested.

15.3.4 Hand-Crank Propelled Wheelchair Carriages

Users of wheelchairs frequently find it necessary to traverse uneven surfaces or surfaces covered by snow or sand. This need surfaced at the 2002 Winter Olympics in Salt Lake City when the University of Utah was contacted by representatives of the Salt Lake Organizing Committee to develop a wheelchair carriage that would facilitate access to snow-covered venues by users of wheelchairs using their own personal wheelchairs. This need was met with two designs.

The first design (model 1) was developed to be quite narrow to allow passage through doors (Figure 15.10). Using removable ramps, the user can propel his/her wheelchair onto the carriage and connect the wheelchair to the carriage. Field testing indicated that the narrow spacing of the tracks greatly limited turning ability.

The second configuration (model 2), seen in Figure 15.11, was designed to incorporate an access "ramp" that is balanced so as to facilitate access to the carriage but then rotates up and locks into place when the user is appropriately situated. Also, this design incorporates an increased track spacing that greatly increased turning ability. The increased width, however, also limits access into most buildings.

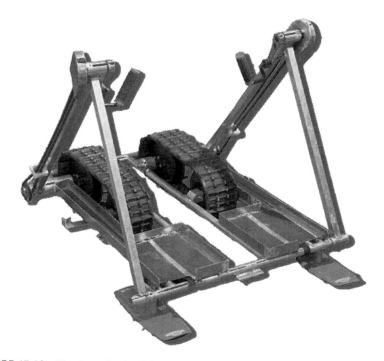

FIGURE 15.10 Hand-crank wheelchair carriage (model 1).

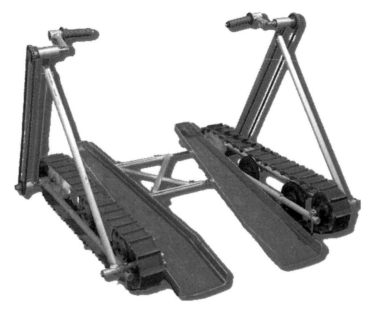

FIGURE 15.11   Hand-crank wheelchair carriage (model 2).

Six volunteer wheelchair users evaluated both wheelchair carriages at a snow-covered venue. In general, they preferred model 2 because of the improved access ramps and increased turning performance. A provisional patent has been requested.

15.3.5   HAND-LEVER PROPELLED WHEELCHAIR

Users of wheelchairs may find it necessary, more efficient, or more convenient to use levers instead of the wheels to propel their wheelchair. In some cases, limited grip strength or mobility affects the ability to grasp and move the wheel. In addition the use of a lever eliminates the user's need to make contact with a dirty wheel. To fulfill this need, a hand-lever propelled wheelchair was developed (Figure 15.12).

This design allows the user to "push" forward with the arms to propel the wheelchair forward or "pull" backward to propel the wheelchair backwards. The push movement requires only that the user contact the lever handle between the thumb and first finger and does not require an actual hand grip. This means that users with limited hand strength can propel the wheelchair. This motion is also more efficient than the forward and down movement required to rotate the wheels directly. The push motion is translated to the wheels through a disk brake that acts as a clutch. When the user pushes forward, the user rotates the forearms slightly to tighten a cable that forces the disk brake calipers to contact, grip the disk, and move the wheel. Since no ratchets are used, the user can easily rotate either wheel in either direction simply by rotating the forearms and pushing on the levers (to go forward) or pulling on the levers (to go backward). The use of the disk brake also provides a braking force proportional to the forearm rotation force, which allows the user to slow or stop the wheelchair gradually, without gripping the wheelchair's wheels with their hands. A provisional patent has been requested.

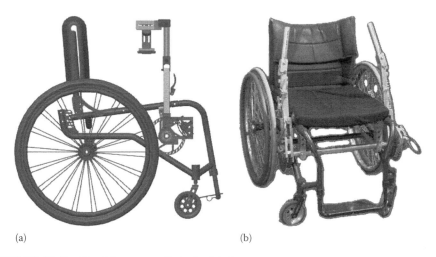

(a) (b)

FIGURE 15.12 Hand-lever propelled wheelchair.

15.4 CONCLUSIONS/RECOMMENDATIONS

Engineers, in collaboration with physicians and other health professionals, can be primary players in the design and development of new technologies to further enhance the lives of people with disabilities. Interdisciplinary research activities at the University of Utah involving the Department of Mechanical Engineering, Department of Physical Medicine and Rehabilitation, Department of Family and Preventive Medicine, Division of Physical Therapy, and Division of Occupational Therapy has resulted in several useful assistive technology devices that have improved the lives of many persons with disabilities. By aiding in their rehabilitation, increasing their mobility and helping them to participate in activities that are encountered in everyday modern life, these devices assist these individuals in leading more fulfilling lives.

REFERENCES

1. Howell, G. et al., Design of a device to exercise hip extensor muscles in children with cerebral palsy, *RESNA Journal of Assistive Technology*, 5(2), 119, 1993.
2. King, E. et al., Evaluation of the hip extensor tricycle in improving gait in children with cerebral palsy, *Developmental Medicine and Child Neurology*, 35, 1048, 1993.
3. Bloswick, D.S. et al., Evaluation of a device to exercise hip extensor muscles in children with cerebral palsy: A clinical and field study, *RESNA Journal of Assistive Technology*, 6(2), 147, 1994.
4. Bloswick, D.S. et al., Testing and evaluation of a hip extensor tricycle for children with cerebral palsy, *Disability and Rehabilitation*, 18(3), 130, 1996.
5. Bloswick, D.S. et al., Development and testing of wheel chairs with lift seat and knee extension propulsion, *Proceedings of the 12th Triennial Congress of the International Ergonomics Association*, 3, 190, 1994.
6. Bloswick, D.S. et al., Maneuverability and usability analysis of three knee-extension propelled wheelchairs, *Disability and Rehabilitation*, 25(4–5), 197, 2003.

16 Enabling Design

Peter Anderberg, Elin Olander,
Bodil Jönsson, and Lena Sperling

CONTENTS

16.1 INTRODUCTION

In order to prevent occupationally related accidents, illnesses and injuries, you would be hard put to find anyone who would argue against equipment in the workplace that was designed for users according to gender, age, body dimensions, and physical and mental capacities. Nor does anyone deny that one of the most stimulating challenges for modern design is to ensure a nondiscriminating approach to the design of products, services, environments, and artifacts, one that can be used by as many people as possible regardless of differences in their ability or situation. This chapter is about uniting the different approaches from the working life and design sectors to achieve an even more fruitful outcome than the one that already exists.

The roots of the expressed need to include a greater number of people as potential users of products, services, and environments can be found in political and ideological endeavors that promote a society for all, and that are seen as prerequisites

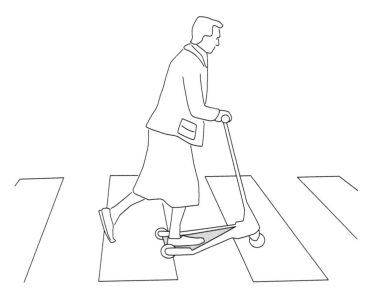

FIGURE 16.1   Elderly people no longer accept the absence of useworthy tools and vehicles.

for democracy. This development is advanced and stimulated by the demographical changes of an aging population [1].

Design involves both functional and emotional aspects. Esthetics includes impressions from all senses. Users with special requirements for personal equipment deserve products of the same (or even higher) esthetic qualities as others. Appealing and pleasant tools and equipment can make people feel welcome, take pride in their work, and promote a positive employee self-image, while at the same time strengthening the company's brand (Figure 16.1).

In many cases, technology developed for disabled people has made its way into the general population (faucets operated by one hand, remote control, low-floor buses, etc.) [2]. What is valuable for disabled persons is often good for the nondisabled majority, but this is not a universal truth. Even less of such a truth is the belief that what profits some disabled people, profits others with different disabilities as well.

In the following discussion, we will elaborate on how design can make a workplace more useworthy [3] for all, including other aspects of daily living. The analysis describes how nondiscriminative design influences function and attitudes as well as control and esthetics. Ethical elements are also discussed.

16.2   NONDISCRIMINATING DESIGN AND INDUSTRIAL DESIGN

A key factor for disabled people to participate fully in society and have control over their presence there is not to be hindered by unnecessarily built-in obstacles in environments and artifacts (Figure 16.2). The principles behind the nondiscriminating design (NDD) approaches—universal design, inclusive design, and design for all—are extremely important for disabled people [4,5] and they are fairly well accepted

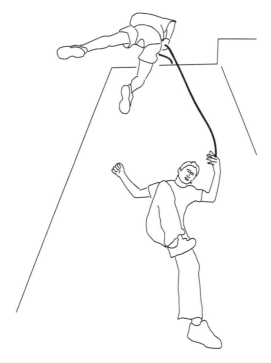

FIGURE 16.2 The ideas and solutions differ considerably if you consider a functional hindrance to be an individual disability or a characteristic of the surroundings.

as a desired goal in design. But to put the principles into practice is not without problems, to say the least. There is no standard disabled person with a standard set of wishes, but rather a multitude of individuals with different abilities, wishes, and personal standards. The concept of Design for Me [6] is introduced along with the other three to make NDD more evident, balance it, complement it, and challenge it.

16.2.1 UNIVERSAL DESIGN, INCLUSIVE DESIGN, AND DESIGN FOR ALL

The differences between universal design, inclusive design, and design for all are ideological, cultural, and historical. Even if they most often may yield similar results, the working approaches differ. At its inner core, Universal Design's ambition is not to distinguish between disabled and able-bodied people or between old and young people [7]. As the American Society on Aging (ASA) elaborates, universal design should be viewed as "a process of ensuring that product and environmental design is compatible with the variation in human capabilities that result from differences among individuals of various ages, cultures, languages, cognitive skills, sizes, shapes, physical conditioning, races, and gender." A product designed to be usable to the greatest extent possible by all ages and abilities, without the need of adaptation or specialized enabling design [8] can be defined as a universal design product.

The Center for Universal Design has developed seven general principles [8,9] used as guidelines when working with the universal design concept in practice as an industrial designer. The principles are (1) equitable to use, (2) flexibility in use, (3) simple and intuitive use, (4) perceptible information, (5) tolerance for error, (6) low physical effort, and (7) size and space for approach and use. There are also four to five recommendations for each principle on how to fulfill the aim.

While the American universal design of the early 1980s, nowadays also frequently used in Japan, aims at nondiscrimination by not explicitly focusing on disabilities, the British inclusive design does the opposite. The rationale behind the latter is one of user inclusion rather than exclusion when designing products, systems, and environments—"what if we design like this, then we would include these user groups as well, rather than exclude them" [1]. Steinfeid and Tauke [10] argue that the term "inclusive design" is preferable to "universal design" because there are no " 'universal solutions' to problems, which meet the needs of all people." The inclusive design approach promotes products that are designed with consideration to all members of society. In particular, the objective is to consider the needs of old and disabled people alongside the younger and able-bodied population to ensure that products are equally appealing and suited to all users, i.e., it could be said to be characterized as a "design for the disabled" approach [1]. Jordan [11] argues that in addition to being morally sensible, inclusive design may lead to market opportunities and financial benefits for companies adopting the concept. The BSI British Standards provides the following definition: "Inclusive Design constitutes a strategic framework and associated processes by which business decisionmakers and design practitioner can understand and respond to the needs of diverse groups of users. The ultimate goal is to develop products and services that can meet the needs of the whole population."

The design for all approach is similar to that of universal design but its background and its geographical area of application is European. The term is most often used in interactive design, striving to make computer program interfaces user-friendly. The Network EIDD described design for all as a philosophy aiming to "improve the life of everyone through design." In the Design for All Declaration (2004), EIDD defines it as design for human diversity, social inclusion, and equality. Design for all is more down-to-earth practice than universal design. Both move away from disability-related issues to largely mainstream issues in design [7].

16.2.2 DESIGN FOR ME AND DESIGN FOR ALL

From the perspective of the designer, design for all means accommodating for a great number of personal solutions. Where design for all is the societal, market, or designer perspective, Design for Me holds the user perspective (Figure 16.3). The user wants his/her functions to work as smoothly as possible and to have control over them themselves. Design for Me is already the predominant design solution when it comes to personal assistance, which is tailor-made to fit the needs of the individual and where full personal control is seen as a prerequisite for high quality of assistance. The same argument holds for technical assistance.

Design for all and Design for Me refer to the same problem complex—the desired functioning of the individual—and are complementary but differ on where the main technological solution is positioned. Design for Me is associated with "stand-alone AT" or "orphan technology" [12] but goes much further. Design for Me consequently

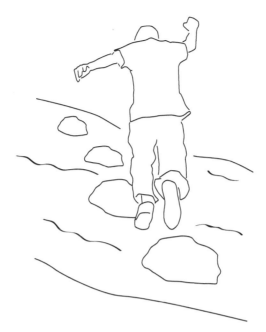

FIGURE 16.3   Design for Me is closely connected to one's own control.

implies, but is not synonymous with, a high degree of individual adaptation. This does not imply that environmental adaptation is unwanted or unnecessary, quite the opposite. It merely points to the fact that greater control over functioning can be achieved in a system where assistance is more personalized, and that assistive technology with high functioning power that follows the individual makes them more independent of environmental changes.

Design for Me also implies a high level of participatory design efforts with a high degree of user involvement in the shaping of the whole support system of technological and personal assistance. In almost all cases, a good design for all facilitates Design for Me. Design for Me can also help in dealing with the design for all paradox: Accommodating for all possible use by all people in a certain situation is impossible. All people do not require the same kind of solutions. The desired solutions are sometimes directly incompatible. Arguments can be raised against relying on individual technological solutions, seemingly associated with the individual model of disability, where the disability is positioned as a defect of the individual. The improvement in functioning of the individual has often been portrayed as promoting a negative, disempowered image of disabled people, rather than seeing the problem as political, social, and environmental.

Even if curb cuts, ramps, and accessible buses no doubt signal a welcoming attitude, and even if the lack of them can be perceived as hostility toward a person in a wheelchair, it could also be argued that in relying on the multitude of necessary adaptations of the environment, both humanmade and natural, disabled people lose control over where they want to go and when. Instead, the sporadic and occasionally implemented adaptations in places decided by others determine where we are allowed to go. With individual solutions the control lies with the individual. It may be argued as well that a high degree of individual control can be a positive attitude shaping element in itself. It is hard to maintain the image of helplessness when an individual has control over the situation. A wheelchair that can climb stairs and drive around in the countryside could prove to be a better solution than having to adapt all buildings and environments in the world. A cell phone is a much better solution than installing stationary telephones on every street corner. The closer to the individual and the more mobile and adaptable, the better the solution often is, at least if the emphasis is on control.

Rather than seeing the difference between Design for Me and design for all as a question of the individual versus the environmental model of disability, it could (somewhat simplified) be seen as a question of weighing attitude versus control aspects of functioning. The question of where the line is drawn between desired use of Design for Me and design for all must be constantly negotiated and problematized in the situations where the assistance is needed. One should not allow design for all to blind oneself to the possibilities of Design for Me. Situated solutions (for Me) represent in themselves one of many possible ways of adapting environments, and it is not fruitful to be too dogmatic. For instance, if I cannot see the blackboard at a distance, I do not demand that it be brought closer to me and only me; I put on my glasses and so would others, while some do not need to. It is the multiple, parallel ways of performing a function that allow Design for Me, just as a selection from a smorgasbord is better than one single dish that contains all different flavors.

16.2.3 INDUSTRIAL DESIGN

Industrial design means the creation/gestalting of useful products intended for mass production, with the aim of adapting them to humans and their environment [13]. "Gestalt" means the total apparition of the product, speaking to us through all our senses, what we hear, see, feel, smell—and even taste. A "gestalt" can be described as an arrangement of separate parts, appearing and working as an entirety (Monö, 1992) [14]. The formulation "useful products" excludes many kinds of artifacts. Products for private as well as professional users are included. "Intended for mass production" means that knowledge is needed about the production system in order to design the product so that it is easy to assemble and economically feasible in the industrial system. "Adapting of products to man" requires knowledge of cognitive as well as physical ergonomics. Products should be esthetically attractive and contribute to user pride. Considering the environment in the design of products means that a life cycle perspective must be applied in industrial design.

Crilly [15] argues that industrial design is characterized not only by the importance of the visual element of the end product but also by the visual output from every phase of the design process when he tries to visualize the designer's intent through consumers response (Figure 16.4). The ability to give form, to realize an idea as a concrete artifact is what distinguishes design from general problem solving [16]. Ilstedt-Hjelm [17] argues that "giving form" is an active process, which implies that there is something there that takes form. Something is expressed through the forms that meet our senses and mind. The product then becomes a sign for a number of denotative and connotative meanings that the users actively construct.

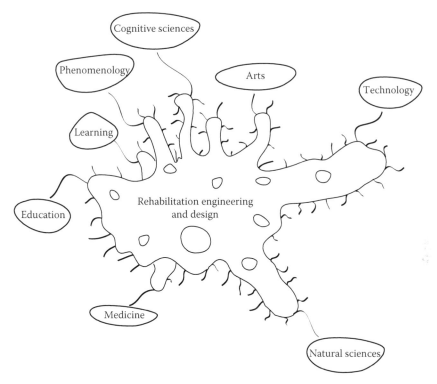

FIGURE 16.4 Rehabilitations engineering and design relates not only to many individual needs, wishes, and dreams but also to many discipline areas.

There are industrial designers who are heavily involved in NDD—we consider ourselves to be members of (or siblings to; all of us are not industrial designers) that group. Many industrial designers have other driving forces than the market (cf. the master's project by Anna Persson [18]) expressing an explicit need for the designer to also be proud of the solutions.

16.3 SITUATED PARTICIPATORY DESIGN

One cornerstone of fruitful design is the necessity of involving users in the design process. This engagement requires not only activating users but also engaging developers themselves in gaining a better understanding of use contexts and situations [19,20].

There are many ways to involve users in a design process. The concept "user-centered design" emerged in the mid-1980s. According to Gould and Lewis, the three main principles of user-centered design are early focus on users and tasks, empirical measurement, and iterative design [21]. Early focus on users and tasks incorporates various methods to examine characteristics of a user group through, for example, user mapping, task analysis, questionnaires, or direct observation. These surveying methods are described in the EU accessibility project Userfit [22] or standard human–computer interaction and human factors literature [23,24].

Empirical measurement is the practice of letting future users use simulations and prototypes and measuring their performance through quantitative feedback including measures of efficiency, number of errors, time to complete tasks, etc. Good descriptions of such test methods may be found in Jeffrey Rubin's *Handbook of Usability Testing* [25]. Iterative design is a standard component in design methods [26] and builds on a cycle of design, testing, and measurements that is repeated as often as needed, starting with early prototypes. Usability engineering [27] builds on the user-centered approach, but attempts to make the process easier to fit into an engineering perspective by focusing on the usability goals as a measure of when the iterative design process may be stopped.

User-centered design may be defined as design for users, design by users, and "design for users with users" [28], depending on the degree of user participation. In design for users, there needs to be no user involvement (Figure 16.5). The strategy "design with and by users" combines ergonomic knowledge with users' expert knowledge in a beneficial way and is part of participatory design.

The benefits and importance of involving users in the design process are many. One of the most important can also be seen as the most trivial. By involving the actual user of the designed product, system or environment, it is much easier to ensure that the design is solving the actual problem or task it is supposed to. The focus on the

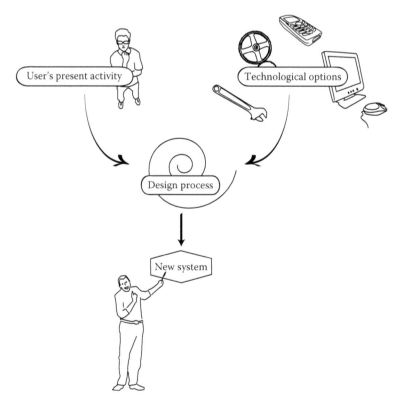

FIGURE 16.5 No element should be withdrawn.

desired function of the user means the person is central and that the technology used is problematized from the individual's wishes concerning the function.

This corresponds to hitting a nail—it is true that you hold the hammer, true that you hit with it, but it is the driving in of the nail that is so central that you hardly notice the hammer. Similarly, both the computer mouse and the cursor are subordinate—it is what is done and what is achieved that matters. The focus is on the action [29]. That is why, in most cases, it is meaningless to measure a person's physical functions without including the use of their available technical aids. This is an area in which the International Classification of Functioning (ICF) needs to be modified [30].

According to Claiborn, there is a "multiplicity of possibilities that go beyond any separation of human and machine. A Paralympian shot-putter, in this view, is not an individual person helped by high-tensile carbon-fiber legs, or a hybrid defined by dual constituent parts, but an athlete capable of multiple boundary-shifting performances" [31].

The quality and height of a pole-vaulter's jump is judged on the height they manage to clear with the pole, not without it. It is of little interest to find out how fast a race car driver is able to walk or run the length of the track because it is the system made up of the driver, the car, and the support team that is the relevant unit to optimize.

Participatory design is closely related to participatory ergonomics. Wilson, a leading researcher and practitioner in this field, described and classified the level of user participation in terms of methods, participants, and process frequency [32]. In "The Swedish Hand Tool Project," a large-scale product development program, interorganizational participation took place in order to increase the knowledge base of hand tool production, distribution, and use [33]. A common understanding was needed in order to bridge information gaps in the chain of central actors: user companies/production units including users of a company providing development opportunities for people with disabilities (assembly workers, production engineers, and purchasers), distributors (salesmen and purchasers), and manufacturers (designers and salesmen), supported by a group of researchers. Participatory approaches to the design of work equipment were compiled and analyzed by Morris et al. [34] in order to promote participation by users and trade unions.

16.4 ETHICS IN DESIGN

Since design is a creative activity, the aim of which is to establish the multifaceted qualities of objects, processes, services, and their systems in entire life cycles, it is also central to the innovative humanization of technologies and to cultural and economic exchange. Design seeks to discover and assess structural, organizational, functional, expressive, and economic relationships, with the task of (Figure 16.6)

- Enhancing global sustainability and environmental protection (global ethics)
- Promoting a win–win situation for final users and market-oriented producers (social ethics), and
- Supporting cultural diversity in a globalizing world (cultural ethics)

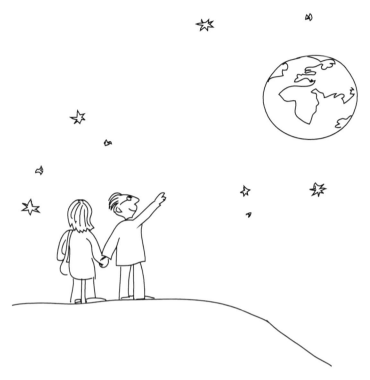

FIGURE 16.6 Ethical considerations have local as well as global sources and impacts.

Most obvious, there are strong elements of ethics in design, both in process and production and in how artifacts later become "actants" in our lives, which means that they influence our lives more or less to the same extent as human beings do. The following is, for the most part, an excerpt from an article by Jönsson et al. entitled "Ethics in the Making" and published in its entirety in *Design Philosophy Papers* [35].

16.4.1 Ethics, Also Outside the Medical Field

Applied ethics in research is no longer regarded as a concern exclusive to the medical field. Exemplars in ethics from other fields such as design are, however, meager, as are relevant practical and design applied guidelines. The more ethically grounded a given area of research is, the greater the chance it can contribute to long-term, meaningful breakthroughs in knowledge. An improved ethics in design can enable a critical questioning that in turn leads to entirely new research questions.

The mere involvement of human subjects and the application of safety provisions in design research do not guarantee it will meet ethical considerations, best practices, or standards. The entire complex interaction with users offers intriguing possibilities, risks, or can result in mediocrity in areas such as: preparation and implementation that is worth the research person's time; respect for their contributions; dignified treatment; feedback in an iterative and interactive process with mutual information and inspiration; and products and processes that are truly influenced by the users.

This reasoning applies to all, but with special distinction to people who are disabled and elderly people. Starting with specific needs as opposed to more general ones (the latter of which result in the necessity for more abstract specifications for the multitudes) can, above, and beyond the ethical dimension, also result in increased innovation and effectiveness for society on the whole. Proceeding from the particular to the general is of considerable value, for ethical reasons as well as for sheer effectiveness.

Involving persons with a variety of disabilities in product development helps to ensure innovative and useworthy products [3]. One of many prerequisites for an ethically sound user involvement is that all participants are aware of the interference taking place in an iterative design process.

An elaboration of ethical aspects in design can be valuable for different stakeholders (user organizations, nongovernmental organizations [NGOs], and the design community) and, of course, for the relevance of resulting products and processes. A more considerate ethical approach could have substantial economical value due to the higher relevance of the results. There has been a considerable increase in the ethical expectations placed on businesses and professions in recent years. Scores of organizations have reacted by developing ethical codes of conduct and professional guidelines to explicitly state their values and principles [36]. Moreover, the drafting of a code of ethics can be seen as an indication of professionalism in an emerging profession [37].

16.4.2 NEED FOR SITUATED ETHICS

Traditionally, medical research and clinically practicing professionals have been in the vanguard of ethical guideline creation, with other research fields involving human subjects and human well-being close behind. Today, the medical disciplines are also frontrunners in combining their work on general ethical principles (autonomy, justice and beneficence, for instance) with research on situated ethics, which is less mechanistic and closer to the context of real people in actual situations and work practices.

Situatedness urges different approaches for different disciplines. The engineering and design sciences with safety, accessibility, and universal design of artifacts and the built environment high on the agenda, cannot lean toward medical exemplars but need to develop their own. An initial difficulty is that the existing key ethical principles, however "universal" they appear to be, originate from medicine. The spirit of the Nuremberg Code, the Helsinki Declaration, and The European Convention (with its explanatory report) is not particularly vitalized in design, to say the least [38–40]. The reason for this is obvious: None of them have been formulated based on experiences from design of civil products for everyday life. Nonetheless, ethical aspects are definitely present in test usages as well as in the influence of the resulting technology in later, everyday use [3]. Ethical design perspectives can also be deduced from The Charter of Fundamental Rights of the European Union ("the right to freedom of expression and information") [41], the Convention on the Rights of the Child [42], and from Citizens Rights and New Technologies: A European Challenge in which the European Group on Ethics in Science and Technologies (EGE) stresses the two basic concepts of dignity and freedom [43]. Accessibility and "design for all" are such fundamental perspectives that they should not be treated separately. They have societal implications for education, information, and participation in social and political processes. *The Principles of Universal Design*, with the approach that environments, services, and products should be designed for use by as many people as possible regardless of situation or ability, is an example of this perspective [44].

You have to have options to make a choice

Hanna was born with a nerve-muscle disease that severely restricts her mobility. At 1½ years of age, she received her first standing support device in order to exercise her muscles and put pressure on her skeleton. In the process of standing, however, she discovered that there was a lot to see from this upright vantage point. Objects in other parts of the room caught her attention. Without the support of her mother's arms, she was suddenly on her own in the world. She wanted to come closer to the objects that she could see at the edge of her upright horizon. Her mother had to move the stationary supporter to the thing that attracted Hanna's attention. "There! There!" she said and pointed. She quickly focused on something else and wanted to move on to it and then the next object and the next. Her mother soon realized that this was not so much about Hanna's wish to interact with different objects: What she actually was out after was the enjoyable feeling of moving around in an upright position. This resulted in the construction of a motorized standing support device that offered Hanna the opportunity to move around in an upright position on her own.

One such device after the other has seen the light of day and enabled Hanna, now a young adult, to gain the identity of a standing—not a sitting—person, including all the existential, physical, and practical effects and side effects involved. One such side effect (that was foreseen) is that Hanna will never master the ability to sit—she will remain a standing or a lying person for the rest of her life. The critical moment is to be found in her early childhood when the people in her surroundings were open-minded enough to start questioning whether a future position as a seated person would be right for Hanna with her "stand-up" ambitions [45,46].

This exemplar might serve as a revelation: What are the ethics (if any) behind the dominating "wheel-chair-for-all" attitude that in no way questions the underlying assumption that somebody who cannot stand up and walk on her own has to live her life primarily as a seated person? In design terms: What are the ethical issues involved in not offering motorized standing supports as an option for mobility injured people? It is easy to understand that an aid in the best of cases does not only fulfill the function it is meant to (to stand up in the example of Hanna); it can also reshape the person's existence and existential terms (Hanna achieved an autonomous, upright mobility). This aspect should be involved in future body technology [47].

16.4.3 DESIDERATA AND "WHERE THE ACTION IS"

In design, the focus might be on "that-which-ought-to-be" (desiderata) versus "that-which-is" (description and explanation) [48]. The concept of desiderata is an inclusive whole of esthetics, ethics, and reason. Desiderata is about what we intend the world to be, which is more or less the voice of design. The greater the difference between the designer's and the user's worlds of concepts, the greater is the need for a user-adjoining and situated design process. You need to immerse yourself in concrete experiences—not only base your understanding on abstract ones. You need to accept and acknowledge the existence of different communities of practice [49]. You need to accept desire as an initiator of change. You need to allow disturbances and not only inform and be informed, but also inspire and be inspired. Designers may be informed and inspired by the users, at the same time as the users are informed and inspired by the designers. Utilizing this two-way information and inspiration in both groups to its full extent has profound ethical implications, while at the same time making the process more efficient and situated.

Still, it is not just a matter of being there, of being situated, but also of grasping the action in its context; not to immediately intellectualize it [50,51]. This is how ethnologists work as well [52]. The question is not really, "What is the situation?" rather, "What do we have to do in order to find out?" By acting, you can capture at an early point many of the factors that you would otherwise have missed [53]. The technology itself can serve as a catalyst and can provoke reflection, answer existing questions while at the same time raising new ones [54].

Example 1

Technology as a challenger/teaser. One reason for choosing to have a robot arm on your wheelchair can be that you know that just by having it there, you will come up with new ways of using it. That is the moment of triumph [3].

Example 2

Learning potential. An "hour rule" time-telling device (measures time in physical length: one row of small lights corresponds to an hour and the lights extinguish as time passes) is more challenging than a door opener. A door opener can be used for opening doors.

But an hour rule can have all kinds of imagined and unimagined uses: structuring, planning, sequencing, etc. Edwin Hutchins started to use the expression "distributed cognition" in the mid-1980s to indicate that the thinking of individuals arises out of an interaction with other people and objects. He had extensive experience in laboratory studies. That was why he could so clearly see that what happened in cockpits and on navigation bridges could not be discovered by observing individuals in a laboratory. Cognitive processes are so strongly influenced by cultural and social phenomena that they neither can nor should be studied under artificial conditions. This is explored extensively in his book, *Cognition in the Wild* [55].

Example 3

Media as mediator. People often learn the best by meeting others with similar problems. When you can identify with someone else, you do not feel alone. If in addition you can meet others who have similar problems but who have come further—good role models—you gain hope in the possibility of achieving a good quality of life yourself. The Internet is a superb meeting place for this. The discussions that arise are often more reflective than conventional ones, which by definition occur in the same place and at the same time [56,57].

A phenomenologically based contribution in the interaction design area is Paul Dourish's book *Where the Action is: The Foundations of Embodied Interaction* [29]. Dourish comes from a computer science background but contributes new perspectives to the philosophy of science and methodological approaches for interaction design. It is based on the acting person and her tools, rather than on rational and disconnected actions. Dourish turns away from the narrow cognitive perspective and abstract representations of the world and to the situated and the embodied interaction between humans and computer systems [*ibid.*, p. 18]. That his approach is phenomenological is clear when he states that our experience of the world is closely tied to the reality of our bodily presence in the world. The same argument holds for our social actions: A conversation between two people is dynamically constructed in response to the present action rather than being abstractly planned in advance. Dourish clearly delineates his idea of embodiment. It should not be understood as the commonplace, physical reality that we exist separately as individuals on this earth, but that we are embodied in a world of artifacts that are constantly interacting [*ibid.*, p. 18]. He maintains that we have to understand that interaction is closely connected to the context in which it occurs, that we need to develop sensitivity to settings and understand how interaction is embodied within these settings (Figure 16.7).

Example 4

Technology in context increases precision. A woman thought her wheelchair-mounted robot arm was too slow. But what exactly does that mean? "Too slow" can refer to speed as well as to acceleration. She thought it was "too slow" when she tried to fry meatballs: They slipped away when she attempted to turn them. In this case, it was the acceleration that was too low. But when she was irritated because

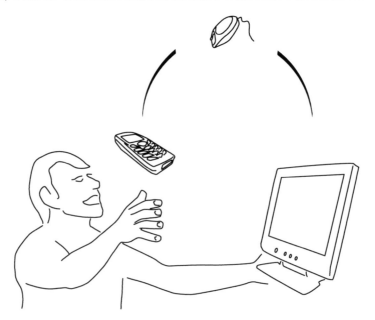

FIGURE 16.7 Hand tools. Capturing female users' expert knowledge revealed their problems in handling a hammer with poor balance.

the arm was "too slow" at pouring sugar in her teacup, it was speed she was referring to. Neither of these needed to be remedied with a stronger motor, which you could have easily concluded if you had not looked at the context. Improving the construction of the grip device technically solved these two problems.

Example 5

Technology as an eye-opener. During a fire drill in a group home, one of the residents explained what he would do if the alarm went off. He would wave a newspaper under the smoke detector. Why? It turned out that every time they toasted bread and the smoke detector went off, that is exactly what the staff member did.

Example 6

Visibility as a tool for empowerment. In the same chapter, you can also read about the man who by moving the photo of Axel from the daily schedule to the staff holiday list could show that he was not particularly fond of Axel. For the personnel, the use of pictures was primarily a way of providing information; for the resident in question, it also became a way to make a point and a wish.

Example 7

Being there without being there. At the Pictorium, a day activity center for adults with cognitive limitation, there was a participant who no one thought could understand pictures. There had many opportunities for him to react to them in the picture-rich setting the center provided, but he had never revealed by facial expression if he was interested or not, or if he understood anything. One day, they were showing a homemade video of the participants involved in a variety of activities. There were two short scenes in which the man in question appeared: one where he was washing dishes, and another in where was showing off his wallet and keys. On both occasions, he demonstrated by gestures, mime, and sounds that these scenes affected him in an entirely different way than anything else on the video. It was apparent that he indeed could identify himself and what he was doing in visual images, which was of great significance for continued work.

16.4.4   INFLUENCE OF USERS ON A PROTOTYPE AND A PROCESS

As already mentioned, the mere involvement of users is not the sole criterion for determining if a design process is ethical or not—it all depends on the spirit and quality of the involvement, the open-mindedness, and eager listening of the participants and, not least of all, the ethics of the result. The resulting artifacts, in turn, are also carriers of ethics and they influence other human beings in a more or less ethical manner.

The tacit knowledge of users can lead to innovative product design. In the Swedish Hand Tool Project [33], users' problems and needs were a common feature of the whole process. The project can be described as a "design for users with users" process [28] since both scientific knowledge about and implicit knowledge of the users were applied. The project started with a kick-off meeting at which all the groups of actors together defined negative values of hand tools that should be

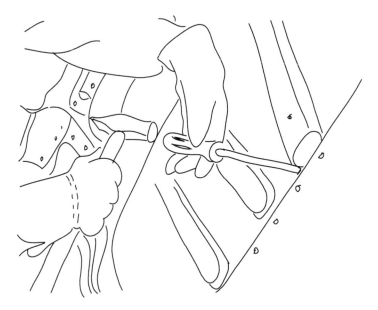

FIGURE 16.8 Interaction design.

avoided in the development of improved products. Aspects of visual esthetics were also included. Questionnaires were sent out to representative workshops of the participating companies: ABB, SAAB Automobile, Samhall, Scania, Volvo Car Corporation, Volvo Car Uddevallaverken AB, Volvo Truck Corporation, and about 30 small- and medium-sized enterprises (SMEs). In the questionnaire, users were asked to describe their worst hand tools in terms of the negative values mentioned and to comment on them (Figure 16.8). They were also asked to describe the use of the tools in terms of body posture, arm positions, and time factors and to estimate how many operators use the tool (e.g., 5 out of 27) as well as to describe the approximate distribution of age and gender. Finally, users were asked to take pictures of the tool and a typical use situation.

Four hundred completed questionnaires were returned. A wide variety of hand tools were represented and classified according to frequency in the participating companies, daily frequency of use and degree of problem. Based on this data, the ten "worst" tools were identified. The representative workshops where these tools were used were then visited. Typical use situations were filmed. The users rated use symptoms on a perceived exertion and pain scale [58] and were interviewed with a customer satisfaction scale. They also provided qualitative comments on their ratings. At the end of each visit, there was a brainstorming session where users and other key people in the workshop wrote down their ideas for improvements. These ideas were then categorized and discussed by the whole group. On the basis of these field studies, user requirements were formulated in qualitative terms for both the selection of products already on the market and for the design and ergonomic evaluation of prototypes. The user requirements for the 10 selected hand tools were accompanied by ergonomic specifications.

The tool identified as causing the most frequent problems was the engineering hammer, an all-round hammer with a wooden handle. The photos as well as the video recordings showed that some female users held the hammer close to its head. When asked why, they replied that in precision work it is efficient to hold the hammer that way and that holding it in its distal part caused wrist pain because of the tool's poor balance. Furthermore, the hammer's professional image was regarded as being rather weak. These were highly important keywords and the starting point for innovation. A well-balanced prototype was designed to be evaluated, along with the original hammer, in an ergonomics laboratory by expert users from industry.

Muscular activity and wrist movements were measured. The eventual symptoms were rated and localized on body and hand maps. The qualities of the product were evaluated with the customer satisfaction scale. The hammer was modified and could then be commercially launched with the user requirements as "ergoments," as were the ergonomic arguments marketed within the project. The hammer is designed at a modular tool. It is possible to assemble parts and handles of various shapes and/or sizes to suit different uses and users. Characteristic qualities of the hammer are optimized distribution of weight, a handle with a diameter that makes it possible to grab in different ways, and grip surfaces that provide comfort and reduce grip force by means of adequate friction. Finally, the hammer is visually appealing. It is a physical representation of the initial user requirements and thus it is no wonder that it is still available at the market.

16.5 FUNCTIONING

Functions are situated in a context, as are obstacles to functions. Functions are located in the space between the individual and his/her surrounding. Functions exist in concrete and well-defined situations but are not a property of the individual. Individuals neither can nor should be classified by the function concept. Thomas [59] makes a distinction between disability and what she calls "impairment effects." Impairment effects are, for example, that blind people (with today's technology) are unable to safely drive a car or that someone in a wheelchair cannot play ice hockey on the local team. This becomes a disability, though, only if driving a car is a condition for obtaining paid employment [60], or if a person in a wheelchair wants to pursue a carrier as a professional hockey player. According to the definition of functions in this chapter, they deal with the effects of impairments in order to reduce disabilities. The interest is in identifying and analyzing the situations where an impairment can lead to a disability and discovering how technology can affect this situation.

It is the experience of function, by the individual in the environment in which technology has been introduced, that is the measure of the function. Functions are thus assessed by how well they correspond to the desired action from the perspective of the individual and not relative to a preconceived norm. It is through long chains of functions that a day and a life are built. From the technological perspective used in this article, it is important to remove the concept of function from a purely mechanistic perspective and put it in a larger context with more variables.

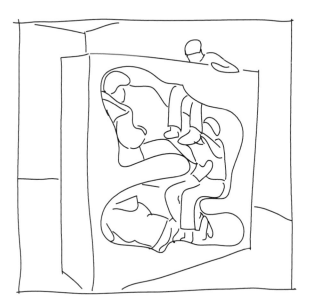

FIGURE 16.9   The function here is more about playing than about sitting.

A focus on functions could bring together the situated and relative perspective of disabilities found in the social model with the more individual and absolute perspective found in rehabilitation and rehabilitation engineering (Figure 16.9).

Sometimes there is a need to problematize space and to discuss functions from an environmental perspective rather than from an individual one. For example, to make sure a building is as accessible for as many people as possible, it can be of interest to discuss functions from a number of hypothetical cases. For each and every one of these, a number of functions are enabled. Together they constitute the function opportunities of the environment.

An important factor to establish is that it is the person involved in the function, the owner of the function, who decides what a good function is. This is referred to as "ownership of the function."

There is a concept in the ICF called "functioning." This is not to be confused with the environmental and situated concept of function described here. Functioning in the ICF is defined as "an umbrella term for body functions, structures, activities, and participation. It denotes the positive aspects of the interaction between an individual (with a health condition) and that individual's contextual factors." Body functions in the ICF definition are the "physiological functions of body systems (including psychological functions)."

The important difference is that function, as described in this article, never refers to bodily functions, but only to the realization of a desired action. Function cannot be assessed as an absolute measure, but only relative to the desired action, and situated in a context with appropriate function support. Functioning in the ICF includes body functions and structures; function as described here is firmly placed in the space between.

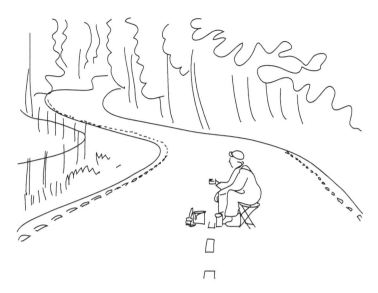

FIGURE 16.10   A line down the middle of the road is a function support for drivers.

16.5.1   Function Support

An important concept to understand when discussing function is the concept of function support. Function support refers to what is needed to perform a function. It can refer to technology or to a person and it is made up of those requirements necessary to perform a function according to the wishes of the function owner. Function support always corresponds to a given function, but a function does not necessarily have dedicated function supports (Figure 16.10).

There are two main categories of function support: technological and human. These two can be combined in a number of ways for the execution of a function. Human function support refers to when another person is a part of the execution. All other supports are classified as technological function supports, including the use of one's own body to perform a function. The difference between using human or technological function support is that the former has a will of its own. This can be a very concrete and tangible problem, something well known to all users of personal assistance. Technology has no will of its own, but is an extension of the user's will. In principle (and in this context), there is no difference between using a wrench or the hand to fasten a screw nut, but having an assistant do it does constitute a difference. There is no difference between walking and driving your own wheelchair, but if your personal assistant (PA) pushes your wheelchair it constitutes a difference in terms of attitude, control, and enabling. In this context, using one's own body is considered to be more similar to using a technical aid, since it is an extension of individual will.

It is inevitable that the use of human function support in the form of personal assistance constitutes a filter to the surrounding world, amplifying or reducing it. Still, the use of human function support is often an unsurpassable system for enabling a function, since the possibilities for adjustment and adaptation to the environment are very high. One big problem with human function support is the loss of control for the user. In a system with technological function support, there is a high level of control, but less flexibility, and thus a lower enabling capacity. The concept of function support is used to ensure that the function involved is looked upon as situated.

16.5.2 DISABILITY "ACE"

Functions and function support can be analyzed by using the disability ACE (Attitude, Control, Enabling). These aspects can be seen as an attempt to integrate important perspectives on functioning into one concept. These factors are derived from and have their base in one of the author's (Peter Anderberg) personal and professional experiences as a rehabilitation engineering professional and personal assistance user.

Attitude concerns how the function is perceived, framed, and socially constructed by others and by oneself in the context where it is used, i.e., to what extent is the function free from or affected by disablist and discrimination attitudes? Attitude is associated with the social model perspectives.

Control focuses on the extent to which the user, the owner of the function, has the power and right to define and execute the function (its choice, development, execution, and financing). Control aspects are closely related to independent living perspectives. It is necessary to clarify that this control must include the right to decline any use of assistive technology or function solutions that for some reason do not fit the needs of the individual user.

Enabling validates how well the constructed implementation of the design, its technology, financing, flexibility, physiognomy, etc., matches the individual's wish to perform the desired actions. Enabling is the traditional approach in rehabilitation technology and design.

16.6 USERS' EMOTIONAL EXPERIENCES OF PRODUCTS

Although functionality always has been, and will remain, an essential precondition for product satisfaction and market success, emotional experiences influence how a product is received. In today's culture, there is evidence of the increasing importance of a product's emotional experience as a driving force of product acquisition and use. Methods for capturing the emotional needs of consumers, incorporating them into the design process and measuring consumer's emotional response are not yet properly developed, and certainly not standardized [61]. Norman [62] argued that if the design does not make sense to users it can cause considerable frustration and there are many artifacts that in Norman's view can be defined as being poorly designed in that sense. One way for the designer to avoid frustration in response to a product is to use a salutogenic approach in design practice. The designer then tries to identify and strengthen those aspects in the artifacts that help the user to cope with adversities (Figure 16.11). The concept salutogenic [63] builds upon a sense of coherence to optimize one's chance of handling a situation or problem and can be divided into three categories: (1) comprehensible—understanding the problem; (2) manageable—having sufficient resources at ones disposal; and

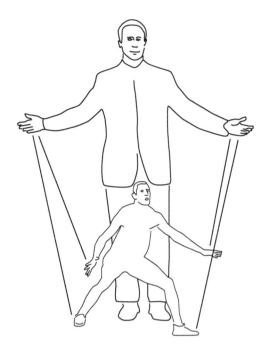

FIGURE 16.11   Who decides? Whose identity is strengthened or threatened?

(3) meaningful—the wish to cope with the problem (which is the most important category). Ilstedt-Hjelm [17] translated Antonovsky's concept into products.
How do you successfully interact with an object? Here "meaningful" stands for the
user's motivation to connect with the object; its degree of emotional significance. If
the user feels meaninglessness when interacting with a product, the feeling might
spread to other parts of life and in the long run hurt the user emotionally, which
can result in burnout or depression. A product that the user does not wish to interact
with will not be considered meaningful for that person, and such a product will
elicit emotions, which will be expressed as unpleasant feelings.

Products that are initially designed to meet both functional and emotional needs
will be experienced positively by the users, contribute to their pride, and even a
strengthened self-concept. Today, assistive products have a low market share compared to ordinary products. Most manufacturing companies do not deal directly with
persons with disability as customers since it is most often other actors who prescribe
and order assistive products for the end user. A person who needs a specific assistive product will have to be satisfied regardless of how they experience its esthetic
or semiotic qualities and simply take what is offered in order to manage the day.
In many cases, younger and able-bodied members of the population benefit from
products that were originally designed for people with some kind of disability.
Examples are the ballpoint pen and the television remote control [11]. In some cases
this effect can work in reverse, with products particularly designed for the able-bodied bringing benefits to disabled users [11]. Jordan mentions the hands-free telephone
and speech technology as examples.

When a user interacts with a product, they will have an experience, a sensation of that interaction through all her senses. Such an experience can last over time, and takes place on both physical and cognitive levels. The boundaries of an experience can be expansive and include the sensorial, the symbolic, the temporal, and the meaningful. A product's sensual values can be divided into how the senses interpret them, i.e., through the visual, audio, or tactile channels. The dominant sense is the visual; what we see frequently reflects our feeling about products. Combined with the tactile sense, they often determine if we like a product or not [13].

It is important to note that human perception is selective. According to Vihma [64], when a person looks at a three-dimensional product the interpretation begins from a detail and proceeds to other details as the person gazes at it (Figure 16.12). The interpretation does not start from a predictable part of the product. The detail may be referred to as an iconic sign. The product's details are then thematized with the help of one's references to the iconic signs. Vihma defines iconic signs as the recognition of similarities between the representational form and the actual object. An iconic sign is bound to culture and to subjective impressions, and can be explained and discussed with other people by relating the interpretation. Different signs merge in a person's experience of a product. Signs do not function separately and individually, but form multilayered references. The complexity of the sign is increased because the references are not stable or fixed qualities of the product.

In a product–user relationship, users may appreciate different product values. Ottosson [65] divides these values into three categories: functional, sensual (perceptual), and image. They are all related to one another. Functional values go hand in hand with good function of products and are, in general, hidden within the product. Sensual values come to us from the surfaces of the product through our senses. Image values represent the appearance we have in our minds of the virtual product.

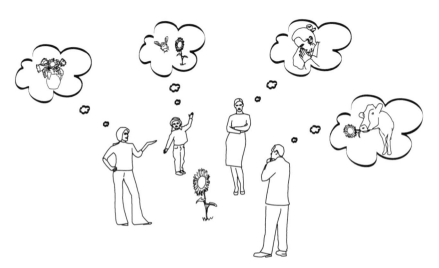

FIGURE 16.12   One single flower yields a manifold of associations.

These values represent characteristics that should present the product to the user at the stage where a potential buyer becomes an owner. Consumers acknowledge soft values—sensual and image values—to a higher degree than only considering the fulfillment of functional values [65] when they are faced with the decision of buying or not buying a product. This is in agreement with Hasdogan [66] who stated that consumers only consider cost, appearance, and brand image, for example, and do not include usability or functionality since they are only potential and not necessarily actual users.

Norman [62] argues that in order to be truly beautiful, wondrous, and pleasurable, a product has to fulfill a useful function, work well, and be usable and understandable. An object that is genuinely beautiful is no better than one that is only pretty if they both lack usability. The design challenge is to make usability and beauty go hand in hand. When dealing with product design, desirable product values can be defined as those qualities within a product that attract the user or make him wish to own the product; qualities that make the user feel a passionate relationship to the product. Avoidable product values will then be such qualities that affect that relationship negatively, break it off, or prevent it from even being established.

For a user to make a long-term attachment to a product, functionality and usability come before esthetics and identity (taste and value). When two products have exactly the same function and usability, the user's taste and value can be more easily expressed. Eikelenberg et al. [67] conclude that comfort and satisfaction cannot be discussed in isolation; they should always be seen as part of an integrative approach. Translated to feelings, these arguments could be expressed as follows: pleasant feelings are associated with both emotional and physical aspects of products and unpleasant feelings with the absence of physical aspects. An unpleasant feeling never stands alone; it is always integrated with a product's functionality. Aboulafia and Bannon [68] distinguish between three feelings related to the time the customer interacts with a product: (1) Affection (short time). This is the immediate response to a design and is therefore especially important in the purchasing situation. (2) Emotion (medium time). (3) Sentiment (long time). This is experienced on a longer term (months/years). Esthetics and emotions are of significant importance in consumers' interaction with any designed artifact. In fact, Norman claims that an attractive appearance, which creates positive emotions and feelings, can help to improve the experience of function and usability [69,70].

A product can be defined by its properties. Properties can be either formal or experiential [11]. Formal product properties are those that can be objectively measured or that have a clear and fairly unambiguous definition within the context of design. Experiential properties, meanwhile, are those that are defined in the context in which the product exists and of the views, attitudes, and expectations of the people experiencing the product. Aspects of a product can be referred to as the product elements. They can be seen as building blocks, which form a product. Formal properties are then manipulations of these elements. Jordan [11] defined six different elements a product can consist of: color, form, product graphics, material, sound, and interaction design. Each of these can be expressed as both formal and experiencing properties, e.g., a form which is sharp and low is considered to make a product faster. The formal property is "pointed" and the experiencing property "speedy."

A product sends out messages formulated in a "language" that we see, hear, or feel. The language consists of signs, product semiotics such as forms, colors, sounds—elements that we associate with esthetics [13]. Product semiotics involves studying the way in which elements relate to one another, how they are organized into wholes, how they are arranged to create harmony, contrast, or dynamism. We use our senses to understand and interpret products. Design semiotics focuses on the artifact as carrier of signs and its capacity to carry and convey a message. From a design semiotic theory perspective, products may be analyzed and explained as a sign. A product should, through its design, convey the intended message to its user. If the user does not understand the product's meaning or function through the design, it becomes inconceivable and may thus produce a negative response in a user situation [71].

Jordan [11] introduced design of pleasurable products as a part of the new human factors by using a product application of Tiger's [72] four categories of pleasure: physio-pleasure, socio-pleasure, psycho-pleasure, and ideo-pleasure. Physio-pleasure has to do with the human body; it covers physical aspects of usability and also the tactile qualities of products. Socio-pleasure refers to the role that the product or service plays in relationships. Psycho-pleasure deals with the cognitive demands of usage as well as the emotional response that a product or service generates. Ideo-pleasure is about our taste and values. If the products and services that we use reflect our taste and values, we will tend to be much more positive about them than if they violate them. When a design team is creating a new product or service they should consider each of the four pleasures.

There is no guarantee that you have access to all your senses. Some people have to manage life without one or more, such as those who have vision and hearing impairments. But most products are designed to be perceived by all the human senses. How will this affect the ability of people with impairments to understand the designer's intent with a product? When designing for users with disabilities, the designer must offer the opportunity to interpret and perceive a product's meaning with different senses on an equal level. One way the designer can achieve this is to consciously use an emotional approach when practicing design. The statement is contradictory since design for emotions and for the user's response to a product seems to be an obvious task for industrial designers. If you design a product, you would like it to be received as a product that most people like and use. You would like the user to respond positively to the product. It is more difficult to understand what it is in the product and the user that results in a specific response. Design for Emotion comprises studying the emotional experiences of users with products, as well as the emotional meanings assigned by users in relation to experience and interaction with products, assessing how emotions vary with different user characteristics and integrating users' emotional expectations into the product development. It acknowledges the fact that the emotion is not a feature of the design, but a subjective experience of the user, owner, or observer of the product [61]. To sum up, products benefits from the designer having a conscious strategy and awareness that emotions are a complex interaction between body and mind, that there are different aspects of a product that may elicit emotions in users, such as esthetics, functionality, brand, and personal associations, that emotions are personal and individual experiences, and different persons express different emotions toward the same situation, event, or physical objects. When you are in a vulnerable situation, like a user of assistive products, the emotional response to those products affects you as a person (identity) and society (norms and values). This makes design for emotion an evident choice of design strategy.

16.7 SPECIAL NEEDS, ENGINEERING, AND DESIGN

We would like to stress that the term "special needs" can be misleading. There are only human needs, more or less possible to satisfy by the individual herself, i.e., more or less in need of tools for their fulfillment. It is not the needs of people with disabilities that are special—but their aids may need to be special. The aids are most often a combination of personal assistance and technological assistance, i.e., cognitive processes are distributed over people, time, and artifacts. As a result, they should not be studied in isolation but in actual interactive situations. Those who assist a person play a key role in the design processes, and the way in which their involvement and knowledge is put to use can make a major difference for the immediate results [73]. They also play a key role in the long run. When a high-tech idea is introduced to a no-tech environment (without even passing through a low-tech one) and finds its place there, almost anything can happen. But there is an ongoing need for a "computer doorman" and a sounding board for evolving ideas. Things start happening when empowerment works and technology always develops more quickly than you imagine. At the same time, it turns out to have unforeseen effects. When, for instance, differently abled people are able to manage long chains of thought themselves through picture representation, one step at a time—many times over, new internal relationship perceptions and whole worlds of concepts are revealed, sometimes causing a revolution for all the persons involved (Figure 16.13).

"One cannot know until one has tried" is the first of the lessons learned over and over again in different contexts [74,75]. We all have an urgent need for guiding principles in order to know how to attempt or at least initiate a complex design process. In addition to the FACE model, we would like to introduce the Security, conText, Experience/memory, and Precision (STEP) method for how to work with and evaluate design for special needs in its context. For an artifact or occurrence to be accessible to a person with cognitive disabilities, it should support the person's awareness of Security, conText, Experience/memory, and Precision (STEP) [76].

The second lesson: "You cannot rely on needs to be formulated by themselves just because they exist. By providing a solution, technology can be a very good way of showing that a problem exists and what it consists of" [77].

The third lesson: To a high degree we are controlled by inner pictures: the end result often turns out to be amazingly like the original picture. Consequently, one has to make one's inner pictures visible, for example, in the form of a mock-up, so that others can see it too, and provide constructive criticism as early as possible.

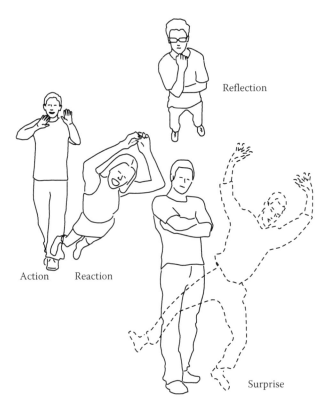

Reflection

Action   Reaction

Surprise

FIGURE 16.13 All reactions, whether expected or surprising, deserve reflection from the practitioners as well as the users.

16.8 ENABLING DESIGN AND REHABILITATION ERGONOMICS AS A WHOLE

Our aim has been to illuminate how a nondiscriminating approach in design may contribute to products that meet users' functional and emotional needs. Innovations often promote the needs of majority groups, while those of underrepresented groups of users, such as women in car assembly and men in nursing or persons with disabilities, are often over looked. Taking their functional and emotional requirements into consideration in design and in the purchasing and supply of equipment will make them feel welcome at work and able to perform their jobs with pride and dignity. The visual design of products is important for the personal identity of employees, and also effects how underrepresented persons are approached by managers and coworkers. Visual design also contributes to the communicated image of the company. Participatory design means involving not only users but other stakeholders such as designers, manufacturers, distributors, and purchasers to learn about user requirements.

The expert knowledge of physical and occupational therapists is most important when designing for users, but these actors can hardly replace users. The contribution to the industrial design process from users is complementary that of professionals.

Both deserve to learn methods that are sensitive to differences in contents, structures, and environments. Taking the needs of a broad range of users into consideration in early phases of design will result in tolerant products that continue to support users in different circumstances and over a long lifetime, thus contributing to a sustainable society. The needs for specific solutions could be reduced as well. Design of system products including a large family of parts with different functional and esthetic characteristics would make it possible to, within the same system, customize solutions for both able-bodied users and persons with disabilities, improving possibilities to meet a variety of functional and emotional needs.

REFERENCES

1. Högberg, D., Ergonomics Integrations and User Diversity in Product Design, PhD thesis, Loughborough University, Leicestershire, 2005.
2. ICTSB Project Team, Design for All. Final Report, 15.05.2000. Available online: http://www.ictsb.org/Activities/design_for_all/Documents/ICTSB%20Main%20Report%20.pdf (accessed Feb. 1, 2007).
3. Eftring, E., The Useworthiness of Robots for People with Physical Disabilities, PhD thesis, Certec, Lund University, Lund, 1999. Available at: http://www.english.certec.lth.se/doc/useworthiness/useworthiness.pdf
4. Aslaksen, F., Bergh, S., Bringa, O., and Heggem, E., *Universal Design Planning and Design for All*. The Norwegian State Council on Disability, Olso, 1997. Available online: http://www.independentliving.org/docs1/nscd1997.pdf (accessed Feb. 1, 2007).
5. Imrie, R. and Hall, P., *Inclusive Design, Designing and Developing Accessible Environments*, Spon Press, London/New York, 2001.
6. Anderberg, P., FACE – Disabled people, Technology and Interne, PhD thesis, Certec, Lund University, Lund, 2006. Available online: http://www.certec.lth.se/doc/face/ (accessed Feb. 1, 2007).
7. Hansson, L., Universal Design—A Marketable or Utopian Concept? PhD thesis, Center of Consumer Science, Göteborg University, Göteborg, 2006.
8. Story, M., Mace, R., and Mueller, J., *The Universal Design File, Designing for People of all Ages and Abilities*, The Center for Universal Design, North Carolina State University, Raleigh, 1998.
9. Preiser, W. and Ostroff, E., *Universal Design Handbook*, McGraw-Hill, New York, 2001.
10. Steinfeid, E. and Tauke, B., Universal designing, In: *Universal Design 17 Ways of Thinking and Teaching*, Christophersen, J., Ed., Husbanken, Oslo, 2002.
11. Jordan, P. W., Inclusive design, In: *Human Factors in Product Design,* Green, W. S. and Jordan, P. W., Eds., Taylor & Francis, London, 1999, 171–178.
12. Seelman, K. D., Universal design and orphan technology: Do we need both?, *Disability Studies Quarterly*, 25(3), 2005.
13. Monö, R., *Design for Product Understanding*, Liber, Stockholm, 1997.
14. Monö, R., *Design for Common Journeys (Design för gemensamma resor)* (in Swedish), Carlssons, Stockholm, 1992.
15. Crilly, N., Products aesthetics representing designer intent and consumer response, PhD thesis, University of Cambridge, Cambridge, 2005.
16. Dahlbom, B., The idea of an artificial science, In: *Artifacts and Artificial Science*, Dahlbom, B., Beckman, S., and Nilsson, G. B., Eds., Almquist & Wiksell, Stockholm, 2002.
17. Ilstedt-Hjelm, S., Making Sense. Design for Well-Being, PhD thesis, NADA, Royal Institute of Technology, Stockholm, 2004.

Ergonomics for Rehabilitation Professionals

18. Persson, A., Kärlek and Industrial Design—I'm Choosing My Life, Master's thesis, Industrial Design Program, Lund University, Lund, 2006.
19. Kirschner, P. A., Buckingham-Shum, S. J., and Carr, C. S., *Visualizing Argumentation. Software Tools for Collaborative and Educational Sense-Making*, Springer-Verlag, London, 2003.
20. Plato, G. and Jönsson, B., *Art and Science – A different convergence, Report, Certec*, Lund University, Lund, 2001. Available online: http://www.certec.lth.se/doc/artand-science/artandscience.pdf (accessed Feb. 1 2007).
21. Gould, J. D. and Lewis, C., Designing for usability: Key principles and what designers think, *Communications of the ACM*, 1985, 28 (3), 300–311. Available online: http://doi.acm.org/10.1145/3166.3170 (accessed Feb. 1, 2007).
22. Poulson, D., Ashby, M., and Richardson, S., USERfit: *A Practical Handbook on User-centred Design for Assistive Technology*, ECSC-EC-EAEC, Brussels-Luxembourg, 1996.
23. Sanders, M. S. and McCormick, E. J., *Human Factors in Engineering and Design*, McGraw Hill, Columbus, OH, 1992.
24. Helander, M. G., Landauer, T. K., and Prabhu, P. V., Eds. *Handbook of Human-Computer Interaction*, 2nd ed., Elsevier Science, New York, 1997.
25. Rubin, J., *Handbook of Usability Testing*, John Wiley & Sons, New York, 1994.
26. Gedenryd, H., How Designers Work—Making Sense of Authentic Cognitive Activities, PhD thesis, Cognitive Studies, no. 75, Lund University, Lund, 1998.
27. Nielsen, J., *Usability Engineering*, The Academic Press Inc., San Diego, CA, 1993.
28. Eason, K. D., User centred design: for users or by users? In: *Proc. 12th Triennial Congress Int. Ergonomics Asso.*, McFadden, S., Innes, L., and Hill, M., Eds., Human Factors Association of Canada, Ontario, 1994, Vol. 1, pp. 78–80.
29. Dourish, P., *Where the Action Is. The Foundations of Embodied Interaction*, MIT Press, Cambridge, MA, 2001.
30. WHO, *International Classification of Functioning, Disability and Health (ICF)*, World Health Organization, Geneva, 2001.
31. Claiborn, L. B., Ditching dualisms: Education professionals view the future of technology and disabilities, *Disability Studies Quarterly*, 25(3), 2005.
32. Wilson J. R., *Participation—A Framework and a Foundation for Ergonomics?* Sage Publications, Newbury Park, CA, 1991.
33. Kardborn, A., Interorganizational participation and user focus in a large-scale product development programme: The Swedish hand tool project. *Journal of Industrial Ergonomics*, 21(5), 369, 1998.
34. Morris, W., Wilson, J., and Koukoulaki, T., *Developing a Participatory Approach to the Design of Work Equipment*, European Trade Union Technical Bureau for Health and Safety, Brussels, 2004.
35. Jönsson, B. et al., Ethics in the making, *Design Philosophy Papers*, 4, 2005.
36. Online Ethics Center for Engineering and Science, Case Western Reserve University, Ohio, 2004. Available online: http://www.cwru.edu/groups/cpe/cpe.html; http://onlineethics.org/ (accessed Feb. 1, 2007).
37. Marjo, R. and Päivi, T., Independent living, technology and ethics, *Technology and Disability*, 15, 205, 2003.
38. *Nuremberg Code*, Washington, DC, 1949–1953. Available at: www.ushmm.org/research/doctors/Nuremberg_Code.htm (accessed Feb. 1, 2007).
39. Helsinki Declaration, 18th World Medical Assembly, Helsinki, June 1964, amended 1975, 1983, 1989. Available at: http://onlineethics.org/reseth/helsinki.html (accessed Feb. 1, 2007).
40. The European Convention, 2003. Available at: http://european-convention.eu.int/ (accessed Feb. 1, 2007).
41. The Charter of Fundamental Rights of the European Union, European Parliament, Nice, 2000. Available at: www.europarl.eu.int/charter/default_en.htm (accessed Feb. 1, 2007).

42. Convention on the Rights of the Child, UNICEF, 2002. Available at: www.unicef.org/crc/crc.htm (accessed Feb. 1, 2007).
43. Citizens Rights and New Technologies: A European Challenge, Report, European Group on Ethics in Science and New Technologies, Brussels, 2000. Available at: http://europa.eu.int/comm/european_group_ethics/docs/prodi_en.pdf (accessed Feb. 1, 2007).
44. Bettye, R. et al., The Principles of Universal Design, Version 2.0, Center for Universal Design, NC State University, Raleigh, 1997.
45. Flodin, E., Assistenter i min lisvärld (Assistants in my lifeworld), in Praktiskt-Pedagogiska Problem (Practical Pedagogical Problems), Halmstad University, Halmstad, no 12, 2000.
46. Flodin, E., Jakten på Instinktivespelaren (Hunt for the Instinctive Player), Master's thesis, Halmstad University, Halmstad, 2000.
47. Tenner, E., *Our Own Devices – The Past and the Future of Body Technology*, Random House, New York, 2003.
48. Edeholt, H., Design Innovation och andra Paradoxer—förändring satt i system (Design, Innovation, and Other Paradoxes), PhD thesis, Chalmers University of Technology, Göteborg, 2004. Available (in Swedish) at: http://webzone.k3.mah.se/k3haed/ (accessed Feb. 1, 2007).
49. Lave, J. and Wenger, E., *Situated Learning: Legitimate Peripheral Participation*, Cambridge University Press, New York, 1991.
50. Mandre, E., Från observation till specialpedagogisk design. Pedagogikens möte med psykiatrin (Designing Remedial Education: Education meets psychiatry), Licentiate thesis, Certec, Lund University, Lund, 1999. English summary available at: http://www.english.certec.lth.se/doc/designingremedial/ (accessed Feb. 1, 2007).
51. Mandre, E., From Medication to Education, PhD thesis, Certec, Lund University, Lund, 2002. Available at: http://www.english.certec.lth.se/doc/frommedicationto/frommedicationto.pdf (accessed Feb. 1, 2007).
52. Jönsson, H., Certecs användarforskning ur ett etnologiskt perspektiv (Certec's user research from an enthnological perspective), Certec, Lund University, Lund, 2000.
53. Suchman, L. A., *Plans and Situated Actions: The Problem of Human–Machine Communications*, Cambridge University Press, Cambridge, 1987.
54. Jönsson, B., Certec's Core, Report, Certec, Lund University, Lund, 1997. Available at: http://www.certec.lth.se/doc/certecscore/ (accessed Feb. 1, 2007).
55. Hutchins, E., *Cognition in the Wild*, MIT Press, Cambridge, MA, 1996.
56. Brattberg, G., Rehabiliteringspedagogik för arbete med långtidssjukskrivna i grupp (Rehabilitation Pedagogics for Working with Groups of People on Long-term Sick Leave), Värkstaden, Stockholm, 2003.
57. Brattberg, G., Väckarklockor (Alarmclocks), Värkstaden, Stockholm, 2004.
58. Borg, G., *Borg's Perceived Exertion and Pain Scales*, Human Kinetics, Champain, IL, 1998.
59. Thomas, C., Disability theory: key ideas, issues and thinkers, In: *Disability Studies Today,* Barnes, C., Barton, L., and Oliver, M., Eds., Polity, Cambridge, 2002.
60. Barnes, C. and Mercer, G., *Disability*, Polity, Cambridge, 2003.
61. ENGAGE, Report of the state of the art, ENGAGE Project, Design for Emotion, 2005. Available at: http://www.emotional-design.org
62. Norman, D. A., Emotion and design—attractive things work better, *Interactions Magazine*, ix(4), 36–42, 2002.
63. Antonovsky, A., *Unrevealing the Mystery of Health, How People Manage Stress and Stay Well*, Josey-Brass, London 1987.
64. Vihma, S., Product as representations – a semiotic and aesthetic study of design products, PhD thesis, University of Art and Design, Helsinki, 1995.

65. Ottosson, S., Dealing with innovation push and market need, Technovation, 24, 279, 2004.

66. Hasdogan, G., The role of user models in product design for assessment of user needs, *Design Studies,* 17, 19, 1996.

67. Eikelenberg, N. et al., Science and design—two sides of creating a product experience, in *Proc. 3rd Int. Conference Design and Emotion,* McDonagh, D., Hekkert, P., van Erp, J., and Gyi, D., Eds., Taylor & Francis Group, London, 2002, 98–103.

68. Aboulafia, A. and Bannon, L. J., Understanding affect in design: an outline of conceptual framework, *Theoretical Issues in Ergonomics Science,* 5, 4, 2004.

69. Norman, D. A., *Psychology of Everyday Things,* MIT Press, Cambridge, MA, 1998.

70. Norman, D. A., *Emotional Design: Why We Love or Hate Everyday Things*, Basic Books, New York, 2004.

71. Wikström, L., The message of products. Methods for valuing the semantic functions of a product from a user perspective. PhD thesis, Chalmers University of Technology, Göteborg, 2002.

72. Tiger, L., *The Pursuit of Pleasure*, Transaction Publishers, Somerset, NJ, 2000.

73. Jönsson, B., Malmborg, L., and Svensk, A., Mobility and learning environments: engaging people in design of their everday environments, Report, Certec, Lund University, Lund, 2002. Available at: http://www.english.certec.lth.se/doc/mobility1/MobilityLearningReport021215.pdf (accessed Feb. 1, 2007).

74. Jönsson, B., Philipson, L., and Svensk, A., *What Isaac Taught Us,* Certec, Lund University, Lund, 1998. Available at: http://www.certec.lth.se/doc/whatIsaac/ (accessed Feb. 1, 2007).

75. Breidegard, B., Att göra för att förstå—konstruktion för rehabilitering (Doing for Understanding—On Rehabilitation Engineering Design), PhD thesis, Certec, Lund University, Lund, 2006.

76. Svensk, A., Design for Cognitive Assistance, Licentiate thesis, Certec, Lund University, Lund, 2001. Available online at: http://www.english.certec.lth.se/doc/designforcognitive/designforcognitive.pdf (accessed Feb. 1 2007).

17 Functional Capacity Evaluation

Megan Davidson

CONTENTS

This chapter will examine the typical content and purposes of functional capacity evaluation (FCE), examine the characteristics of useful tests, and evaluate three widely used FCE test batteries. The focus will be on the clinical applicability of the tests and the valid inferences that can be made from testing. More than 800 tests and measures have been identified that have been used to evaluate work-related disability [1]. These tests range from simple single-question rating scales to measure pain intensity, through to comprehensive test batteries made up of a large number of individual tests. A common criticism of the field has been the proliferation of tests without rigorous testing of the measurement properties of the tests and batteries of tests [2–5].

FCE is generally described as a systematic, comprehensive, and "objective" approach to measurement of a person's ability to perform work-related tasks safely and dependably [6–8]. Isernhagen [9] expands the meaning of the component terms: functional indicating meaningful or useful, capacity meaning maximum ability and evaluation meaning "a systematic approach including observation, reasoning, and conclusion." This recognizes that the FCE is neither value-free nor entirely "objective," but involves clinical reasoning and expertise as part of the process. The FCE may well be made up of a number of measurement procedures, but the resulting evaluation is "a judgement based on a measurement" and is a "judgement of the value or worth of something" [10].

Rather than being solely an evaluation of physical capacity, it may be more helpful to conceptualize FCE as a behavioral assessment in which performance is influenced by multiple factors including a person's beliefs and perceptions [11,12].

FCE is generally considered to have a number of components (Table 17.1) [4–7]. Safety is considered an overriding concern and guidelines for conducting FCE on persons with medical conditions have been published [6]. The final step in the FCE is the report writing in which the evaluator interprets the data and information collected in the preceding steps. The evaluator generally makes recommendations and judgments relating to the purpose of the FCE; for example to determine rehabilitation needs or to make return to work recommendations.

17.1   PURPOSES OF FUNCTIONAL CAPACITY EVALUATIONS

The purpose of the FCE will dictate the extent of effort or cost that is justified. Matheson [1] proposed five types of FCE of increasing complexity requiring increasing time and expense to perform. The briefest FCE evaluates a person's ability to perform specific tasks for the purpose of functional goal setting. Next is FCE for

TABLE 17.1
Typical Components of an FCE

Component	Information Collected
Client/patient interview	Past and current medical history
	Social and vocational history
	Psychological screening
	Patient self-reports of function, quality of life, well-being
Physical examination	Specific to diagnosis (neurological, musculoskeletal, respiratory, etc.)
	Data collected are mainly in impairment domain (strength, flexibility, aerobic capacity, sensory deficits, balance, vision, hearing)
Functional performance	Performance of relevant activities (e.g., lifting, climbing, manual handling)
Interpretation	Comparison of results with normative data, with specific or general occupational demands

disability rating purposes that compares individual performance against normal values and quantifies the person's loss of work capacity. FCE for goal setting or disability rating may take less than 1.5 h. A longer FCE (3–8 h) is required for job matching and occupation matching where the person's adequacy for a particular job or occupation is assessed. The most comprehensive use of FCE is the work capacity evaluation, which may take place over a number of days, and seeks to determine the person's maximum ability for any or all occupations.

The FCE examiner must therefore select tests and measures of specific variables relevant to the particular purpose of the FCE. Given the diversity of purposes for which a FCE is performed, a single lengthy battery of tests applied to all clients is not an efficient approach.

The application of tests in a clinical framework can be performed with three basic purposes in mind: to evaluate an aspect of health status, to predict a future event, or to diagnose a health condition. FCE is used for all three purposes as outlined in Table 17.2.

Testing for evaluative purposes relates to clinical decision-making in that the results of tests may inform rehabilitation decisions by determining the need for a particular type and level of treatment and can be used to monitor response to treatment by quantifying the changes that have occurred during the rehabilitation process. Test results may show a person's condition has stabilized and act as an indicator of a therapy end point if no further improvement is expected. Tests used for evaluative purposes are often called "outcome measures" as they measure the outcomes of health care. Evaluative testing may also inform decision-making about return-to-work recommendations including identifying necessary modifications or adaptations to the working role or environment.

Diagnostic tests are used to determine the probability that a particular disease or condition is present or absent. The correct classification rates determine the utility of a diagnostic test. FCE may be used diagnostically when the intention is to determine the presence or absence of invalidating variables such as submaximal or insincere effort or illness distress [7].

TABLE 17.2
Purposes of FCE

Goal	Objective	Purpose
	i. Determine if physical capacity meets or exceeds work demands	Predictive
Clinical decision-making	i. Justify treatment	Evaluative
	ii. Plan treatment	Evaluative
	iii. Set goals	Evaluative
	iv. Establish baseline status	Evaluative
	v. Monitor progress	Evaluative
	vi. Determine when maximum improvement has been achieved	Evaluative
	vii. Identify persons at risk of poor outcome	Predictive
Patient motivation	i. Alert worker to difference between perceived and actual capacity	Evaluative
	ii. Challenge self-efficacy or fear-avoidance beliefs	Evaluative
Return to work decisions	i. Determine readiness to return to work safely after injury	Predictive
	ii. Determine if physical capacity meets or exceeds work demands	Predictive
	iii. Predict 8-h day endurance	Predictive
	iv. Recommend work restrictions	Evaluative
	v. Identify necessary work modifications	Evaluative
	vi. Determine barriers to return to work	Evaluative
Legal determinations	i. Quantify functional capacities in cases of litigation	Evaluative
Disability determinations	i. Quantify functional capacity in cases of disability	Evaluative
	ii. Identify need for workplace accommodation	Evaluative
Detection of invalidating variables	i. Detection of submaximal or insincere effort	Diagnostic
	ii. Detection of illness distress (e.g., nonorganic signs)	Diagnostic

The characteristics of diagnostic tests and their interpretation is shown in Figure 17.1 and Table 17.3 [13]. Misclassification may have serious consequences, for example, a person incorrectly diagnosed as making an insincere effort may be judged as malingering.

Test result	Target condition: Present	Target condition: Absent	
Positive	a True positives	b False positives	$a + b$
Negative	c False negatives	d True negatives	$c + d$
	$a + c$	$b + d$	$a + b + c + d$

FIGURE 17.1 A two by two "truth" table.

TABLE 17.3

Definition and Calculation of Test Characteristics

Test Characteristic	Definition	Calculation
Sensitivity	The proportion of people who have the target condition who test positive	$a/(a + c)$
Specificity	The proportion of people who do not have the target condition who test negative	$d/(b + d)$
Positive predictive value (PPV)	The proportion of people who test positive who have the target condition	$a/(a + b)$
Negative predictive value (NPV)	The proportion of people who test negative who do not have the target condition	$d/(c + d)$
Positive likelihood ratio	Likelihood of a positive test result in a person with the target condition, compared to the likelihood in a person without the target disorder	Sensitivity/ $(1 -$ specificity$)$
Negative likelihood ratio	Likelihood of a negative test result in a person with the target condition, compared to the likelihood in a person without the target disorder	$(1 -$ sensitivity$)/$ specificity
Accuracy	The proportion of people who were correctly identified as having or not having the target condition	$a + d/$ $(a + b + c + d)$
Prevalence	The proportion of people in the sample who had the target condition	$(a + c)/$ $(a + b + c + d)$

Note: Sensitivity and specificity are read down the columns of the 2 × 2 table, while PPV and NPV are across rows.

When tests are made for a predictive purpose, test results in the present are used to predict a future event. The future event may be framed as a negative event (risk of injury, failure to return to work, sick days, disability) or positive event (sustained return to work, work capacity). The extent to which the test correctly predicts the future event dictates its utility. Screening for risk of some future event (e.g., not returning to work or chronic disability) may be used to determine the type and level of rehabilitation required. The characteristics of predictive tests are the same as for diagnostic tests, with the future event being the "condition" being diagnosed.

FCE tests are predictive when used to determine readiness to return to work or suitability for a particular level of work. The prediction may turn out to be correct: a person judged to be able to return to work successfully does so (true-positive) or a person judged to be unable to return to work does not (true-negative). The prediction may also turn out to be incorrect: a person judged able to return to work fails to successfully do so (false-positive), or the personal judged to be unable to return to work makes a successful return to work (false-negative). Incorrect predictions may have serious consequences for individuals.

Classification of a person as being ready to return to work at a certain level is predicting that they are able to safely undertake the job requirements with a low risk of reinjury. In this case we need to know, given a positive test result (e.g., classified as safe to return to work), the probability that this person will actually achieve a sustained and safe return to work. A test with high sensitivity would ensure that false-negatives were minimized. A test with high specificity would ensure that false-positives were minimized.

17.2 MEASUREMENT ISSUES

A test is "a procedure or set of procedures that is used to obtain measurements (data); the procedures may require the use of instruments" [10]. The terms "test" and "measure" are both used to indicate the procedure used to obtain a measurement.

It is not uncommon for therapists to label a test or measure as "objective" (usually indicating that the therapists are making the observation such as measuring a joint angle) or "subjective" (usually indicating a self-report test such as a pain intensity rating) and to believe that the former is inherently more reliable and valid than the latter. This assumption is misleading as many tests administered by a trained observer, such as tests that require the observer to make categorical judgments, involve arguably subjective judgments.

It is more helpful to consider whether the variable being measured is objective or subjective, rather than the test itself. Objective phenomena—such as weight, height, and range of motion—are directly observable and measurable. Other phenomena that cannot be directly observed, such as pain intensity, quality of life, or depression or anxiety or self-efficacy, may be deemed subjective. Galleleo Gallelei famously said that we should measure what is measurable and make measurable what is not. With subjective phenomena the instruments developed to detect and measure the variables of interest are attempts to make measurable what is not directly measurable. The safety, reliability, validity, and practicality are the characteristics of tests that are pertinent, not whether the variable being measured is subjective or objective.

To judge the clinical utility of any test or measure we need to know the answers to two questions: how close is the observed measurement to the truth? and what valid inferences can be made from the measurement? The first question relates to test reliability, the amount of variability, error or "noise" in the measurement. The second question is about the validity of the test.

Tests are often described as having "excellent reliability," or being "reliable and valid." However, it is misleading to conceptualize tests as having intrinsic qualities of reliability and validity. The reliability and validity of a test relate to the purpose of the test. A test that has sufficient reliability for a particular purpose may not be suitable for another purpose and a test that is valid for making one particular inference may not be valid for making another inference. A test with relatively poor reliability may be sufficient for describing gross differences in function between groups, but would be insufficiently reliable for quantifying a score for an individual that could be compared to norms or to detect meaningful change over time in the variable of interest. In FCE, one may be able to make a valid inference about the change in performance on a lifting task, but it may not be valid to predict workplace performance or future reinjury from that same test.

17.2.1 RELIABILITY

Test reliability is the extent to which different administrations of the test agree between raters or between testing occasions (or between equivalent forms of the same test or parts of a test, although we will not be concerned with this aspect of reliability in this chapter). When a person is tested by different raters or on two occasions (assuming no change in the variable being measured), test results should ideally be identical. In the less than ideal real world, test results should be close enough to ensure that the decision made on the basis of test results would be the same at each test occasion. The reliability of a test is represented by the true variance in a score divided by the true variance plus error. Variance is the standard deviation squared and is a measure of the spread of the scores around the mean. As the only difference in the numerator and denominator is the error variance in the denominator, tests with a large amount of error will yield relatively low reliability coefficients, while those with a small amount of error will yield relative high reliability coefficients. A test with zero error would have a perfect reliability coefficient of 1.00. The closer the coefficient to 1 the smaller the amount of error in the measurement relative to the variability in scores. If there is a very small variability in scores, however, even a small amount of error variance can yield a relatively "poor" correlation coefficient because it represents a higher proportion of the total variance. For this reason researchers usually avoid samples for reliability studies that have a "truncated" or narrow range of scores.

The sources of error in measurement are the test itself, the rater, and the ratee. Even if a test has been reported to have a certain amount of measurement error, this can only be generalized to a clinical setting that utilizes the same instrument in the same standardized manner on similar subjects. Reliability studies on a particular population cannot necessarily be generalized to another population as the variability of scores and error in the new population may be quite different. For this reason, reliability studies on "normal" subjects can usually not be generalized to populations with disease or dysfunction. Measurement error can be minimized clinically by ensuring standardization of all aspects of the test (equipment, time of day, training of raters, instructions to subjects) and by strategies such as averaging multiple administrations of a test.

Commonly reported reliability statistics are percent agreement, kappa, and Spearman's rank-order coefficient for ordinal or "nonparametric" data and Pearson's Product-Moment coefficient, and variants of the intraclass correlation coefficient (ICC) for continuous or "parametric" data. Percent agreement is an overestimate of reliability as many of the agreements may be "chance" agreements. Kappa adjusts for chance agreement. Spearman's rho and Pearson's r are analogous statistics used for ordinal and continuous variables, respectively. Pearson's r and ICCs are used when data are continuous and normally distributed (although the statistics are quite insensitive to violations of the assumption of data type and normality [14]). Where two datasets are systematically different (e.g., when all scores change in the same direction between tests) Pearson's r will overestimate reliability. For this reason, and because it can be used for more than a single pair of observations, the ICC is generally considered the preferred statistic [15,16]. The $ICC_{2,1}$ (the two-way random effects model, where each subject is tested by each rater) should be used when generalizations to other, similar raters is intended [15].

It is common for test reliability to be classified as "weak" and "strong"; or "low," "moderate," and "high"; or "poor," "good," and "excellent" (or even smaller discriminations) based on the magnitude of the reliability coefficient. Further, some authors have proposed cut-points on which to judge whether a test is sufficiently reliable for group or individual data purposes [16]. There is no universal agreement on the cut-points and for the purpose of this chapter, we will take the cut-points of Portney and Watkins [15] that a correlation coefficient or ICC or ≥0.90, or a kappa ≥0.80 is required for making decisions about individual subject scores.

The use of the reliability coefficient to determine if reliability is sufficient for a particular purpose is limited. The coefficient does not express the amount of error in the same unit of measurement as the test and therefore the test user cannot determine whether the magnitude is tolerable for their particular purpose [16]. Rather, the test user needs to know, for a particular measurement, the range within which the true value will fall. In determining change in a variable over time the test user needs to know the magnitude of change in the observed score they would need to measure to be confident that the change is not due to error in the measurement.

A clinically useful expression of measurement error is the standard error of measurement (SEM). The SEM denotes the range within which the observed measurement will actually fall with 68% confidence. When a change score is calculated, the most useful expression of measurement error is the minimum detectable change (MDC), which denotes the magnitude of change that needs to be observed before it can, with a defined level of confidence, be said to exceed measurement error. The confidence level of 90% (MDC_{90}) is has been suggested as an appropriate level for clinical decision-making [17]. In this chapter, the SEM and MDC_{90}, when not reported, have been calculated from studies that report a reliability coefficient and standard deviation of scores by means of Equations 17.1 and 17.2.

$$SEM = sd\sqrt{1-r} \qquad (17.1)$$

where sd is the standard deviation of the scores, and r is the reliability coefficient:

$$MDC_{90} = \pm1.64(SEM\sqrt{2}) \qquad (17.2)$$

Test responsiveness or sensitivity to change is said to be the ability of a test to detect small but meaningful changes over time. This proposed measurement property is problematic in that there is no agreed statistic that can consistently be used to judge responsiveness [18]. The ability of a test to detect change over time can be judged by the MDC (the magnitude of change to be confident that the observed change is greater than measurement error). Whether or not the amount of change is clinically important can be judged against the minimum clinically important difference (MCID), which is the smallest amount of change that would be considered important by patients or other stakeholders [19]. In this chapter, the MCID is estimated, when not reported in the studies, by one-half of a standard deviation of baseline scores [20].

When test scores are used to make a decision with serious consequences for the subject (such as whether or not the person is or is not ready to return to work) or on which compensation decisions are to be made, the reliability of the test is paramount. A test with good reliability will minimize the chance that a different decision would be made by different raters or at different testing occasions.

17.2.2 VALIDITY

Validity is "the degree to which evidence and theory support the interpretations of test scores" [21]. It is important to avoid conceptualizing validity as something inherent to the test and keep in mind that validity relates to the inferences that can be made from the test results. Validity is therefore not something that can be demonstrated "once and for all," but evidence for the validity of particular inferences is provided by a range of study designs that support a logical argument for the intended use of test scores [21].

Evidence for the validity of inferences that can be made from a test score can be derived from many sources. Expert judgments are often used as evidence for face validity and content validity of a test. Evidence for criterion or concurrent validity involves comparison of the test scores with scores on a "gold standard" test. When a test purports to measure a readily observable phenomenon for which a gold standard test exists, evidence for validity is demonstrated in a relatively straightforward manner. For example, the use of results from the modified Schober method (or any other method) to make inferences about lumbar flexion would be supported by a study that demonstrates a strong relationship between test scores with measurements of lumbar flexion taken from plain x-rays.

When the test and gold standard are administered at about the same time it is called criterion validity, and when a test result is used to predict a future event it is called predictive validity. Tests that are used to predict a future event or health state require evidence of predictive validity.

Evidence for construct validity is particularly relevant when the variable or construct of interest cannot be directly observed (such as pain, depression or quality of life). Study designs that provide evidence for construct validity are those that test the expected relationships between test scores to scores on other tests of the same or similar constructs (convergent validity) and tests of different constructs (discriminant validity). Known-groups validity is demonstrated when test scores from groups known or believed to differ on the construct of interest are significantly different.

The measurement property that is termed "responsiveness" is best considered as a form of construct validity that tests the hypothesis that mean scores will change in an expected direction or by a particular magnitude. It is now understood that the many responsiveness indices or "longitudinal validity coefficients" [22] do not yield consistent results and are therefore of limited utility in describing the measurement properties of tests [18,23].

FCE tests are variously defined as measuring "maximum work abilities" [7], the "ability to perform work-related tasks" [6], "current physical abilities in work-related tasks" [24], and the "ability to perform meaningful tasks on a safe and dependable basis" [1]. The positive construct of "ability" can be alternatively framed negatively as "disability."

There is no independent, objective gold standard test of functional capacity. Evaluations of capacity or limitations made by the patient, the doctor, or an FCE evaluator, yield different results and there is no way of knowing which is closest to the "truth." Broewer and colleagues [25] had patients, physicians, and FCE evaluators rate capacity on a consistent scale and found that self-reported disability was worse than physician-rated disability, which was in turn worse than the level of disability estimated by the FCE evaluator. Biases (sources of error) operate in each case and there is no "value-free" method of quantifying a construct in which complex biopsychosocial and behavioral factors are operating.

A body of evidence relating to the construct validity of a test may be available that supports the use of a test as a measure of change in physical performance. At the same time there may be evidence that it cannot validly predict a future event and therefore the use of the test results to make inferences about whether or not a person can return to work without risk of reinjury is not supported.

Validity of tests used for diagnostic and predictive purposes is demonstrated in a properly designed study that quantifies the extent to which test scores correctly classify the persons tested as either having or not having the condition of interest, or as experiencing or not experiencing some future event. As no tests are 100% accurate in their ability to classify correctly, statistics such as sensitivity, specificity, positive and negative predictive values are required to allow quantification of the probability of being correct. Clinical decisions are therefore made on the balance of probabilities that the test result correctly classifies the individual on the variable of interest. "High stakes" tests, where incorrect classification has serious consequences, will generally need very high sensitivity and specificity so that false-positives and false-negatives are minimized. Credible studies of diagnostic test accuracy will assemble an appropriate spectrum of patients, will have blinded and independent persons apply the two tests, and will ensure that all persons have both the index text and the gold standard test [26]. Credible studies of predictive tests will assemble a suitable cohort, will have blinded and independent persons collect the predictor and outcome variables, and will have complete follow-up. For predictive models using multivariate analysis, the utility of the predictive model should be confirmed on a new sample.

17.3   EVIDENCE-BASED FCE

Like all contemporary health care activities, FCE should be based on the best available research evidence. Evidence-based practice has been defined as the "integration of best research evidence with clinical expertise and patient values" [27]. The type of research evidence that is best able to provide answers for specific clinical questions varies with the type of question. The best research evidence is that which seeks to provide the least biased answer (closest to the truth) to the particular research question. Research designs are therefore ranked in a hierarchy of evidence where higher levels of evidence are considered more convincing. In hierarchies of evidence, the highest level of evidence is the systematic review. A systematic review is a rigorous approach to appraising all available primary evidence to answer a specific question. A systematic review differs from a narrative review in that it is itself a research design that seeks to minimize bias. An unbiased review method involves a systematic search for available studies, the application of inclusion and exclusion criteria and critical appraisal of the quality of the included studies by at least two independent reviewers [28].

Few systematic reviews have so far been published in the area of FCE (Table 17.4). Systematic reviewing of research evidence relating to treatment effectiveness has

TABLE 17.4
Systematic Reviews of FCE

Authors	Title
Innes and Straker [2]	Validity of work-related assessments
Innes and Straker [3]	Reliability of work-related assessments
Geusser et al. [29]	Psychosocial factors and FCE among persons with chronic pain
Gouttebarge et al. [24]	Reliability and validity of FCE methods: A systematic review with reference to Blankenship system, Ergos work simulator, Ergo-Kit and Isernhagen work system
Wind et al. [30]	Assessment of functional capacity of the musculoskeletal system in the context of work, daily living, and sport: A systematic review
Shechtman et al. [31]	The use of the coefficient of variation in detecting sincerity of effort: A meta-analysis

had a longer history than systematic reviewing for other types of clinical questions. The Cochrane Occupational Health Field, which aims to gather evidence on the effectiveness of occupational health interventions, at the time of writing (early 2007) listed 40 completed Cochrane systematic reviews and 12 reviews in process that had relevance to the occupational health field.

Earlier in the chapter the purposes of FCE testing were classified as evaluative, predictive, or diagnostic. Because we are interested in a test or set of tests, questions about the reliability and validity of the particular test or tests are relevant. For predictive purposes our question is whether FCE can accurately predict the event of interest (who will/will not return to work successfully, who will/will not experience reinjury). For diagnostic purposes, we could ask if observers can accurately detect maximum patient effort in FCE tasks or if the FCE can correctly determine the level of disability.

It seems that the most valued purpose of the FCE is predictive, i.e., a judgment is made on the basis of testing as to the extent to which the person's capacity exceeds the job demands and, therefore, whether or not the person can return to work in a controlled and safe manner [6].

17.3.1 What Predicts Return to Work and Sick Leave Outcomes?

A number of systematic reviews of prognostic factors have been published since 2000 in the field of occupational disability in low back pain (Table 17.5) or that have a component relating to occupational disability [32]. In these reviews, a large number of demographic, social, psychological, and physical variables are identified as prognostic indicators of sickness absence and return to work. The review by Waddell et al. [33] reported strong evidence for age, psychological distress, job satisfaction, duration of sick leave, employment status, financial incentives, and expectations about return to work as strong predictors of future incapacity for work. A worker's own expectations about returning to work have frequently been identified as a predictor of return to work and duration of sick leave [32–35].

TABLE 17.5

Systematic Reviews of Prediction or Prognosis in Low Back Related Occupational Disability

Authors	Title
Truchon and Fillion [35]	Biopsychosocial determinants of chronic disability and low back pain: A review
Mondloch et al. [32]	Does how you do depend on how you think you'll do? A systematic review of the evidence for a relation between patients' recovery expectations and health outcomes
Linton [37]	Occupational psychological factors increase the risk of back pain: A systematic review
Borge et al. [38]	Prognostic values of physical examination findings in patients with chronic low back pain treated conservatively: A systematic literature review
Crook et al. [39]	Determinants of occupational disability following a low back injury: A critical review of the literature
Pincus et al. [40]	A systematic review of psychological factors as predictors of chronicity/disability in prospective cohorts of low back pain
Waddell et al. [33]	Screening to identify people at risk of long-term incapacity for work
Hartvigsen et al. [41]	Psychosocial factors at work in relation to low back pain and consequences of low back pain; A systematic, critical review of prospective cohort studies
Steenstra et al. [42]	Prognostic factors for duration of sick leave in patients sick listed with acute low back pain: A systematic review of the literature
Kuijer et al. [34]	Prediction of sickness absence in patients with chronic low back pain: A systematic review

The physical demands of work appear to be only a weak predictor of chronic pain and disability [33] and lifting capacity appears to have no predictive value for future low back pain, disability, or return to work [34,36]. There is limited and contradictory evidence that matching physical capacity to job demands reduces future low back pain or work absence [36]. At this point in time, therefore, it appears that the use of the functional capacity component of the FCE for prediction purposes should be made cautiously, if at all. The number of variables operating in the process of injury, rehabilitation, and return to work suggests that a single or even small number of variables will not be found to accurately predict outcomes.

17.3.2 CAN INSINCERE EFFORT BE DETECTED?

A judgment of the sincerity of effort, or maximal effort, or full cooperation of the testee is included in many FCE approaches on the basis that less than maximal effort invalidates the testing process. This is particularly the case where lifting capacity tests are used to classify the level of lifting that will be recommended as suitable for the individual. As the construct of "sincere or maximal effort" is not directly observable methods have been proposed that purport to "diagnose" the underlying presence or absence of the variable. However, there is no good evidence that any of the methods in use are sufficiently accurate to use with confidence [31,43]. Incorrect classification may have such negative consequences for the individual unless a test is available that has a very low rate of false-positives. Individuals who are incorrectly classified as "insincere" or not making a maximal effort may be wrongly denied employment or compensation.

As we have already identified, a large number of biological, psychological, and social variables may impact on the outcome of occupational injuries and rehabilitation. Conceptualizing the FCE process as a behavioral assessment [11,12] and attention to the specific factors that may be delaying a successful outcome for the individual is thought to be a clinically defensible practice [43].

17.4 EVALUATION OF FCE BATTERIES AND TESTS

Table 17.6 lists a number of named test batteries and tests specifically intended to be used to evaluate work capacity. Tests may be administered by a trained observer, or by the person being tested in the form of a self-report questionnaire or test. Pictorial Activity and Task Sort (PATS) instruments are one type of self-report test of work-related functioning [44]. Matheson [44] suggests that PATS instruments may be used to identify inconsistencies between self-report and observed performance on FCE, to target and select FCE tests rather than administer an entire FCE battery, and to monitor response to treatment. PATS tests appear to have a number of advantages over more general activity-limitation questionnaires: they are work-focused and because of the use of pictures can be used more readily than text-based questionnaires for persons with low levels of literacy in English. The latter feature also means a larger number of activities can be rated in a more time-efficient manner than test-based instruments. Importantly, the inclusion of a self-report measure of function provides the individual's perspective on their functional abilities.

Matheson [1] reported a thorough search located over 800 tests and measures relevant to FCE. Reviewers in this field have frequently noted that many tests have little published information available with regard to their measurement properties or the evidence is inadequate [1–5,24,45]. It is therefore no simple matter for the practitioner to select appropriate tests for measuring variables of interest for a particular purpose. The user must decide whether the cost of testing, which can be considerable in FCE, is justified given the inferences that can be made. Low-cost and low-tech tests may be preferred over high-cost and high-tech testing when the purpose is rehabilitation goal-setting and outcome evaluation. A higher cost and higher tech approach may be justified when the purpose of testing is to match a person's ability with critical job demands.

Standards for tests are well established [10,21] so any test being considered for clinical use should be judged against widely accepted criteria (Table 17.7).

It is beyond the scope of this chapter to attempt any comprehensive evaluation of the measurement properties of the large number of tests that have been or are being used for FCE. Three widely used test batteries have been chosen to evaluate

TABLE 17.6
Some FCE Batteries and Tests

FCE Batteries/Tests

Acceptable Maximum Effort (AME)

Accessibility

ARCON

Baltimore (BTE) Work Simulator

Blankenship System

California Functional Capacity Protocol (Cal-FCP)

DOT Residual Functional Capacity Battery

ERGOS Work Simulator

Ergo-Kit FCE

Gibson Approach to Functional Capacity Evaluation (GAPP FCE)

Isernhagen Work Systems (IWS) FCE (now WorkWell FCE)

Key Method Functional Capacity Assessment

LIDO WorkSET Work Simulator

Matheson Work Capacity Evaluation

Pictorial Activity and Task Sorts (perceived capacity)

- RISC Tool Sort (RTS)
- WEST Tool Sort (WTS)
- Loma Linda Activity Sort (LLAS)
- Spinal Function Sort (SFS)
- Hand Function Sort (HFS)
- Activity Card Sort (ACS)
- Generalized Work Function Questionnaire (GWFQ)
- Multidimensional Task Ability Profile (MTAP)

Physio-Tek

Polinsky FCE

Qualitative FCE

PWPE

Singer/New Concepts VES

Smith PCE

Sweat

Valpar Component Work Sample System

WorkAbility Mark III

Work Box

Work-Related Upper Limb Disorders FCE (WRULD-FCE)

WorkHab

in detail: the Isernhagen Work System or WorkWell FCE, the Physical Work Performance Evaluation (PWPE), and the California FCP. This is not to say that these particular tests have measurement properties significantly better or worse than other tests or each other: a head-to-head comparison study would be required to make such a judgment.

TABLE 17.7
Criteria for Assessment of Tests

Criteria	Determination
Safety	When correctly administered, what are the risks of adverse events or injury?
Reliability	To what extent do test results agree when the test is administered:
	• By two raters? (interrater reliability)
	• By the same rater on two occasions? (intrarater or test–retest reliability)
	• At different times of the day?
	What is the impact of testing on subsequent test results? (test reactivity)
	Are results affected by test order?
Validity	To what extent does the test comprehensively sample the construct of interest? (content validity)
	To what extent does the test yield results that:
	• Are consistent with a "gold standard" test? (criterion validity)
	• Correctly predict a future event? (predictive validity)
	• Are consistent with results of other measures of the same construct? (concurrent validity)
	• Discriminate between groups known to differ on the construct? (known groups validity)
Practicality	Are the costs (equipment, training, time of testing and reporting, licensing fees) justified by the purpose of testing?

A comparison of the test content is made in Table 17.8, and a comparison of the equipment and time requirements in Table 17.9. All test systems require a substantial outlay for purchase of equipment, manuals, and training. Cost outlay depends on the particular package purchased from the provider.

17.5 ISERNHAGEN WORK SYSTEMS FCE (WORKWELL SYSTEMS FCE V2)

The Isernhagen Work Systems Functional Capacity Evaluation (IWS-FCE), now called the WorkWell FCE,* was originally developed by Susan Isernhagen two decades ago. It is used in many countries, including the United States, Canada [12,46], and Australia [3]. Testing options are a 1 day protocol that takes 3–4 h, and a 2 day protocol that requires 1 h on the second day. Test administrators must be trained by a WorkWell Systems-approved faculty member.

For the lifting tests, weights are progressively increased with five repetitions at each weight level [47]. Some of the tests (elevated work, kneeling, crouching, sitting, standing) require a position or activity to be maintained for a set time that is considered to be normal. Some tests measure the time taken to perform a number of movement repetitions [48].

---

* WorkWell Systems, 11E Superior Street, Ste 370, Duluth, MN 55802.

TABLE 17.8
Comparison of Content of the IWS, PWPE, and Cal-FCE

	Strength						Sustained Positions								Mobility				Repetitive Movement					Other		
	Lifting low	Lifting high	Carrying bilateral	Carrying unilateral	Pushing	Pulling	Sitting	Standing	Elevated work in	Lowered standing work in	Lowered standing work in sitting	Reclining	Kneeling work	Squatting	Walking	Stairs	Ladder	Crawling	Standing bend	Sitting bend	Standing rotation	Sitting rotation	Squatting	Hand function	Self-reported capacity	Effort
IWS FCE	✓	✓	✓	✓	✓	✓	✓	✓	✓	✓	✓	✓	✓	✓	✓	✓	✓	✓	✓	✓	✓	✓	✓		✓	✓
PWPE	✓	✓	✓	✓	✓	✓	✓	✓	✓	✓	✓		✓	✓	✓	✓	✓	✓			✓	✓	✓	✓		✓
Cal-FCP	✓	✓	✓				✓	✓		✓			✓	✓		✓								✓	✓	✓

Note: IWS also screens balance and hand coordination.

TABLE 17.9

Comparison of Equipment, Time, and Cost

Battery name	Equipment	Time Taken	Cost
IWS FCE	Weight crate, unilateral carry box, free weights and cuff weights, height-adjustable shelving, ladder, stairs, table and chair, overhead work wall system, force dynamometer and adjustable track, heart rate monitor, sphygmomanometer, hand dynamometer, pinch meter, hand coordination test, spinal function sort, foam, stop watch	Testing: 1 day option 3–4 h 2 day option plus 1 h on day 2 Report writing: 20–45 min	Equipment~$2500 Training etc.~$3000– 5000 (depending on number of persons being trained)
PWPE	Adjustable-height shelving, various boxes and containers, free weights, weight sled, step ladder, heart-rate monitor	Testing: 3.5–4.5 h Report: 30 min	Packages start at ~US$5000
Cal-FCP	EPIC lift capacity test: lifting crate and weights, heart monitor, shelves, hand dynamometer, pinch gauge	Testing: 90–120 min Av 84 (sd 17) Total time including report <2 h	Protocol starter set US$500 Equipment~US$4500 EPIC training $350

The level of effort on the lifting and carrying items is judged by the observer as light, moderate, heavy, or maximal on the basis of observations of accessory muscle recruitment, body mechanics, base of support, posture, control, and safety of movement [47,49]. Testing is stopped by the observer if it is determined that maximum effort has been reached, or if further testing is judged to be unsafe [47].

The IWS-FCE battery has approximately 30 test items with the majority having been developed for the battery. Several preexisting tests have been incorporated: hand coordination is measured using the Purdue Peg Board or Minnesota Rate of Manipulation test, walking with the Shuttle Walk Test, and more recently the Spinal Function Sort (SFS) has been added to the WorkWell Systems FCE V2. Only the 18 tests that form the core of the FCE will be evaluated in this chapter.

17.5.1 SAFETY

Test termination in the IWS-FCE occurs if heart rate limits are exceeded of if the tester considers further testing is unsafe, or if the patient is unwilling to continue. One study has reported that a temporary increase in symptoms in people with chronic low back pain is common following a 2.5–3.0 h IWS-FCE protocol, but that exacerbations are short term and a return to pre-FCE levels can be expected [50]. An earlier study reported that when testing lifting and carrying tasks on consecutive days, three of 28 subjects with work-related back pain failed to attend the second day and another three attended but said they could not perform any manual handling testing due to their low back pain [51].

17.5.2 Reliability

In the ISW-FCE the observer makes a judgment, based on criteria, as to the level of effort being made by the person being tested and when a safe maximum lifting level has been reached. Three studies have examined the reliability of raters' judgments of level of effort [49,52,53] and three have examined judgments of safe maximum lifting capacity [51,54,55].

17.5.3 Reliability of Level of Effort

Isernhagen [47] examined reliability of 12 raters' observations of the video-taped performances of the three lifting tasks. Subjects were three males currently receiving workers compensation benefits. The agreement coefficient (kappa) for intrarater reliability of effort categorization as light, moderate, or heavy was 0.68. In the second study [53], five raters tested the lifting and carrying tasks on four healthy subjects. No agreement coefficients were reported and although absolute agreement was 87%–96% between raters and 93%–97% within raters there is no adjustment for chance agreement in these values. In a later study by Reneman et al. [49], nine observers rating the videotaped performance of floor-to-waist lift of 16 patients with chronic low back pain and 15 healthy subjects, reported kappa values of 0.50 and 0.58, respectively, for interrater classification of lift effort as light, moderate, heavy, and maximal. Although all three studies concluded that trained observers can reliably categorize the level of effort in the lifting and carrying tasks, the extent to which this is transferable to other raters in real clinical situations is not clear as all studies used videotaped performances and some used healthy subjects. The kappa coefficients do not exceed the minimum level of .80, which is the minimum for making judgments about an individual's results [15].

17.5.4 Reliability of Safe Maximum Lift

Two studies have explored the extent to which trained observers can reliably determine safe maximum lifting on the floor-to-waist lifting task from videotaped performances [54,55]. In a study of interrater reliability [54], five raters judged as either safe or unsafe the lifting performance of 30 healthy volunteers. Kappa agreement coefficients ranged from .47 to .74 for ratings made without defined criteria for the categories, and .56 to .82 when criteria were defined, demonstrating the importance of explicit criteria in making categorical judgments. In another study [55] five raters judged as either safe or unsafe the lifting performance of 21 patients with chronic low back pain. The kappa value for interrater reliability was .62 in one session and .64 for ratings a day later. Intrarater reliability was .73. Kappa values generally did not exceed the minimum level of .80 and the clinical generalizability of these studies is unclear given the use of videotaped performances and healthy subjects.

A third study (of interrater and test–retest reliability) used a realistic clinical observation by five trained observers to determine safe maximum lifting capacity (in kilograms) of 28 subjects with low back pain performing three lifting and three carrying tasks of the IWS-FCE [51]. Raters observed real-time testing and documented the point at which they would stop the testing due to maximum lift being reached. Subjects were rated on two occasions 2–4 days apart. Intraclass correlation coefficients for interrater reliability ranged from .95 to .98, and test–retest reliability from .78 to .91. Using the minimum acceptable value of .90 for the ICC, the interrater reliability would be judged as acceptable, but the test–retest reliability as marginal at best. The SEM could not be estimated from the data reported in the study. There was a large variation between raters' agreement on the factors limiting lifting, which ranged from kappa .47 to 1.00.

The SEM and the MDC could be calculated from three other studies that have examined the test–retest reliability of the IWS-FCE [56–58] and Reneman et al. [57] who administered 28 IWS-FCE tests to healthy subjects with a 2–3 week interval. The authors considered acceptable reliability as an ICC of at least .75. For the purposes of making judgments for individual patients, we have taken a more stringent cut-point of .90. From this standpoint, only four tests reached these levels of reliability: the floor-to-waist lift (ICC = .95), the two-handed carry (ICC = .90), right-handed carry (ICC = .98), forward bending in standing test (ICC = .93). This study deviated from the usual protocol in that grip strength, hand coordination tests, and sitting and standing tolerance tests were not administered and modifications were made to nine tests. Brouwer et al. [56] used an identical modified testing protocol on 30 patients with low back pain but with a 2-week interval between testing 28 tasks. They reported ICC values between .75 and .87, and kappa values between .25 and 1.00. No tasks had an ICC greater than .90, while four tasks (crawling, crouching, squatting, and rotation to the right in sitting) had a kappa value of least .80. A third study [58] tested two lifting and one carrying tasks on 50 patients with low back pain on two consecutive days and reported ICC values from .77 to .87.

Using the minimum ICC value of .90 as a cut-point does not allow the user to determine if the amount of error is tolerable for a particular purpose. Table 17.10 provides calculations of the SEM, MDC$_{90}$, and MCID derived from the studies. The SEM and MDC$_{90}$ provide an indication of the amount of error in kilograms. The MCID, which is estimated as half the baseline standard deviation, provides an indication of the smallest amount of change (in kilograms) that would be considered clinically important.

From the table, it can be seen that for the floor-to-waist lifting task, the ICC ranged from 0.81 to 0.95. The best estimate of the SEM indicates that the actual value for the test will (with 68% confidence) lie within ±3 kg or at worst ±7 kg. When retesting, a change of at least 8 kg and possibly as much as 16 kg needs to be observed to be 90% confident that this is beyond error in the measurement. The MCID may be as little as 4.7 kg or as much as 9.5 kg.

The differences in estimates of these values are due to the differences in the size of the correlation coefficient, the variability (standard deviation) of scores, and the sample sizes. The greater error in the Brouwer study may at least partly be explained by the 2-week retest period, over which time real changes in capacity may have

TABLE 17.10

Test–Retest Reliability of the IWS FCE Tasks

Task	ICC			SEM			MDC$_{90}$			MCID		
	1	2	3	1	2	3	1	2	3	1	2	3
Floor-to-waist lift (kg)	0.87	0.81	0.95	3.4	6.8	4.3	7.9	15.7	9.9	4.7	7.8	9.5
Waist-to-crown lift (kg)	0.87	0.87	0.89	1.8	2.6	2.0	4.1	6.0	4.6	2.4	3.6	3.0
Short carry 2 hands (kg)	0.77	0.81	0.90	4.3	7.3	6.2	10.1	17.0	14.4	4.5	8.4	9.8
Long carry 2 hands (kg)		0.81	0.84		6.7	6.1		15.5	14.2		7.7	7.6
Long carry R hand (kg)		0.81	0.98		4.9	1.6		11.4	3.8		5.6	5.8
Long carry L hand (kg)		0.81	0.86		4.9	3.8		11.3	8.8		5.6	5.1
Pushing static (kg)		0.75	0.68		5.4	8.4		12.5	19.4		5.4	7.4
Pulling static (kg)		0.78	0.89		6.9	6.2		16.1	14.3		7.4	9.3
Shuttle walk (m)		0.84	0.64		54.6	70.6		126.7	163.9		68.3	58.9
Working overhead (s)		0.36	0.58		71.2	98.1		165.0	227.5		44.5	75.7
Forward bend standing (s)		0.96	0.93		20.8	49.1		48.2	113.9		51.9	92.8
Forward bend sitting (s)		0.72			33.9			78.7			32.1	
Dynamic bending (s)		0.72	0.45		6.2	4.64		14.5	10.8		5.9	3.1
Squatting (s)		0.82	0.54		4.5	2.8		10.4	6.6		5.3	2.1
Rotation standing R (s)		0.60	0.66		5.1	5.3		11.8	12.3		4.0	4.6
Rotation standing L (s)		0.39	0.73		5.4	4.0		12.6	9.2		3.5	3.8
Rotation sitting R (s)		0.64	0.54		5.5	7.2		12.7	17.2		4.6	5.4
Rotation standing L (s)		0.45	0.72		7.8	4.8		18.1	11.1		5.2	4.5

Notes: ICC = Intraclass Correlation Coefficient, SEM = Standard Error of Measurement, MDC$_{90}$ = Minimum Detectable Change (90% confidence), MCID = Minimum Clinically Important Difference.

Study 1 = Reneman et al. (2002), Study 2 = Brouwer et al. (2003), Study 3 = Reneman et al. (2004). Study 1 and 2 sample was chronic low back pain. study 3 were healthy volunteers. The retest periods were study 1: 24 h, study 2: 2 weeks, study 3: 2–3 weeks.

taken place. Two studies have also noted that lifting capacity tends to increase with repeated testing. One study [51] noted that subjects lifting capacity improved significantly between test occasions 2–4 days apart: an average 3.9 kg for the floor-to-waist lift, and 2.5 on the front carrying task. Another study [58] noted an average increase of 1.2–3.1 kg or 6%–9% increase on maximum weight lifted or carried on consecutive days. So it seems that at least some of the increase in lifting capacity on repeated testing is due to a practice or training effect.

A study that considered an immediate test–retest of the forward bend in standing, and the overhead work test in 44 healthy young adults reported Pearson correlations of 0.81 and 0.72 for the two tests, respectively [59]. With such a short retest period and using healthy subjects, this result does not have any direct clinical applicability.

17.5.5 Validity

17.5.5.1 Content Validity

Evidence for the content validity of the ISW-FCE is provided by a comparison of test items with the U.S. Department of Labor's 20 physical demands of work. The ISW-FCE covers 16 of the 20 work demands (the items not covered are feeling, talking, hearing and seeing) [45].

17.5.5.2 Predictive Validity

The predictive validity of the ISW-FCE has been explored in six studies. Three studies have found little or no relationship between IWS FCE test results and future recurrence in people with upper extremity disorders [12] and chronic back pain [60,61]. There is some evidence that better FCE performance, and in particular a higher lifting capacity, is associated with faster recovery in people with upper extremity disorders [12], chronic back pain [61,62], and other, unspecified disorders [63]. However, many of these studies are retrospective and unblinded and provide no usable information as to the clinical applicability of these predictive findings.

17.5.5.3 Diagnostic Validity

The ability of nine observers to determine the presence of submaximal effort in the floor-to-waist lifting task was correct for 85% to 90% of 15 healthy subjects, and 100% of 16 subjects with chronic low back pain [49]. Correct rating of maximal performance was low: 46%–53% in healthy subjects and only 5%–7% of back pain patients. Ratings were of videotaped performances and the "gold standard" of effort were "duration, heart rate and self-rating of performance intensity." The generalizability of the findings to the clinical setting are doubtful given the use of videotaped performances, healthy subjects, and the use of pooled observer data.

17.5.5.4 Construct Validity

Correlations of test results on various aspects of the ISW FCE with self-reported levels of pain and disability have been shown to be weak to moderate [64,65]. Scores on a measure of kinesiophobia showed no significant association with ISW-FCE lifting ability [66]. Performance of the floor-to-waist lift task has been shown to be influenced by self-perceived disability, pain intensity, age and gender, and measures of physical functioning (by observed performance) and self-reported pain and disability appear to provide related, but not strongly correlated, information on physical functioning [11,25]. Weak associations between self-reported pain, disability, and FCE are consistent with other research that has noted the lack of a strong relationship between pain, impairment, and activity limitation [67]. A head-to-head concurrent comparison of the lifting tests in IWS-FCE and the Ergo-Kit FCE in healthy subjects [68] concluded that the two protocols for testing lifting capacity were not sufficiently associated to be used interchangeably. The correlation between the two methods was moderate ($r = .72$), but the difference in maximum average amount of weight lifted was 6.2 kg, which was significant ($p = .000$).

A cross-sectional study [69] examined the "ecological validity" of the static endurance tests of the IWS-FCE (overhead work, crouching, and kneeling) by testing healthy subjects in environments with various levels of noise and requirement to work quickly. They found that the different test conditions that are aspects of a normal work environment did not influence the holding times on the tests.

Performance of the lifting and carrying tests by chronic low back pain patients in The Netherlands, Canada and Switzerland showed substantial differences in maximum weights handled [46]. Patients in the Dutch sample on average lifted the highest weights: 17 kg more than the Canadian sample and 14 kg more than the Swiss. The authors speculated that the differences were due to differences in the testing protocols, patient characteristics, or the context of FCE.

A study of the IWS-FCE [25] found little agreement among estimates made of work-related limitations by patient self-report, clinical examination by a physician, and IWS FCE. The highest levels of limitation were by self-report and lowest levels by FCE. The authors emphasize that in the absence of any "gold standard" tests of limitation, we have no way of knowing which of these methods is closest to the truth. Possible explanations for the differences are a desire to please (to do well when a health professional is testing) or underestimating capacity on the self-report. This is consistent with the phenomenon that self-reports of activity limitation are higher when completed independently than when completed by face-to-face to interview [70,71]. Again, we have no way of knowing which should be considered the gold standard. The different perspectives on functioning provided by observational and self-report methods supports the inclusion in the latest version of the WorkWell FCE of the SFS, a self-report measure of work capacity.

17.6   PHYSICAL WORK PERFORMANCE EVALUATION

The PWPE was developed in the early 1990s by Lechner and colleagues [72] and is available from ErgoScience Inc.* The system is said to be used widely in a number of countries, including the United States, Canada, and Australia [73]. The PWPE comprises 36 tests arranged in six sections evaluating dynamic strength, position

---

* ErgoScience Inc. 15 Office Park Circle, suite 214, Birmingham, AL 35223.

tolerance, mobility, fine motor skills, coordination, balance, and endurance. On the basis of number of repetitions, heart rate, duration of tasks, and observed physical signs, a "safe level of work" is determined for each task. For the strength, position tolerance and mobility sections (21 tests) the worker is categorized into one of six levels of work ability: unable to work, sedentary, light, medium, heavy, and very heavy work. An overall level of physical work ability is also made. Balance and coordination are screened, not comprehensively evaluated. Endurance is projected from changes in heart rate response and performance. The rater also makes a judgment of the level of participation or cooperation of the person being tested as "self-limiting," "full participation," or "overextending." This judgment is made by comparing the subject's perception of maximum effort with observed physical signs such as use of accessory muscles and trunk alignment. Physical signs are also used to evaluate when maximum function is reached. Testing is terminated when the examiner judges a maximal safe effort has been reached [72].

17.6.1 SAFETY

The PWPE protocol requires screening for cardiovascular problems and instruction on "correct" lifting technique prior to testing [72]. No studies of safety have been published in the peer-reviewed literature.

17.6.2 RELIABILITY

Two published studies have examined interrater reliability of the PWPE [72,73] and two test–retest reliability [74,75]. Lechner et al. [72] examined interrater reliability for pairs of physical therapists (from a total of 11) simultaneously assessing 50 patients with musculoskeletal disorders. Durand et al. [73] had five experienced raters and 41 patients with low back pain. Tuckwell et al. [75] had a single rater administer three tests from each section, with a 2-week interval between testing, on 24 subjects with stable musculoskeletal conditions. Brassard et al. [74] tested 30 healthy workers. Table 17.11 shows the kappa statistics for ordinal data (agreement on the level of work and cooperation).

The study by Lechner et al. [72] yielded interrater agreement of 0.80 or more for judgments of subject cooperation for all items in the mobility section, for three of the position tolerance items and only waist-to-eye level lift and unilateral carrying in the dynamic strength section. These findings were not replicated in the study by Durand et al. [73] who reported much lower kappa values for most of the tasks. In that study only three tasks, all in the position tolerance section, reached the 0.80 minimum: sitting, elevated work in standing, and kneeling. Interrater reliability for rating level of work reached 0.80 in the Lechner study for only the unilateral carry task, while in the Durand study kappa values of at least 0.80 were reported for 9 of the 21 tests.

The raters in both studies were trained and experienced therapists. In neither study were the raters absolutely independent as both were present at testing with one performing the testing and the other as a "silent observer" and kappa values may therefore have been overestimated. It is important to note that a slightly different kappa statistic was used in each study, confounding a direct comparison between the studies.

TABLE 17.11

Comparison of Reliability Studies for the PWPE (Kappa Statistics)

| | Interrater | | | | Test–Retest | |
| | Cooperation | | Level of Work | | | |
	Lechner	Durand	Lechner	Durand	Tuckwell	Brassard
Dynamic Strength						
Floor-to-waist lift	0.79	0.62	0.78	0.72	0.77	
Waist-to-eye level lift	**0.83**	0.36	0.77	0.66		
Bilateral carry	0.67	0.32	0.75	**0.84**	0.75	
Unilateral carry	**0.80**	0.42	**0.88**	0.73		
Push	0.67	0.25	0.62	**0.82**	0.75	
Pull	0.56	0.60	0.68	0.79		
LOW rating for section			0.74	**0.81**		0.49
Position Tolerance						
Sitting		**1.00**		0.76	0.38	0.35
Standing		0.66		**0.84**	0.60	0.50
Elevated work—standing	0.71	**0.82**	0.67	**0.80**		0.44
Lowered work—standing	0.71	0.68	0.69	**0.83**		0.45
Kneeling	0.77	**0.81**	0.56	**0.83**	0.70	0.05
Lowered work—sitting	**0.82**	0.34	0.60	0.72		0.09
Squatting	**0.84**	0.55	0.59	0.65		0.20
Reclining reach	**0.87**	0.64	0.66	0.76		0.36
LOW rating for section			0.54	0.72		0.48
Mobility						
Walking	**0.97**	0.66	0.50	**0.84**	0.37	0.67
Crawling	**0.83**	0.64	0.75	0.78		**0.83**
Climbing ladder	**0.95**	0.38	0.63	0.47		**0.83**
Climbing stairs	**0.81**	0.66	0.70	**0.80**	0.19	0.63
Repetitive squatting	**0.87**	0.63	0.33	0.70	0.60	0.67
Repetitive trunk rotation—standing	**0.90**	0.48	0.64	0.54		0.34
Repetitive trunk rotation—sitting	**0.87**	0.65	0.58	0.37		0.44
LOW rating for section			0.58	0.54		0.52
Overall LOW				0.76		0.43

Note: Lechner $n = 50$, musculoskeletal disorders, Durand $n = 41$ low back pain, Tuckwell $n = 24$ musculoskeletal disorders, Brassard $n = 30$ healthy workers. Lechner used free-marginal kappa, Durand unweighted kappa, Tuckwell weighted kappa. Values of 0.80 or greater are shown in bold type.

The inter and intrarater reliability of the maximum lifting capacity on the floor-to-waist lift from two pilot studies of 10 subjects each were reported as $ICC_{3,1}$ 0.97 and 0.94, respectively, in a report on the effect of lumbosacral supports on abdominal muscle strength [76]. These values may not be generalizable to other raters [15].

TABLE 17.12
Test–Retest Reliability PWPE Dynamic Strength Section

Task	ICC	Lower	Upper	SEM	Lower	Upper	MDC_{90}	Lower	Upper	MCID
Floor-to-waist lift (kg)	.88	.76	.94	6.74	4.76	9.53	15.63	11.05	22.10	9.73
Waist-to-eye level lift (kg)	.81	.64	.90	6.32	4.59	8.70	14.66	10.63	20.18	7.25
Bilateral carry (kg)	.81	.63	.90	8.72	6.32	12.17	20.22	14.67	28.22	10.00
Unilateral carry (kg)	.79	.61	.89	6.76	4.89	9.21	15.68	11.35	21.36	7.38
Push (kg)	.82	.66	.91	5.75	4.07	7.90	13.33	9.43	18.32	6.78
Pull (kg)	.91	.83	.96	5.25	3.50	7.22	12.18	8.12	16.73	8.75

Source: Brassard, B., et al., *Can. J. Occup. Ther.—Revue Canadienne d Ergotherapie*, 73, 206, 2006.
Note: Lower and upper bounds of SEM and MDC_{90} are calculated from the lower and upper bounds of the ICC.

In a study of test–retest reliability of level of work ratings, [75] none of the coefficients reached 0.80 and three of the nine tasks examined (stair climbing, sitting, and walking) had values less than 0.40. In the Brassard study, only two tasks had kappa values higher than 0.80. The use of observed physical signs in the judgment criteria has been proposed as a factor contributing to poor interrater reliability [72,73] and use of fluctuations in pain and self-limiting behavior to poor test–retest variability [75].

Calculations of the SEM, MDC_{90}, and MCID from the Brassard study (Table 17.12) show that for the floor-to-waist lift, the true score may be within ±6.74 kg of the observed score, an improvement of 15.6 kg would be needed to be 90% confident of exceeding measurement error, and a change of around 10 kg would typically be considered clinically important. The reader should keep in mind, however, that the subjects in the Brassard study were healthy and these values may not necessarily be generalizable to a clinical population.

17.6.3 Validity

17.6.3.1 Content Validity

The PWPE battery includes the 20 physical work demands of the *Dictionary of Occupational Titles* [72].

17.6.3.2 Predictive Validity

In the first report of the PWPE, Spearman rho correlations between actual and predicted levels of work were reported as ranging from 0.41 ($p = .002$) to 0.55 ($p < .01$) [72]. While 14%–18% were reported as working above the level predicted by the PWPE, it is not stated what proportion was working at or below the predicted level of work. This study was cross-sectional and can only loosely be considered as predictive. It is more usefully an indicator of convergent validity.

A later study by the test developers, reported only as an abstract [77], predictive validity of the PWPE evaluated in 30 subjects undertaking a work-hardening program. Baseline PWPE results were used to tailor the work-hardening program to the individual, and at the end of the program the participants were retested only on those tasks that were targeted by the intervention. Return to work predictions were made at the conclusion of the program and workers were followed up 3 and 6 months later to determine their work status. Agreement between predictions at program completion and work status at both follow-up points was 87%. The authors noted that external factors had prevented return to work for all the individuals who had not returned to work, but who had been predicted to do so.

The sensitivity, specificity and positive and negative predictive values have not yet been reported for the PWPE. Without this information derived from a property designed study, it is not possible to determine the extent to which RTW predictions based on the PWPE can accurately predict return to work or any other outcome of interest.

17.6.3.3   Diagnostic Validity

In the PWPE, the evaluator makes a judgment of subject participation or cooperation by comparing the subject's self-perception of maximum ability to the rater's observations of physical signs [72]. No studies have yet demonstrated the diagnostic validity of the judgment of subject cooperation in the PWPE.

17.6.3.4   Construct Validity

Little published evidence exists to support the construct validity of the PWPE. The therapist's judgment of overall level of work is moderately associated with actual work level (rho = .41 to .55) [72]. Isokinetic strength and anthropometric variables have been shown to be strongly predictive (R^2 = .61 to .88) of safe lifting maximum lifting capacity in the floor-to-waist task [78].

17.7   CAL-FCP

The Cal-FCP* was developed for the Industrial Medical Council in California [79] and is intended to "measure the work consequences of soft tissue musculoskeletal injury" specifically within the California disability determination model [80]. The evaluation is conducted 30 days postinjury in cases where the worker remains off work or continues in active treatment. The protocol, which takes on average 84 (sd 17) min to complete [80], evaluates pain, self-perceived functional capacity, and observed functional capacity (Table 17.13). The sequence of testing allows sitting and standing tolerance to be evaluated.

When testing lifting capacity the subject is asked after each lift cycle whether or not they would be able to perform the lifting task on a "safe and dependable basis eight to twelve times per day" [81]. The evaluator makes a rating of effort on the

---

* Available from EPIC, 188 Woodlands Place Court, St. Charles, MO 63303.

TABLE 17.13
Tests in the Cal-FCP Battery

Test	Description
Structured interview	Current functional abilities compared to premorbid ability
Health Questionnaire and physical exam	Screening for cardiovascular risk factors, resting blood pressure and heart rate
Spinal Function Sort (SFS) or	Self-reported ability to perform work activities. SFS has 50 cards with pictured tasks. Person indicates on 5-point rating scale their current ability to perform the task: able, only slightly restriction, restricted, very restricted, almost unable and unable. Total summed score is the Rating of Perceived Capacity (RPC). RPC scores range 0–200.
Hand Function Sort (HFS)	HFS has 62 items. Rating scale is as for SFS
Pain drawing 0–10 cm VAS pain ratings	Information concerning symptoms: ocation and type of pain; intensity and frequency of worst pain; intensity and frequency of usual pain
Job Demands Questionnaire	Self-reported job demands
Lateral Pinch Test	Pinch strength using B&L Pinch Gauge
Power Grip Test	Grip strength using JAMAR hand dynamometer
Standing range of motion (Static Position Tolerance Tests)	Observed ability to assume and maintain postures for 15 s each (stand and reach to shoulder and eye level, stoop and reach to knee level, crouch and reach to knee level, kneel and reach to knee level). Rated as able, slightly, moderately or very restricted, or unable.
EPIC Lift Capacity Test (ELC)	Isoinertial, progressive test of lift capacity. 3 tests: knuckle-to-shoulder, floor-to-knuckle, floor-to-shoulder each tested for infrequent lift capacity (1 rep per cycle) and frequent lift capacity (4 reps per cycle). Relative Acceptable Weight is calculated for Test 3 (max weight divided by body weight). % Normal lift capacity from tables by age.
Carry 100 ft	Ability to carry weight 100 ft at 3 miles per hour. Weight increased in 10 lb increments until maximum load used in ELC Test 3 is reached. Rated as no restriction, slight, moderately or very restricted, or unable.
Climbing 10 ft	Step up/down 8 in. step for 15 cycles, 1 step per second, while carrying maximum load able to lift in ELC Test 3. Rated as no restriction, slight, moderately or very restricted, or unable.

ELC tests, as "reliable," "questionable," or "unreliable" on the basis of observable behaviors during lifting [80]. An overall rating of test effort as "sincere" or "insincere" is made for the Cal-FCP as a whole.

Interpretation of Cal-FCP results is via a decision algorithm that results in classification of the worker as having no disability or one of eight categories of disability with a corresponding recommendation of the recommended level of work. Category A has 10% lost work capacity and no very heavy lifting is recommended, through to 70% lost work capacity for Category H for which sedentary work is recommended [79].

Testing of the measurement properties has not occurred for all components of the Cal-FCP (Table 17.14) and in this chapter only the ELC and Function Sort components will be considered in detail.

17.7.1 SAFETY

Lifting capacity is not tested on persons using heart-rate limiting medications, or who have a resting heart rate of more than 90 bpm, or resting blood pressure greater

TABLE 17.14
Overview of Key Reliability and Validity Studies for each Test in the Cal-FCP

Test	Reliability	Validity
Structured interview	No studies located	No studies located
Health Questionnaire and physical exam	No studies located	No studies located
Spinal Function Sort (SFS), or	Gibson and Strong [82] Matheson et al. [83]	Gibson and Strong [82]
Hand Function Sort (HFS)	No studies located	Matheson et al. [84] Sufka et al. [85] Robinson et al. [86]
Pain drawing	No studies located[a]	No studies located[a]
VAS pain ratings	No studies located[b]	No studies located[b]
Job Demands Questionnaire	No studies located	No studies located
Lateral Pinch Test: B&L Pinch Gauge	Mathiowetz et al. [87]	Mathiowetz et al. [87] Mathiowetz et al. [88] Harth and Vetter [89]
Power Grip Test JAMAR hand dynamometer	Nitschke et al. [90] Mathiowetz [91]	Harth and Vetter [89] Mathiowetz [91] Boadella et al. [92] Smith et al. [93]
Standing range of motion	No studies located	No studies located
EPIC Lift Capacity test (ELC)	Matheson [94] Matheson et al. [81] Matheson et al. [95]	Jay et al. [96]
Carry 100 ft	No studies located	No studies located
Climbing 10 ft	No studies located	No studies located

Note: Only studies published in peer-reviewed journals were considered.

[a] See Carnes and colleagues' systematic review on the use of pain drawings as a psychological screening tool [97].

[b] For this particular set of pain rating scales. For studies of VAS scales see Downie et al. [98] Ogon et al. [99].

than 159/100 mmHg, or who have other risk factors [81]. Lift testing is terminated if any one of seven end points is reached, including exceeding heart rate limits, reaching 8 on the 10-level perceived load scale (i.e., a rating of the load as "very heavy"), achievement of load guideline or target load, or poor lifting technique. The end point of each test may therefore be terminated by either the evaluator or the subject [81].

An absence of new injuries or exacerbations has been reported after administering the ELC test to healthy and disabled persons [81] and the whole Cal-FCP protocol to workers with soft-tissue musculoskeletal injuries [80].

17.7.2   VALIDITY: ENTIRE TEST BATTERY

17.7.2.1   Content Validity

Test battery content was selected on the basis of criteria related to safety, reliability, validity, practicality and utility, and to allow categorization using the California Schedule for Rating Permanent Disabilities [79].

17.7.2.2   Predictive Validity

No studies of the predictive validity were found for any component of the Cal-FCP test battery.

17.8   EPIC LIFT CAPACITY TEST

17.8.1   RELIABILITY

Only one study has reported the interrater reliability of the rating of sincere effort (ICC = 0.83, ICC model not stated) for two evaluators' ratings of six subjects with musculoskeletal problems [96].

Two articles, both by the test developers, have been published on the test–retest reliability of the Maximum Acceptable Weight achieved in the ELC tests. The first article [81] reported three studies: one of 26 healthy male adults, one of 318 healthy adults, and one of 14 adults with chronic disability following spinal and lower extremity injuries. Raters in the larger study were 65 professionals undertaking certification for the ELC testing. The retest period was 5–14 days and in the sample of disabled individuals, a different rater was used on the two test occasions. The second article [94] reported the results of 110 professionals rating 531 healthy adults during their certification training. The retest period was 5–17 days.

The test–retest reliability coefficients and corresponding SEM, MDC_{90}, and MCID have been calculated from data provided in the report (Tables 17.15 and 17.16). These values are an expression of the measurement error of the tests in kilograms. The SEM indicates the range within which a person's true score will fall (i.e., the observed value plus or minus the SEM) with 68% confidence. The MDC_{90} indicates the magnitude of change in kilograms that would need to be observed

TABLE 17.15
ELC Test–Retest Reliability of Mean Maximum Acceptable Weight (kg) in Healthy Adults

Task	Reliability Coefficient			SEM			MDC_{90}			MCID		
	1	2	3	1	2	3	1	2	3	1	2	3
1. Knuckle-to-shoulder 1/cycle	.90	.93	.94	2.59	1.88	1.76	6.01	4.36	4.09	4.10	3.55	3.60
2. Floor-to-knuckle 1/cycle	.92	.88	.91	2.18	2.98	2.55	5.05	6.91	5.91	3.85	4.30	4.25
3. Floor-to-shoulder 1/cycle	.92	.93	.94	2.28	1.88	1.75	5.28	4.36	4.06	4.03	3.55	3.58
4. Knuckle-to-shoulder 4/cycle	.86	.91	.92	2.39	1.88	1.74	5.55	4.35	4.03	3.20	3.13	3.08
5. Floor-to-knuckle 4/cycle	.88	.91	.89	2.48	2.30	2.45	5.74	5.32	5.69	3.58	3.83	3.70
6. Floor-to-shoulder 4/cycle	.92	.91	.84	1.92	1.92	2.64	4.46	4.45	6.12	3.40	3.20	3.30

Notes:　ICC = Intraclass Correlation Coefficient, SEM = Standard Error of Measurement, MDC_{90} = Minimum Detectable Change (90% confidence), MCID = Minimum Clinically Important Difference.

Study 1 = Matheson et al. [81], n = 26 healthy males, retest 5–17 days, reliability coefficient is Pearson' r.
Study 2 = Matheson et al. [81], n = 290 healthy adults, retest 5–17 days, reliability coefficient is ICC1,1.
Study 3 = Matheson [1], n = 531 healthy adults, retest 5–14 days, reliability coefficient is ICC (model not stated).

TABLE 17.16

ELC Test–Retest Reliability of Mean Maximum Acceptable Weight (kg) in Adults with a Chronic Musculoskeletal Disorder

Task	Pearson r	SEM	MDC_{90}	MCID
1. Knuckle-to-shoulder 1/cycle	.95	1.30	3.01	2.90
2. Floor-to-knuckle 1/cycle	.93	1.93	4.48	3.65
3. Floor-to-shoulder 1/cycle	.94	1.69	3.92	3.45
4. Knuckle-to-shoulder 4/cycle	.86	1.87	4.34	2.50
5. Floor-to-knuckle 4/cycle	.82	2.46	5.71	2.90
6. Floor-to-shoulder 4/cycle	.82	1.36	3.15	1.60

Note: Sample was 14 paid volunteers unemployed due to chronic disability (8 spine and 6 lower extremity) [81].

before one could be 90% confident that the change exceeded measurement error. The MCID is an estimate of the smallest amount of change that would be considered clinically important.

For example, for test 3 (floor-to-shoulder lift, 1 rep per cycle), the observed value will be correct within a range either side of the value equivalent to the SEM. When measured across time, for example when using the ELC to determine outcomes of a rehabilitation or work-hardening program, once the change exceeds the MDC_{90} the therapist can be 90% confident that this represents change beyond error in the measurement. So an individual whose maximum acceptable weight on test 3 was 10 kg would need to improve this by at least 4 or 5 kg at follow-up before this could, with 90% confidence, be said to be actual improvement and not just measurement error. Improvements less than the MDC_{90} cannot be dismissed as being explained entirely by measurement error, however, the more the magnitude of change falls short of the MDC_{90} the lower the confidence that it is real change. A change of about 3.5–4 kg would typically be considered to be clinically important. The reader should keep in mind that the values for healthy subjects cannot necessarily be generalized to a clinical population, and the values for the disabled group is drawn from a very small sample.

The test developers have also explored the ELC test reactivity—the extent to which practice with the test influences the apparent improvement in performance [95]. Fifty-five people with low back problems were randomized into two groups and underwent the same rehabilitation program. One group was tested before and after, while the other group was tested only at the end of the program. While the pre–post group improved significantly on the ELC test, there were no differences between the ELC test results of the two groups. This suggests that there is no detectable learning effect of a single ELC test administered 8 weeks before a second test. The issue of test reactivity is an important one where improvements may be attributable to a learning effect rather than to actual improvements in the variable being measured.

17.8.2 Validity

17.8.2.1 Diagnostic Validity

To test the accuracy of judgments of effort rating by five experienced evaluators, 41 adults with musculoskeletal disorders were instructed to make a sincere maximal effort, or to give an insincere effort of 50% of maximum [96]. Raters used physical responses (blood pressure and heart rate), observed behaviors (postures, movements) and the results of the SFS or Hand Function Sort (HFS; which have inbuilt reliability checks) to arrive at an overall test effort rating of "sincere" or "insincere." Participants were randomized to the submaximal effort ($n = 20$) or full effort ($n = 28$) group and the evaluators were said to be blind to group membership, although the success of blinding was not reported.

The study reported overall accuracy of 86.8% for the raters' ability to correctly identify maximal and submaximal effort. The positive and negative predictive values reported were 94.4% and 80%. The corresponding prevalence (53%), sensitivity (80%), specificity (94%), positive likelihood ratio (13), and negative likelihood ratio (0.2) could be calculated from the information provided in the study. The consequences of incorrectly judging a person as making an insincere effort are probably greater then incorrectly judging a person as making a sincere effort. In this study only one person was incorrectly judged as insincere, while four persons were incorrectly judged as sincere. Figure 17.2 shows the numbers being correctly and incorrectly identified as sincere or insincere effort. Of the 17 persons judged as insincere only one was incorrectly judged. Of the 21 persons judged as sincere four were incorrectly judged. The results of this study can be clinically interpreted as meaning that, when the prevalence of insincere effort is 53%, the post-test probability that a person who is rated as making an insincere maximal effort is actually making an insincere effort is 94% and the post-test probability that a person who is rated as making a sincere effort is actually making a sincere effort is 80%.

Clinicians must be aware that as the prevalence of insincere effort cannot be known these post-test probabilities cannot be extrapolated to clinical practice. For example, if the real prevalence (pretest probability) of insincere effort was 10%, then a positive test result (person judged to be making an insincere effort), the post-test probability of the person actually being insincere would be only 60%.

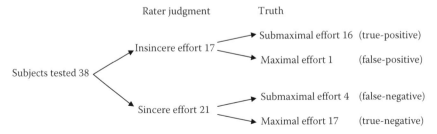

FIGURE 17.2 Diagnostic validity of the rating of effort during the ELC test from Jay et al. [96].

In another study [100] 90 subjects with chronic low back pain were randomized to a 100% or 60% effort group. The PILE lifting protocol was used, which is similar to the ELC, and overall rating of effort was based on 17 signs. A single-blinded evaluator conducted the FCE, although the success of blinding was not reported. In this study, the tester judged 53 subjects to be making a submaximal effort and of these, 16 were incorrectly classified. This means that 30% of people who were judged as not making a maximal effort were incorrectly classified, and 19% of people judged to be making a maximal effort were incorrectly classified. Until sufficient, quality studies of the diagnostic validity of tests are available clinicians should be very cautious about making judgments of sincerity of effort.

17.8.2.2   Construct Validity: ELC

Expected gender and age differences on lift capacity have been reported on 64 adults with work-related musculoskeletal disorders [80]. The same study reported no significant differences between males and females on the percentage loss of lift capacity, nor did gender or age affect the disability rating. Those rated as making "questionable" effort had lower scores on the SFS and greater percentage loss of lift capacity than those rated as making a "reliable" effort.

In a sample of 530 healthy adults age, resting heart rate and body weight were significantly associated with lift capacity, and body weight had the strongest correlation (ICC = .84 to .94) [94]. This was seen as evidence for the calculation of relative acceptable weight by dividing maximum acceptable weight lifted by body weight. Associations were also found between variables expected to be related: pinch and grip strength were significantly and moderately correlated ($r = .63$ and .67 on the right and left, $p < .0001$), the SFS was moderately correlated with ELC test # 3 ($r = .58$), relative acceptable weight ($r = .59$) and the lost work capacity rating ($r = .67$).

17.9   SPINAL FUNCTION SORT

17.9.1   RELIABILITY

Two studies have appeared in the peer-reviewed literature on the reliability of the SFS [82,83]. The split-half reliability ($r = 0.98$) and 3-day test–retest reliability ($r = .85$) for the SFS was reported in a sample of 180 people with back pain [83]. Test reactivity was identified in the same study with subjects' SFS scores improving significantly when tested before and after FCE. Subjects with chronic disability (more than 360 days) improved 2%, while those with injury of less than 90 days duration improved by 14%. This systematic increase in workers' self-evaluated work capacity following FCE may indicate a change in self-efficacy that occurs after the person performs the various work-related tasks, but this has not been tested.

In a sample of 42 people with chronic back pain the internal consistency of the test was 0.98, test–retest reliability (ICC) on a subset of 14 subjects over 4–14 days was 0.89 [82]. The SEM could be calculated as 13 points, the MDC_{90} 31 points and the MCID 20 points. The score range of the SFS is 0 to 200 points.

17.9.2 VALIDITY

The study by Gibson and Strong [82] also tested the construct validity of the SFS. Expected correlations were demonstrated between SFS and measures of pain, perceived disability, self-efficacy, and expectations of return to work. SFS scores were not related to chronicity of back pain. Evidence for known groups validity is found in a study where back pain patients who exhibited a centralization of pain phenomenon had better SFS scores than those who did not [85] and in another study [86] scores for people with back pain were on average worse in the group who had undergone back surgery.

17.10 HAND FUNCTION SORT

Only one report of the measurement properties of the HFS has been published and this is a retrospective data review of 126 cases of adults with musculoskeletal impairments [84]. Principal components analysis of the 62-item test show one major factor explaining more than 50% of variance and two minor factors [84]. Scores on the HFS were significantly different for groups with and without upper extremity impairments [84]. Total HFS score and some category scores were significantly and moderately to strongly related to grip strength of the dominant hand [84]. There is no published evidence for the reliability of the HFS.

17.11 CONCLUSIONS

The large number of tests and batteries of tests that are available for FCE pose a challenge to the clinician to select tests and measures that are appropriate for a particular purpose. For even long-established and widely used FCE protocols gaps in the evidence relating to reliability and validity persist. At present, there is limited evidence that accurate predictions about future events can be made on the basis of FCE. It is also doubtful that judgments made about a person's sincerity of effort during testing can be made with acceptable accuracy. The consequences of testing should be kept in mind when making inferences from FCE test results. Where the consequences of decisions made on the basis of test results are "high stakes" then test accuracy is paramount. Testing of ability to perform work-related activities should be seen only as part of a comprehensive evaluation of the range of biopsychosocial variables that are relevant for the specific purpose for which the FCE is being conducted.

REFERENCES

1. Matheson, L., The functional capacity evaluation, in *Disability Evaluation*, Andersson, G., Demeter, S., and G, S., Eds. Mosby Yearbook, Chicago, IL, 2003.
2. Innes, E. and Straker, L., Validity of work-related assessments. *Work*, 13, 125, 1999.
3. Innes, E. and Straker, L., Reliability of work-related assessments. *Work*, 13, 107, 1999.
4. Jones, T. and Kumar, S., Functional capacity evaluation of manual materials handlers: a review. *Disabil Rehabil*, 25, 179, 2003.
5. King, P.M., Tuckwell, N., and Barrett, T.E., A critical review of functional capacity evaluations. *Phys Ther*, 78, 852, 1998.
6. Hart, D.L., Isernhagen, S.J., and Matheson, L., Guidelines for functional capacity evaluation of people with medical conditions. *JOSPT*, 18, 682, 1993.

7. Rondinelli, R.D. and Katz, R.T., *Impairment Rating and Disability Evaluation*. W.B. Saunders, Philadelphia, PA, 2000.
8. Tramposh, A.K., The functional capacity evaluation: Measuring maximal work abilities. *Occup Med*, 7, 113, 1992.
9. Isernhagen, S.J., Contemporary issues in functional capacity evaluation, in *The Comprehensive Guide to Work Injury Management*, Isernhagen, S.J., Ed. Aspen Publishers, Gaithersburg, MD, 1995, p. 410.
10. Rothstein, J., Campbell, S.K., Echternach, J.L., Jette, A.M., Knecht, H.G., Rose, S.J., Standards for tests and measurements in physical therapy practice. *Phys Ther*, 71, 589, 1991.
11. Gross, D.P. and Battie, M.C., Factors influencing results of functional capacity evaluations in workers' compensation claimants with low back pain. *Phys Ther*, 85, 315, 2005.
12. Gross, D.P. and Battie, M.C., Does functional capacity evaluation predict recovery in workers' compensation claimants with upper extremity disorders? *Occup Environ Med*, 63, 404, 2006.
13. Davidson, M., The interpretation of diagnostic tests: A primer for physiotherapists. *Aust J Physiother*, 48, 227, 2002.
14. Havlicek, L.L. and Peterson, N.L., Effect of the violation of assumptions upon significance levels of the Pearson r. *Psychol Bull*, 84, 373, 1977.
15. Portney, L.G. and Watkins, M.P., *Foundations for Clinical Research: Applications to Practice*. Appleton & Lange. Norwalk, CT, 1993.
16. Streiner, D.L.N., Norman, G.R., *Health Measurement Scales. A Practical Guide to their Development and Use*. 2nd edn. Oxford University Press, Oxford, 1995.
17. Stratford, P.W. and Binkley, J.M., Measurement properties of the RM-18: A modified version of the Roland-Morris Disability Scale. *Spine*, 22, 2416, 1997.
18. Terwee, C.B., et al., On assessing responsiveness of health-related quality of life instruments: Guidelines for instrument evaluation. *Qual Life Res*, 12, 349, 2003.
19. Wright, J.G., The minimal important difference: Who's to say what is important? *J Clin Epidemiol*, 49, 1221, 1996.
20. Norman, G.R., Sloan, J.A., and Wyrwich, K.W., Interpretation of changes in health-related quality of life: The remarkable universality of half a standard deviation, *Med Care*, 41, 582, 2003.
21. American Educational Research Association, A.P.A., National Council on Measurement in Education, Standards for Educational and Psychological Testing, Washington, DC, 1999.
22. Finch, E., et al., *Physical Rehabilitation Outcome Measures*. Canadian Physiotherapy Association. Hamilton, Ontario, 2002.
23. Murawski, M.M. and Miederhoff, P.A., On the generalizability of statistical expressions of health related quality of life instrument responsiveness: A data synthesis. *Qual Life Res*, 7, 11, 1998.
24. Gouttebarge, V., et al., Reliability and validity of functional capacity evaluation methods: A systematic review with reference to Blankenship system, Ergos work simulator, Ergo-Kit and Isernhagen work system. *Int Arch Occup Environ Health*, 77, 527, 2004.
25. Brouwer, S., et al., Comparing self-report, clinical examination and functional testing in the assessment of work-related limitations in patients with chronic low back pain. *Disabil Rehabil*, 27, 999, 2005.
26. Greenhalgh, T., Papers that report diagnostic or screening tests. *BMJ*, 315, 540, 1997.
27. Sackett, D.L., et al., *Evidence-Based Medicine. How to Practice and Teach EBM*, 2nd edn. Churchill Livingstone, Edinburgh, 2000.
28. Greenhalgh, T., Papers that summarise other papers (systematic reviews and meta-analyses). *BMJ*, 315, 672, 1997.
29. Geisser, M.E., et al., Psychosocial factors and functional capacity evaluation among persons with chronic pain. *J Occup Rehabil*, 13, 259, 2003.

30. Wind, H., et al., Assessment of functional capacity of the musculoskeletal system in the context of work, daily living, and sport: A systematic review. *J Occup Rehabil*, 15, 253, 2005.
31. Shechtman, O., et al., The use of the coefficient of variation in detecting sincerity of effort: A meta-analysis. *Work*, 26, 335, 2006.
32. Mondloch, M.V., Cole, D.C., and Frank, J.W., Does how you do depend on how you think you'll do? A systematic review of the evidence for a relation between patients' recovery expectations and health outcomes. *CMAJ*, 165, 174, 2001.
33. Waddell, G., Burton, A.K., and Main, C.J., *Screening to Identify People at Risk of Long-Term Incapacity for Work. A Conceptual and Scientific Review*. The Royal Society of Medicine Press, London, 2003.
34. Kuijer, W., et al., Prediction of sickness absence in patients with chronic low back pain: A systematic review. *J Occup Rehabil*, 16, 439, 2006.
35. Truchon, M. and Fillion, L., Biopsychosocial determinants of chronic disability and low-back pain: A review. *J Occup Rehabil*, 10, 117, 2000.
36. Waddell, G. and Burton, A.K., Occupational health guidelines for the management of low back pain at work: Evidence review. *Occup Med (Oxf)*, 51, 124, 2001.
37. Linton, S.J., Occupational psychological factors increase the risk of back pain: A systematic review. *J Occup Rehabil*, 11, 53, 2001.
38. Borge, J.A., Leboeuf-Yde, C., and Lothe, J., Prognostic values of physical examination findings in patients with chronic low back pain treated conservatively: A systematic literature review. *J Manipul Physiol Ther*, 24, 292, 2001.
39. Crook, J., et al., Determinants of occupational disability following a low back injury: A critical review of the literature. *J Occup Rehabil*, 12, 277, 2002.
40. Pincus, T., et al., A systematic review of psychological factors as predictors of chronicity/disability in prospective cohorts of low back pain. *Spine*, 27, E109, 2002.
41. Hartvigsen, J., et al., Psychosocial factors at work in relation to low back pain and consequences of low back pain: A systematic, critical review of prospective cohort studies. *Occup Environ Med*, 61, e2, 2004.
42. Steenstra, I.A., et al., Prognostic factors for duration of sick leave in patients sick listed with acute low back pain: A systematic review of the literature. *Occup Environ Med*, 62, 851, 2005.
43. Lechner, D.E., Bradbury, S.F., and Bradley, L.A., Detecting sincerity of effort: A summary of methods and approaches. *Phys Ther*, 78, 867, 1998.
44. Matheson, L.N., History, design characteristics, and uses of the pictorial activity and task sorts. *J Occup Rehabil*, 14, 175, 2004.
45. Lechner, D., Roth, D., and Straaton, K., Functional capacity evaluation in work disability. *Work*, 1991, 38, 1991.
46. Reneman, M.F., et al., Material handling performance of patients with chronic low back pain during functional capacity evaluation: A comparison between three countries. *Disabil Rehabil*, 28, 1143, 2006.
47. Isernhagen, S.J., Hart, D.L., and Matheson, L.M., Reliability of independent observer judgments of level of lift effort in a kinesiophysical functional capacity evaluation. *Work*, 12, 145, 1999.
48. Kuijer, W., et al., Matching FCE activities and work demands: An explorative study. *J Occup Rehabil*, 16, 469, 2006.
49. Reneman, M.F., et al., Testing lifting capacity: Validity of determining effort level by means of observation. *Spine*, 30, E40, 2005.
50. Reneman, M.F., et al., Symptom increase following a functional capacity evaluation in patients with chronic low back Pain: An explorative study of safety. *J Occup Rehabil*, 16, 197, 2006.
51. Gross, D.P. and Battie, M.C., Reliability of safe maximum lifting determinations of a functional capacity evaluation. *Phys Ther*, 82, 364, 2002.

52. Isernhagen, S.J., Functional capacity evaluation: Rationale, procedure, utility of the kinesiophysical approach. *J Occup Med*, 2, 157, 1992.

53. Reneman, M.F., et al., The reliability of determining effort level of lifting and carrying in a functional capacity evaluation. *Work*, 18, 23, 2002.

54. Gardener, L. and McKenna, K., Reliability of occupational therapists in determining safe, maximal lifting capacity. *Aust Occup Ther* J, 46, 110, 1999.

55. Smith, R.L., Therapists' ability to identify safe maximum lifting in low back pain patients during functional capacity evaluation. *J Orthop Sports Phys Ther*, 19, 277, 1994.

56. Brouwer, S., et al., Test–retest reliability of the Isernhagen Work Systems Functional Capacity Evaluation in patients with chronic low back pain. *J Occup Rehabil*, 13, 207, 2003.

57. Reneman, M.F., et al., Test–retest reliability of the Isernhagen Work Systems Functional Capacity Evaluation in healthy adults. *J Occup Rehabil*, 14, 295, 2004.

58. Reneman, M.F., et al., Test–retest reliability of lifting and carrying in a 2-day functional capacity evaluation. *J Occup Rehabil*, 12, 269, 2002.

59. Reneman, M.F., et al., Measuring maximum holding times and perception of static elevated work and forward bending in healthy young adults. *J Occup Rehabil*, 11, 87, 2001.

60. Gross, D.P. and Battie, M.C., The prognostic value of functional capacity evaluation in patients with chronic low back pain. Part 2: Sustained recovery. *Spine*, 29, 920, 2004.

61. Gross, D.P. and Battie, M.C., Functional capacity evaluation performance does not predict sustained return to work in claimants with chronic back pain. *J Occup Rehabil*, 15, 285, 2005.

62. Gross, D.P., Battie, M.C., and Cassidy, J.D., The prognostic value of functional capacity evaluation in patients with chronic low back pain. Part 1: Timely return to work. *Spine*, 29, 914, 2004.

63. Matheson, L.N., Isernhagen, S.J., and Hart, D.L., Relationships among lifting ability, grip force, and return to work. *Phys Ther*, 82, 249, 2002.

64. Gross, D.P. and Battie, M.C., Construct validity of a kinesiophysical functional capacity evaluation administered within a worker's compensation environment. *J Occup Rehabil*, 13, 287, 2003.

65. Reneman, M.F., et al., Concurrent validity of questionnaire and performance-based disability measurements in patients with chronic nonspecific low back pain. *J Occup Rehabil*, 12, 119, 2002.

66. Reneman, M.F., et al., Relationship between kinesiophobia and performance in a functional capacity evaluation. *J Occup Rehabil*, 13, 277, 2003.

67. Waddell, G., *The Back Pain Revolution*. 2nd edn. Churchill Livingstone, Edinburgh, 2004.

68. Ijmker, S., Gerrits, E.H., and Reneman, M.F., Upper lifting performance of healthy young adults in functional capacity evaluations: A comparison of two protocols. *J Occup Rehabil*, 13, 297, 2003.

69. Reneman, M.F., et al., Functional capacity evaluation: Ecological validity of three static endurance tests. *Work*, 16, 227, 2001.

70. Lyons, R.A., et al., SF-36 scores vary by method of administration: implications for study design. *J Public Health Med*, 21, 41, 1999.

71. Hoher, J., et al., Does the mode of data collection change results in a subjective knee score? Self-administration versus interview. *Am J Sports Med*, 25, 642, 1997.

72. Lechner, D.E., et al., Reliability and validity of a newly developed test of physical work performance. *J Occup Med*, 36, 997, 1994.

73. Durand, M.-J., et al., The interrater reliability of a functional capacity evaluation: The physical work performance evaluation. *J Occup Rehabil*, 14, 119, 2004.

74. Brassard, B., et al., Test–retest reliability study of the Physical Work Performance Evaluation. *Can J Occup Ther—Revue Canadienne d Ergotherapie*, 73, 206, 2006.

75. Tuckwell, N.L., Straker, L., and Barrett, T.E., Test–retest reliability on nine tasks of the Physical Work Performance Evaluation. *Work*, 19, 243, 2002.

76. Smith, E.B., et al., The effects of lumbosacral support belts and abdominal muscle strength on functional lifting ability in healthy women. *Spine*, 21, 356, 1996.

77. Lechner, D.E., et al., Predictive validity of a functional capacity evaluation: The physical work performance evaluation. *Phys Ther*, 76, S81, 1996.

78. Prim, J.F., et al., Factors influencing the lifting ability of healthy females 20 to 35 years of age (abstract). *Phys Ther*, 73, S51, 1993.

79. Mooney, V. and Matheson, L.N., *Objective Measurement of Soft Tissue Injury. Examiner's Manual*. Industrial Medical Council State of California, California, 1994.

80. Matheson, L.N., et al., Standardized evaluation of work capacity. *J Back Musculoskel Rehabil*, 6, 249, 1996.

81. Matheson, L.N., et al., A test to measure lift capacity of physically impaired adults. Part 1-Development and reliability testing. *Spine*, 20, 2119, 1995.

82. Gibson, L. and Strong, J., The reliability and validity of a measure of perceived functional capacity for work in chronic back pain. *J Occup Rehabil*, 6, 159, 1996.

83. Matheson, L.N., Matheson, M.L., and Grant, J., Development of a measure of perceived functional ability. *J Occup Rehabil*, 3, 15, 1993.

84. Matheson, L.N., Kaskutas, V.K., and Mada, D., Development and construct validation of the Hand Function Sort. *J Occup Rehabil*, 11, 75, 2001.

85. Sufka, A., et al., Centralization of low back pain and perceived functional outcome. *J Orthop Sports Phys Ther*, 27, 205, 1998.

86. Robinson, R.C., et al., Improvement in postoperative and nonoperative spinal patients on a self-report measure of disability: The Spinal Function Sort (SFS). *J Occup Rehabil*, 13, 107, 2003.

87. Mathiowetz, V., et al., Reliability and validity of grip and pinch strength evaluations. *J Hand Surg [Am]*, 9, 222, 1984.

88. Mathiowetz, V., et al., Grip and pinch strength: Normative data for adults. *Arch Phys Med Rehabil*, 66, 69, 1985.

89. Harth, A. and Vetter, W.R., Grip and pinch strength among selected adult occupational groups. *Occup Ther Int*, 1, 13, 1994.

90. Nitschke, J.E., et al., When is a change a genuine change? A clinically meaningful interpretation of grip strength measurements in healthy and disabled women. *J Hand Ther*, 12, 25, 1999.

91. Mathiowetz, V., Comparison of Rolyan and Jamar dynamometers for measuring grip strength. *Occup Ther Int*, 9, 201, 2002.

92. Boadella, J.M., et al., Effect of self-selected handgrip position on maximal handgrip strength. *Arch Phys Med Rehabil*, 86, 328, 2005.

93. Smith, G.A., et al., Assessing sincerity of effort in maximal grip strength tests. *Am J Phys Med Rehabil*, 68, 73, 1989.

94. Matheson, L.N., Relationships among age, body weight, resting heart rate, and performance in a new test of lift capacity. *J Occup Rehabil*, 6, 225, 1996.

95. Matheson, L.N., et al., A test to measure lift capacity of physically impaired adults. Part 2-Reactivity in a patient sample. *Spine*, 20, 2130, 1995.

96. Jay, M.A., et al., Sensitivity and specificity of the indicators of sincere effort of the EPIC lift capacity test on a previously injured population. *Spine*, 25, 1405, 2000.

97. Carnes, D., Ashby, D., and Underwood, M., A systematic review of pain drawing literature: Should pain drawings be used for psychologic screening? *Clin J Pain*, 22, 449, 2006.

98. Downie, W.W., et al., Studies with pain rating scales. *Ann Rheum Dis*, 37, 378, 1978.

99. Ogon, M., et al., Chronic low back pain measurement with visual analogue scales in different settings. *Pain*, 64, 425, 1996.

100. Lemstra, M., Olszynski, W.P., and Enright, W., The sensitivity and specificity of Functional Capacity Evaluations in determining maximal effort: A randomized trial. *Spine*, 29, 953, 2004.

18 Accommodation through Improved Design

Steven F. Wiker

CONTENTS

18.1 INTRODUCTION

Often we think of accommodation as an effort aimed at helping someone overcome legally defined physical, sensory, or mental impairments by modifying the design of physical layouts, tools, equipment, or job task(s). In other cases one attempts to enable an individual to perform activities of daily living to meet the requisite occupational responsibilities. Reasonable accommodation is a material component in legislation that aims to help impaired individuals to integrate into the mainstream of society as fully functional and integrated citizens. What constitutes impairment and how reasonable accommodation efforts may be are continuing processes that are typically resolved through societal processes. All of us have some degree of impairment when compared against a more capable individual, and we are all impaired, to some extent, by less than ideal layouts, equipment, tools, or task designs that have been poorly conceived.

The thesis of this chapter is that design-induced impairments are often eliminated, or sufficiently mitigated, by application of appropriate ergonomic design principles. A corollary is that poorly designed jobs, equipment, tools, or environments often result in accidents and injuries that impair individuals and force return-to-work efforts (i.e., accommodation for those who have permanent job-induced impairments). If good design is used, not only do we enhance the accommodative nature of the workplace, but we act to prevent future accidents, injuries, and impairments that often lead to additional accommodation effort.

18.2   BACKGROUND

18.2.1   MAGNITUDE OF CHALLENGE

Approximately 43 million adults (age 18 years and older), or 20.9% of the adult population, in the noninstitutionalized U.S. population were found to possess disabilities. This estimate was reduced to 27 million persons, or 18.8% of the population for individuals between 18 and 64 years of age (Harris et al., 2005). Workers with less education and lower incomes (Chirikos and Nestel, 1989; Harris et al., 2005) or who are older than 45 years are more likely to experience or possess impairments that result in disability.

Approximately, 23% of legally defined disabled people reported that their impairments resulted from injuries or accidents on the job, and 13% attributed their disabilities to poor working conditions (U.S. Department of Health and Human Services, 1980). Musculoskeletal and cardiovascular conditions, which included impairments due to bad backs, arthritis, heart ailments, and hypertension, were the most common problems among people reporting disability (Lando et al., 1982).

18.2.1.1   Consequences of Poor Design

The Americans with Disabilities Act of 1990 and the World Health Organization's classification of impairments, disabilities, and handicaps (WHO, 1980) posit the argument that impairment or disability is not a necessary consequence of physiological impairment or functional limitation. Employment and disability benefits are, thus, based upon impact of the impairment on functioning rather than existence of a quantifiable physiologically-based loss.

In addition employers must comply with statutes prohibiting employment discrimination on the basis of disability. Employers must consider on an individual basis whether a job applicant with a disability can perform the job with reasonable accommodation. Job standards that exclude all people with any impairment, or that exclude people with a specific impairment, cannot be set unless those standards are crucial to the performance of the job. Accommodation aims to enable impaired individuals to perform essential functions of the job. Reasonable accommodations are intended to ensure that the worker is capable of performing a particular job and that they are not denied that job because of design impediments that are unrelated to performance (e.g., the inability to pass through a doorway that is not compliant with building codes). To do this, an employer is expected to determine when accommodation that preserves the applicant's or worker's employability is reasonable and when such accommodation is not possible. Failure to accommodate may constitute discrimination.

Employers also face issues with returning workers to their jobs after workplace injuries or illnesses. Typically, rehabilitation efforts are focused upon restoration of job-related abilities and are financed through a variety of sources such as state and federal vocational rehabilitation, workers compensation, social security death index (SSDI), and private health insurance. In most cases following a significant injury, workers will be attempting to return to work with some degree of permanent impairment. The probability that individuals that have impairments are at greater risk of future injury in hazardous jobs is material. Successful return to work by workers with severe impairments is low (Mudrick, 1987), resulting in greater costs for the employer.

Employers of workers or job applicants with impairments face accommodation concerns in terms of direct or immediate costs of reasonable accommodation. However, poor design imposes far greater insidious costs associated with compromised productivity, quality, and increased risk of safety and health hazard consequences.

18.2.2 Design-Induced Accommodation Challenges

Often poor design of jobs, equipment or workplaces, impair performance, safety, and health of all workers. If that is the case, improved design can increase productivity and quality of work for all workers, including those who are impaired. Accommodation requirements are often eliminated or mitigated if designs follow ergonomic design principles.

Pheasant (1988) cataloged five engineering design fallacies associated with use of anthropometric data. Designers often suffer from one or more of the following fallacies:

- This design is satisfactory for me; thus, it will therefore be satisfactory for everybody else.
- This design is satisfactory for the average person—it will therefore be satisfactory for everybody else.
- The variability in human beings is so great that it cannot possibly be catered for in any design; however, since people are so wonderfully adaptable, it does not matter anyway.
- Ergonomics is expensive and since products are actually purchased on appearance and styling, ergonomics considerations may be conveniently ignored.
- Ergonomics is an excellent idea. I always design with ergonomics in mind—but I do it intuitively and rely on my common sense so I do not need tables of data.

Until designers understand the impact of their design errors, it will be difficult to materially improve accommodation across the board. In most respects, problems created by inadequate consideration of human engineering design principles lead to insidious impairments in the general population and exacerbates the effects of impairments of individuals that are labeled as "disabled."

Overcoming design flaws typically requires focal attention to human requirements for

- Ability to lift, carry or otherwise move everyday objects
- Eyesight (even when wearing glasses or contact lenses), speech, or hearing
- Manual dexterity
- Memory, learning, concentration, understanding
- Mobility
- Perception of the risk of physical danger
- Physical coordination
- Hydration, sustenance, and continence issues
- Environmental tolerance
- Others

Efforts that lead to accommodation through proper engineering design are essentially the same as those that are used to address accommodation of humans with material impairments. Rigorous application of the accommodation process at the beginning and throughout the design process not only reduces the frequency and intensity of individual accommodation efforts, but also serves to promote both an expansion of the labor pool and market share of usable products and services.

18.2.3 WHY DESIGNERS OFTEN MAKE ACCOMMODATION MORE DIFFICULT

From the problems of designer philosophies described in the preceding discussion, there are a number of studies that have shown that multiple population stereotypes exist for any given design and that minority perspectives can be held by large segments of the human population (see Sanders and McCormick, 1993 for examples of these problems). Thus, one cannot presume that one's personal view of "common sense" matches that of the majority of individuals who are intended users of the design.

In fact, designers and engineers who create new, or modify existing designs are adept at thinking "outside of the box" and achieve breakthroughs because they use approaches, analyses, or resources in a manner that are unusual in nature. Unique education, training, experience, and skills, by their nature, are not likely to operate entirely within what is deemed the realm of "common sense."

If product designs rely upon an individual designer's intuitive "common sense," then we are likely to encounter accidents and related problems due to a mismatch between the designer's and user's mental models, expectations, and performance capabilities. To overcome this problem, one must accept that individuals vary in their knowledge, belief systems, training, experience, skills, and physical and mental capacities to use designs or to use them without significant error and frustration. Essentially, the need for accommodative design is broad and should be addressed in all design processes and considerations.

Integrating human engineering requirements for any design should be determined at the outset and throughout the design development process. Integrating good human engineering design in the early stages of design reduces costs, the likelihood that post hoc modifications will have to be made, and the breadth of user populations or market share of products that will be restricted. When early involvement of ergonomists in the design process does not occur, usability, functionality, safety, and accommodation feasibility are compromised.

Other problems develop when "quick fixes" are made to designs for a variety of reasons. Typically neither the original designers nor ergonomists are involved in such design modifications, and unintended problems arise. For example, it may be less expensive to use a different colored dye in polymers that are used to construct a product. The color of the product is changed. The color for labels on the product may no longer offer the contrast sensitivity needed, and operators may confuse controls, reducing functionality and potentially introducing a safety hazard.

Sometimes designers forget to consider the capabilities and limitations of their intended and unintended user populations when they are making decisions about design parameters. For example, direction of reading symbols or icons cannot be assured if a product is to be used internationally. Some cultures read from right-to-left, top-to-bottom, left-to-right, and so forth. Reliance upon single coding paradigms that rely upon visual detection and recognition of labels, instructions, or other visually dependent coding systems are likely to pose problems. This clearly is a problem when individuals with low vision, or who are blind, must use designs that rely solely upon visual perception for information transmittal. Failure to understand impaired population capabilities and limitations makes designs difficult to use and often unsafe.

Designers often forget that they are not designing a single product, piece of equipment, task method, or working or living environment; instead, they are designing a component that functions within a larger system. This situation can result in abrupt mismatches or transitional problems that can impose significant burdens upon those with material impairments. For example, a well-designed full-sized automobile becomes a problem when the community allocates and designs parking spaces and stalls for small vehicles with few exceptions. Hours may be required each week to find parking for the vehicle, and to complete longer walk distances to a facility of interest. Moreover, carrying heavy loads for longer distances can pose additional risks. While the vehicle may be properly designed as a unit, within the community context, it degrades user efficiency and increases risk of musculoskeletal injury.

Project managers often misjudge the initial amount of effort that may or may not be required to engineer equipment, products, processes, and environments that are functional and safe when they require interaction with humans. Nearly all engineering curricula do not require engineers or other professions to take coursework that facilitates integration of ergonomic design principles in the design process. Good ergonomic design can only be achieved through rigorous analysis, and comprehensive manipulation of appropriate design principles early in design phases. This effort takes time, incurs cost, and if not used wisely, can result in production of significant upstream flaws that cannot be overcome without significant cost and rework. If design problems cannot be overcome, the performance goals or usability of the design will be constrained.

Simply providing textbooks, design handbooks, and focused ergonomic design standards for use by the design team is not always helpful. The leading design guidance is often too general, and does not specifically address populations with material single or combined sensory, cognitive, and motor impairments. Research used to create "normative" data sets has only received scant funding and the knowledge-base for designers interested in meeting the needs of impaired populations is sparse. Ergonomists, vocational rehabilitation specialists, and relevant scientific and clinical specialists have much to do to provide enhanced guidance to the design community. At present, the best predictor of design effectiveness is through valid testing and evaluation with appropriate diversity in the test population.

18.3   SCOPE

It would be pretentious to assume that a short chapter can fully address all theoretical foundations, methodologies, and tactics that are used by human engineering professionals in promoting universal and safe designs. No attempt has been made to comprehensively summarize a wealth of knowledge, methodologies, or approaches to ergonomic design. There are many excellent sources of such information that the reader can pursue for detailed information or to learn of such methods—including many of the chapters in this book. Additional reference and specific design guidance is provided in the bibliography section of this chapter.

The intent of this chapter is to illustrate the ergonomic design process and to highlight basic design issues that have material impact upon in preventing or mitigating the need for specific accommodation. A general approach is recommended to help tackle major problems that are likely to be encountered. One cannot rely solely on recommendations, guidelines, checklists, or standards to eliminate accommodation problems or hazards. Guidelines are often too broad or too specific within the context of a particular human–machine–task–environment system to provide material support. A systems approach to design and evaluation is proposed to enhance the universal characteristics of design and soften challenges facing accommodation efforts. Any specific accommodation efforts should follow the same general design process with greater specific focus upon the individual user's capabilities and limitations.

18.4   ACCOMMODATION THROUGH ERGONOMIC DESIGN PROCESS

Ergonomic design, development, and implementation of accommodating systems follow a standard process. Designers typically need to

- Understand the objectives and goals of the system and their impact upon the human's roles and performance requirements
- Understand human performance capabilities or limitations that are relevant for shaping of the particular system's design, functional allocation between humans and machines, and identification of potential risks for system failure, safety and health problems
- Evaluate prototype human–machine–task–environment system performance
- Determine if human–machine system performance meets design criteria
- Determine if other relevant ergonomic design standards are complied with

Designs in complex systems are fluid and one usually follows the above steps in an iterative and sometimes a heuristic manner. Often one may capitalize on previous designs, documentation, and test results. At each step of the process, judgment is highly dependent on the skill and expertise of the analyst or analysts. Use of handbooks, standards, and design guidelines will help guide many design decisions. However, testing of designs is obligatory to insure that design requirements and objectives are met when a variety of users with a variety of impairments are included within the intended design population.

Ergonomists tend to follow a systematic process for design development, review, and validation. The general process followed is outlined in the following sections.

18.4.1   Understand System Performance Objectives and Constraints

Without a clear understanding of the system's objectives and design constraints, one cannot determine which designs or design options are appropriate for anticipated user populations, desired staffing levels, training and skills of the user population, performance envelopes, safety and health considerations, and other useful information for the design team.

Performance specifications delineate the goals and performance requirements for a design or a system. Specifications are typically prepared by a team that is involved in the development of a system. They itemize functions, define parameters, and spell-out design constraints. The design team creates or responds to a "design-to" specification that states system performance requirements and user capability requirements.

If performance objectives and constraints are not clear at the outset of the project, this usually results in difficulties in meeting project time and cost milestones and avoiding design-induced usability constraints. Time constraints promote cutting corners, increasing the risk of inadvertent design flaws and greater accommodation problems.

The specification typically translates the user's operational needs into system functions and requirements, allocates those requirements to subsystems, and allocates general functions to operators and service personnel. Beyond expected or required functional allocations, the specifications do not address specific requirements in terms of human performance beyond gross statements about personnel requirements (e.g., to be used by airline pilots, firefighters, general public, etc.).

System requirements must be project-specific, and requirements should be written in a verifiable form. If the requirements are too broad, the design team will face great difficulty proving that they have met their goals. Establishing requirements in operationally defined and verifiable manner provides a common perspective and basis of understanding among the design team and its sponsors or customers.

The objective at this stage of design is to determine how the system design specifications map onto human performance requirements or demands. Here the designer should determine what the user population's performance envelopes are, and provide feedback on these aspects to the design team; particularly if the requirements are unreasonable.

18.4.2 DETERMINING HUMAN INTERFACE REQUIREMENTS

Once the ergonomic and team understands the functional flow of work performed within or by the system, a greater understanding is required of the actual tasks performed by the human and how they interact with tools, equipment, other humans, their environment, and so forth. This information is a prerequisite to begin mapping functional demands upon human perceptual, cognitive, and motor performance requirements.

Human activity analysis may include a variety of analytical tools to help define human performance requirements for an existing or future system design using

- Function allocation
- Function and operational flow analysis
- Decision action analysis
- Action information analysis
- Task analysis
- Timeline analysis
- Link analysis
- Simulation
- Controlled experimentation
- Workload assessment

18.4.3 FUNCTIONAL FLOW ANALYSIS

Functional flow analysis is a procedure for decomposing a system design into functional elements and for identifying the sequences of functions or actions that must be performed by a system. Starting with system objectives, functions are identified and described iteratively with higher top-level functions being progressively expanded into lower levels containing more and more detailed information. As demonstrated in Figure 18.1, functions or actions are individually and hierarchically numbered in a way that clarifies their relationship to one another and permits traceability of functions throughout the entire system. This information helps the design team understand the phases and sequence or flow of activities within each phase.

Functional flow diagrams help design teams understand where nodes, or transition of work from one node to the next, can pose difficulties for individuals who have impaired performance capacities. For example, if an individual can fly an airplane but suffers an impairment that prohibits their ability to perform the aircraft fueling operation, the pilot will have to rely upon airport workers to complete that operation. The pilot may be able to fly an aircraft without difficulty, but would not be able to fly into and takeoff from fields that require pilots to fuel their planes without assistance.

Higher level functions are carried out to such additional levels of detail as required. The entire spatial and organizational flow of the worker is easy to understand. Moreover, the need for individuals or teams to move with or respond to the flow becomes apparent. Some teams prefer to identify the function's output on the connecting arrow to the next function, and add additional inputs to the next function.

Connector blocks are used to link functional flows from one page to the next and arrows enter function blocks from the left, and exit from the right. Thus, the flow is from top to bottom, then left to right on the diagram. Functions that are subordinate to the general function are placed below it as shown, and so show the normal sequence of system functions, left to right, and, if necessary, down. Whenever arrows join or split, their junctions are shown with "and," "or," and "and/or" gates in circles. The "and" gate requires that all the following or preceding functions must be performed first. The "or" gate requires that only one of preceding functions must be performed to move forward.

For each of the functions, the team can add the need for decisions phrased as questions with binary choices. Each function is a short verb–noun combination with occasional adjectives or other modifiers. For example, one decision in setting up audiovisual apparatus might be "Projector status OK?" This can be decomposed into lower-level decisions such as "Power On?", "Projection Mode Properly Set?", and "Projector Connected to Computer?"

Each decision is placed in a diamond symbol and is phrased as a question that may be answered with a binary, yes/no response. Function blocks and decision diamonds are given reference numbers as is done with functional flow diagrams.

18.4.4 OPERATIONAL ANALYSIS

An operational analysis is another analytical model that is used by industrial engineers to describe the sequential flow of tasks or work over time. This method is designed to obtain information about situations or events that will confront workers in a linear manner. If conditional changes occur, one can bend the operational analysis

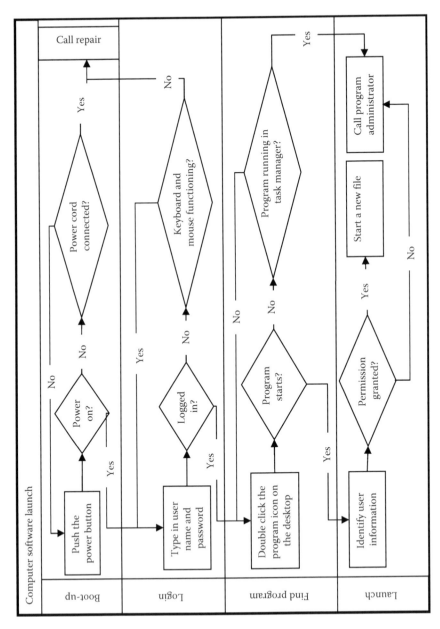

FIGURE 18.1 Example of a functional flow diagram showing activities, sequences or flows of functions.

somewhat to handle that problem. However, if conditionally-mediated sequences are encountered, the functional flow diagram is a better model for describing work.

Scenarios and anticipated operations are created and assumptions and operating environments are documented. Scenarios should be sufficiently detailed to convey an understanding of all anticipated operations and should cover all essential system functions (e.g., failures, both hard and soft, and emergencies).

Operational analyses are typically driven by the system performance objectives and requirements. Scenarios are usually developed by knowledgeable experts that include procedures, equipment use, environmental constraints, and potential rare or unanticipated outcomes. The scenarios are delineated to sufficient detail to allow designers and analysts to work together on design formulation or assessment.

From an accommodation standpoint, the operational analysis provides an interactive description of the human constraints and requirements. For example, Figure 18.2

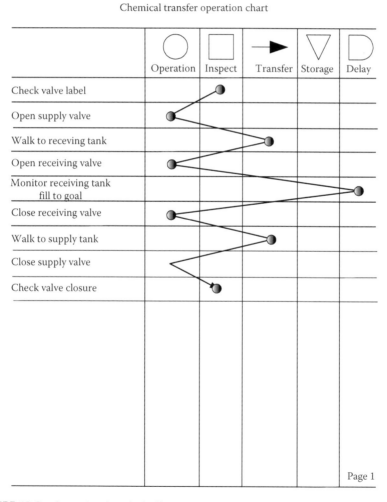

FIGURE 18.2 Operational analysis diagram symbology. (From Wiker, S.F., Importance of Human Factors Engineering in Promotion of Safety, in Haight, J. (Ed.) *Safety Professional's Handbook*, 2008. With permission.)

shows how often one must walk from point to point, and when delays will occur (e.g., environmental conditions, skill and training requirements, etc.), performance envelopes that can affect system performance, and failure modes and effects that have to be considered when specifying ergonomic design requirements. Thus, the team that produces the operational analysis should be experienced with the technology, the operations addressed, and content experts should be participants—including human engineering experts.

Typically workers with impairments encounter problems with operations, inspections, and worker-accompanied transfers or storage activities. Delays often allow catch-up or work-ahead times for workers who fall behind or who need extra time to complete their work due to impairments.

18.4.5   TASK ANALYSIS

Task analysis is the first step in taking a systematic approach to design. Task analysis can focus on both what actually happens in the workplace now, or can be used as a tool to specify the design of a new system. It provides a detailed description of how goals are accomplished so that designers can provide means of enhancing human performance.

Analysis involves a systematic breakdown of a function into its underlying tasks, and tasks into subtasks or elements. The process creates a detailed task description of both manual and mental activities, task and element durations, task frequency, task allocation, task complexity, environmental conditions, necessary clothing and equipment, and any other unique factors involved in or required for one or more humans to perform a given task. Estimates are made of the time and effort required to perform tasks; perceptual, cognitive, and motor performance demands, training requirements, and other information that is needed to support other system development activities.

To decide what type of information should be collected and how it should be gathered, it is necessary to identify the focus of the analysis, and what the results will be used for. One cannot collect all task information, but just sufficient information to allow you to address your specific objectives (see Tables 18.1 and 18.2). For example, if one is designing a new job, modifying an existing job, or developing job training requirements, information that is relevant to task design usually becomes apparent and should be used to structure the task analysis.

Like functional diagrams, task analyses use hierarchical number systems to help the analyst understand the organizational relationships among subtasks, tasks, and jobs. Once a task or subtask is numbered, it holds that number for the remainder of the design project.

18.4.6   LINK TASKS TOGETHER

Link analysis is a method for arranging the physical layout of instrument panels, control panels, workstations, or work areas to meet certain objectives. For example, to reduce total amount of movement, increase accessibility, time to complete a task, or to recognize when simultaneous access to equipment becomes infeasible. A link is any useful connection between a person and a machine or part, two persons, or two parts of a machine.

Different types of links can be noted. For example, if an operator must walk to a supervisor to obtain permission to initiate an operation, or to consult with regarding

TABLE 18.1

Tasks Analysis Information That Is Typically Gathered

Task Information	Description
Task and subtask structure	An organized, often hierarchical listing of the activities involved in a task with tasks and subtasks numbered accordingly
Importance or priorities of subtasks	Assessment of the criticality of subtasks from a performance or safety perspective
Frequency of subtasks	Frequency of occurrence of subtasks under different conditions
Sequencing of subtasks	Order of occurrence of subtasks under different conditions
Decisions required	Part of the sequencing may be based on a decision needed to choose the branch of activity and thus a given set of subtasks
Trigger conditions for subtask execution	Execution of a subtask may depend upon the occurrence of a particular event or a decision made in during a previous task or subtask
Objectives	Performance objectives are provided including the importance to the overall mission
Performance criteria	Human performance criteria are delineated such as perceptual requirements, psychomotor performance, accuracy constraints, etc.
Information required	Information that must be provided at each level of task or subtask that must be attended or used by the operator
Outputs	Information, products or other results of human effort that result from the subtask
Knowledge and skills required	Information and skills that the user utilizes in decision making and task performance

a problem, that activity represents a person–person link. If the operator returns to actuate the machine tool's cycle lever to press a metal part that represents a person–machine link. When the pressed part is automatically transferred to a conveyor, that event represents a machine–machine link.

The steps involved in a link analysis are the following:

- List all personnel and items to be linked
- Determine frequencies of linkages among operators, tools, machines, etc.
- Classify the importance of each link
- Calculate frequency-importance values for each link
- Sort link frequency-importance product values to focus on links with greatest cost
- Fit the layout into the allocated space minimizing linkage values
- Evaluate the new layout against the original objectives

TABLE 18.2

Potential Methods or Data Collection Required for Task Analysis

Data Collection Method	Description
Direct and videotape observations	Use of time study or work sampling methods to develop job descriptions and psychomotor demands.
Interviews and questionnaires	Interview workers or operators to determine the sequence of operations, tasks, subtasks, and hazards and difficulties they encounter in the performance of their job or task.
Focus group	Discussion with a group of typically 8 to 12 people, away from work site. A moderator is used to focus the discussion on a series of topics or issues. Useful for collecting exploratory or preliminary information that can be used to determine the questions needed for a subsequent structured survey or interview.
Interface surveys	A group of methods used for task and interface design to identify specific human factors problems or deficiencies, such as labeling of controls and displays. These methods require an analyst to systematically conduct an evaluation of the operator–machine interface and record specific features. Examples of these methods include control/display analysis, labeling surveys, and coding consistency surveys.
Existing documentation	Review any existing standard datasets from production engineering departments or other industries, operating manuals, training manuals, safety reports, and previous task analyses.
Link analysis	A method for arranging the physical layout of instrument panels, control panels, workstations, or work areas to meet certain objectives, for example, to reduce total amount of movement or increase accessibility. The primary inputs required for a link analysis are data from activity analyses and task analyses and observations of functional or simulated systems.
Work sampling analysis	A method for measuring and quantifying how operators spend their time. Random or uniform sampling of activities are then aggregated over some appropriate time period, for example, a day, and activity-frequency tables or graphs are constructed, showing the percentage of time spent in various activities.
Checklists	Use a structured checklist to identify particular components or issues associated with the job. Available for a range of ergonomic issues, including workplace concerns, human–machine interfaces, environmental concerns.
Job Safety Analysis (JSA)	Using JSA one can identify what behaviors in an operation are safe and correct. This analysis can be performed during task analysis. For each task or subtask, the analyst determines how the task should be performed and potential unsafe or hazardous methods. See chapters providing greater detail on JSA methods and benefits.

TABLE 18.2 (continued)
Potential Methods or Data Collection Required for Task Analysis

Data Collection Method	Description
Critical incident analysis	Critical incidents can lead to accidents or system failures. This information is typically gained from human operators who supply first-hand accounts of critical incidents which are accidents, near-accidents, mistakes, and near-mistakes they have made when carrying out some operation. The critical incident technique only identifies problems—not solutions. The percentages of errors found in a critical incident study do not necessarily reflect their true proportions in operational situations, because the incidents are dependent on human memory and some incidents may be more impressive, or more likely to be remembered than others. To be useful, the incidents must be detailed enough (a) to allow the investigator to make inferences and predictions about the behavior of the person involved, and (b) leave little doubt about the consequences of the behavior and the effects of the incident. The ergonomic then groups incidents into categories that have operational relevance: Mistakes and near-mistakes in reading an indicator, Mistakes and near-mistakes in using a control, Mistakes and near-mistakes in interpreting a label, Mistakes and near-mistakes in navigating to a hospital room. The analyst then uses human-factors knowledge and experience to hypothesize sources of difficulty and how each one could be further studied, attacked, or redesigned to eliminate it. Studies are usually necessary to find ways of mitigating or eliminating those problems where elimination cannot be achieved based upon first principles alone.
Fault tree analysis	Some analysts use fault tree analysis in conjunction with critical incident, task analysis or job safety analysis or failure modes and effects analyses. Event Trees, starting from a problem root such as equipment or other form of failure, follow through a path of subsequent system events to a series of final outcomes. This is also a probabilistic analysis that gives rise to likely failures and consequences that should be considered in the design of equipment, layouts, human capability demands, and so forth.
Failure modes and effects analysis (FMEA)	FMEA is a method used to understand the consequences resulting from a failure within a system. Humans can be considered components that can fail for various reasons, and following FMEA methods, outlined in other chapters of this text, one can examine opportunities for eliminating or softening failure impacts. Typically, FMEA is used during functional flow, task, workload, linkage, and other ergonomic analyses. It helps in ergonomic analyses to determine what scenarios need to be interrupted by increasing the reliability of human–machine system performance.

Evaluation of various workplace or equipment arrangements can be made to assess move distances traversed during typical or unusual operations, the crowding of activities, and opportunities to cluster equipment to expedite operation. The evaluation should also consider adjustment or operation of multiple machines, or the need for concurrent or rapid sequential inspection of operational states. Linkage analysis also concentrates focus upon human interactions with one another and hardware. This information is often critical in identifying unnecessary hurdles that confront those with and without physical impairments (Figure 18.3).

18.4.7 WORKLOAD ASSESSMENT

General workload assessment can also be performed at this point using timeline analysis. Timeline analysis follows naturally from task and linkage analysis. Here one is concerned with the scheduling and loading of activities upon individual operators. Charts are produced showing sequences of operator actions, the times required for each action, and the time at which each action should occur. The method produces plots of the temporal relationships among tasks, the durations of individual tasks, and the times at which each task is, or should be, performed.

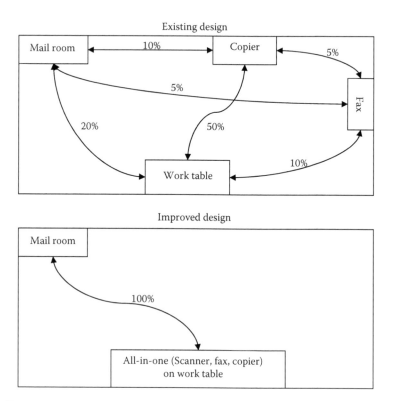

FIGURE 18.3 Example of linkage analysis showing relationships among office equipment placement and movement of the individual among office machines with a poorly laid out office.

Activity	Turn on ignition	Drive in city	Drive on highway	Exit highway	Park	Cell phone use	Exit car
			Sequence of activities				
Pre-trip inspection	1						
Monitor mirror		1	1	1	1	1	
Monitor gauges		1	1			1	
Seat belt	1						
Radio		1	1				1
GPS programming	1						1
GPS following			1	1			
Traffic light		1					
Exit sign			1	1			
Speed limit		1	1	1		1	
Unlock vehicle	1						
Lock vehicle							1
Open window	1						
Close window			1				1
Check street name		1					
Pick up cell						1	
Workload	5	6	7	4	1	4	4

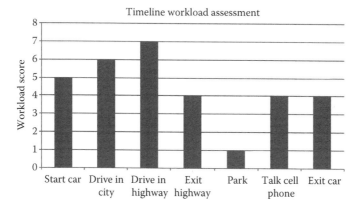

FIGURE 18.4 Example of workload timeline analysis in which simultaneous activities are counted as the workload metric.

Figure 18.4 shows that one can integrate times from separate task analyses to show overlapping activities of two or more persons. The greatest estimated concurrent workload occurs during the driving on highway phase. This information serves to focus upon activities that can challenge the physical or cognitive capacities of individuals with impairments.

18.4.8 FUNCTIONAL ALLOCATION

Results from task analyses and workload timelines are often considered when making functional allocation decisions among workers, workers and machines, and machines. Functional allocation is a procedure for assigning each system function, action, and decision to hardware, software, and humans. There are many approaches one can take to allocation decisions. They can range from "Fitts' Lists" of machine versus human performance capacities, to "line balancing" algorithms, and results from expert, worker, and other inputs.

Professional judgment is involved in selecting criteria to be considered, and in determining the weights to be assigned to allocation criteria. In general, nearly all allocation decisions will have to address at least the following decision criteria:

- Implementation constraints
- Maintainability and support logistics
- Number of personnel required
- Performance capability
- Personnel selection and training costs
- Political considerations
- Power requirements
- Predicted reliability
- Safety
- Technological feasibility

18.4.9 ANALYSIS OF SIMILAR SYSTEMS

If possible, consider designs and analyses of like systems to help you understand important design issues that have been considered in the past, and which may be quite satisfactory for your current problem. If you can gain access to reports, tests and evaluations, interviews of users of such designs, and any history of accidents or accident investigation reports, you will be able to capitalize on the work of previous design teams.

One should be careful that they do not blindly accept the previous design without considering the differences between your current design requirements and those of the previous project. Antecedent systems often provide better initial insights into operation and maintenance of the proposed design, skills and training, and a history of usability or safety problems. If you are intending to use the design in different environments, with expanded user populations, under more stressful operating environments, then previous designs may not be adequate and will require modification.

18.4.10 PRELIMINARY FOCUS GROUPS

Focus groups can help one to assess user needs, perspectives and concerns early in the design process. This is particularly true when one is designing for populations that possess individuals with one or more impairments, or when impairments are induced by fatigue or boredom. Focus group membership should be a representative of the intended user group, and small enough to encourage equal opportunity for expression of opinions and insights (e.g., 5 to 10 members) about design issues and user needs. If one cannot capture all of the inputs desired by a small focus group, then multiple focus groups should be considered. Preliminary focus groups can be much less formal than subsequent group meetings where greater moderation, and more focal or structured query, is needed for specific issues. Designers cannot fully understand all aspects of accommodation and should capitalize upon inputs from communities that they are trying to accommodate, or envelop, within their design.

18.4.11 ALLOCATE ROLES, RESPONSIBILITIES, AND PERFORMANCE REQUIREMENTS

Accommodating designs determine specific roles of humans in meeting the system design objectives and requirements, and reduce human performance demands as much as practicable. Determining how performance demands are to be functionally allocated among human, machines, and software often helps the design team shift overly challenging human demands onto machines, or to eliminate problematic performance demands altogether.

Documenting the basis for task allocation, performance demands, and safety responsibilities among the mosaic of humans, firmware, and software not only assists in development of accommodating designs, it will serve as the basis for proving that some accommodations are not reasonable or feasible. It is better to perform and document these actions during job design or analysis stages and provide it for future consideration in accommodation decisions, rather than performing limited post hoc analyses on a case-by-case basis. Superficial post hoc analyses are often not successful in defending decisions to not accommodate and invite expensive legal debate.

18.4.12 PERFORM ACTUAL OR SIMULATED TASK ANALYSIS

Activity analyses are typically performed using functional, decision and action flow methods, simulation and mockup analysis, along with examination of similar systems and use of focus groups. The information gained is used to understand human performance requirements and the need for allocated responsibilities. Job safety analyses can also be performed during task analysis to determine sources of accidents and failure modes and their effects. For individuals with impairments, direct offline testing or in workplace probationary evaluation are often considered the most valid methods for determining the acceptability of the accommodation effort. That may or may not be the case depending upon the job, the individual applicant's impairments, and other factors.

18.4.13 DETERMINE DESIGN QUESTIONS OR PROBLEMS ENCOUNTERED

It is inevitable that design questions or problems will highlight themselves during task allocation efforts. Questions will arise regarding the best method to couple humans to workplaces, equipment, tools, and tasks within the context of the working environment, and to envelop performance capabilities afforded by the user population and individual of interest. This process can be used to backchain through the design process when populations with material impairments are expected to participate with the technology and associated occupational activities.

It is important to develop concise definitions of design questions or problems to scope the design effort. By bounding the question, or solution space, one enables development of responsive answers in a time- and cost-efficient manner. Knowing when one has obtained a functional answer to the designer's question(s) signals one to stop with confidence and move on to the next question. It also makes validation of the recommendations more straightforward and efficient.

18.4.14 Understand the Design Questions

Interrelating design questions with system performance requirements is critical. If these steps are decoupled, one can recommend a design that optimally addresses the design question within a particular subsystem but results in a suboptimal system performance. Design recommendations for controls, displays, seat design, and cockpit layout that enable a race car and its driver to traverse a race track at maximum vehicle capacity will proffer little or no performance advantage, prove overly costly, and might promote inappropriate operation on highly trafficked downtown city streets. Use of alternative designs or augmentative technologies that may degrade elements of job performance may be entirely acceptable if delays are less than inherent job slack times that cannot be removed, or if the design expedites other elements of the job. Whether changes in design elements are acceptable or not must be addressed within the context of the performance objectives.

18.4.15 Select Candidate Design Concepts for Evaluation and Testing

Accommodation considerations should play a material role in selecting the best design option. While universal design is the goal, the final design selected may not necessarily be the most universal design. This can be an acceptable outcome when the potential use or employment of impaired individuals is unlikely, the performance losses of underutilized universal design are high (which is rare), and options for specialized modification have not been eliminated by the design.

Experimentation in laboratory or field conditions is usually required to performance test design options. Analysis, presentation, and interpretation of results are requisite for the collective design team. Testing must be time and cost frugal, but experimental findings should have adequate statistical power to found rational decisions. Depending upon the nature of the questions or problems addressed, testing and evaluation may iterate until a satisfactory design state is achieved using performance selection or utility metrics.

If multiple performance factors must be addressed, the design team should determine weights to be assigned to each performance metric. The sum of the product of weighted or valued performance metrics is often employed to rank design options using a multiattribute utility model or other forms of decision support paradigms.

As with products liability protection paradigms, all the documents that are generated or that were consulted, and those that were used in design decisions in the development of the system should be archived. Any tailoring of information used from standards should be documented. Ambiguously worded requirements in standards should be reworded or operationally defined so that the design team's interpretations of the guidelines are clear. This information will be used to evaluate accommodation policies, as well as options for creating accommodations for applicants with impairments.

Disputes in almost all matters related to design result from some combination of miscommunication, misunderstanding, ignorance of facts and design issues, and technological limitations at the time of design or request for accommodation. Keeping the documentation and making nonproprietary information readily available saves costs associated with documentation requests for accommodation, for disputing claims, or when needed for embracing new technologies. This information is also very important when periodic design reviews are conducted for evaluation of design improvements.

18.4.16 DOCUMENT AND JUSTIFY RECOMMENDED DESIGN FEATURES OR OPTIONS

Documentation of standards relied upon, rationale for tailoring standards to address the design question, testing methods, data, analyses, findings, interpretations of findings, and rationale for recommendations must be documented thoroughly. This is the norm for good engineering design and is requisite for expanding and easing accommodation of impaired workers or injured workers who wish to return to work.

Computer programs, drawings, or mockups and detailed reports should be delivered for use and archiving. The number of reports, detail that is required, and structure of reports can vary from project to project. However, most ergonomic design reports include:

- Human factors system function and operator task analysis
- Human factors design approach
- Human factors test or simulation plans
- Procedural, data documentation, and analysis reports
- Personnel and training plans

18.4.17 MAP PERFORMANCE REQUIREMENTS ONTO A HUMAN USER

For each system function assigned to the human, the analyst should work bottom-up in specifying perceptual, cognitive, and motor demands that must be met to achieve required task performance using specific displays, controls, workplace configurations, and all the other design variables that affect operator performance and safety. Often, stipulating design requirements must support design trade-offs. The ergonomist must convey to the design team where trade-off decisions are likely to occur, and the consequences of such trade-offs.

One cannot simply cite specific standards or sections of standards and expect designers to read and fully understand ergonomic design guidance. Dumping a stack of textbooks, design handbooks, or relevant standards upon the design team's table and expecting them to understand the information in a fast-paced design process is very unrealistic and invites errors. Instead, knowledgeable professionals must meter out information as needed and provide clear trade-off consequences, or conduct preliminary analyses, to help direct designs along a successful path. The professional should provide a range of specifications with consequences described in a manner that the design team can understand and consider in making design decisions.

It is also a mistake to allow designers to try to use disparate standards or design handbooks in which they cherry-pick what they believe is important or relevant design information. When inexperienced designers are confronted with only general recommendations, such information can be interpreted in different ways, some of which may not result in systems that are easily usable and, thereby, accommodating.

Finally, some demands or requirements placed upon the human user do not have well-defined answers or specifications. This can be frustrating to those who are: (1) under time constraints to arrive at a recommendation for the design team, or (2) design team members who are in holding patterns awaiting input from the ergonomists or professionals. Sometimes the design team cannot wait for development of specifications and must move forward. This can pose problems if there is no opportunity to correct decisions at a later time.

18.4.18 ARE ACCEPTABLE STIMULI PRESENTED TO THE USER?

Rarely are studies performed to determine sensory thresholds for populations that are classified as impaired. For example, low-vision impairments are not homogenous within the affected group. Low-vision can result from reduced visual acuity, asymmetric dysfunction of the retinae, poor contrast sensitivity, severe myopia, etc.. Thus, analysts will normally design work based upon "normative" population thresholds and use multipliers while considering the potential negative impact of excessive stimulus intensity.

For example, audible alarms can be raised to reduce problems for those with hearing deficits. However, the sound pressure levels for an alarm that an automobile's gas has reached a given level cannot be so loud that it creates a startle reaction in drivers. Thus, the analyst should consider presenting stimuli to more than one sensory modality (e.g., auditory, visual, haptic, etc.) to reduce the impact of those with specific sensory impairment (e.g., auditory cues work for those who are blind, visual cues work for those who are deaf, haptic cues work for those who are both blind and deaf, etc.).

Presuming that one or more of the stimuli are presented, one must insure that the perceivable stimuli have sufficient signal-to-noise ratios to insure adequate detection of stimuli as intended. The following sections address the use of psychophysical, signal detection, and information theory methods to promote effective communication of stimuli by all users; including those with impairments.

18.4.19 STIMULUS INTENSITY ADEQUATE?

A psychometric function describes the relationship between a sensed physical stimulus and the perceived intensity of that stimulus. Change in perceived intensity with change in actual physical intensity obeys a power function. Thus, one will experience different perceptual intensity changes in response to variations in actual stimulus intensity depending upon the type of stimulus used (see Figure 18.5).

The particular stimulus modality that is selected is often task and socially motivated. However, when given an option, analysts should select stimulus modes that produce a wide range of perceived intensity with variation in the physical stimulus. The greater the power exponent, the more likely the user population is going to be able to discriminate differences or material changes in the stimulus intensity. See Table 18.3 for a limited example of power function exponents for various stimuli.

The psychometric function detection behavior can be characterized as a sigmoid function with the cumulative percentage of correct responses (or a similar value)

Perceived intensity = k(physical intensity)**power

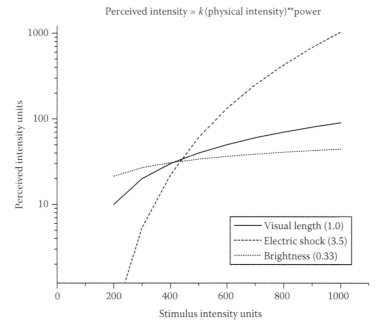

FIGURE 18.5 Impact of stimulus mode upon perceived stimulus intensity with change in physical stimulus intensity change based upon power exponent noted in legend. (From Wiker, S.F., Importance of Human Factors Engineering in Promotion of Safety in Haight, J. (Ed.). *Safety Professional's Handbook*, 2008. With permission.)

displayed on the ordinate and the physical parameter on the abscissa. If the stimulus parameter is very far toward one end of its possible range, the person will always be able to respond correctly. Towards the other end of the range, the person never perceives the stimulus properly and correct responses become a function of chance.

TABLE 18.3
Various Stimulus Power Function Exponents for Several Stimuli

Stimulus	Power Exponent	Description
Brightness	0.50	Brief flash brightness
Heaviness	1.45	Lifted weights
Lightness	1.20	Reflectance of gray papers
Loudness	0.67	Sound pressure of 3000 Hz tone
Muscle force	1.70	Static contractions
Pressure on palm	1.10	Static force on skin
Vibration	0.60	Amplitude of 250 Hz on finger
Vibration	0.95	Amplitude of 60 Hz on finger
Visual area	0.70	Projected square
Visual length	1.00	Projected line

Source: Stevens, S.S., *Psychol. Rev.*, 64, 153, 1957.

In between, there is a transition range where the user has an above-chance rate of correct responses, but does not always respond correctly.

The inflection point of the sigmoid function or the point at which the function reaches the middle between the chance level and 100% is usually taken as sensory threshold. A stimulus that is less intense than a human's sensory threshold will not elicit reliable sensation. Psychophysicists who study the relationship between physical stimuli and their subjective correlates, or percepts, have established thresholds for various stimuli that are used by designers.

Several different sensory thresholds have been developed for use by designers:

Absolute threshold (AL): The lowest level at which a stimulus can be detected 50% of the time. This is a measure of practical importance in that it is the smallest amount of energy that can be sensed by a typically young adult human, who is focused upon the source of the stimulus in the absence of other stimuli, 50% of the time. Absolute thresholds are generally determined by plotting detection rates against stimulus intensity or characteristics.

Recognition threshold (RL): The level at which a stimulus can not only be detected but also recognized fifty percent of the time.

Differential threshold (DL): The level at which an increase in a detected stimulus can be perceived 50% of the time. This threshold for intensity adjustment is often referred to as the just noticeable difference (JND). Designers often want to use detection of change in stimulus intensity as a code or indication in the state of performance of the machine, tool, product, alarm, or other informative signal. These thresholds are referred to as difference thresholds or limens (DLs), and refer to the amount of increase that is required in the physical intensity of a sensed stimulus before one can detect a JND. This magnitude depends upon the starting stimulus intensity.

Terminal threshold (TL): The level beyond which a stimulus is no longer detected 50% of the time. The upper end of the detectable stimulus range results from an inability of sense organs to respond to increased stimulus intensity, or to respond when such exposures are injurious. Some upper thresholds are set by consensus because we cannot safely study such exposures without injuring humans.

Thresholds, or Limens, are determined at the midpoint of a cumulative detection probability threshold because the inflection point of the function provides the greatest resolution of sensory response to changes in the stimulus.

Equal increments of physical energy do not produce equal increments of sensation between lower and upper stimulus thresholds. Often designers anticipate that increments in stimulus intensities of signals can be arbitrarily used between lower and upper bounds of stimulus intensities with equivalent results; that is usually not the case. For a given type of stimulus, the DL, at a given stimulus intensity, complies with an approximate fraction referred to Weber's law or fraction. For example, for a stimulus with a Weber fraction of 0.10, one must only increase the stimulus by 10% to detect a JND. For a stimulus intensity of 10, the JND is 1; however, when the stimulus is increased to 100, the stimulus must be increased by 10 units to produce a JND.

For many sensory modalities, the JND is an increasing function of the base level of current level of stimulus intensity. The ratio of the JND or delta I and the current stimulus intensity is roughly constant. Measured in physical units, we have

$$K = \frac{\Delta I}{I}$$

where

K is the ratio, fraction or constant for that particular type of stimulus and often referred to as the Weber fraction or constant,

I is the intensity of stimulation, and

ΔI is the change in stimulus intensity from the level I.

Designers often overestimate the percentage of detections, and that such values are only useful when the human is intensely attending the stimulus. A rule of thumb is that if one wants detection at 95% or 99%, the 50% detection threshold can be multiplied approximately by 2 and 3 respectively. However, if the operator is not intensely focused on the stimulus, or the stimulus is dynamically changing or moving, threshold multiples of 10 or greater may be required to achieve intended design objectives. Standards, handbooks, or testing may be required to find stimulus intensities that meet design requisite performance objectives. Acceptable values should be determined by test and evaluation when populations with multiple partial sensory impairments are expected to receive and use the sensory stimuli ensembles.

Confusion in design can occur when designers wish users to detect changes in a stimulus intensity level. While there are a large number of JNDs for any given stimulus (see Table 18.4), JNDs represent relative change detection capabilities, most stimuli that are presented in a manner that does not allow relative comparison, can only produce 7 ± 2 absolute detection levels. For example, if intensity of a pure tone is presented as a cue or alarm for severity of oil temperature, perhaps one would use only two levels of sound power level to cue the vehicle operator. Attempting to use many levels of any given stimulus intensity to provide absolute cues will not be successful, particularly in populations with limited ranges of sensory perception. If designed poorly, users will confuse the signals and respond inappropriately (see Tables 18.4 and 18.5).

Many investigators have contributed to our understanding of the specific types and ranges of physical energy, typically referred to as stimuli, which fall within human perceptual capabilities. Mowbray and Gebhard (1958) and Van Cott and Warrick (1972) have cataloged much of the early work. Today, many design guidelines and standards publish topically relevant thresholds for use by designers and engineers.

As mentioned earlier, one must also take care to control the upper end of a stimulus intensity. If the stimulus intensity is too great, the user can not only experience an alerting and stressful reaction, but also experience sensory stimulus fatigue-based impairments and concomitant changes in psychometric function and threshold specifications.

18.4.20 VISUAL ACUITY PROBLEMS

Of all human senses, vision is probably the most important for system design. It is often quoted that as much as 80% of the information we receive from machines and systems comes to us by way of our eyes. There are many issues to be considered when specifying the importance and nature of visual imagery. However, visual

TABLE 18.4
Relative Discrimination of Physical Intensities and Frequencies

Sensation	Number of JNDs
Brightness of white light	570 discriminable intensities of white light.
Hues at medium intensities	128 discriminable wavelengths at medium intensities.
Flicker frequencies between 1–45 Hz with on/off cycles of 0.5	375 discriminable interruption rates between 1 and 45 interruptions per second at moderate intensities and an on/off cycle of 0.5.
Loudness of 2000 Hz tones	325 discriminable intensities for pure tones of 2000 Hz
Pure 60 dBA tones between 20 and 20,000 Hz	1800
interrupted white noise	460 discriminable interruption rates between 1 and 45 interruptions per second at moderate intensities and an on/off cycle of 0.5.
Vibration	15 discriminable amplitudes in chest region with broad contact vibrator within an amplitude range of 0.05–0.5 mm.
Mechanical vibration	180 discriminable frequencies between 1 and 320 Hz.

Source: Van Cott, H.P. and Warrick, M.J., 1972. Man as a system component. In Van Cott, H.P. and Kinkade, R.G. (Eds.), *Human Engineering Guide to Equipment Design* (Rev. ed.)(p. IP-39). Washington, DC: Government Printing Office; Mowbray, H.M. and Gebhard, J.W.,1958. *Man's Senses as Informational Channels (Report No. CM-936)*. Silver Spring, MD: Applied Physics Laboratory, The Johns Hopkins University.

TABLE 18.5
Number of Absolutely Identifiable Sensations

Sensation	Number Identifiable
Brightness	3 to 5 with white light of 0.1–50 mL
Hues	12 or 13 wavelengths
Interrupted white light	5 or 6 rates
Loudness	3 to 5 with pure tones
Pure tones	4 or 5 tones
Vibration	3 to 5 amplitudes

Source: Van Cott, H.P. and Warrick, M.J., 1972. Man as a system component. In Van Cott, H.P. and Kinkade, R.G. (Eds.), *Human Engineering Guide to Equipment Design* (Rev. ed.) (p. IP-39). Washington, DC: Government Printing Office; Mowbray, H.M. and Gebhard, J.W.,1958. *Man's Senses as Informational Channels (Report No. CM-936)*. Silver Spring, MD: Applied Physics Laboratory, The Johns Hopkins University.

acuity or target size, contrast, and magnitude of illumination of visual stimuli are minimal questions that need to be addressed when considering accommodation of human visual impairment.

Visual activity refers to the ability to see spatial detail and recognize image features. Usually visual acuity is specified in minutes of arc; the angle subtended by the object viewed. For objects less than $10°$ of arc, we can use a small angle tangent approximation to estimate visual arc:

Visual angle (minutes of arc) = $(57.3)(60)L/D$

where
   L is the size of the object measured perpendicularly to the line of sight and
   D the distance from the front of the eye to the object.

Visual acuity may be classified in the following categories:

- Detection, merely detecting the presence of something
- Vernier, detecting misalignment
- Separation, detecting the separation or gap between parallel lines, dots or squares
- Form, identifying shapes or forms

Physical and physiological factors affect visual acuity. Illumination, contrast, time of exposure, and color are typically important determinants of visual acuity. Engineering design handbooks provide significant guidance on the impact of various combinations of these factors (Woodson, Tillman, and Tillman, 1992).

Designers use visual thresholds. However, unless otherwise specified, thresholds are set at 50% detection rates when the observer is focused or waiting for the presentation of the stimulus. Visual arc thresholds are increased by multiples to obtain adequate recognition thresholds. Usually, such multiples are determined for various tasks by experimentation. If the observer has lower visual acuity than the unimpaired population, then additional multiples may be required.

Visual impairments can materially increase the size or visual angle requirements for objects, text, or discriminating features to be detected. Inverting the Snellen ratio and multiplying the required visual acuity for normal vision can extend recognition for those who have say, 20:400 vision (e.g., multiply the visual acuity value by 400/20 or 20).

Operator age may also materially affect contrast sensitivity and color quality. Designers should understand that visual detection and recognition is dependent upon both the targets' contrast and the amount of illumination of the target. If illumination is reduced at dusk, inside buildings, or in vehicles at night, one may have to increase the size of the target for any given level of contrast (see Figure 18.6).

Vibration and hypoxia, reduced oxygen content in the brain brought on by ascent to high altitudes or the inhalation of certain kinds of gases, also reduce acuity. Pilots who breathe pure oxygen at high altitude at night frequently report dramatic increase in their color vision.

Moreover, if the designer relies only upon color as a differentiating code for stimuli or information, reduction in illumination shifts vision from color to black

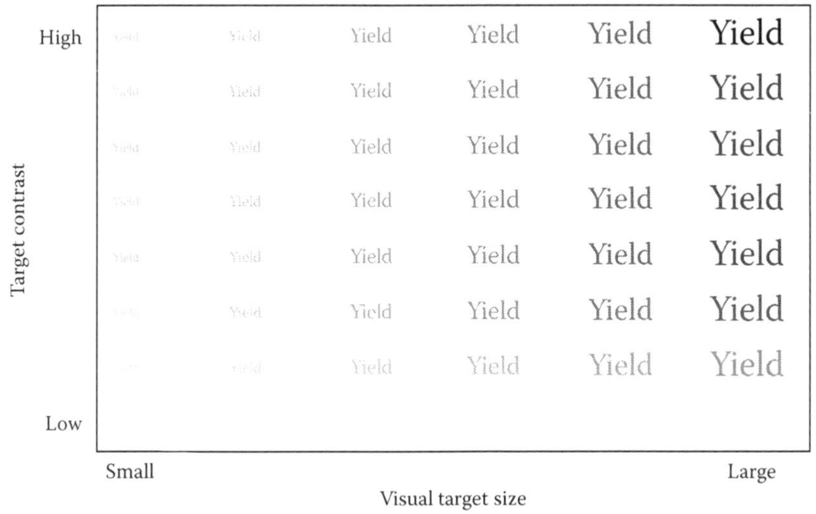

FIGURE 18.6 Example of impact of target contrast and illumination upon spatial frequency or visual acuity. (Note change in visibility of words under different levels of illumination showing the importance of contrast and size of visual targets under different levels of illumination). (From Wiker, S.F., Importance of Human Factors Engineering in Promotion of Safety in Haight, J. (Ed.) *Safety Professional's Handbook*, 2008. With permission.)

and white and color cues will be difficult to discriminate. Color perception is also affected by the characteristics of the target (spectral content, luminance), the environment in which it is viewed, and the observer (Israelski, 1978). About 8% of men and less than 1% of women have some degree of color vision deficiency. Color vision will be particularly problematic if the individual's visual contrast sensitivity or illumination levels are low and rod vision subordinates cone vision.

The type of illumination used can also materially affect color perception and discrimination. Two colors that appear identical in tungsten light may appear entirely different in daylight. High-pressure sodium lighting distorts almost all colors. Designers often fail to consider that material variations in illumination characteristics can influence color detection across a wide range of operational environments. This is true when individuals have some degree of color blindness or pathos that dims light impinging upon the retina.

18.4.21 AUDITION PROBLEMS

Hearing is very important for human operators because it allows communication by way of speech, and to attend to a variety of auditory cues such as bells, buzzers, beeps, horns, sirens, and other sounds that do not require visual attention. Designers often rely upon auditory signals for alerting multiple operators when visual stimuli cannot be relied upon.

Audition is a complex sensory system that defies comprehensive description in this document. However, one can describe a process that most ergonomists go through in assessing the acceptability of speech or auditory display design.

First, the objective is that displayed information should match generally accepted selection criteria for auditory displays:

- Message is simple and short
- Message calls for immediate action
- Message will not be referred to later
- Message deals with events in time
- Operator's visual system is overloaded
- Illumination is poor
- Job requires movement away from a visual display
- Stimulus is acoustical in nature

Discrimination among frequencies and temporal sound patterns is much more reliable than attempting to discriminate between increases in sound intensity of a pure tone. To avoid ambiguity, systems should use no more than about six different auditory signals. Use of previously learned signals is preferred, and increasing repetition rate of pulses rather than amplitudes should be used to convey urgency.

Intelligibility of speech within a noise field is related to the signal-to-noise ratio. Noise in occupational environments, during emergencies or storms, and situations can mask speech if it is not sufficiently greater in sound power level than the noise field. Normal speech averages about 65 dBA, if one must shout the sound power level reaches 100 dBA.

Measuring the percentage of correct words transmitted from a speaker to a listener, one arrives at a speech intelligibility score (e.g., percent correct). Speech intelligibility decays when the signal-to-noise ratio narrows across the voice spectrum. If one measures the one-third octave band sound power level (SPL) of the actual or expected noise field and overlays the SPL of the speech then difference in between speech and noise decibel values becomes the signal-to-noise ratio for speech. For the purposes of the articulation index (AI) if the power of noise exceeds the SPL of speech, the signal-to-noise ratio is set to zero.

Weighting the differences in SPLs across the frequency spectrum and summing the weighted differences provides the AI:

$$AI = \frac{W_i}{30dB} \sum_{i=1}^{5} (dBA_{Speech} - dBA_{Noise} + 12dB)$$

where
W_i is the weight for the ith frequency band
dBA_{speech} the sound power level of speech at the ith frequency band, and
dBA_{noise} the sound power level of noise at the ith frequency band.

The weighting factors for each frequency band are provided in Table 18.6.

One can also take the average dBA readings for one-third octave bands at 500, 1000, and 2000 Hz center frequencies and use that average as the speech interference level (SIL) metric. Once the SIL is determined, then one can use Figure 18.7 to determine if worker proximity and vocalization capacity are adequate for transmitting spoken messages in various noise fields.

TABLE 18.6

Weighting Coefficients for Articulation Index Frequency Bands

Frequency (Hz) Band (i)	Weighing Factor (W_i)
250	0.072
500	0.144
1000	0.222
2000	0.327
4000	0.234

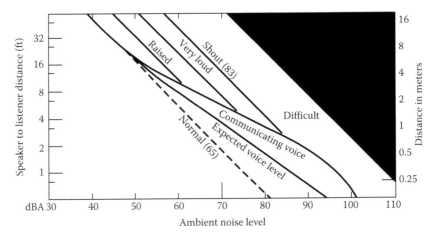

FIGURE 18.7 Effect of SIL and the functional relationship between proximity of speaker-listeners and required speech sound power level. (Adapted from J.C. Webster, Speech Interference by Noise, *Proceedings,* Inter-Noise 74, Institute of Noise Control Engineering, p. 558).

Intelligibility can be enhanced by designing verbal messages by using the following pointers:

- Make it simple and redundant
- Use a reduced vocabulary set with simple words
- Phrases used have contextual meaning (e.g., pilots hear "Cleared to Land" on final approach)

Many designers seem to assume that users of their systems will have adequate hearing. Unfortunately, hearing impairments are ubiquitous, increase with age, and far too often develop occupationally with exposure. Unimpaired young operators can converse comfortably at 55 dBA. At 50 years of age, speech sound power must average 67 dBA, and at age 85 years, loud speech is required in moderate noise fields (e.g., about 85 dBA) (Coren, 1994).

Since designers usually have no control over who will use their systems, most systems should be designed with the expectation that they will be used by persons with hearing difficulties. Providing volume controls so that listeners can pick their own listening levels is one important design option. These approaches will make auditory signal design more accommodating. One may have to consider using multiple coding strategies to overcome limited auditory capabilities. Of course, augmentive technologies may be required by hearing-impaired users to insure that acoustic information is received, or they may require use of alternative sensory modes for displaying information or cues (e.g., visual or vibratory cues).

18.4.22 ARE SIGNALS DETECTED AS EXPECTED?

One cannot presume that if a stimulus is suprathreshold, it will be detected in a dependable manner. As shown in Figure 18.8, observers can detect the presence (Hits) and absence of suprathreshold stimuli (Correct Rejections). However, they can also miss signals (Misses), and report the presence of a stimulus when it is absent (false alarms). The magnitude of each of these outcomes depends upon the observer's expectations regarding the presence of signals, their sensorial or perceptual sensitivity (d'), and their decision criterion (beta).

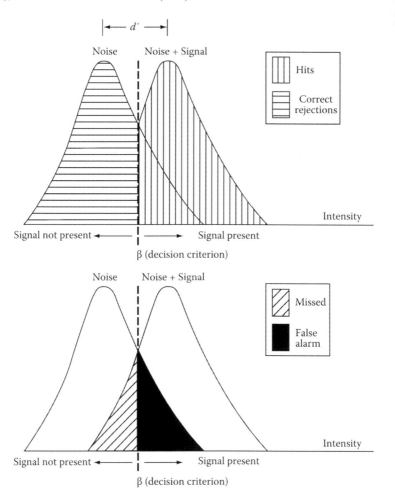

FIGURE 18.8   General stimulus signal detection behaviors given a user's stimulus sensitivity (d') and their decision criterion (β or beta) used to determine whether the stimulus is signal or noise.

The beta used by an observer is the magnitude of the physical stimulus intensity at which point the observer will uniformly report the presence of a stimulus and absence if the intensity falls below that criterion. The observer's sensitivity, or inherent ability to detect the signal, can change as they age, with fatigue, and other factors that can degrade sensation. The observer's response criterion (beta) can also change based upon their expectation of the presence of the signal and values and costs associated with judgments. If beta changes, in the face of a constant d', material differences will result in the operators accurate reporting of the presence of signal and their false alarm (FA) rate (see Figures 18.9 and 18.10).

Individuals with sensory impairments that affect the dimension of a stimulus presented, suffer decrements in the d' or sensitivity. Impairments that reduce operator sensitivity (d') can also affect their positioning of beta. As will be shown in the next few paragraphs, beta is influenced by perceived incidence rate of targets and the values and costs of their placement of beta.

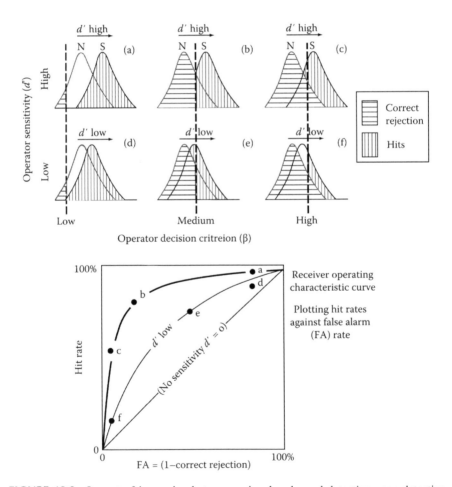

FIGURE 18.9 Impact of increasing beta upon signal or hazard detection upon detection performance when operator sensitivity (d') is constant.

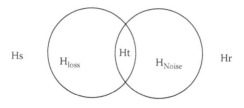

$$Ht = Hs + Hr - Hsr$$

FIGURE 18.10 General model showing that information sent (Hs) and which is also received (Hr) is deemed as transmitted information (Ht) with an ideal design producing two overlapping diagrams demonstrating perfect transmission.

One can attempt to improve the observer's beta by providing accurate information about the probability of signal and noise, and the values of making Hit, Correct Rejection, and the positive magnitude of creating false alarms and misses. By adjusting the theoretical optimal beta by a payoff matrix, one can modulate observer signal detection theory (SDT) performance:

$$\beta_{Optimal} = \frac{P(N)}{P(S)} * \frac{V_{CR} + C_{FA}}{V_{Hit} + C_{Miss}}$$

As shown by the equation above, and demonstrated in Table 18.7, one can easily bias the observer's response criterion by changing their perception of the prevalence of signals and the values and costs of their decisions. The observed beta for an observer is the ratio of the ordinal probabilities of signal and noise at the decision criterion. Thus, if the beta is large, criterion is shifted to the right (i.e., physical stimuli must be substantial before the observer will report the presence of a signal). If the beta is small, the criterion is shifted to the left and small physical stimuli intensities will result in conclusions that signals are present.

Errors in signal detection can provoke unanticipated behaviors because cues to initiate behaviors are missed, or inappropriate behaviors occur when cues are absent. Signal detection performance depends upon the observer's (1) expectation of a signal, (2) their response criterion (beta), and (3) observational sensitivity to the stimulus (d').

One can compute the observed operator's sensitivity or d' by estimating the distance between signal plus noise distribution (SN) and the noise distribution (N) in units of z-scores. The z-scores are determined by determining the miss and FA rates and finding the z-scores from the means of each distribution to the response criterion.

Another method to evaluate an observer's d' and beta involves plotting the hit rate against the FA rate for various signal detection trials in which different frequencies of signals or payoff matrices are used to shift betas. The result is a receiver's or observer's operating characteristic curve. The greater the distance of the curve from the diagonal, the greater the signal-to-noise ratio and the greater the observer's capacity to detect the signal. Betas are determined by the tangent to the curve at the empirical plot point.

A receiver operating characteristic (ROC) curve allows one to compare an observer's d' and beta simultaneously by plotting hit rates against FA rates for various betas that are changed by altering the probability of signals, the payoff matrix, or allowing the observer to select different confidence levels for each decision about the presence of a

TABLE 18.7

Different Values for the Locus of Optimal Physical Intensity or Optimal Beta Given Different Perceived Probabilities for Signals and Values and Costs for Decision Outcomes

Probability of Signal and Noise		Values ($)		Costs ($)		
Noise	Signal	Hit	Correct Rejection	Miss	False Alarm	
0.9	0.1	100	100	100	100	9
0.9	0.1	100	100	100	100	9
0.9	0.1	100	100	100	100	9
0.9	0.1	100	100	100	100	9
0.9	0.1	1000	10	1000	10	0.09
0.9	0.1	1000	10	1000	10	0.09
0.9	0.1	10	1000	10	1000	900
0.9	0.1	10	1000	10	1000	900
0.1	0.9	100	100	100	100	0.11
0.1	0.9	100	100	100	100	0.11
0.1	0.9	100	100	100	100	0.11
0.1	0.9	100	100	100	100	0.11
0.1	0.9	1000	10	1000	10	0.0011
0.1	0.9	1000	10	1000	10	0.0011
0.1	0.9	10	1000	10	1000	11.11
0.1	0.9	10	1000	10	1000	11.11

signal or hazard. The ROC can be used to compare the d' values for different equipment designs, among observers for personnel selection or impact of ambient and potentially masking phenomena (e.g., fog, rain, or darkness) upon the driver's capacity.

When performing tests to determine whether or not an impaired applicant can perform work that involves SDT (e.g., quality control inspector), it is important that the applicant has a clear instruction set addressing the incidence of defectives as well as the costs and values of the four possible decision outcomes. Using a paradigm in which the operator is tested repeatedly with different purported flaw incidence and different values and costs for decisions, one can rapidly create a ROC without having to worry about where the applicant actually places their betas for each of the trials. The ROC plot can be compared against requisite performance ROC to determine whether or not the applicant can meet minimal signal detection performance requirements; regardless of where the applicant set their betas during the application or screening tests.

An example of this paradigm is provided in Figure 18.9, observers a, b, and c have greater d' or sensitivities, than f, e and d, all of which do not share the same beta or decision criterion. Some observers are very liberal in that they seek to increase hit rates at the expense of increased false alarms (e.g., a and d) while others are very conservative in their decision criterion (e.g., f and c) where greater intensities of signals are needed before they are willing to claim the stimulus is a signal. The conservative betas reduce hits and false alarms.

The importance of understanding SDT is that one can anticipate significant differences in human detection of a signal or communication given differences depending upon the perceived expectancy of the signal and the values and costs associated with their performance. A designer should understand that simply because a stimulus is suprathreshold, it does not guarantee that the human will accurately respond to signals or correctly reject their presence. To enhance accommodation of the design for all, stimulus–noise ratios should be increased, and the observer should clearly understand what the signal should look like. Costs and values associated with decision outcomes should also be very clear to the user.

Operator sensitivity can be improved by using magnifiers, structured light presented at angles to induce shadows of surface flaws, use of haptic exploration of the surface with fingers, x-rays, and other augmenting schemes that collectively enhance detection of the flaw. Providing static examples of flaws for inspectors to make side-by-side comparisons can be helpful, particularly if memory problems exist, or incidence of particular flaws is very low and recall needs reinforcement.

18.4.23   IS THE INFORMATION CONFUSING THE OPERATOR OR USER?

Even if the operator reliably receives the stimuli, they can confuse stimuli that are very similar in nature or perception, or ambient noise can mask attributions and produce miscommunications. This can occur frequently when sensory imagery received by the observer is incomplete or differential due to impaired sensory or motor capacities. Discriminating features may be lost among sensory coding schemes that lead to confusion and noise in interpretation of the imagery. If one cannot detect a small dot, a small cross element, then an observer may not be able to discriminate among an "i," "t," and an "l."

If an operator's task requires the identification or classification of information, the sensory task has transitioned into perceptual task. The goal is to receive (Hr) all information that is sent (Hs). If that occurs, then the two circles in the Venn diagram below will superimpose and all information is transmitted (Ht) with no loss (H_{loss}) and no noise (H_{noise}). With loss of information some of the sent information is lost, and noise is classified as information, which was received but that was not sent.

To determine the amount of information that was transmitted, we calculate the information that was sent, received, and that was collectively noise and loss. Information is computed in terms of bits. If we have a single event i, we can determine the information sent by that stimulus using the formula provided in Figure 18.10.

If we have a large number of events with each possessing a different probability of occurrence, we can compute the average amount of information presented to the observer by the following formula:

$$Hs_{average} = \sum_{i=1}^{N} P_i \log_2 \left[\frac{1}{P_i} \right]$$

where

$Hs_{average}$ is the average information presented and
P_i is the probability of presentation or incidence of code or symbol.

Incidence of send and received symbols can be computed for 1000 presentations of each stimulus

	Weather symbols				
Response					Sums
Thunderstorm	900	0	0	0	900
Thunderstorm and rain	100	0	300	300	700
Visible lightening	0	500	400	300	1200
Thunderstorm and hail	0	500	300	400	1200
Sums	1000	1000	1000	1000	4000

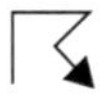

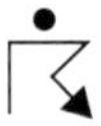

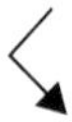

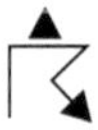

	Weather symbols					
Response	Symbol A	Symbol B	Symbol C	Symbol D	Sums	Bits
Symbol A	0.23	0.00	0.00	0.00	0.23	0.48
Symbol B	0.03	0.00	0.08	0.08	0.18	0.44
Symbol C	0.00	0.13	0.10	0.08	0.30	0.52
Symbol D	0.00	0.13	0.08	0.10	0.30	0.52
Sums	0.25	0.25	0.25	0.25	1.00	
Bits	0.50	0.50	0.50	0.50		

$$H_s = 2.00 \text{ bits}$$
$$H_r = 1.97 \text{ bits}$$
$$H_{sr} = 3.15 \text{ bits}$$
$$H_t = 0.81 \text{ bits}$$

FIGURE 18.11 Example of a confusion matrix demonstrating failure of warning symbols to consistently warn about the appropriate hazard.

For example, if we wish to evaluate four symbols or codes that have been proposed for thunderstorm, thunderstorm and rain, visible lightening and thunderstorm and hail, we can evaluate the transmittal of intended information using a confusion matrix shown in Figure 18.11. The incidence of symbols sent, the incidence of symbols received, and the incidence of sent and received symbols can be computed for 1000 presentations of each stimulus.

The distribution of responses provided by the subjects showed that the thunderstorm symbol produce 900/4000, or 23% of the 4000 presentations resulting in about a half bit of information:

$$0.49 \text{bits} = (.23) \log_2 \left[\frac{1}{.23} \right]$$

By computing the average information sent ($H_s = 2.0$ bits), information received from the marginal probabilities of the rows ($H_r = 1.97$), and the information content inside the matrix ($H_{sr} = 3.15$ bits), we can determine the information that is transmitted ($H_t = H_s + H_r - H_{rs} = 0.81$ bits). In the example above, we find that the lost information ($H_s - H_t = 2.00 - 0.81 = 1.19$ bits) is due both to confusion and noise ($H_r - H_t = 1.97 - 0.81 = 1.16$ bits).

Designers of icons, symbols, or other types of information that must be presented to users often become too close to their design, or fail to understand that sensory impairments can "filter" discriminating features of stimuli, and expect no confusion. For example, use of differences in contrast may be effective for some populations, those with low visual contrast sensitivity, may not be able to use that coding element to discriminate among stimulus cues. Diming a symbol to indicate a state change may not be recognized by someone with a low-vision impairment in which contrast sensitivity is poor.

Conducting confusion matrix studies, one can determine which symbols or sensory stimuli are confusing, ferret out what features, or general affordance, that fail to discriminate among similar symbols. For example, the skull and cross-bones icon was only confused with the biohazard by 10% of the observers, if we can determine why the confusion exists (or at least make adjustments in the imagery that resolve the confusions), we can prevent misunderstandings that can have performance, safety, or health consequences, and that may impede accommodation.

It is not necessary to remove all confusions if the resulting behaviors and impacts are equivalent. Providing feedback to the user that their interpretation was incorrect may be sufficient to retrain the user with every mistake. For example, if an impaired worker reliably detects but confuses the symbology shown in the table above, but each symbol or icon requires the same precautions, then the consequences are nil.

18.4.24　Have You Relied Too Heavily Upon an Affordance?

Gibson (1966) described an affordance as an objective property of an object, or a feature of the immediate environment, that indicates how to interface with that object or feature. Norman (1988) refined Gibson's definition to refer to a perceived affordance, one in which both objective characteristics of the object are combined with physical capabilities of the actor, their goals, plans, values, beliefs, and interests. An affordance is a form of communication that conveys an intended purpose and operation of a device or a message, as well as behaviors that are to be avoided. This is a powerful design element that can be useful if used wisely, and punishing if it motivates inappropriate or undesired behaviors. Cognitive dissonance may also develop and lead one to use of the object in manner that was neither expected, nor promoted by the affordance.

An example of a positive affordance is offered by the steering wheel of a new car. One may have never driven the car before, but the design of the steering wheel and the actor's previous experiences lead them to expect that rotation of the wheel to right when rolling will cause the car to veer to the right. An undesired affordance could be produced by exit path flashing illumination lighting that creates an illusion of movement in a direction that is opposite to that which is desired.

Often impaired individuals have limited sensory portals to detect information that, collectively, produces the desired affordance. If the designer is relying heavily upon development of an affordance to produce a desired perception, they may have to create the affordance with cues that still convey the desired information. A classic example of this problem is demonstrated by turning off the sound for a suspenseful scene in which the music is used to convey to the viewer that the victim is at extreme risk. The director attempts to show how much danger the poor soul is in by presenting ominous music and sounds, and how unknowing the victim is by their facial and gestural behaviors that suggest that everything is normal. When the sound is off, the scene presents a state of normality and the presence of a hazard cue is gone. Turn off the screen brightness and turn up the volume and you are left with a sense of monition—without any sense that an unknowing victim exists. This demonstration shows how compelling both visual and auditory information can be in generating the intended affordance. For individuals who are deaf, subtitles might have to be used to warn them that the assailant is in the closet and is ready to pounce.

In sum, affordances can be very powerful influences in the receipt and interpretation of sent stimuli, and if not evaluated through tests and evaluation procedures, can lead to unexpected outcomes if the intended meaning(s) are not developed.

18.4.25 ARE THE COGNITIVE DEMANDS ACCEPTABLE?

Cognitive demands include handling information that is received from the sensory system, attended to, used with human memory to learn and support decision making and selection of responses.

18.4.26 HUMAN MEMORY LIMITS

Memory is requisite for detection of problems, diagnostics, handling protocols, and learning new material. Deficits in sensory, short-term memory (STM) or long-term memory (LTM) are often direct or indirect causes for human performance failures and constraints in accommodating affected individuals.

To memorize information it has to be actively encoded. Sensory information flows into through senses continually. However, only the information to which we pay material attention to and that has meaning to us are candidates for successful memory store (Shiffrin, 1988). Any design elements or work processes that disrupt our attention or our understanding of the meaning of the information that we are attending will act to inhibit development of learning and memory.

Sensory memories are limited buffers for sensory input. Visual iconic sensory memory is briefly present for visual stimuli and aural stimuli produce echoic sensory memory. Other sensory inputs have brief sensory memory periods as well. Stimuli captured by sensory memory must move rapidly into STM through attention. If the stimuli are not attended, the STM essentially filters that information and it decays away. If sensory impairments exist, the cocktail of sensory input is changed and subsequent use of the "filtered" input can have performance consequences.

Transfer of sensory stimuli into information that can be used at "higher" processing stages is often referred to as encoding. Three principal encoding methods have been proposed:

- Structural (encoding with emphasis on the physical structural characteristics of the stimulus)
- Phonemic (encoding with emphasis on the sounds of the words or phenomena)
- Semantic (encoding with emphasis on the meaning)

Working memory is the next stage and serves as the "workbench" for reinforcement of the encoded sensory memory of interest, and for temporary recall of the information under process. Elaboration of encoded information occurs when it is associated with other information. Elaboration can include visual imagery that adds richness to the material to be remembered and often connects information from other sensory modalities. Finally, the imagery is usually made self-referent in that the individual attempts to make the information relevant to their life history and personal learning history.

Three stages of memory storage are generally accepted: sensory store, short-term store, and long-term store. Sensory store retains the sensory images for periods of time that are just long enough to develop a perception (< 200 ms). Short-term memory can retain information for about 20–30 s without rehearsal of that information. If the information is verbally rehearsed or the image that must be maintained is continually or episodically refreshed after short intervals, then STM can last as long as the reinforcing or rehearsal behavior continues. Short-term memory appears to be limited in the number of items that it can functionally maintain at any given time (e.g., 7 ± 2 items; Miller, 1956). Yet if those items are packed into "chunks," and smaller "chunks" are packed into larger "chunks," then limitations can appear to wane.

Short-term memory has been referred to as a simple rehearsal buffer that is vulnerable to decay in rehearsal or displacement with incoming information into the first-in-first-out buffer. It may be more complex, but that metaphor is effective guidance for designers who are concerned about whether or not information conveyed to the user can be stored or associated with long-term store.

If information is sufficiently rehearsed, made semantically relevant, or can be integrated into long-term store associations, it may be permanently stored in LTM. Transition of STM into LTM requires rehearsal and development of associative "hooks" to bring the information into the LTM semantic structure. Rehearsal can be simple recitation of the material in STM (e.g., maintenance rehearsal), or elaborative in which the meaning of information is developed and associated with relevant components of LTM. Elaborative rehearsal appears to develop LTM in a much more effective manner, presumably because greater numbers of associations are established and the "bigger" picture of the information is established.

Long-term memory can be divided into declarative (explicit) and procedural (implicit) memories (Anderson, 1976). Declarative memory requires conscious recall and is often referred to as explicit memory because it consists of information that is explicitly stored and retrieved.

Declarative memory consists of semantic memory (meaning of information independent of context) and episodic memory (information that is contextually specific—dependent upon the time and place that the information was gathered such as the birth of your child (e.g., sensations, emotions, and personal associations of a particular place or time)). Memory of autobiographical events within one's own life is generally viewed as a subset of episodic memory.

Procedural or implicit memory is based upon implicit learning of operations or sequences—not based on the conscious recall of information. Learning motor skills is a component of procedural memory that requires motor rehearsal.

Long-term memory appears to attempt to build associations that are organized into either clusters (i.e., related material), conceptual hierarchies of items (e.g., leaders vs. followers, inputs vs. outputs), and semantic networks (i.e., less structured associations or relationships between nodes of facts or concepts), schemas (i.e., clusters of knowledge about an event or object abstracted from prior experience with the object), and scripts (i.e., schema which organizes our knowledge about things or activities).

Even if LTM is permanent, a wealth of evidence shows that retrieval may not be successful or accurate. Retrieval requires selection of appropriate cues or "pointers" to information maintained within LTM. Cues may be contextual or mood-based. Contextual cues are relevant to the information that we are attempting to recall.

For example, if we are attempting to construct an equation for the circumference of a circle and wish to recall the value of π, information that we have retained about circles is "made available." The set of memories associated with circles is made available, and we can find the memorized value of the constant (hopefully).

On the other hand, cues that create an emotional state or sense of being may enable access to memories that are linked with that sensation. Odors of coffee and soft guitar music may return memories related to previous experiences associated with those phenomena.

Memories recalled appear to be reconstructions (Bartlett, 1932) that can be influenced by current information or cues (e.g., errors in eyewitness recall produced by misleading questions (Loftus, 1979)). If information cannot be maintained in STM long enough, it cannot be used to pull information from long-term store. The information is no longer available to help assemble percepts or associative structures that are used in assessment and decision making, or for developing more complex associations that are used to bring the information into long-term store.

Cognitive impairments, various diseases, and situational or task-design interference cause disturbance in STM retention, rehearsal or refreshment of working memory. Interference can be sensory, redirection of attention, or trying to remember too much at a given moment. Sometimes development of strong stimuli that produce cognitive focus or tunnel vision can preclude gathering as much information into working memory as expected.

Long-term storage may be classified as episodic memory (storage of events and experiences in a serial form) or as semantic memory (organization record of associations, declarative information, mental models or concepts, and acquired motor skills). Information from STM is stored in LTM through rehearsal. Rehearsal of information, concepts, and motor activities enhances transfer into LTM. Learning is most effective if it is distributed across time.

Accommodation for memory impairment requires one provide sufficient opportunity for the user to focus upon sensory memory allow entry and rehearsal in STM, or to establish associations that allow the user to recall information from long-term store. Designers can rely too heavily upon learning and recall on the part of the operator to prevent errors in sequences of operations to support choice, diagnostic, or predictive decisions.

Designing down memory demands is always a good idea. Furthermore, reducing task strain and burden to support working memory can promote accurate recall and sequencing of information that are needed to make good decisions or to operate machines and tools, perform tasks properly, and many other activities for everyone. Memory aids can be in the form of: aids such as use of checklists and task performance histories, increased display times, electronic to do lists, attentional cues, chunking large amounts of information into smaller acronyms, or chunks that can be "unpacked" and contextual cues.

18.4.27 DESIGN IN MEMORY AIDS

Memory aids are used by all of us and can be of particular importance for individuals who have memory impairment. Memory aids can be built into the design of equipment (e.g., controls are placed in linear sequence of operation so that the user does not have to remember which control to operate after the previous control—they simply make adjustments one control after another along a line of placement). Other aids can be cognitive tools that are provided to new trainees (e.g., pilots are taught mnemonics and acronyms to remember operations and sequence of operations when flying planes in case they lose their checklists or are subjected to stressful emergencies). Typically, designers develop acronyms and mnemonics to assist users in remembering associations and sequences to reduce risk of recall error and cognitive burdens.

Acronyms. Acronyms are words that represent titles, sequences, or number sequences of alphanumeric letters that code underlying information. For example, acronyms are often used to remember university names (e.g., WVU, West Virginia University), or checklists (e.g., GUMPS: Check Gas, Undercarriage, Manifold Pressure, Propeller and Seatbelts before landing).

Mnemonics. Mnemonics are techniques for remembering information that is otherwise quite difficult to recall. Using mnemonics one can cue recall of lists, sequences of operations, and other information that is often difficult to remember. Use of vivid imaginative effort for construction and use of mnemonic increases the likelihood that it will be recalled and used.

Method of Rhyme mnemonics are used to recall information. For example, "i before e, expect after c, or when sounded like 'a' as in neighbor and weigh." Pilots are trained with a rhyme, "High to low, look out below!" The latter rhyme refers to a warning that changes in barometric pressure can lead to incorrect altimeter readings (e.g., reduction in barometric pressure will indicate that the aircraft's altimeter will read higher than true).

Mnemonics help workers remember the associations and interrelationships among items. Associations can be remembered by creating imagery of

- Placing things on top of one another
- Crashing or merging things together
- Wrapping items around one another
- Linking them using the same color, smell, shape, or feeling

Location Mnemonics. Location mnemonics can be used to guide recall of spatial organization or sequences of information. You use the journey method by associating information with landmarks on a journey that you know well. Several methods have been used to reinforce memory and learning about sequences, associations, and clusters of unlinked information.

Method of Loci, or the ancient Roman room technique, is an ancient and effective way of remembering information where its structure is not important. The Roman room technique is similar to the journey method. It works by pegging images coding for information to known things, in this case to objects in a room. The Roman room technique is most effective for storing lists of unlinked information, while the journey method is better for storing lists of ordered items. One can create rooms within rooms and objects within each room are used to recall information. For example, to remember the following number 808360202 one can create a map of the country of area codes and move from the Hawaiian Coast, West Coast, and East Coast telephone area codes.

When designers cannot eliminate the need for unassisted memory, they should consider offering acronyms and mnemonics as training aids. These tools can be used to support recall of procedural sequences, options available, phone numbers, etc.

18.4.28   Does the Design Support Human Decision Making?

Humans are not consistently rational decision makers. Many decisions are based upon heuristics or rules of thumb that are developed based upon past experiences. In other cases decisions can be flawed because of innate limitations in human decision making capacities.

A decision is a process that one uses to reduce uncertainty. Three classes of decision are (1) choosing from among options, (2) predicting an outcome, or (3) diagnosis. The cognitive burden imposed by this activity is derived from having to recall or maintain a set of attributes or facts and their values in terms of the nature of the decision. Metaphorically, one can view a complex decision as a long regression equation with many terms and coefficients. The greater the number of terms and coefficients, the more difficult the cognitive burden becomes and the greater the likelihood that the decision will not be ideal. Choice decisions typically are easier to make than prediction decisions because predictions often require additional mental algebra.

Diagnosis typically produces the greatest burden because the individual often has to back chain from a current state to an array of possible etiologies—requiring that one recalls many potential "regression equations" along with their coefficients and properties. If one is in the early stages of diagnosis of, say circuit faults, there may be hundreds of sources for such faults. Further data gathering is required until the solution space can be adequately narrowed. Even when adequately narrowed, the potential solution space may be very large and can exceed human capacity to handle without high risk of error.

Often designers do not consider the impact of their design upon human decision making burden. Stressful epochs, aging, or mental impairment, individually or collectively serve to impair the rate and quality of human decision making. Often designs force too many decisions, bias decisions from choice to toward diagnosis, and increase the level of mental algebra that is imposed upon the user or worker.

Attributes or facts may take time to obtain and do not always arrive in an optimal or expected sequence or time frame. This means that decision makers may have to arrive at conclusions or make decisions without all of the facts—or choose to reduce their decision stress by making decisions early before one has to gather and consider additional information. Initial attributes or weights associated with those attributes can also decay with time when the decision maker must wait for additional information.

Decisions based upon an incomplete or erroneous attribute-weighting matrix often occur. Matching of weights to attributes may be out of phase, and early assessments based upon limited facts can lead to inappropriate initial hypotheses that, based upon prior experience or workload issues, are inappropriately adhered to. Initial hypotheses can serve as filters for new information in that the decision maker pays attention to only incoming facts that support their initial guess. Thus, from experience decision makers attempt to arrive at decisions quickly to reduce their cognitive workload.

As the cognitive workload increases, decision envelopes change, or working memory is challenged, or organic impairments constrain decision making capacity, decision makers gravitate toward decision making strategies that reduce their cognitive performance demands. This process often leads to error. Some of the types of design-mediated decision errors are summarized in the following paragraphs.

When in doubt, correlate. Often when challenged, decision makers seek causality by correlation. This is a particular problem when individuals cannot attend much information when making decisions. For example, engines do not run without gasoline. The engine cannot start; therefore, the gasoline tank is empty. Obviously, that is not the only explanation for gasoline engine not starting. However, those with cognitive impairment may gravitate to simple correlations and not be able to move cognitively outside of the box without some assistance from the designer (e.g., provide a list of potential reasons why the vehicle will not start).

Rules of thumb or heuristic approaches to decision making are also used to simplify the process. Heuristics rely upon a subset of attributes and exclude the need to for further data gathering. In most cases, copy machines fail to execute the copy command when paper needs to be reloaded into the machine. There are other reasons why the copy command may not function (e.g., paper jam, inadequate toner, power loss, etc.). Without a message to the operator why the failure has occurred, most operators will begin sequences of activities aimed at adding paper to the copy machine. Rules of thumb are useful, but when they produce inappropriate behaviors, then the designer should intervene with a clear error message explaining the nature of the fault and how to overcome the problem.

Humans are not objective statistical or computational machines. Statistical assessment of data is usually by intuition rather than calculation and it leads to errors in assigning weights to attributes. Humans tend to linearize curvilinear relationships and, thus, over or underestimate future behaviors of systems. Humans also tend to overestimate variability when means or ranges in sampled data are greater, and they dislike arriving at estimates that are near the extremes (i.e., they behave conservatively when estimating proportions). Estimates of means can be significantly influenced by the frequency of occurrence of a particular value (e.g., while the mean may be 20, there were 6 values of 4 while no other number was repeated, the mean must be close to 4). Humans do not use Bayes' rule very well; the probability of some event changes based upon existence or probabilities of prior events. Failure to correctly statistically characterize probabilities and magnitudes leads to a false perception of reality that can provoke an inappropriate decision.

When in doubt, choose conservative decision outcomes. Essentially, regress toward the "mean" even if that is inappropriate. Most rules-based or bureaucratic administrative systems promote use of rules to apply to a problem to reduce decision stress for workers who do not have the education, training or skills to solve problems directly. They prefer simple characteristics that allow selection of a rule, regardless of whether or not it is appropriate. Designers often expect too much analytical capacity from a user population and essentially design in errors when users have options to always pursue most conservative or rules-based options.

Humans bias their decisions based upon either primacy or recency factors. First impressions can take hold and bias all subsequent information gathering and weighting. Or, a recent negative experience can shift the bias toward recent information, negating prior data or experiences. Either bias can provoke errors in assessments and decisions. First impressions of workers are often incorrect, and a recent error that leads to a significant negative outcome (e.g., accident) does not necessarily reflect the worker's history of safe behavior.

Divide and conquer in the face of overwhelming data and choices. Throwing too much information at a human often forces the individual to seek a quick decision. They seek to accept a small set of hypotheses (usually less than three or four hypotheses) and attend information that principally supports one or more of their initial guesses. Ease of recall of an initially feasible hypothesis may be used to filter additional information, or the worker can rely upon heuristics, primacy bias, and other biasing behaviors to control their mental workload in decision making.

Reliable or highly diagnostic sources can be over weighted by the decision maker, resulting in inappropriate selection of hypotheses and data gathering. A coworker who has expertise in the operation and minor repair of copy machines may be sought out for assistance with every electromechanical piece of equipment in the facility, leading to overburden of that worker and errors when their expertise is limited. Second opinions and verification through testing, experimentation, simulation, or other objective measurements should be used to check expert opinions. One should also provide those opportunities when the expert is a machine, a gauge, or computer display. Humans often believe that computers do not make mistakes when, in fact, they do. Providing expertise or guidance from a computer to its user and multiple diagnostic checks can help those who need basic assistance with making choices, predictions or diagnostics.

Overconfidence in one's ability to make decisions. We can be lucky and have performed well as decision makers in the in past. If we become overly confident, then we can bias our perspectives and expectancies and produce a poor decision. Cognitively impaired individuals may elect to stay within their zone of operating confidence. By limiting their experiences, they may find that their operational history is very consistent and it leads to reinforcement of highly constrained but ritualistically successful performance. When an outlier situation develops that appears to fall within their zone of confidence, they will quickly respond with decisions that may be very inappropriate.

Designers can improve performance by indicating to the operator or user that the current situation is statistically novel and work with the user by providing checklists or diagnostic guidance that allows management-by-consent problem resolution processes. Assisted problem-solving will help users recognize that the problem may fall out of their expertise and require collaborative intervention with the machine, technicians, or supervisors.

Negative consequences outweigh positive consequences. If all benefits and costs result in a zero-sum gain, the decision maker is likely to select outcomes that are risk aversive or avoid costs rather than pursue gains. This may be particularly true with workers who have impairments and who are very concerned with performing their jobs without negative outcomes that might indicate that they cannot handle the job.

Confirmation and negative information bias. Once we believe a worker believes that they have the answer, they tend to develop "cognitive tunnel vision" and resist attending information that contradicts their assessment or belief.

To help the decision maker avoid poor decisions and negative consequences such as accidents, injuries or losses, the designer should

- Train the decision maker so they understand what is causal and what is not
- Reduce decision options as much as feasible
- Perform statistical computations and mathematical operations for the decision maker and present them in a persistent manner for reinspection and reevaluation
- Remind the decision maker of all attributes that exist or that have been encountered to prevent exclusion
- Provide memory aids like checklists, diagnostic fault trees, and so forth to reduce the cognitive burden that promotes cognitive shortcutting

18.4.29 REDUCE MENTAL WORKLOADS

Presuming that component activities can be performed in a serial fashion effectively, one may still encounter accommodation problems when one or more tasks must be performed concomitantly.

Wickens proposed a multiple-resource theory for workload assessment and control in which different resources exist for different modalities (Wickens, 1984). Auditory and visual processing resources, central processing resources, and different motor resources are required for the performance of psychomotor tasks. Resources are classified by type and have dedicated channels. If one designs work that must pass through one particular type of channel, they can experience resource limitation problems, degraded performance, physiological strain, and other negative outcomes. By redesigning a task that inputs do not share a signal channel and outputs can use multiple channels, one can increase workloads, to a point, without running into resource allocation constraints. Wickens is careful to point out that workload design is a little more complicated than my simplified characterization of the theory. However, the general principles appear to work well.

The multiple resource model is presented as elements. The processing stage addresses sensory encoding and perception, central and response processing. The second element addresses input and response modes. The auditory, visual, and tactile modality draw upon different resources and cross-modal time-sharing can be better performed than intramodal time-sharing. One can listen to the radio and track the position of their car in a lane concurrently much better than they can listen to the radio and listen to instructions about when and how much to turn the steering wheel, with their eyes closed, to maintain lane position. The third element is the processing mode which can be verbal or spatial in nature. Overburdening a particular channel or switching between encoding, processing, and response modalities has negative consequences in terms of mental workload. There are a wealth of studies and supplementary discussions on the nuances of human workload that cannot be adequately addressed here. However, the general concept of unbalanced or excessive use of resources creates problems in mental workload and, thereby, promotes performance decrements, strain, and increases the likelihood of adopting shortcut behaviors that are unsafe.

From an accommodation perspective, the multiresource model argues that if impairments exist in one or more channels, one should consider dividing the task sensory, cognitive, and output demands across other available channels. For example, if a worker does not have visual sensory capacity, using the auditory channel may be a solution. However, loading all work into the auditory channel alone can overwhelm the channel capacity of the worker and force slowed or serial processing of information. Use of a combination of haptic and auditory sensory feedback and verbal and manual control would be better than forcing all work to be handled by auditory input and verbal output.

Typically, concomitant task timeline analysis is used to estimate the mental workload (i.e., task time-sharing). Balancing task timelines helps to reduce mental workloads amongst and within workers. Timeline-based mental workload models must be evaluated with actual workloads. You can use time-sharing information to help adjust task sequencing and design to reduce mental workloads; however, you have to test the impact of joint task workloads to determine if they are acceptable or not. There are no a priori models that allow one to determine whether mental workloads are acceptable save through actual testing.

18.4.30   MENTAL WORKLOAD ASSESSMENT

The underlying rationale for workload measurement is that humans have many but limited resources for performing work. When one or many underlying resources are overallocated, performance suffers and psychological and physiological stress develop. Absolute workload assessments can be made when directly measuring primary and secondary tasks that burden the same resource pool. Relative resource demand assessment can be made when using comparative evaluation of indirect measures such as physiological strain. Which type of workload measurement should be used depends upon a number of factors. This is particularly true when considering cognitively impaired individuals who may overload sensory channels, who have limited working memory capacity, or who are using greater mental resources in general to perform any given task. Individuals with material impairments will experience high mental workloads and will, accordingly, suffer in performance, sense of control, and mental fatigue. Excessive mental workloads are problematic and should be reduced as much as practicable, regardless of the degree of impairment of the user or operator.

A number of metrics have been developed for assessment of mental workload. No single metric is ideal because they vary in their sensitivity, diagnosticity, primary-task intrusion, implementation requirements (e.g., availability of equipment, expense, and other logistical constraints), and operator acceptance (e.g., certain operator populations are very resistant to admitting any problems with their ability to handle task demands in fear of ordinal ranking for choice opportunities in the future—other operators may not honestly respond—putting honest responders at a disadvantage if the information was available to decision makers). Sensitivity is an index of the responsiveness of the metric to changes in workload. Diagnosticity is the ability to discern the type or cause of workload, or the ability to attribute it to an aspect or aspects of the operator's task (Wierwille and Eggemeier, 1993).

Primary task intrusion occurs when measurement of the workload metric interferes with task performance and, thereby, gives false indications of workload problems. Secondary tasks can be used to assess remaining resource capacity after primary task requirements are made and the primary and secondary tasks share the same resources. Sometimes subjects switch primary and secondary task priorities when they know that only secondary task performance is being measured. Self-report measures taken after completion of the task and most physiological measures seem to degrade primary-task performance the least (Eggemeier et al., 1991).

The reader should understand that substantial arguments and cautions exist for use of mental workload metrics in the literature and a book would be required to adequately address those elements. There is no reliable decision algorithm for selection of one or more metrics beyond the selection criteria noted above, the nature of the tasks performed, the nature of the operator population, and the nature of questions that have to be addressed in the assessment.

Errors have occurred in past measurement of mental workload, resulting in operators being put at risk. Often errors develop because designers have used inappropriate metrics (based upon the selection criteria noted above) or have not corroborated outcomes of a single metric (e.g., failed to use a battery of metrics). For example, one may measure primary performance and find no decrement, concluding that mental workloads are adequate. Yet such performance may have been achieved at extreme effort producing psychological and physiological strain. With time, that situation will cause degradation of performance.

Another example is relying simply upon a physiological metric because it is objective. Physiological metrics are integrated measurements that reflect totality of workload exposure; they often have lag times and do not offer much diagnostic value. Personality structure can influence stress responses and one can miss resource overloads in individuals who may not share concern about performance decrements.

Self-report tools offer great value, but they are subject to cooperation of the operator. Poorly described procedures, neophyte operators, or managerial factors (e.g., If I report problems with this new system and others don't, will I be at a future disadvantage for selection to use the new system?). Designers who are strong advocates of their design are not necessarily the individuals who should design, present, or assess outcomes of self-report mental workload tools to operators.

Often mental workload is found to be high or inadequately considered in the design of the original system, or a result of modifications that are made without adequate evaluation of the impact of the add-on equipment, task, or responsibilities. Complex systems are typically designed concurrently with separate design teams working on components of a design. Often teams work too independently and fail to understand that ergonomic designs that are appropriate for their components are not when all components are merged and integrated into an operational system. Often the visual, auditory, and motor resources are overtaxed during certain performance scenarios, particularly when handling system malfunctions or complex problems. Mental workload assessments in component design may be useful at those levels; however, failing to replicate mental workload assessment at design completion or integration stages can be disastrous—particularly if systematic tests are not performed within an acceptable scope of failure modes.

18.4.31   ARE MOTOR PERFORMANCE DEMANDS EXCESSIVE?

Motor response or performance can be classified as discrete, continuous, sequential discrete, open-loop movements, or closed-loop continuous movements. These activities are mediated by reaction time components. Recommended textbooks in the reference sections have excellent and in-depth reviews of human reaction time and motor performance. The following sections address sources of errors that designers have encountered when designing or evaluating the impact of their designs upon motor performance requirements and capabilities.

18.4.32   ARE ANTICIPATED REACTION TIMES REALISTIC?

Time taken by operators to detect and physically start a response to some external event or input, a change in a traffic light, or hazard signal, is grossly referred to as reaction time. Reaction times are not static within operators; fatigue, attention or vigilance decrement, stress, aging, cognitive or motor impairments and other factors can influence reaction time. Reaction time is also influenced by the number signals or events the operator has to attend. The Hick–Hyman law demonstrates that if one increases, the number events that must be attended, that the information content in that response is increased, and with increased information processing, one will encounter increased latencies in response times.

Reaction time has been classified as simple, disjunctive, or choice. Most reaction time data have been collected under ideal laboratory conditions where subjects are extremely focused on the reaction time task. As time-sharing increases reaction times will increase, sometimes demonstrably (e.g., McClelland, Simpson, and Starbuck, 1983). Designers often err in performing restricted laboratory or field tests of reaction times and presume that such times will hold when the operator is exposed to many time-sharing activities; those times will probably be very inaccurate. For such situations, the designers should carefully consider the consequences of long response latencies. If such outcomes are problematic, then design interventions will be needed (e.g., computer-assisted vigilance, engineer in soft failures, increased operator training and awareness, etc.).

18.4.33 ARE OPEN-LOOP PERFORMANCE OR DISCRETE MOVEMENT TIMES REALISTIC?

Open-loop motor tasks occur when one moves the hand, limb, head, or performs a muscular effort in which feedback is not or cannot be used to guide or track the movement trajectory. For example, a discrete rapid movement of a hand to a control location. Fitts' law provides an open-loop motor performance prediction model based upon the concept that different movement amplitudes to different endpoint or target accuracy constraints produce different information processing demands for humans. Human information processing rate capacity is limited and, thus, one can anticipate that longer times will be required to perform longer movements, or more precise movements, because more information must be processed within a channel capacity constrained motor system.

Fitts (1954) demonstrated a reliable relationship between movement times and task indexes of difficulty that were characterized in terms of bits of information:

$$MT = a + b \log_2 (2 \, A/W)$$

where

a and b are regression model coefficients,
A the amplitude or move distance, and
W the move endpoint accuracy requirement or target width.

The above model argues that the human's motor information processing capacity is limited. There are different degrees of molecularization of this model (Wiker et al., 1989). Thus, if the forearm and hand information processing rate is 100 ms/bit (index of difficulty (ID) (bits) = $\log_2(2A/W)$), then asking one to produce manual or control movements that require 80 ms/bit is infeasible. Keeping the information processing rate well below the individual's motor information capacity is requisite for effective accommodation. The above relationship is empirically determined by measuring the individual's information processing capacity and comparing it against the task-required performance.

For example, a computer touch screen requires one to move 10 cm to select an option that is defined by a 1 cm button and the designer has allocated 2 s to perform this task. This produces an ID of $\log_2$ (2(10 cm)/1 cm) = 4.3 bits. The processing rate is 4.3 bits/2 s or 465 ms/bit. Testing of an individual with a tremor-based neurological disorder shows that their maximum functional ID is 3 bits, and their information processing rate limit for a forearm hand movement is 500 ms/bit. To accommodate this individual's performance constraints, the designer can reduce the movement distance, increase the effective diameter of the target button, or increase the duration of time that is allocated to the task. The designer does not want to slow task performance and decides to enlarge buttons to allow an effective 4 cm target size. The new ID becomes 2.32 bits with a requisite information processing rate of 861 ms/bit. This design change allows the individual to perform the button actuation within the required time envelop.

The designer should evaluate the motor performance demands within the context of many other variables, including mental workload, but at least in the example above, they have eliminated a performance constraint for the impaired worker. Reducing the ID for control or manual assembly tasks to a minimum will improve performance for everyone and reduce the percentage of individuals with neuromotor impairments who cannot be accommodated by the design. If the motor performance demands cannot be reduced to acceptable levels, the model above serves as a quick check or confirmation that alternative accommodation strategies may be in order (e.g., voice-activated selection and execution of the button option). Documenting the motor ID and ms/ID task demands will allow the vocational rehabilitation professionals to rapidly determine whether or not a client can perform the motor tasks or will have to use some form of augmenting technology to perform the job.

18.4.34 Manual Tracking or Closed-Loop Performance Demands Excessive?

Closed-loop tracking tasks occur when one drives a vehicle, aims at a target, or performs any task in which motor behavior is adjusted to control an error. Tracking can be pursuit (e.g., the operator sees both the target and target tracking feature (e.g., roadway, cursor, gun site, etc.) or compensatory (e.g., only the magnitude and direction of error is presented and the operator is asked to null the displayed error) in nature. Pursuit tracking is an easier task because the operator can see and forecast movement of the target.

Tracking performance is materially affected by control order. Zero-order controllers produce displacement outcomes in response to control displacement. First-order controls increase response velocity in correspondence to the magnitude of the control's displacement. Second-order controls increase response acceleration in correspondence to the magnitude of control displacement. Third-order controls relate the magnitude of jerk response to control displacement. In general, zero and first-order controls produce best results and reduce mental workload demands. When higher order controls are used, they are difficult to master and to achieve desired results—in most, but not all cases.

In addition to control order, designers often introduce response lags into the system that can result in overcontrolling, phase errors, control system instability, and other problems (see Figure 18.12). Often poorly designed controls create control–display response incapability (e.g., tillers on sailboats vs. steering wheels, the operator moves the tiller to the left to make the vessel turn right) that result in tracking mistakes, lost time, and accidents. Individuals with impairments introduce additional response lags that make marginally-stable control-response systems unstable. Reducing impact of response delays increases performance for everyone and can tolerate greater degrees of impairment.

Controls often have to have their gain's set. The magnitude of the response per unit change in control displacement. High-gain controls can be useful when large responses are needed to catch up with the target. However, high-gain controls are very problematic once the target is close and fine positioning (e.g., need for low-gain control status) is required to acquire and hold onto the target.

The operator's effective bandwidth in tracking tasks can be reduced when control deadspace (e.g., control slack or movement before underlying response is engaged) or control backlash (e.g., control "kick-back at the end of movement within the deadspace). If the required bandwidth exceeds the operator's bandwidth

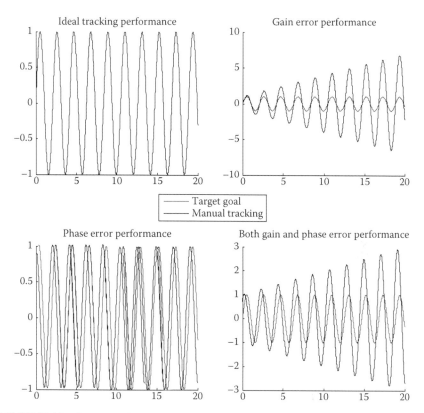

FIGURE 18.12 Example of tracking task error showing the relationship between phase and gain errors on tracking.

capacity, phase and gain errors can occur and, thereby, make the device or system uncontrollable.

If the recipe for the control design (e.g., gain, bandwidth, deadspace, backlash, momentum or inertia, compensatory vs. pursuit, and other characteristics) is not matched well with the assigned task, operator performance can be significantly challenged or lost. Matters only get worse when multiaxis or dual limb tracking tasks are required.

Far too often ergonomists are brought in to resolve tracking task problems in which designers thought they were helping the operator by introducing variable gain, variable control order, and dual tracking opportunities—often letting the operator switch rapidly between modes. Whether or not such designs are helpful must be determined by realistic performance testing. Bode plots of phase gain errors in tracking behavior can give absolute and relative tracking performance capacity. As gains of any magnitude are coupled with large phase errors, the system is less controllable.

Designers often inherit control systems within the context of their new system design. Mental workloads and capacities to handle inherent tracking demands can differ materially from one system to another. Thus, looking at similar systems and planning on the control design, which has been acceptable in the antecedent system, does not guarantee that the design will be acceptable in a new application where perceptual, cognitive, and motor demands are quite different. Only thorough testing in the context of system failures can one determine if the control system design is satisfactory for populations with a variety of sensory, cognitive and/or motor impairments.

In sum, avoid tracking tasks in the design of products, equipment, or job processes wherever possible. Tracking tasks are challenging for everyone and if they can be avoided, do so. If the system must track, attempt to allow the human to supervise the machine-automated tracking behavior. If the machine cannot track the target, it is very likely that the human will not behave much better.

If tracking must be supervised, provide pursuit tracking displays to improve situational awareness on the part of the supervising operator. If the human must take over for a machine, then attempt to reduce control orders and gains as low as feasible. Anticipate that the tracking task will fail and permit soft failure effects.

For example, rather than ask a human to trace along edges of dark ship on lighter water to determine its length and beam, allow the operator to select the image and have the computer do an edge-detection analysis to perform the operation length and width geometric computation. If the algorithm makes a mistake (e.g., traces the superstructure of the vessel), allow the user to lower the threshold or command a "second" best edge-detection effort. The information may have to be gathered from a set of discrete edge-detection trials (one trial provides a good indication of the beam, another gives a good estimate of the length). However, even with four discrete edge-detection trials, performance could be much faster and more accurate than asking a human with a material intentional tremor disorder to either trace edges or to use a pen to tap on loci needed to compute the desired dimensions (Figure 18.12).

18.4.35　Anthropometric Requirements Met?

In the past, the principal problem confronting accommodation was providing access to workplaces, community resources, infrastructure, or other societal phenomena. Those challenges have not been resolved entirely at this moment; however, significant progress is being made in that arena. There are a number of sources of information that one can use to design doorways, traffic passages, workstations, and other areas for wheelchair access and functional reach (Woodson et al., 1992).

It is important to understand that just providing clearance-based and mobility access to a work area is not sufficient to accommodate individuals given the variety of impairments that exist in our society. One must also consider the concept of functional and social access. Social access addresses the integration of an impaired individual within the work unit.

Fully integrated accommodation within a work unit enables and facilitates team-based work, embedded training, and social interplay that are important for working relationships. Providing isolated but equal performance options in which the individual is separated from their coworkers, compromises performance and growth of the team as well as the individuals within the team.

Social isolation can occur even if the individual is working within the same area if accommodation forces the individual to use radically different methods to perform their work. For example, if an individual must use voice control for nearly every aspect of their work, coworkers are likely to be disturbed by the running or repetitive verbal discourse. Coworkers might elect to use headsets to listen to music to mask out the "noise," or avoid that area of the workplace to escape the distraction. Coworkers might also request that a noise-limiting cubical be used to isolate the interference. Both example "interventions" serve to isolate the worker from coworkers. When accommodation strategies are considered, those which avoid social isolate should be pursued.

Access anthropometry is addressed in stages. First, design for clearance and maneuverability not only for the impaired individual, but for their interplay with coworkers (e.g., passage ways should allow side-by-side movement with coworkers while discussing issues, or passing coworkers or others in passageways without forcing anyone to change their normal patterns of movement to permit passage clearance). This consideration should be extended from primary ingress/egress to emergency exit passages as well. Examples of detailed design guidance provided in standards and design handbooks are provided in Figure 18.13.

Once clearance access is provided, the designer should insure that visual access of displays, controls, and other sites that the worker is expected to view are, indeed, accessible. Functional reach (i.e., ability to reach and functionally perform the requisite task such as reach and operate a crank control with adequate strength and precision) must be assessed and corrected if problems are encountered. Often designs that compel high force actuations are poor designs for everyone, more so for individuals who have functional limitations that are imposed by neuromotor disorders, or because they are in a wheelchair, they must use strength-compromising postures (e.g., overhead or extended reaches where arm strength can be significantly reduced) (Figure 18.14).

Organization of control layout. The designer should consider constraints that are imposed by anthropometric clearance and limited movement capacity of the user, as well as sensory and motor impairments. Designers attempt to lay out equipment and control panels to enhance convenience, accuracy, speed, or strength capacity of the user. Classically, several control and equipment layout paradigms have been used. They include importance of use, frequency of use, sequence of use, and functional groupings. The schema that is best depends upon the design and other criteria that must be evaluated by the designer.

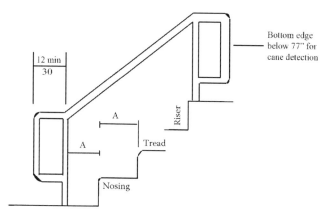

FIGURE 18.13 Example of ramp and stair design guidance that is available within standards and guidelines. (Modified from Wiker, S.F., Importance of human factors engineering in promotion of safety, Haight, J. (Ed.)., *Safety Professional's Handbook*, 2008. With permission.)

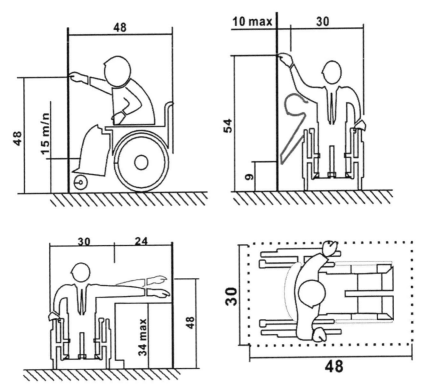

FIGURE 18.14 Example of clearance and reach anthropometry guidance for individuals using wheelchairs. (Wiker, S.F., Importance of human factors engineering in promotion of safety, Haight, J. (Ed.)., *Safety Professional's Handbook*, 2008. With permission.)

Importance principle. Important equipment should be placed in the most convenient locations. Importance is determined by how critical a piece of equipment is in terms of achieving the task or goals of the system. As shown in Figure 18.15, the most important controls are placed in the primary control zone to ease access and speed of access, secondary or less important controls are successively placed outboard of the primary control zone. Emergency equipment or controls should be placed near the primary zone for easy access (typically in the secondary control zone). One should remember that the primary control zone may have to be re-centered and re-sized for different forms of impairment.

Frequency of use. If controls have equivalent importance then placement of controls should be based upon frequency of use. One can organize the control placement following Figure 18.15 but substitute frequency or importance in setting primary and secondary zones for equipment and control placement. Some impairments markedly reduce physical capacity to perform frequent movements without developing fatigue. If that is the case, then positioning controls within high-strength zones for

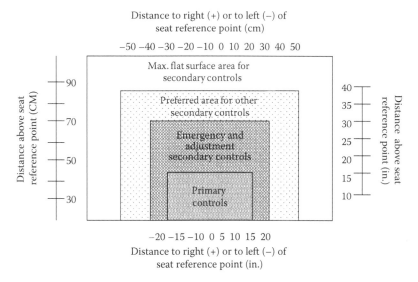

FIGURE 18.15 Control layout schema based upon the principle of importance. (Wiker, S.F., Importance of human factors engineering in promotion of safety, Haight, J. (Ed.)., *Safety Professional's Handbook*, 2008. With permission.)

the impaired worker may be required. One may also have to change control operation using other modalities (e.g., voice control, etc.) or by augmentive technologies.

Sequence of use. Where possible controls should be laid out to capitalize upon sequence of use. For example, if a set of toggle switches or buttons must be actuated in a specific sequence, it helps to sequentially position the controls so that the operator can move along a line of actuation. This speeds actuation and provides a memory aid as well.

Functional grouping. Each of the aforementioned control layout principles can also be used within functional groupings of controls. For example, all engine, radio, illumination, and other controls that can be functionally clustered are grouped. Within the group of controls, one can use importance, frequency, or sequence of use design principles for further layout guidance.

These design principles become increasingly more important when users have functional limitations and must control the amount of muscular activity or effort in operating a machine or performing tasks. Poor layouts increase performance times, actuation errors, and can produce unnecessary fatigue or discomfort.

Many constraints to accommodation due to functional anthropometry problems can be addressed effectively if designs reduce clearance or access problems, permit short reaches for seated operators, and controls selected are low-force and provide simple linear actuation movements (e.g., avoid wheeled-control valves and opt for machine actuated push buttons to close or open the valve). If the controls are poorly positioned, require high-force actuation, require high-frequency operation, and have other poor anthropometric layout for the population at large, then matters only worsen for workers who have one or more impairments.

18.5   DESIGN USING APPROPRIATE ERGONOMIC STANDARDS, CODES, AND REGULATIONS

Standards, codes, and guidelines provide design information in a methodological manner (e.g., MIL-STD 1472D, NASA-STD-3000, and ANSI/HFS 100-1988). Most standards are classified as specification standards where specific guidance is provided. The guidance may not yield the best design outcome. However, it should yield, if applied properly, an acceptable design. Performance standards do not provide cookbook types of guidance. Instead, performance standards help the designers understand what the requisite performance criteria are for an area of application. There are a number of areas where research is developing toward standards for guiding design for individuals or populations who are impaired (Carbonell, 1999; Cremers and Neerincx, 2004; Dukarskii and Rubin, 1994; Fanshawe, 1999; Gulliksen, Andersson, and Lundgren, 2004; Jones and Tamari, 1997; King, Evans, and Blenkhorn, 2004; Mace, 1998; McCullagh, 2006; Morita, 2001; Pastel, Wallace, and Heines, 2007; Rodriguez, Domingo, Ribera, Hill, and Jardi, 2006; Schulman et al., 2005; Sears, Lin, and Karimullah, 2002; Vanderheiden and Tobias, 1998; Zimmermann, Vanderheiden, and Al Gilman, 2002).

Standards result from consensus among content experts from industrial firms, trade associations, academia, technical societies, labor organizations, consumer organizations, and government agencies. Failure to pay heed to standards and codes may be disastrous, particularly if a product, machine, or system is ever involved in a product liability law suit. Anyone who fails to consider standards, codes, or guidelines in their professional safety life is often simply asking for an accident, injury, death or loss of property and, subsequently, a costly tutorial in tort law.

One may deviate from standards or guidelines, however, justification for such deviation will have to be strong and demonstrate a better and safer design as a result. Given that standards are consensus-based, that is a code word for the lowest common agreement. Designs may need to improve the performance or specifications depending upon a number of factors. While exceeding standards may need justification to the design team and those who authorize expenditures, falling below the standard is usually not acceptable.

Equally important is that it is often impossible for an evaluator or inspector, who typically is not trained in human factors, to decide whether a design does, or does not, meet a performance standard. In a perfect world there would be no opportunity for ambiguity or misinterpretation of ergonomic design standards. That is simply not the case. Asking designers to interpret ergonomic standards without help is usually a bad idea.

Moreover, standards have to be "tailored" or used with multifaceted design demands and constraints. Trade-off decisions have to be made such that the intent of the standard is met. Sometimes, standards present apparently contradictory or congruent information when, if fact, they are not. Moreover, not all requirements of a specification or performance standard have to be "met" or designed to. Designers may spend significant amounts of time attempting to resolve apparently incongruent advice or requirements with a standard, a set of building codes, or set of federal regulations. Terrible mistakes occur when a designer latches onto a specification, uses it, and fails to detect that there is an overriding specification in a separate standard that they do not have access to.

Finally, standards, codes, and regulations cannot be used by anyone effectively if they do not understand the system's performance objectives, requirements, and design from a top-down perspective. Myopic use of the information provided in standards, design handbooks, building codes, and other consensus-based design guidance is an opportunity for misapplication of the standard.

Design checklists have their place. However, far too often checklists are published without any validation or assurance that the design is effective and safe if no problems are highlighted, or that problems exist if one or more questions result in problematic responses. In truth, design checklists are more of a screening tool to grab attention of someone with appropriate education, skills, and expertise to rule out problems with more thorough analyses.

Design checklists query for binary responses on issues that are typically univariate in nature. Far too often design problems represent interactions among a variety of design features. Additive responses may not provide any valid insight to the true magnitude of a problem or the acceptability of a design. While design checklists can be used to help detect the possibility of a problem, they offer no protection, one way or another, if used blindly and improperly.

18.6 OTHER CONSIDERATIONS

18.6.1 Training Team Design Members

Short courses addressing the general utility of ergonomic or universal design are useful. An intense course over a couple of days or hours cannot be expected to provide designers with the capacity to apply accommodation principles in the design of complex human–machine systems. While designers will become sensitive to general concepts, they will not be able to evaluate engineering trade-off decisions or address specific questions that are challenging.

That said, sensitivity training for team members across disciplines is always beneficial in that it serves to enhance collaborative interaction and appreciation for problems in their colleague's domains of expertise. Of course, ergonomists must be prepared to provide design recommendations that are well-defended and tutorial in nature. Designers are not happy about altering their preliminary, intended, or extant designs without solid justification. Constructing well-documented and thorough justifications for improvements in designs serves both to gain acceptance and to provide on-the-job training for the design team. Helping the design team learn why design principles are applicable often helps integrate such principles in future preliminary designs, expediting ergonomic review and hopefully reducing the need to design changes.

Finally, any design efforts require interaction and learning from intended user populations for the design. Use of focus groups that include a variety of intended-users with a variety impairments is extremely beneficial. The focus groups catch needs for design improvements and serve to educate all design team members concerning usability issues and preferences from direct experience with their impairments.

18.6.2   Do You Need to Select and Train Your Personnel?

Nearly all systems require some level of personnel selection and training. The nature of personnel selection is determined by the perceptual, cognitive, and motor performance demands that have been imposed by allocation of tasks within the human–machine system. Since other chapters deal with these requirements, I will only reinforce the need for ergonomists to insure that personnel selection factors are considered and carefully matched to the system's design requirements and behaviors. This is particularly important when attempting to accommodate potential users who are impaired situationally or chronically.

Training often is used to relax personnel selection criteria and pressures. The more complex and difficult the system is to operator, the greater the likelihood that it will need personnel with greater education, training, skills, and other capacities. Training programs are likely to be more extensive as well. As extensive training requirements develop, the level of accomodation for users who are impaired decays. Whenever possible, developing or selecting designs that reduce or eliminate needs for training will serve to increase the accomodation of those with impairments.

From a safety perspective, training programs should envelop operator understanding and recognition of hazards, safe behaviors, and failure response or emergency protocols. After recognizing a danger, individuals must act to protect themselves against an accident and possible harm. One must know what actions are correct and safe and one must complete the action required. Knowing the appropriate action and performing it correctly requires training, practice, and reinforcement through design and use of appropriate warnings, labels, and other hazard–response communications.

Even the best selection and training programs typically do not select personnel with the exact skills needed to operate new systems, or produce consistently desired responses. Training helps to reduce the risk of accidents and the impact or severity of accidents. Far too often, however, ergonomists are confronted with heavy reliance on the part of designers to use personnel selection and training to handle design problems. Moreover, many accident investigations produce conclusions that personnel selection and training must be improved to reduce risk of future accidents. These outcomes are code words for poor design that requires selection of humans with greater capacities or more training and practice to operate with greater margins of safety.

18.6.3   Understand the Level of Effort

Documentation is requisite in ergonomic design and justification, particularly when systems under development are large, may require years to produce, and one can anticipate the need for future modifications or updates based upon changes in system requirements, technology, or user populations. One must document all analyses, preliminary studies, tests and evaluations, and how standards were tailored or shaped in their application for the project. It is not unusual for design and engineering team members to move on and off of the project, thus, requiring documentation review by the relieving team members or project managers.

Documentation is also requisite for investigators of accidents or disputes that involve accidents or failure to reasonably accomodate individuals with impairments.

If project performance objectives change, previous documentation can aid in understanding the implications of making such changes, or where additional testing and evaluation will be required.

Methodical analysis, documentation, and communication with design team members are time consuming. Given the initial cost of ergonomic contributions, one must insure that outcomes make the initial investment and subsequent modifications cost-effective—starting over with ergonomic evaluation of complex systems is untenable.

18.7 CONCLUDING REMARKS

It is possible to design safe and effective systems that accommodate a wide range of human impairments. Ergonomic design principles work to improve the marriage between humans, their machines, tasks, and operating environments. If the design is appropriate, performance is enhanced for everyone, accidents are prevented, and severity of consequences of failures or accidents is mitigated—including prevention of new postaccident impairments. While there is a cost associated with accommodation of individuals to particular jobs and workplaces, the insidious costs of weak design that produces insidious decrement in everyone's performance, safety, and health, are far greater. Everyone benefits from broader application of ergonomic design principles and reasonable integration of impairment accommodation into the initial design of workplaces, equipment, tools, and tasks.

BIBLIOGRAPHY

TEXTBOOKS AND DESIGN HANDBOOKS

Boff, K. R., Kaufman. L., and Thomas. J. P. (Eds.) 1986. *Handbook of Perception and Human Performance*. Volume I: Sensory Processes and Perception. Volume II: Cognitive Processes and Performance. New York: John Wiley & Sons.

Boff, K. R. and Lincoln, J. E. (Eds.) 1999. *Engineering Data Compendium: Human Perception and Performance*. Wright-Patterson Air Force Base, OH: Harry G. Armstrong Aerospace Medical Research Laboratory.

Chapanis, A. 1959. *Research Technique's in Human Engineering*. Baltimore, MD: The Johns Hopkins University Press.

Meister, D. 1971. *Human Factors: Theory and Practice*. New York: John Wiley & Sons.

Salvendy, G. (Ed.) 1997. *Handbook of Human Factors and Ergonomics*. New York: John Wiley & Sons.

Sanders, M. and McCormick, E. J. 1993. *Human Factors in Engineering and Design* (7th ed.). Hightstown, NJ: McGraw-Hill.

Taylor, J. H. 1973. Vision. In J. F. Parker, Jr., and V. R. West (Eds.), Bioastronautics Data Book (pp. 611–665). Washington, DC: Scientific and Technical Information Office, National Aeronautics and Space Administration.

Van Cott, H. P. and Kinkade, R. G. (Eds.) 1972. *Human Engineering Guide to Equipment Design*. (Rev. ed.). Washington, DC: Government Printing Office.

Wickens, C. D. 1992. *Engineering Psychology and Human Performance*. New York: HarperCollins.

Woodson, L., Tillman, P., and Tillman, B. 1992. *Human Factors Design Handbook*. New York: McGraw-Hill.

Useful General Design Standards

A through listing of all standards related to human factors engineering and ergonomics can be obtained via the International Ergonomics Association's website (http://www.iea.cc/standards). Ergonomists use the following standards regularly:

MIL-STD-1472D. This military standard, titled Human Engineering Design Criteria for Military Systems, Equipment and Facilities. It is available free from the Navy Publishing and Printing Service Office, Standardization Document Order Desk, 700 Robbins Avenue, Building #4, Section D, Philadelphia, PA 19111–5094.

NASA-STD-3000. A multivolume compendium, "Man- Systems Integration Standards." It is available from the National Aeronautics and Space Administration, Lyndon B. Johnson Space Center, Houston, TX 77058.

Building and Construction Codes

The National Electrical Safety Code and Life Safety, BOCA National Building Code and the BOCA National Mechanical Codes have a large number of design requirements that are based upon ergonomic research.

OSHA Standards

These are standards, prepared by the Federal Occupational Safety and Health Administration, address safe design and are often upon ergonomic design principles:

29 CFR Parts 1900 to 1927 Department of Labor. Washington, DC: Office of the Federal Register, National Archives and Records Administration.

Recommended Journals

Applied Cognitive Psychology
Applied Ergonomics
Aviation, Space, and Environmental Medicine
Ergonomics
Ergonomics in Design
Human Computer Interaction
Human Factors
IEEE Transactions on Systems, Man, and Cybernetics
International Journal of Industrial Ergonomics
Proceedings of Human Factors and Ergonomics Society

Citations and Recommended Readings

Aasman, J., Mulder, G., and Mulder, L. J. M. 1987. Operator effort and the measurement of heart-rate variability. *Human Factors*, 29, 161–170.

Adams, J. A. 1982. Issues in human reliability. *Human Factors*, 24, 1–10.

Bailey, R. W. 1982. *Human Performance Engineering: A Guide for System Designers*. Englewood Cliffs, NJ: Prentice-Hall.

Barnes. R. M. I. 1949. *Motion and Time Study* (3rd ed.). New York: John Wiley & Sons.

Bartlett, F. C. 1932. *Remembering: A Study in Experimental and Social Psychology.* Cambridge: Cambridge University Press.

Blanchard, B. S. and Fabrycky, W. J. 1990. *Systems Engineering and Analysis.* Englewood Cliffs, NJ: Prentice-Hall.

Brenner., M., Doherthy, E. T., and Shipp, T. 1994. Speech measures indicating workload demand. *Aviation, Space, and Environmental Medicine*, 65, 21–26.

Broadbent, D. E. 1958. *Perception and Communication.* London: Pergamon.

Carbonell, N. 1999. Multimodality: A Primary Requisite For Achieving an Information Society For All, Munich, Germany.

Chapanis, A. 1980. The error-provocative situation: A central measurement problem in human factors engineering. In W. E. Tarrants (Ed.), *The Measurement of Safely Performance* (pp. 99–128). New York: Garland STPM Press.

Chapanis. A. 1988. Words, words, words revisited. *International Review of Ergonomics.* 2, 1–30.

Cooper, M. D. and Phillips, R. A. 1994. Validation of a safety climate measure Proceedings of the British Psychological Society: 1994 Annual Occupational Psychology Conference. Birmingham, Jan 3–5.

Cooper, M. D., Phillips, R. A., Sutherland, V. J., and Makin, P. J. 1994. Reducing accidents using goal- setting and feedback: A field study. *Journal of Occupational & Organisational Psychology*, 67, 219–40.

Coren, S. 1994. Most comfortable listening level as a function of age. *Ergonomics*, 37(7), 1269–1274.

Cremers, A. H. M. and Neerincx, M. A. 2004. Personalisation Meets Accessibility: Towards the Design of Individual User Interfaces For All, Vienna, Austria.

Crossman, E. R. F. W. 1959. A theory of the acquisition of speed skill. *Ergonomics*, 2, 153–166.

Cushman, W. H. and Rosenberg, D. J. 1991. *Human Factors in Product Design.* Amsterdam: Elsevier.

DI-CMAN-K8008A Feb. 29. 1988. Data Item Description: System Segment Specification. Washington, DC: Department of the Air Force.

DI-HFAC-80740A. 26 May 1994. Human Engineering Program Plan. Washington, DC: Department of Defense.

DI-HFAC-80743A. 26 May 1994. Human Engineering Test Plan. Washington, DC: Department of Defense.

DI-HFAC-80744A. 26 May 1994. Human Engineering Test Report. Washington, DC: Department of Defense.

DI-HFAC-80745A. 26 May 1994. Human Engineering System Analysis Report. Washington, DC: Department of Defense.

DI-HFAC-80746A. 26 May 1994. Human Engineering Design Approach Document- Operator. Washington, DC: Department of Defense.

DI-HFAC-80747A. 26 May 1994. Human Engineering Design Approach Document- Maintainer. Washington, DC: Department of Defense.

DOD-HDBK-761A Sept. 30, 1989. Human Engineering Guidelines for Management Information Systems. Redstone Arsenal, AL: U.S. Army Missile Command.

DOD-HDBK-763. 27 Feb. 1987. Human Engineering Procedures Guide. Washington, DC: Department of Defense.

Dukarskii, S. M. and Rubin, G. J. 1994. The Universal Software For Design, Development and Maintenance of Automated Classifiers, Moscow, Russia.

Eggemeier, F. T. and Wilson, G. F. 1991. Performance-based and subjective assessment of workload in multi-task environments. In D. L. Damos (Ed.), *Multiple-Task Performance* (pp. 217–278). London: Taylor & Francis.

Eggemeier, F. T., Wilson, G. F., Kramer, A. F., and Damos, D. L. 1991. Workload assessment in multi-task environments. In D. L. Damos (Ed.)., *Multiple-Task Performance* (pp. 207–216). London: Taylor & Francis.

Fanshawe, D. G. J. 1999. Making It Easy for All [User Interface Design for the Disabled], Munich, Germany.

Fitts, P. M. 1954. The information capacity of the human motor system in controlling the amplitude of movement. *Journal of Experimental Psychology*, 47(6), 381–391.

Geldard, F. A. 1953. *The Human Senses*. New York: John Wiley & Sons.

Gibson, J. J. 1966. *The Senses Considered as Perceptual Systems*. Boston, MA: Houghton Mifflin.

Gopher, D. and Braune, R. 1984. On the psychophysics of workload: Why bother with subjective measures? *Human Factors*, 26, 519–532.

Gordon. S. L. 1994. *Systematic Training Program Design: Maximizing Effectiveness and Minimizing Liability*. Englewood Cliffs, NJ: Prentice-Hall.

Green, A. E., (Ed). *High Risk Safety Technology*, New York: Wiley, 1982.

Grose, V. L., *Managing Risk: Systematic Loss Prevention for Executives*. Englewood Cliffs, NJ: Prentice-Hall, 1988.

Gulliksen, J., Andersson, H., and Lundgren, P. 2004. Accomplishing universal access through system reachability - A management perspective. *Universal Access in the Information Society*, 3(1), 96–101.

Harris, B. H., G. Hendershot, et al. 2005. A Guide to Disability Statistics from the National Health Interview Survey, Employment and Disability Institute Collection. Ithaca, New York: Cornell University.

Hart, S. G. and Wickens, C. D. 1990. Workload assessment and prediction. In H. R. Boohe (Ed.), MANPRINT: *An Approach to Systems Integration* (pp. 257–296). New York: Van Nostrand Reinhold.

Hicks, T. G. and Wierwille, W. W. 1979. Comparison of five mental workload assessment procedures in a moving-base driving simulator. *Human Factors*, 21, 129–143.

Hill, S. G., Iavecchia, H. P., Byers, J. C., Bittner, A. C., Zaklad, A. L., and Christ, R. E. 1992. Comparison of four subjective workload rating scales. *Human Factors*, 34, 429–439.

Hockey, G. R. J. 1986. A state control theory of adaptation and individual differences in stress management. In G. R. J. Hockey, A. W. K. Gaillard, and M. G. H. Coles (Eds.), *Energetics and Human Information Processing* (pp. 285–298). Dordrecht, The Netherlands: Martinus Nijhoff Publishers.

Hoeks, L. T. M. 1995. The pupillary response as a measure of mental processing load: With application to picture naming. PhD Thesis, Nijmegen, the Netherlands: University of Nijmegen.

Huey, B. M. and Wickens, C. D. (Eds.) 1993. *Workload Transition*. Washington, DC: National Academy Press.

Hughes, P. K. and Cole, B. L. 1988. The effect of attentional demand on eye movement behaviour when driving. In A. G. Gale, M. H. Freeman, C. M. Haslegrave, P. Smith, and S. P. Taylor (Eds.), *Vision in Vehicles—II* (pp. 221–230). Amsterdam: North-Holland.

Humphrey, D. G. and Kramer, A. F. 1994. Toward a psychophysiological assessment of dynamic changes in mental workload. *Human Factors*, 36, 3–26.

Hyndman, B. W. and Gregory, J. R. 1975. Spectral analysis of sinus arrhythmia during mental loading. *Ergonomics*, 18, 255–270.

Hyönä, J., Tommola, J., and Alaja, A.-M. 1995. Pupil dilation as a measure of processing load in simultaneous interpretation and other language tasks. *The Quarterly Journal of Experimental Psychology*, 48A, 598–612.

Israelski, E. W. 1978. Commonplace human factors problems experienced by the colorblind—a pilot questionnaire survey. In *Proceedings of the Human Factors Society 22nd Annual Meeting* (pp. 347–351). Santa Monica, CA: Human Factors Society.

Itoh, Y., Hayashi, Y., Tsukui, I., and Saito, S. 1990. The ergonomic evaluation of eye movement and mental workload in aircraft pilots. *Ergonomics*, 33, 719–733.

Johnson, A. K. and Anderson, E. A. 1990. Stress and arousal. In J. T. Cacioppo and L. G. Tassinary. *Principles of Psychophysiology* (pp. 216–252). Cambridge: Cambridge University Press.

Jones, E. R., Hennessy, R. T., and Deutsch, S. (Eds.) 1985. *Human Factors Aspects of Simulation*. Washington, DC: National Academy Press.

Jones, K. E. and Tamari, I. E. 1997. Making our offices universally accessible: guidelines for physicians. *CMAJ*, 156(5), 647–656.

Jordan, P. W. and Johnson, G. I. 1993. Exploring mental workload via TLX: The case of operating a car stereo whilst driving. In A. G. Gale, I. D. Brown, C. M. Haslegrave, H. W. Kruysse, and S. P. Taylor (Eds.), *Vision in Vehicles–IV* (pp. 255–262). Amsterdam: North-Holland.

Jorna, P. G. A. M. 1992. Spectral analysis of heart rate and psychological state: A review of its validity as a workload index. *Biological Psychology*, 34, 237–257.

Kantowitz, B. H. 1987. Mental workload. In P. A. Hancock (Ed.), *Human Factors Psychology*. (pp. 81–121). Amsterdam: North-Holland.

Kantowitz, B. H. 1992. Selecting measures for human factors research. *Human Factors*, 34, 387–398.

Kaufman, J. E- and Haynes, H. (Eds.) 1981. *IES Lighting Handbook: Reference Volume*. New York: Illuminating Engineering Society of North America.

King, A., Evans, G., and Blenkhorn, P. 2004. WebbIE: A browser for visually impaired people, Cambridge, UK.

Kirwan, B. 1987. Human reliability analysis of an offshore emergency blowdown system. *Applied Ergonomics*, 18, 23–33.

Kirwan, B. and Ainsworth, L. K. 1992. *A Guide to Task Analysis*. London: Taylor and Francis.

Kryter, K. D. 1972. Speech communication. In H. P. Van Cott and R. G. Kinkade (Eds.), *Human Engineering Guide to Equipment Design* (pp. 161–226). Washington, DC: Government Printing Office.

Kurke, M. I. 1961. Operational sequence diagrams in system design. *Human Factors*, 3, 66–73.

Lando, H. A. 1982. A factorial analysis of preparation, aversion, and maintenance in the elimination of smoking. *Addictive Behaviors*, 7(2), 143–154.

Loftus, E. F. 1979. *Eyewitness Memory*. Cambridge, MA: Harvard University Press.

Lowrance, W. W. 1976. *Of Acceptable Risk*. Los Altos, CA: William Kaufmann.

Mace, R. L. 1998. Universal design in housing. *Assistive Technology*, 10(1), 21–28.

MANPRINT Apr. 17, 1987. Manpower and Personnel Integration (MANPRINT) in Material Acquisition Process (Army Regulation 602-2). Washington, DC: Department of the Army.

Martin, D. K. and Dain, S. J. 1988. Postural modifications of VDU operators wearing bifocal spectacles. *Applied Ergonomics*, 19, 293–300.

May, J. G., Kennedy, R. S., Williams, M. C., Dunlap, W. P., and Brannan, J. R. 1990. Eye movement indices of mental workload. *Acta Psychologica*, 75, 75–89.

McAfee, R. B. and Winn, A. R. 1989 The use of incentives/feedback to enhance workplace safety: A critique of the literature. *Journal of Safety Research*, 20, 7–19.

McCullagh, M. C. 2006. Home modification. *American Journal of Nursing*, 106(10), 54–63; quiz 63–54.

Meijman, T. F. 1989. *Mentale belasting en werkstress. Een arbeidspsychologische benadering (Mental Workload and Workstress. A Workpsychological Approach)*. Assen, The Netherlands: van Gorcum.

Meister, D. 1989. *Conceptual Aspects of Human Factors*. Baltimore, MD: The Johns Hopkins University Press.

Miller, G. A. 1956. The magical number seven plus or minus two: Some limits on our capacity for processing information. *Psychological Review*, 63(2), 81–97.

MIL-STD-1472D March 14, 1989. Military Standard: Human Engineering Design Criteria for Military Systems, Equipment and Facilities. Washington, DC: Department of Defense.

MIL-H-46855B April 5, 1984. Human Engineering Requirements for Military Systems, Equipment and Facilities. Redstone Arsenal, AL: U.S. Army Missile R&D Command.

MIL-STD-490A June 4, 1985. Specification Practices. Washington, DC: Department of Defense.

MIL-STD-499A(USAF) May 1, 1974. Military Standard: Engineering Management. Washington, DC: Department of Defense.

MIL-STD-1521B June 4, 1985. Technical Reviews and Audits for Systems. Equipments, and Computer Software. Washington, DC: Department of Defense.

MIL-STD-1472D March 14 1989. Human Engineering Resign Criteria for Military Systems, Equipment and Facilities. Washington, DC: Department of Defense.

Morita, H. 2001. Standardization of universal design in Japan. *Sanyo Technical Review*, 33(3), 16–23.

Mowbray, H. M. and Gebhard, J. W. May 1958. *Man's Senses as Informational Channels (Report No. CM-936)*. Silver Spring, MD: Applied Physics Laboratory, The Johns Hopkins University

Muckler, F. A. and Seven, S. A. 1992. Selecting performance measures: "objective" versus "subjective" measurement. *Human Factors*, 34, 441–455.

Norman, D. A. and Bobrow, D. G. 1975. On data-limited and resource-limited processes. *Cognitive Psychology*, 7, 44–64.

Norman, D. A. 1988. The *Psychology of Everyday Things*. New York: Basic Books.

Nygren, T. E. 1991. Psychometric properties of subjective workload measurement techniques: implications for their use in the assessment of perceived mental workload, *Human Factors*, 33, 17–33.

O'Donnell, R. D. and Eggemeier, F. T. 1986. Workload assessment methodology. In K. R. Boff, L. Kaufman, and J. P. Thomas (Eds.), *Handbook of Perception and Human Performance. Volume II, Cognitive Processes and Performance* (pp. 42/1–42/49). New York: Wiley.

Pastel, R., Wallace, C., and Heines, J. 2007. RFID cards: A new deal for elderly accessibility, Beijing, China.

Pelsma, K. H. (Ed.) 1987. *Ergonomics Sourcebook: A Guide to Human Factors Information*. Lawrence, KS: The Report Store, A Division of Ergosyst Associates, Inc.

Pheasant, S. 1988. *Bodyspace*. London: Taylor & Francis.

Price, H. H. 1985. The allocation of functions in systems. *Human Factors*, 27, 33–45.

Risk Assessment in the Federal Government. *Managing the Process,* Washington, DC: National Academy of Sciences, National Academy Press, 1983.

Rodriguez, E. P. G., Domingo, M. G., Ribera, J. P., Hill, M. A., and Jardi, L. S. 2006. Usability for all: Towards improving the e-learning experience for visually impaired users, Linz, Austria.

Roscoe, A. H. 1992. Assessing pilot workload. Why measure heart rate, HRV and respiration? *Biological Psychology*, 34, 259–287.

Roscoe, A. H. 1993. Heart rate as psychophysiological measure for in-flight workload assessment. *Ergonomics*, 36, 1055–1062.

Rouse, W. B., Edwards, S. L., and Hammer, J. M. 1993. Modelling the dynamics of mental workload and human performance in complex systems. *IEEE Transactions on Systems, Man, and Cybernetics*, 23, 1662–1671.

Rowe, W. D. 1983. *Evaluation Methods for Environmental Standards*. Boca Raton, FL: CRC Press.

Schulman, C. I., Namias, B. J., Rosales, O., Pizano, L. R., Ward, C. G., and Namias, N. 2005. A portable, universal patient positioning and holding system for use in the burn patient 'The Burnwalter'. *Burns*, 31(5), 647–649.

Sears, A., Lin, M., and Karimullah, A. S. 2002. Speech-based cursor control: Understanding the effects of target size, cursor speed, and command selection. *Universal Access in the Information Society*, 2(1), 30–43.

Shiffrin, R. M. and Czerwinski, M. P. 1988. A model of automatic attention attraction when mapping is partially consistent. *Journal of Experimental Psychology: Learning, Memory, and Cognition*, 14(3), 562–569.

Stevens, S. S. 1957. On the psychophysical law. *Psychological Review*, 64(3), 153–181.

Swain, A. D. and Gutlman, H. K. Aug, 1983. Handbook of Human Reliability Analysis with Emphasis on Nuclear Power Plant Applications. Report NUREG/CR-1278,

Teigen, K. H. 1994. Yerkes-Dodson: A law for all seasons. *Theory & Psychology*, 4, 525–547.

Thomson, J. R. 1987. *Engineering Safety Assessment: An Introduction*. New York: Wiley.

Thorsvall, L. and Åkerstedt, T. 1987. Sleepiness on the job: Continuously measured EEG changes in train drivers. *Electroencephalography and Clinical Neurophysiology*, 66, 502–511.

Tversky, A. and Kahneman, D. 1974. Judgment under uncertainty: Heuristics and biases. *Science*, 185, 1124–1131.

Van Cott, H. P. and Warrick, M. J. 1972. Man as a system component. In H. P. Van Cott and R. G. Kinkade (Eds.), *Human Engineering Guide to Equipment Design* (Rev. ed.) (p. IP-39). Washington, DC: Government Printing Office.

Vanderheiden, G. and Tobias, J. 1998. Barriers, incentives and facilitators for adoption of universal design practices by consumer product manufacturers. *Proceedings of the Human Factors and Ergonomics Society*, 1, 584–588.

Vivoli, G., Bergomi, M., Rovesti, S., Carrozzi, G., and Vezzosi, A. 1993. Biochemical and haemodynamic indicators of stress in truck drivers. *Ergonomics*, 36, 1089–1097.

WHO (1980). *International Classification of Impairments, Disabilities, and Handicaps: A Manual of Classification Relating to the Consequences of Disease*. Geneva: World Health Organization.

Wickens, C. D. 1984. Processing resources in attention. In R. Parasuraman and D. R. Davies (Eds.). *Varieties of Attention*. (pp. 63–102). London: Academic Press.

Wickens, C. D. 1991. Processing resources and attention. In D. L. Damos (Ed.), *Multiple-Task Performance* (pp. 3–34). London: Taylor & Francis.

Wickens, C. D. 1992. *Engineering Psychology and Human Performance*. New York: HarperCollins.

Wiener, E. L. 1987. Application of vigilance research: Rare, medium, or well done? *Human Factors*, 29, 725–736.

Wierwille, W. W. and Eggemeier, F. T. 1993. Recommendations for mental workload measurement in a test and evaluation environment. *Human Factors*, 35, 263–281.

Wiker, S. F., Langolf, G. D., and Chaffin, D. B. 1989. Arm posture and human movement capability. *Human Factors*, 31(4): 421–442.

Wilson, G. F. and Eggemeier, F. T. 1991. Psychophysiological assessment of workload in multi-task environments. In D. L. Damos (Ed.), *Multiple-Task Performance* (pp. 329–360). London: Taylor & Francis.

Woodson, W. E., Tillman, B., and Tillman, P. 1992. *Human Factors Design Handbook: Information and Guidelines for the Design Of Systems, Facilities, Equipment, and Products for Human Use* (2nd ed.). New York: McGraw-Hill.

Zimmermann, G., Vanderheiden, G., and Al Gilman, S. D. 2002. Prototype implementations for a universal remote console specification, Minneapolis, MN.

Index

Printed and bound by CPI Group (UK) Ltd, Croydon, CR0 4YY

18/10/2024

01776243-0018